Cognitive Neuro-rehabilitation, Second Edition

Evidence and Application

Edited by

Donald T. Stuss,

Gordon Winocur

Ian H. Robertson

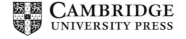

CAMBRIDGE
UNIVERSITY PRESS

CAMBRIDGE UNIVERSITY PRESS

Cambridge, New York, Melbourne, Madrid, Cape Town, Singapore, São Paulo, Delhi, Dubai, Tokyo, Mexico City

Cambridge University Press
The Edinburgh Building, Cambridge CB2 8RU, UK

Published in the United States of America by Cambridge University Press, New York

www.cambridge.org
Information on this title: www.cambridge.org/9780521518031

© Cambridge University Press 2008

First edition © Cambridge University Press 1999
This edition published 2008
Paperback Edition 2010
Reprinted 2011

Printed in the United Kingdom at the University Press, Cambridge

A catalog record for this publication is available from the British Library

ISBN 978-0-521-51803-1 Paperback

Contents

The plates are to be found between pages 78 and 79.

Contributors

Claude Alain
Rotman Research Institute at Baycrest,
University of Toronto,
Toronto, ON, Canada

Amy F. T. Arnsten
Department of Neurobiology,
Yale University School of Medicine,
New Haven, CT, USA

Lars Bäckman
Karolinska Institute,
Stockholm, Sweden

Malcolm A. Binns
Rotman Research Institute at Baycrest,
Toronto, ON, Canada

Sandra E. Black
Heart and Stroke Foundation Centre for Stroke Recovery
LC Campbell Cognitive Neurology Research Unit
Sunnybrook Research Institute
Rotman Research Institute at Baycrest
Division of Neurology, Department of Medicine,
Sunnybrook Health Sciences Centre,
University of Toronto,
Toronto, ON, Canada

S. Thomas Carmichael
Program in Neurorehabilitation and Neural Repair,
Department of Neurology,
David Geffen School of Medicine,
University of California,
Los Angeles, CA, USA

Keith D. Cicerone
Department of Neuropsychology,
JFK Johnson Rehabilitation Institute,
Edison, NJ, USA

Maurizio Corbetta
Department of Neurology, Radiology, Anatomy and
Neurobiology,
Washington University School of Medicine,
St. Louis, MO, USA

Bruce Crosson
VA RR&D Brain Rehabilitation Research Center, and
Department of Clinical and Health Psychology,
University of Florida Health Science Center,
Gainesville, FL, USA

Jeffrey L. Cummings
UCLA Alzheimer's Disease Center,
University of California,
Los Angeles, CA, USA

Deirdre R. Dawson
Kunin-Lunenfeld Applied Research
Unit at Baycrest,
University of Toronto,
Toronto, ON, Canada

Michael deRiesthal
VA Medical Center,
Gainesville, FL, USA

Roger A. Dixon
Department of Psychology,
University of Alberta,
Edmonton, AB, Canada

Laura Eggermont
Department of Clinical Neuropsychology,
Vrije Universiteit Amsterdam,
Amsterdam, The Netherlands

Kirk I. Erickson
Beckman Institute for Advanced Science and Technology,
University of Illinois,
Urbana, IL, USA

Anthony Feinstein
Neuropsychiatry Program,
Sunnybrook Health Sciences Centre,
University of Toronto,
Toronto, ON, Canada

Susan M. Fitzpatrick
James S. McDonnell Foundation,
St. Louis, MO, USA

Fu Qiang Gao
Heart and Stroke Foundation Centre for Stroke Recovery,
LC Campbell Cognitive Neurology Research Unit,
Sunnybrook Health Sciences Centre,
Toronto, ON, Canada

Douglas D. Garrett
Rotman Research Institute at Baycrest,
Department of Psychology,
University of Toronto,
Toronto, ON, Canada

Omar Ghaffar
Neuropsychiatry Program,
Department of Psychiatry,
Sunnybrook Health Sciences Centre,
University of Toronto,
Toronto, ON, Canada

Robbin Gibb
Department of Neuroscience,
Canadian Centre for Behavioral Neuroscience,
University of Lethbridge,
Lethbridge, AB, Canada

Elizabeth L. Glisky
Department of Psychology,
University of Arizona,
Tucson, AZ, USA

Martha L. Glisky
Evergreen Hospital Medical Center,
Kirkland, WA, USA

Leslie J. Gonzalez Rothi
VA Brain Rehabilitation Research Center,
Gainesville, FL, USA

Cheryl L. Grady
Rotman Research Institute at Baycrest,
Departments of Psychiatry and Psychology,
University of Toronto,
Toronto, ON, Canada

Carol Greenwood
Kunin-Lunenfeld Applied Research
Unit at Baycrest,
University of Toronto,
Toronto, ON, Canada

Gerri Hanten
Department of Physical Medicine and Rehabilitation,
Baylor College of Medicine,
Houston, TX, USA

Richard G. Hunter
Harold and Margaret Milliken Hatch Laboratory of
Neuroendocrinology,
The Rockefeller University,
New York, NY, USA

Masud Husain
Institute of Neurology and Institute of
Cognitive Neuroscience,
University College London,
London, UK

Narinder Kapur
Addenbrooke's Hospital,
Cambridge, UK

Bryan Kolb
Canadian Centre for Behavioral Neuroscience,
University of Lethbridge,
Lethbridge, AB, Canada

Arthur F. Kramer
Beckman Institute for Advanced Science and Technology,
University of Illinois,
Urbana, IL, USA

Susan A. Leon
VA Brain Rehabilitation Research Center,
Gainesville, FL, USA

Harvey S. Levin
Department of Physical Medicine and Rehabilitation,
Baylor College of Medicine,
Houston, TX, USA

Brian Levine
Rotman Research Institute at Baycrest,
University of Toronto,
Toronto, ON, Canada

Nadina Lincoln
Institute of Work Health and Organisations,
University of Nottingham,
Nottingham, UK

Thomas W. McAllister
Department of Psychiatry,
Dartmouth-Hitchcock Medical Center,
Lebanon, NH, USA

Edward McAuley
Department of Kinesiology and Community Health
University of Illinois
Urbana, IL
USA

Bruce S. McEwen
Harold and Margaret Milliken Hatch Laboratory of
Neuroendocrinology,
The Rockefeller University,
New York, NY, USA

David M. Morris
Department of Physical Therapy,
University of Alabama at Birmingham,
Birmingham, AL, USA

Stephen E. Nadeau
Brain Rehabilitation Research Center,
Malcolm Randall DVA Medical Center,
Gainesville, FL, USA

Roshan das Nair
School of Psychology,
University of Nottingham,
Nottingham, UK

Matthew Parrott
Kunin-Lunenfeld Applied Research Unit,
Baycrest,
Toronto, ON, Canada

Jennie Ponsford
School of Psychology, Psychiatry and
Psychological Medicine,
Monash University,
Clayton, Victoria, Australia

George P. Prigatano
Barrow Neurological Institute,
St. Joseph's Hospital – CHW,
Phoenix, AZ, USA

Joel Ramirez
LC Campbell Cognitive Neurology Research Unit,
Sunnybrook Health Sciences Centre,
Toronto, ON, Canada

John M. Ringman
UCLA Alzheimer's Disease Center,
University of California,
Los Angeles, CA, USA

Ian H. Robertson
Trinity College Institute of Neuroscience, and
School of Psychology,
Trinity College Dublin, Ireland

Amy D. Rodriguez
Department of Communicative Disorders,
University of Florida,
Gainesville, FL, USA

John C. Rosenbek
Department of Communicative Disorders,
University of Florida,
Gainesville, FL, USA

Bernhard Ross
Rotman Research Institute at Baycrest,
University of Toronto,
Toronto, ON, Canada

Erik Scherder
Department of Clinical Neuropsychology,
Vrije Universiteit Amsterdam, and
Institute of Human Movement Sciences,
Rijksuniversiteit Groningen, The Netherlands

Victoria Singh-Curry
Institute of Neurology and Institute of Cognitive Neuroscience,
University College London,
London, UK

Trudi Stickland
Hotchkiss Brain Institute,
Faculty of Medicine,
University of Calgary,
Calgary, AB, Canada

Donald T. Stuss
Rotman Research Institute at Baycrest,
University of Toronto,
Toronto, ON, Canada

Edward Taub
Department of Psychology,
University of Alabama at Birmingham,
Birmingham, AL, USA

Gary R. Turner
Rotman Research Institute at Baycrest,
Toronto, ON, Canada

Harry V. Vinters
Department of Pathology and Laboratory Medicine
(Neuropathology),
UCLA Medical Center,
University of California,
Los Angeles, CA, USA

Samuel Weiss
Hotchkiss Brain Institute,
Faculty of Medicine,
University of Calgary,
Calgary, AB, Canada

John Whyte
Moss Rehabilitation Research Institute,
Elkins Park, PA, and
Department of Rehabilitation Medicine,
Thomas Jefferson University,
Philadelphia, PA, USA

Barbara A. Wilson
MRC Cognition and Brain Sciences Unit,
Cambridge, UK

Gordon Winocur
Rotman Research Institute at Baycrest,
University of Toronto,
Toronto, ON, Canada

J. Martin Wojtowicz
Department of Physiology,
Faculty of Medicine,
University of Toronto,
Toronto, ON, Canada

Preface

The field of cognitive neurorehabilitation has advanced notably in several ways since the publication, in 1999, of the first edition of *Cognitive Neurorehabilitation: A Comprehensive Approach*. The science has improved. This is particularly evident in the methods of treatment; in understanding the different factors that might affect successful outcome; in the expanded use of neuroimaging modalities to understand the limitations and benefits of neurorehabilitation; and in the understanding of the potential pathophysiological mechanisms in different patient groups that are key to the development of new procedures. Our overall objective in editing this new and expanded volume remains in essence the same as the first: summarize the latest developments in cognitive neuroscience research related to cognitive neurorehabilitation; review the principles that form the platform of successful interventions; and synthesize new findings about the rehabilitation of cognitive changes in different populations.

Cognitive Neurorehabilitation, Second Edition: Evidence and Application provides understanding of *why* cognitive neurorehabilitation may or may not work; *how* to use different neuroimaging methods to evaluate the efficacy of interventions; *what* personal and external factors impact rehabilitation success; *how* biological and psychopharmacologic changes can be understood and treated; *how* to treat different disorders such as language and memory; and *where* the field is going in research and clinical application.

Cognitive Neurorehabilitation, Second Edition: Evidence and Application is intended to be a comprehensive reference volume for those interested in the scientific base of cognitive neurorehabilitation, and will include the most up-to-date information for the practicing clinician. The book is an expanded edition, with five major sections compared with four in the first edition, and 32 chapters compared with 22 in the first. More importantly, as reflected in the title, this is a totally new volume, not just a "second" edition. The content is much more comprehensive in scope, containing information not present in the first edition. Chapters that were present in the first edition have been significantly updated to reflect current knowledge. For example, there are state-of-the-art reviews of the principles underlying successful neurorehabilitation, the methods and value of neuroimaging, and new neurorehabilitation procedures. Some important chapters in the first edition on clinical programs and services were not included in the second edition because of our desire to emphasize the neuroscience underpinnings of neurorehabilitation.

The volume consists of six Parts, each organized and prefaced by its section editor(s): (I) *Principles of cognitive neurorehabilitation*, extending from the basics of neuroplasticity to principles of compensation, incorporating all levels of evidence currently available; (II) *Application of imaging technologies*, an overview of the use of structural and functional neuroimaging procedures including MRI, ERPs and MEG; (III) *Factors affecting successful outcome*, with chapters discussing the impact of internal and external factors including mood, self-awareness, exercise and diet; (IV) *Pharmacologic and biological approaches*, covering the rationale for pharmacologic strategies as well as practical examples related to different disorders, and current advances in promoting neural regeneration and stem cell research; (V) *Behavioral/neuropsychological approaches*, summarising the strengths and weaknesses of therapies targeting motor and various types of cognitive disorders (e.g., attention, aphasia, neglect, "executive", memory); and (VI) an *Overview*, evaluating the current status of rehabilitation through the lens of neuroscience research, and suggesting the future of cognitive rehabilitation.

This second edition maintains positive features of the first edition, including summary bullet points throughout the chapters; the scientific emphasis; the content organization. Within each chapter, there are highlights of different sections to provide the reader, especially students, with key summaries of the content. The topics broadly cover subject matter important to cognitive rehabilitation, from basic anatomy and chemistry, to rehabilitative methods, to consideration of psychosocial factors. The overall organization of the book and the structure of each chapter were designed so that the volume would also be a suitable textbook at the graduate level. The book is not, however, a practical "cookbook" of what to do for different neurorehabilitation healthcare professionals.

There are also many new features. We have added chapters that reflect the changes in knowledge, thinking and approaches in the last decade. We have included information not presented in other neurorehabilitation books: e.g., variability of performance; mechanisms underlying success and failure in rehabilitation of executive dysfunction; the role of neurogenesis in brain recovery; the potential of stem cell research. We have added color figures which should highlight in a striking visual manner the most important information, especially in neuroimaging.

We tried to reach four primary audiences (reflected in the type of contributors).

(a) Healthcare professionals actively involved in rehabilitation. This includes clinical psychologists, neuropsychologists, occupational therapists and to some degree physiotherapists. For this group, our goal was to provide a reference for clinicians to evaluate the scientific basis of treatment.

(b) Rehabilitation physicians actively involved in cognitive neurorehabilitation. Neurologists, physiatrists and psychiatrists will find the information important in guiding their referrals, and in evaluating the quality of service provided.

(c) Students. For all graduate programs interested in the scientific basis of cognitive rehabilitation, the information in this second edition should be indispensable. Although there is value for undergraduate courses, the book was geared to a higher level.

(d) Researchers in rehabilitation. Our goal was to provide scientific information to help researchers in cognitive rehabilitation gain new background information and insights. We also hope that the book will serve as a creative ferment to stimulate new research. And, finally, we hope to convince cognitive neuroscientists that, indeed, there is "science" in cognitive neurorehabilitation.

A secondary market goal was that some of the information provided would be of interest and value to healthcare workers involved in neurorehabilitation, but not necessarily in the front lines of research or clinical care (e.g., social workers, hospital administrators). Such professionals play a critical role in all aspects of rehabilitation medicine and contribute significantly to the process of knowledge transfer.

We hope that we have to some degree achieved our stated objectives, and that this volume will directly or indirectly improve the lives of those whom we try to help through cognitive neurorehabilitation. We thank all the authors who contributed to this second edition.

Particular thanks go to Susan Gillingham, who did all the organisation work. Without Susan, *Cognitive Neurorehabilitation, Second Edition: Evidence and Application* would not have come to fruition.

We are pleased to dedicate this second edition of *Cognitive Neurorehabilitation* to the many patients who have given their time and effort to participate in the many research projects that have advanced the science, in the hope that maximum benefit may come to similar individuals in the future.

Donald T. Stuss,
Gordon Winocur and
Ian H. Robertson

Principles of cognitive neurorehabilitation

Introduction to Section 1

Gordon Winocur

Cognitive neurorehabilitation is predicated on two fundamental principles: (1) that the brain has within it an inherent plasticity that enables it to recover from damage that gives rise to cognitive impairment, and (2) that individuals have the capacity to make behavioral adjustments necessitated by changing circumstances. At the same time, the development of the field rests on recognition of and adherence to other essential principles. Foremost are those principles that guide the conduct and assessment of research that ultimately fuels the development of successful rehabilitation programs. Too often, these principles receive insufficient attention and, as a result, the foundations on which treatment programs rest can be a little shaky. It is appropriate then that the first section of this book, which is intended to be comprehensive and broader in scope than the first edition, is devoted to some of the over-riding principles that are central to cognitive neurorehabilitation, and to its continued development as a form of clinical practice within rehabilitation medicine.

The first two chapters cover neuroplasticity and the brain's potential for reorganization in ways that make optimal use of residual resources in promoting cognitive recovery. Kolb and Gibb review principles that govern brain plasticity and factors that affect its expression following regional damage. In describing some of the cellular and physiological mechanisms underlying plasticity, Kolb and Gibb make the important point that the level of analysis must depend on the questions being asked. This has important implications for cognitive

neurorehabilitation. For example, an understanding of alterations at the neuronal or neurotransmitter level are critical to the development of pharmacological therapies, whereas an appreciation of reorganisation of neural circuitry through neuroimaging, may be more relevant to designing behavioral therapies that invoke the use of appropriate strategies. The chapter broadly reviews research that demonstrates that brain plasticity is influenced by a wide range of factors that include age, etiology of damage, and type of experiences. Kolb and Gibb end with the interesting observation that brain plasticity may not always work in the patient's interest and cite, as an example, counter-productive changes that occur in relation to developmental disorders. This is important for cognitive neurorehabilitation because brain-damaged individuals often develop maladaptive responses and their neurophysiological imprint must be overcome for rehabilitation to proceed successfully.

In their chapter, Hunter and McEwen focus on the relationship between adverse life experiences and chronic dysregulation of the neuroendocrine axis which, combined, increase the risk of various diseases (e.g., type 2 diabetes, stroke), that include cognitive impairment as part of their symptomatology. Attention is directed to stress-induced abnormal release of adrenal steroids (e.g., cortisol) and their toxic effects on brain regions such as the hippocampus. In contrast, there may be benefits from treatment with gonadal steroids (e.g., androgens, estrogens). Hunter and McEwen acknowledge the controversy in this area but also remind us of the considerable evidence linking such treatment to positive effects on dendritic growth and synaptic function in the hippocampus. Under some circumstances, the authors suggest, this form of cognitive therapy may be warranted. Hunter and McEwen assess the potential for pharmacologic treatment of cognitive problems that are related to metabolic disorders and, in line with other contributors (e.g., Kolb and Gibb; Dawson and Winocur; Dixon, Garrett and Bäckman) stress the importance of combining such interventions with a healthy lifestyle, physical exercise, and a psychosocial environment that is both stimulating and supportive.

Consistent with the brain's capacity for reorganization is the principle of compensation, whereby cognitive abilities are recovered through a combination of adaptive changes in brain function and behavior. Dixon *et al.* provide a lucid account of conditions that give rise to compensatory approaches and the mechanisms by which compensation is mediated. On a cautionary note, they point out that, because of constraints and diminished resources resulting from damage to functional systems, successful compensation in one area may entail losses in other areas. Because these losses may have negative consequences, they must be taken into account in rehabilitation programs aimed at promoting compensation. As well, Dixon *et al.* emphasize the important interplay between compensation that occurs between neural and behavioral levels, and the need for them to influence each other if optimal benefits are to be achieved. The authors cite several studies of behavioral training-induced cognitive improvements and, importantly, provide related evidence that such improvements are accompanied by stable and long-lasting biological changes. Dixon *et al.* further underscore the importance of compensation to rehabilitation practice by arguing for the universality of the process and its relevance to different types of injury and abnormality.

Ultimately, progress in neurorehabilitation practice will flow from quality research and this is the focus of Rodriguez and Rothi's thought-provoking chapter. The authors acknowledge the randomized control trial (RCT) as the gold standard in rehabilitation research. At the same time, they argue that exploratory studies have a rightful place in the investigative process and, properly conducted, can even help to shape RCTs, rendering them more informative in the larger picture. A substantial portion of the chapter is devoted to Rothi's multistage model for conducting neurorehabilitation research. According to the model, in the initial *discovery* stage, clear hypotheses are proposed and evaluated at the basic science level. This stage might involve animal models or normal humans but, in the second, *translation* stage, the research is extended to the targeted populations. The third, *innovation*, stage entails exploratory clinical study using the principles established in stages 1 and 2. At this point, a treatment should be ready for a phase I clinical trial (*evaluation/formalization stage*), in which optimal conditions are created for demonstrating a treatment effect. A positive outcome would lead to a more rigorous phase II trial (*efficacy stage*) that would take into account effect sizes and possibly involve multiple sites. A phase III clinical trial (*effectiveness stage*) would then be conducted to establish the full potential of the treatment program. Finally, it is necessary to consider issues related to delivery of the program and its impact, taking into account practical considerations such as costs and benefits.

Cicerone takes on a similar cause in his probing chapter. He too acknowledges the important advances made through RCTs and, like Rodriguez and Rothi, argues that there are important benefits to be derived from other approaches. He suggests, for example, that observational studies may be even more useful than RCTS in certain situations – such as evaluating behaviors that have a relatively low rate of occurrence, or in assessing naturally occurring services. Cicerone's position is that we need more *good* RCTs in neurorehabilitation research and, to achieve that, investigators must strive to avoid design pitfalls which occur all too frequently. As examples, he cites unsuccessful randomization, failure to employ double-blind designs and masked-outcome assignments, and inadequate long-term follow-up. Moreover, it is important to be cognizant of the need to report fully all relevant procedures, provide information on treatment compliance and

treatment integrity, and, in the interest of repro-
ducibility, to use accessible outcome measures.
The chapters by Cicerone and Rodriguez and Rothi
contain important messages and provide a valuable road-map for conducting scientifically rigorous rehabilitation research that ultimately will
lead to improved treatment programs and better
outcomes.

As Kolb and Gibb point out in their chapter, a
critical consideration in evaluating cognitive neurorehabilitation programs is in the selection of outcome measures and this is the focus of Lincoln
and Nair's chapter. They begin by emphasizing
the need to distinguish between impairments
induced by brain damage and changes in functional
performance – neurorehabilitation may be effective
in improving performance without necessarily
affecting the fundamental impairment. If assessment focused exclusively on cognitive impairment
(as measured by standard cognitive tests), the benefits of the program may not be fully appreciated or
even detected. In selecting cognitive instruments
for measuring outcome, Lincoln and Nair emphasize established criteria (e.g., reliability, validity,
sensitivity to program-induced change and practicality) and, in addition, remind us that not all tests
are well suited for assessing outcome. Some are
better suited as screening or diagnostic instruments.
They go on to review strengths and weaknesses of
assessment techniques in various cognitive domains
(e.g., attention, memory, executive function). The
authors also underscore the need for ecologically
valid tests but caution that sometimes such tests
(e.g., the Rivermead Behavioral Memory Test) only
indirectly measure performance in everyday activities. Finally, they point out that, although participation in a wide range of activities in a social context is
the ultimate aim of cognitive neurorehabilitation,
few measures of participation rate actually exist,
and that progress in this area must be considered a
research priority.

In Chapter 3 of this section, Stuss and Binns bring
into focus the fundamental principle of behavioral
variability, as it applies to cognitive neurorehabilitation. It is well established that cognitively
impaired patients can be extremely variable in the
expression of their cognitive problems. It follows
that variability should be taken into account routinely in assessing recovery or the effects of cognitive neurorehabilitation. Yet, it is not and, as Stuss
and Binns point out, to assess outcome in a single
snapshot in time, runs the risk of masking benefits
or, conversely, giving an exaggerated impression of
improvement. Because it is so tempting to mistakenly conclude positive effects following a single
assessment, Stuss and Binns label variability as a
"silent disorder." Their highly enlightening chapter
is particularly informative on intra-individual variability, which typically receives less attention than
inter-individual variability. They discuss various
ways of measuring intra-individual variability (e.g.,
between-task scatter; within-task dispersion), as
well as mediating factors (e.g., structural – fatigue,
rhythmic changes; task demands; personality; age).
They also provide insights into possible mechanisms and, in the process, distinguish between frontal lobe-mediated, general control processes, and
damage-specific control processes that are said to
be regulated by brain regions associated with the
functions affected. The chapter ends with a description of individual cases that dramatically make the
authors' point that variability is a critical index of
cognitive impairment that must be factored into
neurorehabilitation programs and treatment
assessment. It remains to be seen, of course, whether
variability measurement will prove practical in diagnosis and in assessing outcome. Nevertheless, in
convincingly showing that increased variability is
an inherent part of the pathology associated with
cognitive impairment and the recovery process,
Stuss and Binns have made a strong case for investigating the possibilities.

1

Principles of neuroplasticity and behavior

Bryan Kolb and Robbin Gibb

Introduction

Behavioral neuroscience spent much of the twentieth century seeking the fundamental rules of cerebral organization. One underlying assumption of much of that work was that there is constancy in cerebral organization and function, both between and within mammalian species (e.g., Kaas, 2006). One unexpected principle to emerge, however, was that although there is much constancy in cerebral functioning, there is remarkable variability as well. This variability reflects the brain's capacity to alter its structure and function in reaction to environmental diversity, thus reflecting a capacity that is often referred to as *brain plasticity*. Although this term is now commonly used in psychology and neuroscience, it is not easily defined and is used to refer to changes at many levels in the nervous system ranging from molecular events, such as changes in gene expression, to behavior (e.g., Shaw & McEachern, 2001). The relationship between molecular or cellular changes and behavior is by no means clear and is plagued by the problems inherent in inferring causation from correlation. Nonetheless, we believe that it is possible to identify some general principles of brain plasticity and behavior. As we do so we will attempt to link these principles to potential clinical implications.

Assumptions underlying brain plasticity

As we consider the principles of brain plasticity, we need to consider five underlying assumptions that will color our perspective.

Brain plasticity takes advantage of a basic, but flexible, blueprint for cerebral organization that is formed during development

The process of brain development is a remarkable feat of nature. Billions of neurons and glia must be generated, they must migrate to their correct locations, and they must form neuronal networks that can underlie functions that range from as simple as postural reflexes to complex thought. Although a complete genetic blueprint for neuronal organization might be possible for a simple creature like the nematode *Caenorhabditis elegans*, which has a total of 302 neurons, it is not remotely possible for the mammalian brain to have a specific blueprint (Katz, 2007). The best that nature can be expected to do is to produce a rough blueprint of cerebral organization that must be shaped by experience in order for animals to exploit specific ecologies, including cultures. The disadvantage of such flexibility is that it is possible to make errors, but this problem is certainly outweighed by the advantage of having a brain that can learn complex motor or perceptual skills that could scarcely have been anticipated by evolution thousands or even millions of years before.

Cerebral functions are both localized and distributed

One of the great issues in the history of brain research relates to whether functions are discretely localized in the brain (for a review, see Kolb & Whishaw, 2001). The resolution to this debate was important because the degree of localization of

Cognitive Neurorehabilitation, Second Edition: Evidence and Application, ed. Donald T. Stuss, Gordon Winocur and Ian H. Robertson. Published by Cambridge University Press. © Cambridge University Press 2008.

function places constraints on the potential extent of functional plasticity. The more distributed a function, the greater the likelihood that the neural networks underlying the function will be flexible after a brain injury. As we enter the twenty-first century it is clear that functions are at once localized and distributed. Consider language. Although there are discrete language zones in the cortex, language is much more distributed across the cortex than would have been expected from the classical neurologists (e.g., Geschwind, 1972). But there are limits to distributed functions, especially in the sensory systems. For example, information coming to the occipital lobe travels from the eye to subcortical areas, then to Visual area 1 (V1) where it is processed, and then is sent on to other visual regions such as V2 and on to V3 etc. If V1 is only partially damaged, V2 will still receive some input and can function, albeit not normally. Further, after partial damage, neural networks in V1 and V2 could reorganise and possibly facilitate some type of functional improvement. But if V1 is completely (or substantially) damaged, downstream visual areas, such as V2, will not be provided with appropriate inputs and no amount of reorganization in V2 could generate functional recovery. The partial localization of functions thus places significant constraints upon plasticity and recovery of function.

3. Changes in the brain can be shown at many levels of analysis

Although it is ultimately the activity of neuronal networks that controls behavior, and thus changes in neuronal network activity that are responsible for behavioral change, there are many ways to examine changes in the activity of networks. Changes may be inferred from global measures of brain activity, such as in the various forms of *in vivo* imaging, but such changes are far removed from the molecular processes that drive them. Changes in the activity of networks likely reflect changes at the synapse but changes in synaptic activity must result from more molecular changes such as modifications in channels, gene expression, and so on. The problem in studying brain plasticity is to choose a surrogate marker that best suits the question being asked. Changes in potassium channels may be perfect for studying presynaptic changes at specific synapses that might be related to simple learning in invertebrates (e.g., Kandel, 1979; Lukowiak *et al.*, 2003; Roberts & Glanzman, 2003) but are impractical for understanding sex differences in language processing. The latter might best be studied by *in vivo* imaging or postmortem analysis of cell morphology (e.g., Jacobs *et al.*, 1993). Neither level of analysis is "correct." The appropriate level must be suited for the research question at hand.

One convenient surrogate for synaptic change in laboratory studies of brain and behavior is dendritic morphology. In this type of study entire neurons are stained with a heavy metal (gold, silver or mercury) and the dendritic space is calculated (Figure 1.1). It is assumed that by knowing the space available for

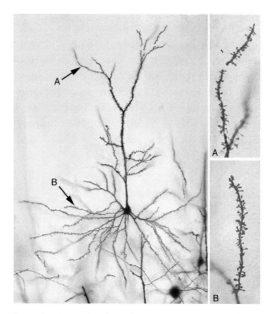

Figure 1.1. Example of a Golgi-Cox stained pyramidal cell from layer III of the parietal cortex of the rat. A. Higher power magnification showing spines on an apical branch. B. Higher power magnification showing spines on a basilar branch. (Photograph courtesy of Grazyna Gorny.)

synapses it is possible to infer associations between synaptic organization and behavior – notwithstanding the problems inherent in correlational studies discussed below. The studies of Jacobs and Scheibel (Jacobs *et al.*, 1993; Jacobs & Scheibel, 1993) provide a good example. These researchers examined the dendritic morphology of pyramidal neurons in postmortem brains of people whose educational and employment history was known. Comparison of synapse numbers in the posterior speech zone of people with university education, high-school education, or less than high-school education showed that there were progressively more synapses on the neurons from brains with more education. The study cannot tell us why this correlation is present but it tells us that there is some relationship between experience and synaptic organization.

To be functionally meaningful, changes reflecting brain plasticity must persist for at least a few days

Changes in neuronal activity related to brain plasticity may be of limited duration, perhaps in the order of seconds or milliseconds. While such changes are interesting in their own right, we are focusing our attention on longer-lasting changes that persist for at least a few days. This is a practical assumption as we think about how experiences might be related to chronic behavioral changes seen after brain injury or with addiction.

Correlation is not a four-letter word

By its very nature, behavioral neuroscience searches for neuronal correlates of behavior. Some of these changes are directly associated with behavior but others are more ambiguous. Consider an example. If an individual is given a psychoactive drug we may see an obvious acute behavioral change such as increased motor activity. If the drug is taken repeatedly, we may see that there is an escalating increase in the drug-dependent hyperactivity, a phenomenon referred to as *drug-induced behavioral sensitisation*. If we were to look for changes in the brain

that were related to the observed sensitization we might find a change in synapse number in some discrete brain region such as the nucleus accumbens (NAcc). Both the behavioral change and the synaptic change are correlates of the drug administration. But what is the relationship between the behavioral and synaptic change? We can conclude that the drug caused the behavioral change but it is less clear that the drug directly caused the neuronal change. Perhaps the behavioral change caused the neuronal change or maybe both were related to some other change in the brain. Thus, a common criticism of studies trying to link neuronal changes to behavior is that "they are only correlates." This is true but it is hardly a reason to dismiss such studies. The task is to try to break the correlation by showing that one change can occur without the other. The presence of such evidence would disconfirm causality but, unfortunately, the failure to break the correlation is not proof of causation. Ultimately the proof would be in showing how the synaptic changes arose, which would presumably involve molecular analysis such as a change in gene transcription. For many studies this would be an extremely difficult challenge and often impractical. It is our view that once we understand the "rules" that govern neuronal and behavioral change, we will be better able to look for molecular changes. Furthermore, we argue that a certain level of ambiguity in the degree of causation is perfectly justifiable at this stage of our knowledge. Understanding the precise mechanism whereby the synaptic changes might occur is not necessary to proceed with further studies aimed at improving functional outcome.

Principles of brain plasticity

Although it is presumptuous to try to identify basic principles of brain plasticity when so much is still unknown, we believe that the progress over the past decade allows us to begin to identify some of the rules underlying brain plasticity. These principles should be seen as a work in progress that will undoubtedly be expanded and further demonstrated over the next decade.

When the brain changes, this is reflected in behavioral change

The primary function of the brain is to produce behavior but behavior is not constant. We learn and remember, we create new thoughts or images, and we change throughout our lifetime. All of these processes require changes in neural networks. It follows that whenever neural networks change, behavior, including mental behavior, will also change. A corollary of this principle is that in order to change behavior we must change the brain. This latter idea is especially important as we search for treatments for brain injuries or diseases.

Plasticity is found in all nervous systems and the principles are conserved

Even the simplest animals, such as the nematode *C. elegans*, can show simple learning that is correlated with neuronal plasticity (e.g., Rose & Rankin, 2001). Similarly, there is now an extensive literature showing neuronal and other changes in invertebrates such as sea snail *Aplysia* during simple learning, including associative learning. Furthermore, it now has become clear that both simple and complex nervous systems show both pre- and postsynaptic changes and that the changes are remarkably similar (e.g., Rose & Rankin, 2001). There is reason to believe, for example, that there are NMDA-like changes in learning in both mammals and invertebrates (e.g., Roberts & Glanzman, 2003). The details of the postsynaptic second messengers may differ in simple and complex systems but the general principles appear to be conserved across both simple and complex animals.

The brain is altered by a wide range of experiences

Virtually every experience has the potential to alter the brain, at least briefly. It now has been shown that a wide variety of experiences can also produce

Table 1.1. Factors affecting the synaptic organization of the normal brain

Factor	Reference
Sensory and motor experience	Greenough & Chang, 1989
Task learning	Greenough & Chang, 1989
Gonadal hormones and stress hormones	Stewart & Kolb, 1988
Psychoactive drugs (e.g., stimulants, THC)	Robinson & Kolb, 2004
Neurotrophic factors (e.g., NGF, bFGF)	Kolb *et al.*, 1997
Natural rewards (e.g., social interaction, sex)	Fiorino & Kolb, 2003
Aging	Kramer *et al.*, 2004
Stress	McEwen, 2005
Anti-inflammatories (e.g., COX-2 inhibitors)	Silasi & Kolb, 2007
Diet (e.g., choline)	Meck & Williams, 2003
Electrical stimulation: kindling	Teskey *et al.*, 2001
Long-term potentiation	Ivanco *et al.*, 2000
Direct cortical stimulation	Teskey *et al.*, 2004

enduring changes, ranging from general sensory-motor experience to psychoactive drugs to electrical brain stimulation (see Table 1.1). The bulk of these studies have used morphological techniques such as electron microscopy or Golgi-like stains and have shown that experience-dependent changes can be seen in every species of animals tested, ranging from fruit flies and bees to rats, cats and monkeys (for a review see Kolb & Whishaw, 1998). Consider a few examples.

When animals are placed in complex environments rather than simple laboratory cages, within 30 days there is about a 5% increase in brain weight and cortical thickness, an increase in cortical acetylcholine and neurotrophic factors (e.g., nerve growth factor (NGF), brain-derived neurotrophic factor (BDNF), fibroblast growth factor-2 (FGF-2)), as well as changes in physiological properties of neurons such as those measured in studies of long-term potentiation (LTP) (for a review see Kolb & Whishaw, 1998). Although most studies have focused on neocortical changes, similar changes can also be seen in hippocampus and striatum (e.g., Comery *et al.*, 1996; Juraska, 1990). The anatomical and physiological changes are associated with improved performance on tests of both motor and cognitive behaviors and although the data are correlational, it is generally assumed that the morphological changes are responsible for the facilitation in behavior.

Experience-dependent changes in the brain do not require procedures as intense as complex housing, however. Increased social experience selectively increases synapses in the orbital frontal cortex (Fiorino & Kolb, 2003; Hamilton *et al.*, 2003). We have also seen that tactile stimulation either in infancy or adulthood alters cells in sensorimotor cortex (e.g., Gibb & Kolb, submitted a,b). This latter treatment has also been used in animals with cortical injuries to stimulate dendritic growth and facilitate functional recovery Although there is little evidence that exercise can enhance plasticity in the normal brain, there is growing evidence that it can facilitate plastic changes in the injured lab animal and human brain (e.g., Gibb *et al.*, 2005; Kramer *et al.*, 2006).

A final example can be seen in the effects of psychoactive drugs. Robinson & Kolb (1999a) showed that repeated doses of amphetamine or cocaine given to rats produced a persisting increase in dendritic length and spine density localized to the medial prefrontal cortex (mPFC) and NAcc but not to adjacent sensorimotor cortical regions. It now appears that repeated doses of all psychoactive drugs, including prescription drugs, change neuronal morphology. The details of drug-induced morphological changes vary with the drug but the general principle is that psychoactive drugs alter neuronal morphology in the cerebrum and this can be seen both in dendritic measures as well as in a variety of more molecular measures (for a review, see Hyman *et al.*, 2006). Once again, the relationship between the behavioral changes, such as drug-induced behavioral sensitization, and the altered neuronal networks has yet to be proven but there is little doubt that the chronic effects of drug use are not neutral to cerebral functioning. The ability of drugs to alter neuronal morphology may be important for rehabilitation because drugs can be combined with behavioral treatments such as rehabilitation therapy, including cognitive therapy (e.g., Gonzalez *et al.*, 2006).

Taken together the examples described above illustrate the power of experience in modulating cerebral networks and in facilitating remodeling stimulated by behavioral therapies. Although experience is likely more effective in remodeling neural networks as they are repairing after injury, improvement still can occur late after injury (e.g., Hodics *et al.*, 2006). Psychomotor stimulants may provide a powerful way of reinstating cerebral plasticity late after injury to facilitate the effectiveness of behavioral therapies.

Plastic changes are age-specific

When weanling, adult or senescent rats were placed in a complex environment, we had anticipated that we would find larger changes in the younger animals but to our surprise, we found a qualitative difference in the neuronal response to the same experience. Thus, whereas rats at all ages showed an increase in dendritic length and branching in neocortical pyramidal cells after complex housing, rats placed in the environments as infants showed a *decrease* in spine density whereas young adult or senescent rats showed an *increase* in spine density (Kolb *et al.*, 2003a). A similar drop in spine density was found in later studies in which newborn rats were given tactile stimulation with a soft brush for 15 min, three times daily over the first 10 days of life (Kolb & Gibb, submitted).

The obvious question is whether the behavioral effects to the complex housing are the same depending upon the age at experience. Our early results suggest that there is an advantage in both cognitive and motor tasks and that it does not matter when the experience occurred. There are clearly different ways to organize neuronal networks to enhance both motor and cognitive behaviors. This point is important as we consider treatments for brain dysfunction – there may be many ways to facilitate recovery.

Early events, including prenatal events, can influence the brain throughout life

Our finding that early *postnatal* experiences could alter neuronal organization led us to ask if *prenatal* experiences might also alter cerebral organization. In one study pregnant dams were placed in complex environments for 8 hours a day prior to their pregnancy and then throughout the 3 week gestation. (In different studies the dams were in the environments during the day or night but it made no difference.) Analysis of the adult brains of their infants showed a *decrease* in dendritic length and an *increase* in spine density in adulthood (Gibb *et al.*, submitted). We were surprised both that there was a large effect of *prenatal* experience and that it was qualitatively different than experience either in the juvenile period or in adulthood. More recently we have shown that a variety of *prenatal* experiences alter brain organisation in adulthood including prenatal tactile stimulation (i.e., stimulation of the pregnant dam), exercise during pregnancy, prenatal stress and psychoactive drugs. All of these experiences also chronically alter motor and cognitive functions, with the precise effect varying with the different experiences (for a review see Kolb *et al.*, in press).

Although we do not know how these *prenatal* changes might influence the effect of *postnatal* experiences, it is clear that prenatal experiences produce chronic effects on brain organization and behavior. One is reminded here of the idea of cognitive (or neural) reserve as being key factors in the onset of dementias (e.g., Stern, 2006). Might early life events influence cognitive reserve in adulthood or senescence?

Plastic changes are area dependent

Although we are tempted to expect plastic changes in neuronal networks to be fairly general, it is becoming clear that many experience-dependent changes are highly specific. The clearest examples can be seen in neuropsychological studies in which animals are trained on cognitive or motor tasks. For example, rats trained on a visuospatial task show specific changes in visual cortex whereas rats trained on motor tasks show specific changes in motor cortex (e.g., Greenough & Chang, 1989; Kolb & Cioe, submitted; Withers & Greenough, 1989). Such task-dependent specific changes are reasonable in view of the relative localization of functions in the cortex. But not all area-dependent changes are so easily predicted. Consider two examples.

We noted above that the effect of psychoactive drugs appeared to be selective to regions that receive dopaminergic innervation. We therefore were surprised to find that the orbitofrontal cortex (OFC), another region that receives dopaminergic innervation, showed drug-induced changes that are opposite to those in mPFC and NAcc (Robinson & Kolb, 2004). Thus, whereas psychomotor stimulants *increased* dendritic length and spine density in the mPFC, they *decreased* the same measures in the OFC. The contrasting effects of these drugs on the two prefrontal regions are puzzling given the similarity in thalamic and other connections of the two regions (e.g., Uylings *et al.*, 2003). Curiously, there also are differential effects of gonadal hormones on the two prefrontal regions as well: mPFC neurons have more synaptic space in males whereas OFC neurons have more space in females (Kolb & Stewart, 1991). Although we do not yet know what such differences mean behaviorally, there can be little doubt that the differential response of two such similar cortical regions to drugs and hormones must be important in understanding their functions.

Plastic changes are time-dependent

There is growing evidence that plastic changes are not constant and can change over time. The clearest example comes from drug studies. For example, although there are large increases in spine density and dendritic length 2 weeks after cessation of cocaine administration, these changes slowly disappear over a

4-month period (Kolb *et al.*, 2003b). In contrast, when rats are given morphine and the brains are examined immediately after drug cessation, there is an increase in dendritic arborization in NAcc (Ballesteros-Yáñez *et al.*, 2006) but a month later the changes are just the opposite (Robinson & Kolb, 1999b). One reason for the time-dependent effects of the drug exposure may be that behavior is changing as the animals are first in withdrawal and then adapt to the drug's absence.

Time-dependent plasticity also can be seen in response to repeated electrical brain stimulation. Repeated low intensity stimulation can slowly lead to the development of spontaneous seizures, a phenomenon known as *kindling* (Teskey, 2001). The development of seizures is correlated with changes in dendritic length and spine density that normalize a month after cessation of electrical stimulation (Teskey *et al.*, 2001). Curiously, the stimulation also produces physiological changes that do not change. In this case it appears that the experience (i.e., the electrical stimulation) produces both dendritic and physiological change but the two are not related.

The possibility that there are different chronic and transient experience-dependent changes in cerebral neurons is consistent with genetic studies showing that there are different genes expressed acutely and chronically in response to complex environments (Rampon *et al.*, 2000). The difference in how transient and persistent changes in neuronal networks relate to behavior is unknown.

Brain injury produces plastic changes that vary with etiology

Although we may be able to point to a specific proximal cause of a brain injury, such as a stroke, the end result of brain injury is not the result of a single causative event. Rather, there is an initial event followed by a cascade of cellular events that can seriously compromise the injured brain as well as brain regions that were not directly injured. Such post-injury changes may be rapid, such as changes in pH or ionic balance that can occur within seconds or minutes after an injury, or they may be slower such as the production of glia that migrate to the injured tissue. Of more interest, however, are the longer-term changes in neuronal networks that underlie the emerging post-injury functions. The nature of these changes varies with the cause of the injury.

The adult brain can be injured in numerous ways, including especially stroke, head trauma, and neurosurgical excision for disease. The literature on functional recovery and rehabilitation quite reasonably has assumed that after the initial post-injury period, patients with different types of brain injuries are likely to benefit similarly from treatments. However, this presumption rests on the assumption that the reparative processes that spontaneously begin after injury are similar for different types of injuries. A study by Gonzalez & Kolb (2003) leads us to question this assumption.

These authors gave rats equivalent lesions of the sensorimotor cortex but produced the damage either by arterial occlusion, vascular stripping or surgical suction. The behavioral outcomes were similar in three groups, with severe chronic motor symptoms in the contralateral limbs. Similarly, the infarct volumes were essentially identical across the groups. What was surprising, however, was when the authors examined the morphology of neurons in the striatum and perilesional area they found that each group was different (see also Szele *et al.*, 1995). For instance, the brains with suction lesions showed atrophy of dendritic fields, whereas the brains of animals with vascular stripping lesions showed reconfigured fields with increased dendritic arborization. We hasten to note, however, that the behavioral recovery within the different groups was comparable, at least with the behavioral measures that the authors employed. This finding is reminiscent of the evidence showing that perinatal experiences can have different effects on brain organization but similar effects on behavior.

One message from the Gonzalez and Kolb study is that capacity for treatment-induced recovery is likely not equivalent after injuries with differing etiologies because the brain is changing differently with different etiologies. This conclusion has obvious implications for rehabilitation of human patients although we are unaware of any direct studies on this issue.

Neuronal plasticity following brain injury varies with age

It has been known since the time of Broca that children seem to have a better outcome after early injury than adults, but we are just beginning to understand why this might be so. The first systematic studies on the comparative effects of early brain injury were done by Margaret Kennard, who studied the effects of motor cortex lesions in infant monkeys. Her seminal observation was that the animals with early lesions showed better recovery of motor functions than those with injuries in adulthood (e.g., Kennard, 1942). Although there was later support for the Kennard findings that "earlier is better" (e.g., Akert et al., 1960), other studies in monkeys were less supportive (Goldman, 1974). It was not until age was systematically varied in studies in rats and cats that the relationship between age at injury and functional outcome became clearer.

We have examined the behavior of adult rats that had focal injuries to the mPFC, motor, temporal, posterior parietal, or posterior cingulate cortex at postnatal days 1, 4, 7, 10, or 90 (i.e., adult). The overall result was that regardless of the location of injury, the functional outcome was always best after injury during the second week of life, which in the rat is a time of intense cerebral synaptogenesis and glial formation. A similar pattern of results can be seen in parallel studies of the effects of cortical lesions in kittens by Villablanca and his colleagues (e.g., Schmanke & Villablanca, 2001; Villablanca et al., 1993), although because the rat and cat develop at different rates the precise ages are different in the two species. The key point here is that birth date is irrelevant – it is the stage of neural development that is important.

But what brain changes account for the age effects? In principle, there are three ways that an injured brain could compensate for lost tissue: (1) reorganisation of existing neuronal networks; (2) development of novel networks; and (3) regeneration of the lost tissue. All three occur after early brain injury. We consider each briefly.

The first studies on anatomical compensations after early brain injury focused on connectivity after unilateral damage to the motor system (e.g., Castro, 1990; D'Amato & Hicks, 1980; Villablanca & Gomez-Pinilla, 1987; Whishaw & Kolb, 1988). The general finding was that if there is perinatal damage to the cortex that normally gives rise to the cortico-bulbar and corticospinal pathways, the intact pathway on the opposite side sprouts new connections both to subcortical motor regions of the damaged hemisphere as well as through an enlarged ipsilateral corticospinal pathway. These new pathways are believed to underlie the better motor outcomes of the early injuries. Parallel findings are seen in the sensory systems as novel pathways develop after damage to primary visual cortex (see a review by Payne & Lomber, 2001). Curiously, however, novel pathways are not always beneficial. We have found that damage to the mPFC in the first week of life results in many anomalous networks but this is correlated with poor outcome on various measures of cognitive function (Kolb et al., 1994). In general, however, the development of novel networks provides one explanation for the Kennard effect.

Another way to make inferences about neuronal network remodeling is to examine dendritic morphology after early injuries. The overall result of these studies is that when functional outcome is good, there is an increase in dendritic arborization and spine density in pyramidal neurons in the remaining cortical mantle (e.g., Kolb et al., 1992, 1994; Kolb & Whishaw, 1989). In contrast, when functional outcome is poor, there is an atrophy of dendritic arbor and spine density. The emergence of the beneficial compensatory changes in dendritic organization takes several weeks and is correlated with an emergence of the improved cognitive function (Kolb & Gibb, 1993).

The idea that the generation of new tissue might be possible after cerebral injury in postnatal mammals was slow to develop and faced considerable skepticism (e.g., Altman, 1962). There now is compelling evidence that new neurons can be formed after injury (see Chapter 22 by Stickland, Weiss & Kolb, this volume) and especially after neonatal injury (Kolb *et al.*, 1998). For example, rats with mPFC lesions around postnatal day 10 show a spontaneous regeneration of much of the lost tissue. Removal of the tissue removes the functional recovery and blockade of the tissue regrowth prevents the recovery (e.g., Dallison & Kolb, 2003; Kolb *et al.*, 1998). Although the spontaneous regeneration can occur after mPFC lesions such regeneration is uncommon, but it can be induced by infusion of FGF-2 after cortical injury on day 10 (e.g., Monfils *et al.*, 2006). Again in these studies the removal of the new tissue leads to a return of the functional deficits and prevention of the regrowth prevents the functional recovery.

The effect of age on post-injury plasticity is likely not only relevant during development. Teuber (1975) reported that brain-injured soldiers also showed a benefit of being younger: 18-year-olds fared better than 25-year-olds who fared better than older soldiers. It is generally assumed that plastic changes are less likely to occur as the brain ages but this has not been well studied and there is little doubt that even senescent animals can show considerable cortical plasticity (e.g., Kolb *et al.*, 2003a; Kramer *et al.*, 2004). There still needs to be systematic studies of cerebral plasticity and behavior throughout the lifespan in both normal and brain-injured animals.

Experience-dependent changes interact

As animals travel through life they have an almost infinite number of experiences that could alter brain organization. There are virtually no experimental studies attempting to determine how a lifetime's experiences might interact. We attempted to address this question in a series of studies in which animals received psychoactive drugs before placement in complex environments (Hamilton & Kolb, 2005; Kolb *et al.*, 2003b; Li *et al.*, 2005). We hypothesized that because the mPFC and NAcc were so profoundly altered by the drugs, they might show less (or no) change in response to the housing experience. To our surprise, not only did the mPFC and

NAcc show no response to the experience, but neither did any other cortical regions. For example, pyramidal neurons in the parietal cortex, which normally show large experience-dependent change but little drug-dependent change, showed no response to the complex housing after prior experience with amphetamine, cocaine, or nicotine. An obvious question was whether prior experience with complex housing would interfere with drug-dependent changes. It does. Animals given complex housing experience prior to repeated doses of nicotine show a much attenuated response to the drug.

Another example of interactions in experience-dependent changes can be seen in the sexually dimorphic response of cortical and hippocampal neurons to complex housing. Juraska (1990) has shown that whereas occipital cortex neurons show increased dendritic arbor in response to complex housing in males, there are no such changes in females. In contrast, females show increased dendritic arbor in hippocampus whereas males do not.

One of the most common experiences of everyday life is stress. In view of the significant effects of stress on dendritic morphology and neurogenesis (see Chapter 4 by Hunter & McEwen, this volume) it seems likely that stress will interact with other experience-dependent changes. We have found, for example, that prenatal stress will block the normal recovery from cortical injury in the second week of life (Gibb & Kolb, unpublished).

Finally, we note that prenatal exposure to experiences described above interact with later postnatal brain injury to produce differential changes in neuronal networks and correlated functional recovery. For instance, rats given prenatal experience via their mother's exposure to tactile stimulation or complex housing show an attenuated effect of the later experience to perinatal brain injury and in some instances show almost complete recovery that is correlated with enhanced dendritic changes (Gibb *et al.*, submitted). In contrast, rats exposed to stress or fluoxetine prenatally show an exaggerated behavioral effect of the same perinatal brain injuries and the poor outcome is correlated with an apparent blockade of post-injury compensatory changes (Day *et al.*, 2003).

Experience differentially affects the normal and injured brain

We initially assumed that a given experience would produce similar changes in the normal and injured brain although there might be quantitative differences in the two conditions. It is now becoming clear that the same experience can sometimes have the opposite effect in the normal and injured brain. One example is tactile stimulation during infancy: there is a decrease in spine density in otherwise normal animals but an increase in cortically injured animals (Kolb & Gibb, submitted). Preliminary studies show similar paradoxically different effects of other treatments such as complex housing and psychoactive drugs. This type of finding has important implications for the development of rehabilitative treatments so we need to understand *why* the effects are different in the normal and injured brain.

Understanding normal plasticity gives us a key to fixing the abnormal brain

It is our working hypothesis that as we learn more about how the normal brain can be changed by experience we will be able to apply this knowledge to the injured brain. This strategy is proving to be successful and Tables 1.2 and 1.3 summarize examples of developing treatments for damage to adult and infant brains, respectively. The general conclusion from this literature is that many, but not all, factors that produce dendritic reorganization and functional benefit in the normal brain can provide benefit after brain injury in both adults and infants. The greatest benefit to lab animals with injury at any age is clearly complex housing. As noted earlier, complex housing leads to increases in various growth factors, and includes social stimulation, sensory stimulation, and increased motor activity. It is likely the combination of all of these factors that provides the large benefit. A key feature too is that there are 24 hours of stimulation 7 days a week, rather than an hour or so twice a week as might be more likely with typical therapy given to human brain-injured patients. Although it would be ideal

Table 1.2. Factors enhancing recovery of the injured adult brain

Factor	Reference
Complex housing	Biernaskie & Corbett, 2001
Olfactory stimulation	Gonzalez & Kolb, 2006
Psychoactive drugs (e.g., stimulants)	Sutton *et al.*, 1989
Neurotrophic factors (e.g., nerve growth factor)	Kolb *et al.*, 1997
Anti-inflammatories (e.g., COX-2 inhibitors)	Silasi & Kolb, 2007
Electrical stimulation	Teskey *et al.*, 2004
Inosine	Chen *et al.*, 2002
Antibodies to No-Go	Papadopoulos *et al.*, 2006

Table 1.3. Factors enhancing recovery from early brain injury

Factor	Reference
Post-injury complex housing	Kolb & Elliott, 1987
Post-injury tactile stimulation	Gibb & Kolb, submitted b
Prenatal complex housing	Gibb *et al.*, submitted
Prenatal tactile stimulation	Gibb & Kolb, submitted a
Gonadal hormones	Kolb & Stewart, 1995
Neurotrophic factors (e.g., fibroblast growth factor-2)	Comeau *et al.*, 2007
Diet (e.g., choline; vitamins/ minerals)	Halliwell *et al.*, submitted
Olfactory stimulation	Gonzalez & Kolb, 2006

to provide human patients with some type of equivalent therapy this would likely be impractical for most health care systems to provide. Furthermore, placing animals or human patients with severe motor deficits in complex environments is likely to be quite stressful so we need to look at alternate treatments. To date, the most promising treatments include the use of psychomotor stimulants such as amphetamine (Sutton *et al.*, 1989) or nicotine (Gonzalez *et al.*, 2006). Clinical trials with amphetamine have given uneven results, likely because of differences in lesion size. Laboratory studies suggest that whereas rats with small lesions show a significant benefit of amphetamine, those with large lesions do not (Goldstein & Davis, 1990). Nicotine may prove to be more effective as it induces widespread changes in neuronal morphology in the normal brain and preliminary laboratory studies do show that nicotine is much more effective than amphetamine in treating animals with large cortical strokes (Moroz & Kolb, 2005).

One additional treatment that is proving to be effective in treating both laboratory animals and stroke patients is direct cortical electrical stimulation (Kleim *et al.*, 2003; Teskey *et al.*, 2003). An obvious extension of the electrical stimulation studies is the combination of the stimulation with other factors such as sensory or motor therapies or psychomotor stimulation, although to our knowledge this has not yet been tried. We note too that pre-injury experiences may interact with post-injury treatments. Recall the complex interactions of experience and drugs discussed above. In one preliminary study we did show that prior exposure to nicotine blocked the effectiveness of post-injury nicotine treatment, a result reminiscent of the drug/environment studies (Gonzalez & Kolb, unpublished observations).

In sum, we believe that there is considerable potential in treating brain injury with factors that are known to enhance brain plasticity in the normal animal. It is likely that combinations of treatments will prove the most effective. We do note too, however, that it is quite likely that injuries of different etiologies will respond differently to specific factors.

The relative strength (and duration) of plasticity is related to relevance of the event to the animal and the intensity or frequency of the events

Although most experiences must be repeated for us to learn, some experiences need only be encountered once and there is long-term change in behavior. One example is food aversions that are related to a single incidence of illness, a phenomenon referred to as *taste aversion conditioning*. If animals are presented with a novel taste that is paired with illness, there is an immediate and permanent aversion to the taste. This learning requires only a single trial.

The key point is that food-related illness is highly relevant to the animal and the brain is clearly prepared to make certain associations (Yamamoto *et al.*, 1994). A parallel example can be seen in imprinting in fowl (e.g., Lorenz, 1970), which is a process where an organism learns, during a sensitive period, to restrict its social preferences to a class of objects. Horn and his colleagues have shown that there are immediate changes in a part of the chick's hyperstriatum after visual imprinting. A variety of rapidly occurring changes have been demonstrated including an *increase* in dendritic length but a *decrease* in spine density, increased glutamatergic excitatory transmission, increased NMDA receptor density, increased immediate early gene expression, and other postsynaptic molecular changes (e.g., Horn 1998; Horn *et al.*, 2001; Solomonia *et al.*, 2005). An important feature of the Horn experiments is that although the most effective stimuli for the changes are fowl, in the absence of fowl there are still changes, thus suggesting flexibility in the innate imprinting system.

The intensity of stimuli can be manipulated in other models by varying drug doses, time in complex housing, duration of electrical stimulation, etc. For example, drug studies show that low doses of psychomotor stimulants produce more restricted changes in dendritic arborization than higher doses (e.g., Diaz-Heijtz *et al.*, 2003) whereas additional doses of psychomotor stimulants produce escalating increases in spine density (Kolb *et al.*, 2003b). Similarly, although animals may show increased dendritic material in cortical pyramidal cells after only a few days of complex housing, the increases are much larger after longer durations (e.g., Greenough & Chang, 1989).

One interesting aspect of electrical stimulation is that whereas high frequency (25–200 Hz) stimulation will produce enhanced postsynaptic potentiation (i.e., long-term potentiation), low frequency stimulation (3 Hz) will produce reduced potentiation (e.g., Cain, 2001; Teyler, 2001). The different forms of stimulation lead to the activation of different postsynaptic signaling pathways and a host of different plastic changes (e.g., Teyler, 2001).

Finally, a recent meta-analysis of physiotherapy after stroke has concluded that the duration and intensity of post-stroke therapy has a direct effect on recovery on tests of daily living (Kwakkel *et al.*, 2004). These studies had no measure of brain changes but the behavioral benefits of the therapy provide a fairly strong suggestion that the treatment did alter cerebral organization.

Brain plasticity is not always a good thing

To this point we mostly have emphasized the plastic changes in the brain that can support improved motor and cognitive function. But plastic changes can also interfere with behavior. For example, it is reasonable to propose that some of the maladaptive behavior of drug addicts could result from drug-related changes in prefrontal neuronal morphology (Robinson & Kolb, 2004). Another example can be seen in schizophrenia.

Schizophrenia is a developmental disorder in which the brain begins to show abnormalities in morphology and behavior in late adolescence. The abnormalities include reduced volumes of the frontal and temporal lobes as well as increased ventricular volume. Morphological analysis of neurons in the prefrontal cortex of postmortem brains of schizophrenic patients shows a reduction in dendritic arborization and spine density (Black *et al.*, 2004). The cause of these changes is poorly understood but one hypothesis is that the changes are in response to some developmental abnormality in the hippocampus (Lipska & Weinberger, 2002). Analysis of hippocampal neurons in postmortem tissue from schizophrenics shows disorganised organization of pyramidal cells that could result from some sort of brain perturbation or genetic abnormality (Conrad *et al.*, 1991). The precise cause is difficult to study in human postmortem tissue but it is possible to manipulate the hippocampus in developing laboratory animals. Behavioral studies of laboratory animals with small ventral hippocampal lesions (or hippocampal inactivation) in infancy show adult functional disorders that are reminiscent of animals with adult prefrontal injury (Lipska & Weinberger,

2002). Anatomical studies of similar animals show reduced dendritic arborisation and spine density similar to what has been seen in human schizophrenic patients (Flores *et al.*, 2005). Such changes are not seen in rats with similar injuries in adulthood. It thus appears that both the behavioral and morphological effects of the small ventral hippocampal injury only occur after a perturbation in infancy. This perturbation is proposed to lead to plastic changes in the developing prefrontal cortex that lead to behavioral abnormalities in adulthood. One prediction of this model is that the structural abnormalities in the frontal lobe should not progress in adulthood but likely would remain static. This appears to be the case (Pantelis *et al.*, 2005).

There are many other examples of pathological plasticity including pathological pain (Baranauskas, 2001), pathological response to sickness (Raison *et al.*, 2006), epilepsy (Teskey, 2001), and dementia (Mattson *et al.*, 2001). One goal is to find ways to block or reverse pathological plasticity, although this is likely to prove difficult.

Postscript

We have tried to identify a set of principles that describe the "rules" that define experience-dependent changes in brain and behavior. Our choice of literature used to define the principles is obviously biased and somewhat arbitrary but we believe that we have provided a framework that others may find useful in designing treatments for motor and cognitive rehabilitation.

REFERENCES

Akert, K., Orth, S., Harlow, H. F., & Schiltz, K. A. (1960). Learned behavior of rhesus monkeys following neonatal bilateral prefrontal lobotomy. *Science*, **132**, 1944–1945.

Altman, J. (1962). Are new neurons formed in the brains of adult mammals? *Science*, **30**, 1127–1128.

Ballesteros-Yáñez, I., Ambrosio, E., Benavides-Piccione, R. *et al.* (2006). The effects of morphine self-administration on cortical pyramidal cell structure in addiction-prone Lewis rats. *Cerebral Cortex*, **17**, 238–249.

Baranauskas, G. (2001). Pain-induced plasticity in the spinal cord. In C. A. Shaw & J. C. McEachern (Eds.), *Toward a Theory of Neuroplasticity* (pp. 373–386). Philadelphia, PA: Psychology Press.

Biernaskie, J., & Corbett, D. (2001). Enriched rehabilitative training promotes improved forelimb motor function and enhanced dendritic growth after focal ischemic injury. *Journal of Neuroscience*, **21**, 5272–5280.

Black, J. E., Kodish, I. M., Grossman, A. W., Klintsova, A. Y., Orlovskaya, D., Vostrikov, V., Uranova, N., & Greenough, W. T. (2004). Pathology of layer V pyramidal neurons in the prefrontal cortex of patients with schizophrenia. *American Journal of Psychiatry*, **161**, 742–744.

Cain, D. P. (2001). Synaptic models of neuroplasticity: What is LTP? In C. A. Shaw & J. C. McEachern (Eds.), *Towards a Theory of Neuroplasticity* (pp. 118–129). Philadelphia, PA: Psychology Press.

Castro, A. (1990). Plasticity in the motor system. In B. Kolb & R. Tees (Eds.), *Cerebral Cortex of the Rat* (pp. 563–588). Cambridge, MA: MIT Press.

Chen, P., Goldberg, D., Kolb, B., Lanser, & Benowitz, L. (2002). Axonal rewiring and improved function induced by inosine after stroke. *Proceedings of the National Academy of Sciences of the United States of America*, **99**, 9031–9036.

Comeau, W. L., Hastings, E., & Kolb, B. (2007). Pre- and postnatal FGF-2 both facilitate recovery and alter cortical morphology following early medial prefrontal cortical injury. *Behavioural Brain Research*, **180**, 18–27.

Comery, T. A., Stamoudis, C. X., Irwin, S. A., & Greenough, W. T. (1996). Increased density of multiple-head dendritic spines on medium-sized spiny neurons of the striatum in rats reared in a complex environment. *Neurobiology of Learning and Memory*, **66**, 93–96.

Conrad, A. J., Abebe, T., Austin, R., Forsythe, S., & Scheibel, A. B. (1991). Hippocampal pyramidal cell disarray in schizophrenia as a bilateral phenomenon. *Archives of General Psychiatry*, **48**, 413–417.

Dallison, A., & Kolb, B. (2003). Recovery from infant medial frontal cortical lesions in rats is reversed by cortical lesions in adulthood. *Behavioural Brain Research*, **146**, 57–63.

D'Amato, C. J., & Hicks, S. P. (1980). Development of the motor system: Effects of radiation on developing corticospinal neurons and locomotor function. *Experimental Neurology*, **70**, 1–23.

Day, M., Gibb, R., & Kolb, B. (2003). Prenatal fluoxetine impairs functional recovery and neuroplasticity after

perinatal frontal cortex lesions in rats. *Society for Neuroscience Abstracts*, **29**, 459.10.

Diaz Heijtz, R., Kolb, B., & Forssberg, H. (2003). Can a therapeutic dose of amphetamine during pre-adolescence modify the pattern of synaptic organization in the brain? *European Journal of Neuroscience*, **18**, 3394–3399.

Fiorino, D., & Kolb, B. (2003). Sexual experience leads to long-lasting morphological changes in male rat prefrontal cortex, parietal cortex, and nucleus accumbens neurons. *Society for Neuroscience Abstracts*, **29**, 402.3.

Flores, G., Alquicer, G., Silva-Gómez, A. B., Zaldivar, G., Stewart, J., Quirion, R., & Srivastava, L. K. (2005). Alterations in dendritic morphology of prefrontal cortical and nucleus accumbens neurons in post-pubertal rats after neonatal excitotoxic lesions of the ventral hippocampus. *Neuroscience*, **133**, 463–470.

Geschwind, N. (1972). Language and the brain. *Scientific American*, **226**, 76–83.

Gibb, R., & Kolb, B. (submitted a). Prenatal tactile stimulation alters brain and behavioral development and facilitates recovery from perinatal brain injury.

Gibb, R., & Kolb, B. (submitted b). Tactile stimulation that facilitates functional recovery after perinatal cortical injury is mediated by FGF-2.

Gibb, R., Wegenast, W. A., & Kolb, B. (2005). Intensity of maternal exercise during pregnancy predicts functional and anatomical outcome of offspring following perinatal brain injury. *Society for Neuroscience Abstracts*, **31**, 835.17.

Gibb, R., Gonzalez, C. L. R., & Kolb, B. (submitted). Complex environmental experience during pregnancy facilitates recovery from perinatal cortical injury in the offspring.

Goldman, P. S. (1974). An alternative to developmental plasticity: Hererology of CNS structures in infants and adults. In D. G. Stein, J. J. Rosen, & N. Butters (Eds.), *Plasticity and Recovery of Function in the Central Nervous System* (pp. 149–174). New York, NY: Academic Press.

Goldstein, L. B., & Davis, J. N. (1990). Influence of lesion size and location on amphetamine-facilitated recovery of beam-walking in rats. *Behavioral Neuroscience*, **104**, 320–327.

Gonzalez, C. L. R., & Kolb, B. (2003). A comparison of different models of stroke on behaviour and brain morphology. *European Journal of Neuroscience*, **18**, 1950–1962.

Gonzalez, C. R., & Kolb, B. (2006). Olfactory stimulation stimulates recovery from neonatal frontal injury in rats. *Unpublished observations*.

Gonzalez, C. L. R., Gharbawie, O. A., & Kolb, B. (2006). Chronic low-dose administration of nicotine facilitates recovery and synaptic change after focal ischemia in rats. *Neuropharmacology*, **50**, 777–787.

Greenough, W. T., & Chang, F. F. (1989). Plasticity of synapse structure and pattern in the cerebral cortex. In A. Peters & E. G. Jones (Eds.), *Cerebral Cortex, Vol.* **7** (pp. 391–440). New York, NY: Plenum Press.

Halliwell, C. Tees, R., & Kolb, B. (Submitted). Prenatal choline treatment enhances recovery from perinatal frontal injury in rats.

Hamilton, D. A., & Kolb, B. (2005). Differential effects of nicotine and complex housing on subsequent experience-dependent structural plasticity in the nucleus accumbens. *Behavioral Neuroscience*, **119**, 355–365.

Hamilton, D. A., Silasi, G., Pellis, S. M., & Kolb, B. (2003). Experience-dependent synaptogenesis in motor, occipital, and orbitofrontal cortex of the rat. *Society for Neuroscience Abstracts*, **29**, 198.11.

Hodics, T., Cohen, L. G., & Cramer, S. C. (2006). Functional imaging of intervention effects in stroke motor rehabilitation. *Archives of Physical Medicine and Rehabilitation*, **87**, *Suppl.* 12, S36–S42.

Horn, G. (1998). Visual imprinting and the neural mechanisms of recognition memory. *Trends in Neurosciences*, **21**, 300–305.

Horn, G., Nicol, A. U., & Brown, M. W. (2001). Tracking memory's trace. *Proceedings of the National Academy of Sciences of the United States of America*, **98**, 5282–5287.

Hyman, S. E., Malenka, R. C., & Nestler, E. J. (2006). Neural mechanisms of addiction: The role of reward-related learning and memory. *Annual Review of Neuroscience*, **29**, 565–598.

Ivanco, T., Racine, R. J., & Kolb, B. (2000). The morphology of layer III pyramidal neurons is altered following induction of LTP in somatomotor cortex of the freely moving rat. *Synapse*, **37**, 16–22.

Jacobs, B., & Scheibel, A. B. (1993). A quantitative dendritic analysis of Wernicke's area in humans. I. Lifespan changes. *Journal of Comparative Neurology*, **327**, 83–96.

Jacobs, B., Schall, M., & Scheibel, A. B. (1993). A quantitative dendritic analysis of Wernicke's area in Humans. II. Gender, hemispheric, and environmental factors. *Journal of Comparative Neurology*, **327**, 97–111.

Juraska, J. (1990). The structure of the rat cerebral cortex: Effects of gender and environment. In B. Kolb & R. C. Tees (Eds.), *Cerebral Cortex of the Rat* (pp. 483–506). Cambridge, MA: MIT Press.

Kaas, J. (2006). *Evolution of Nervous Systems*. New York, NY: Elsevier.

Kandel, E. (1979). *Behavioral Biology of Aplysia*. San Francisco, CA: Freeman & Co.

Katz, P. S. (2007). Evolution and development of neural circuits in invertebrates. *Current Opinion in Neurobiology*, **17**, 59–64.

Kennard, M. (1942). Cortical reorganization of motor function. *Archives of Neurology*, **48**, 227–240.

Kleim, J. A., Bruneau, R., Vandenberg, P., MacDonald, E., Mulrooney, R., & Pocock, D. (2003). Motor cortex stimulation enhances motor recovery and reduces peri-infarct dysfunction following ischemic insult. *Neurological Research*, **25**, 789–793.

Kolb, B., & Cioe, J. (submitted). Contrasting effects of motor and visual learning tasks on dendritic arborization and spine density in rats.

Kolb, B., & Elliott, W. (1987). Recovery from early cortical damage in rats. II. Effects of experience on anatomy and behavior following frontal lesions at 1 or 5 days of age. *Behavioural Brain Research*, **26**, 47–56.

Kolb, B., & Gibb, R. (1993). Possible anatomical basis of recovery of function after neonatal frontal lesions in rats. *Behavioral Neuroscience*, **107**, 799–811.

Kolb, B., & Gibb, R. (submitted). Tactile stimulation after posterior parietal cortical injury in infant rats stimulates functional recovery and altered cortical morphology.

Kolb, B., & Stewart, J. (1991). Sex-related differences in dendritic branching of cells in the prefrontal cortex of rats. *Journal of Neuroendocrinology*, **3**, 95–99.

Kolb, B., & Stewart, J. (1995). Changes in the neonatal gonadal hormonal environment prevent behavioral sparing and alter cortical morphogenesis after early frontal-cortex lesions in male and female rats. *Behavioral Neuroscience*, **109**, 285–294.

Kolb, B., & Whishaw, I. Q. (1989). Plasticity in the neocortex: mechanisms underlying recovery from early brain damage. *Progress in Neurobiology*, **32**, 235–276.

Kolb, B., & Whishaw, I. Q. (1998). Brain plasticity and behavior. *Annual Review of Psychology*, **49**, 43–64.

Kolb, B., & Whishaw, I. Q. (2001). *Fundamentals of Human Neuropsychology, Fifth Edition*. New York, NY: Worth.

Kolb, B., Gibb, R., & van der Kooy, D. (1992). Cortical and striatal structure and connectivity are altered by neonatal hemidecortication in rats. *Journal of Comparative Neurology*, **322**, 311–324.

Kolb, B., Gibb, R., & van der Kooy, D. (1994). Neonatal frontal cortical lesions in rats alter cortical structure and connectivity. *Brain Research*, **645**, 85–97.

Kolb, B., Gorny, G., Cote, S., Ribeiro-da-silva, & Cuello, A. C. (1997). Nerve growth factor stimulates growth of cortical pyramidal neurons in young adult rats. *Brains Research*, **751**, 289–294.

Kolb, B., Gibb, R., Gorny, G., & Whishaw, I. Q. (1998). Possible regeneration of rat medial frontal cortex following neonatal frontal lesions. *Behavioral Brain Research*, **91**, 127–141.

Kolb, B., Gibb, R., & Gorny, G. (2003a). Experience-dependent changes in dendritic arbor and spine density in neocortex vary qualitatively with age and sex. *Neurobiology of Learning and Memory*, **79**, 1–10.

Kolb, B., Gorny, G., Li, Y., Samaha, A.-N., & Robinson, T. E. (2003b). Amphetamine or cocaine limits the ability of later experience to promote structural plasticity in the neocortex and nucleus accumbens. *Proceedings of the National Academy of Sciences of the United States of America*, **100**, 10523–10528.

Kolb, B., Halliwell, C., & Gibb, R. (in press). Factors influencing neocortical development in the normal and injured brain. In M. S. Blumberg, J. H. Freeman, & S. R. Robinson (Eds.), *Developmental and Comparative Neuroscience: Epigenetics, Evolution, and Behavior*. New York, NY: Oxford University Press.

Kramer, A. F., Bherer, L., Colcombe, S. J., Dong, W., & Greenough, W. T. (2004). Environmental influences on cognitive and brain plasticity during aging. *Journals of Gerontology: Series A; Biological Sciences and Medical Sciences* **59**, 940–957.

Kramer, A. F., Erickson, K. I., & Colcombe, S. J. (2006). Exercise, cognition, and the aging brain. *Journal of Applied Physiology*, **101**, 1237–1242.

Kwakkel, G., van Peppen, R., Wagenaar, R. C., Wood Dauphinee, S., Richards, C., Ashburn, A., Miller, K., Lincoln, N., Partridge, C., Wellwood, I., & Langhorne, P. (2004). Effects of augmented exercise therapy time after stroke: a meta-analysis. *Stroke*, **35**, 2529–2539.

Li, Y., Kolb, B., & Robinson, T. E. (2005). Psychostimulant drugs alter the effect of complex housing on synaptic plasticity in ca1 pyramidal neurons. *Society for Neuroscience Abstracts*, **31**, 1032.4.

Lipska, B. K., & Weinberger, D. R. (2002). A neurodevelopmental model of schizophrenia: neonatal disconnection of the hippocampus. *Neurotoxicology Research*, **4**, 469–475.

Lorenz, K. (1970). *Studies on Animal and Human Behavior*. Cambridge, MA: Harvard University Press.

Lukowiak, K., Sangha, S., Scheibenstock, A., Parvez, K., McComb, C., Rosenegger, D., Varshney, N., & Sadamoto, H. (2003). A molluscan model system in the search for the engram. *Journal of Physiology – Paris*, **97**, 69–76.

Mattson, M. P., Duan, W., Chan, S. L., & Guo, Z. (2001). Apoptotic and antiapoptotic signaling at the synapse: From adaptive plasticity to neurodegenerative disorders. In C. A. Shaw, & J. C. McEachern (Eds.), *Toward a Theory of Neuroplasticity*. Philadelphia, PA: Psychology Press.

McEwen, B. S. (2005). Glucocorticoids, depression, and mood disorders: structural remodeling in the brain. *Metabolism*, **54**, (*Suppl. 1*), 20–23.

Meck, W. H., & Williams, C. L. (2003). Metabolic imprinting of choline by its availability during gestation: implications for memory and attentional processing across the lifespan. *Neuroscience and Biobehavioral Reviews*, **27**, 385–399.

Monfils, M.-H., Driscol, I., Kamitakahara, H., Wilson, B., Flynn, C., Teskey, G. C., Kleim, J. A., & Kolb, B. (2006). FGF-2-induced cell proliferation stimulates anatomical, neurophysiological and functional recovery from neonatal motor cortex injury. *European Journal of Neuroscience*, **24**, 739–749.

Moroz, I. A., & Kolb, B. (2005). Amphetamine facilitates recovery of skilled reaching following cortical devascularization in the rat. *Society for Neuroscience Abstracts*, **30**, 669.6.

Pantelis, C., Yücel, M., Wood, S. J., Velakoulis, D., Sun, D., Berger, G., Stuart, G. W., Yung, A., Phillips, L., & McGorry, P. D. (2005). Structural brain imaging evidence for multiple pathological processes at different stages of brain development in schizophrenia. *Schizophrenia Bulletin*, **31**, 672–696.

Papadopoulos, C., Tsai, S-Y, Cheatwood, J. L. *et al.* (2006). Dendritic plasticity in the adult rat following middle cerebral artery occlusion and Nogo-A neutralization. *Cerebral Cortex*, **16** (4), 529–536.

Payne, B. R., & Lomber, S. G. (2001). Reconstructing functional systems after lesions of cerebral cortex. *Nature Reviews Neuroscience*, **2**, 911–919.

Raison, C. L., Capuron, L., & Miller, A. H. (2006). Cytokines sing the blues: inflammation and the pathogenesis of depression. *Trends in Immunology*, **27**, 24–31.

Rampon, C., Jiang, C. H., Dong, H., Tang, Y. P., Lockhart, D. J., Schultz, P. G., Tsien, J. Z., & Hu, Y. (2000). Effects of environmental enrichment on gene expression in the brain. *Proceedings of the National Academy of Sciences of the United States of America*, **97**, 12880–12884.

Roberts, A. C., & Glanzman, D. L. (2003). Learning in aplysia: looking at synaptic plasticity from both sides. *Trends in Neurosciences*, **26**, 662–670.

Robinson, T. E., & Kolb, B. (1999a). Alterations in the morphology of dendrites and dendritic spines in the nucleus accumbens and prefrontal cortex following repeated treatment with amphetamine or cocaine. *European Journal of Neuroscience*, **11**, 1598–1604.

Robinson, T. E., & Kolb, B. (1999b). Morphine alters the structure of neurons in the nucleus accumbens and neocortex of rats. *Synapse*, **33**, 160–162.

Robinson, T. E., & Kolb, B. (2004). Structural plasticity associated with exposure to drugs of abuse. *Neuropharmacology*, **47**, Suppl. 1, 33–46.

Rose, J. K., & Rankin, C. H. (2001). Behavioral, neural circuit, and genetic analyses of habituation in *C. elegans*. In C. A. Shaw & J. C. McEachern (Eds.), *Toward a Theory of Neuroplasticity* (pp. 176–192). Philadelphia, PA: Psychology Press.

Schmanke, T. D., & Villablanca, J. R. (2001). A critical maturational period of reduced brain vulnerability to injury. A study of cerebral glucose metabolism in cats. *Developmental Brain Research*, **131**, 127–141.

Shaw, C. A., & McEachern, J. C. (2001). *Toward a Theory of Neuroplasticity*. Philadelphia, PA: Psychology Press.

Silasi, G., & Kolb, B. (2007). Chronic inhibition of cyclooxygenase-2 induces dendritic hypertrophy and limited functional improvement following motor cortex stroke. *Neuroscience*, **144**, 1160–1168.

Solomonia, R. O., Kotorashvili, A., Kiguradze, T., McCabe, B. J., & Horn, G. (2005). Ca^{2+}/calmodulin protein kinase II and memory: Learning-related changes in a localized region of the domestic chick brain. *Journal of Physiology* **569**, 643–653.

Stern, Y. (2006). Cognitive reserve and Alzheimer disease. *Alzheimer Disease and Associated Disorders*, **20**, Suppl. 2, S69–S74.

Stewart, J., & Kolb, B. (1988). The effects of neonatal gonadectomy and prenatal stress on cortical thickness and asymmetry in rats. *Behavioral and Neural Biology*, **49**, 344–360.

Sutton, R. L., Hovda, D. A., & Feeney, D. M. (1989). Amphetamine accelerates recovery of locomotor function following bilateral frontal cortex ablation in cats. *Behavioral Neuroscience*, **103**, 837–841.

Szele, F. G., Alexander, C., & Chesselet, M.-F. (1995). Expression of molecules associated with neuronal plasticity in the striatum after aspiration and thermocoagulatory lesions of the cerebral cortex in adult rats. *Journal of Neuroscience*, **15**, 4429–4448.

Teskey, G. C. (2001). Using kindling to model the neuroplastic changes associated with learning and memory, neuropsychiatric disorders, and epilepsy. In C. A. Shaw, & J. C. McEachern (Eds.), *Toward a Theory of Neuroplasticity* (pp. 347–358). Philadelphia, PA: Psychology Press.

Teskey, G. C., Hutchinson, J. E., & Kolb, B. (2001). Cortical layer III pyramidal dendritic morphology normalizes within 3 weeks after kindling and is dissociated from kindling-induced potentiation. *Brain Research*, **911**, 125–133.

Teskey, G. C., Flynn, C., Goertzen, C. D., Monfils, M.-H., & Young, N. A. (2003). Cortical stimulation improves skilled forelimb use following a focal ischemic infarct in the rat. *Neurological Research*, **25**, 794–800.

Teskey, G. C., Flynn, C., Goertzen, C. D., Monfils, M. H., & Young, N. A. (2004). Cortical stimulation improves skilled forelimb use following a focal ischemic infarct in the rat. *Neurological Research*, **25**, 794–800.

Teuber, H.-L. (1975). Recovery of function after brain injury in man. In *Outcome of Severe Damage to the Nervous System, Ciba Foundation Symposium 34*. Amsterdam, NL: Elsevier North-Holland.

Teyler, T. J. (2001). LTP and the superfamily of synaptic plasticities. In C. A. Shaw, & J. C. McEachern (Eds.), *Toward A Theory of Neuroplasticity* (pp. 101–117). Philadelphia, PA: Psychology Press.

Uylings, H. B. M., Groenewegen, H. J., & Kolb, B. (2003). Do rats have a prefrontal cortex? *Behavioural Brain Research*, **146**, 3–17.

Villablanca, J. R., & Gomez-Pinilla, F. (1987). Novel crossed corticothalamic projections after neonatal cerebral hemispherectomy. A quantitative autoradiography study in cats. *Brain Research*, **410**, 219–231.

Villablanca, J. R., Hovda, D. A., Jackson, G. F., & Infante, C. (1993). Neurological and behavioral effects of a unilateral frontal cortical lesion in fetal kittens. II. Visual system tests, and proposing an "optimal developmental period" for lesion effects. *Behavioural Brain Research*, **57**, 79–92.

Whishaw, I. Q., & Kolb, B. (1988). Sparing of skilled forelimb reaching and corticospinal projections after neonatal motor cortex removal or hemidecortication in the rat: support for the Kennard doctrine. *Brain Research*, **451**, 97–114.

Withers, G. S., & Greenough, W. T. (1989). Reach training selectively alters dendritic branching in subpopulations of layer II-III pyramids in rat motor-somatosensory forelimb cortex. *Neuropsychologia*, **27**, 61–69.

Yamamoto, T., Shimura, T., Sako, N., Yasoshima, Y., & Sakai, N. (1994). Neural substrates for conditioned taste aversion in the rat. *Behavioral Brain Research*, **65**, 123–137.

2

Principles of compensation in cognitive neuroscience and neurorehabilitation

Roger A. Dixon, Douglas D. Garrett and Lars Bäckman

Introduction

Since the first version of this chapter (Dixon & Bäckman, 1999), the concept of compensation has garnered increasing attention at both the behavioral (cognitive) and biological (neural) levels. It remains a focal and fruitful concept to pursue within the theoretical and applied cognitive neurosciences, and has gathered substantial momentum with regard to conceptualization, definition, classification and application. Several key components of compensation identified previously remain relevant, whereas others require modification and elaboration given new theoretical and empirical developments. Recent findings broaden the perspective on the existence and role of compensation in neurorehabilitation, whether as an outcome of specific insult (e.g., stroke), or of a more gradual accumulation of neural damage (e.g., mild cognitive impairment or Alzheimer's disease). In this chapter we have revised and updated our earlier contribution. Although the structure and key issues remain the same, the new version reflects recent empirical and conceptual advances.

We began our earlier chapter by describing selected aspects of the long history of the concept of compensation (see Bäckman & Dixon, 1992; Dixon & Bäckman, 1999). Historically, compensation has been regarded as an elegant, hovering principle of balance, a natural "sublime law" (Ralph Waldo Emerson's term) of regression or egression to the norm, a tendency to return to normalcy from deficit or deviance. There is an intrinsic and dynamic balance suggested in many early passages: for losses there are corresponding gains and for gains there may be corresponding losses. Accordingly, a key feature of compensation in the cognitive neurosciences is the notion that, for brain injuries or neurodegenerative deficits, there may be ways to recover some degree of function. Often the early notions of compensation portray the human organism, the human brain and human lifespan development as a dynamic, variable, adaptive, and self-correcting system. How well does this view represent the empirically based theoretical views of compensation emerging in such specialty areas as cognitive aging, cognitive neuroscience and cognitive neurorehabilitation? Do principles of compensation operate similarly for all deficits, regardless of type (e.g., typical aging decrements, traumatic brain injury, neurodegenerative), severity (e.g., mild, severe), or duration? What are the specific mechanisms of compensation and how do they operate? Is compensation enacted spontaneously or automatically, and/or as the result of effort or training? What defines a "deficit" in cognitive performance or neurological integrity, and what deficits constitute opportunities for compensation? Can these deficits, opportunities and the compensatory mechanisms themselves be identified empirically and classified conceptually?

The chapter begins with a definition and several principles of compensation as they apply to selected domains within contemporary cognitive neuroscience and rehabilitation. We apply these principles to the related areas of compensation for

Cognitive Neurorehabilitation, Second Edition: Evidence and Application, ed. Donald T. Stuss, Gordon Winocur and Ian H. Robertson. Published by Cambridge University Press. © Cambridge University Press 2008.

organic memory impairment and compensatory brain change.

Concept of compensation in cognition and neuroscience

- The term *compensation* is used by a wide range of literatures, including neurosciences, neurological disorders, acquired speech and language disorders, sensory injuries or deficits, cognitive aging, and others.
- Common to these literatures is the notion that compensation refers to a process of overcoming losses or deficits through one of several identifiable mechanisms.

Broadly, the term compensation refers to a process through which deficits or losses are moderated. Although there are some differences across areas of research, the concept converges upon several identifiable themes. For earlier reviews (e.g., Bäckman & Dixon, 1992; Dixon & Backman, 1999), scores of articles pertaining to compensation were collected. The use of the term was traced back to Emerson in the early 1900s, and through a rapid acceleration after the 1960s. Brandtstädter & Wentura (1995) located even earlier homologous usages of compensation in eighteenth century philosophy. For example, they quoted Formey, an eighteenth century observer, as remarking that, "for man, there is never gain without loss, and no loss without gain . . . compensation everywhere" (Brandtstädter & Wentura, 1995, p. 83). Examples of early literature in clinical sciences include Adler's (1927) view of compensation in personality as a crucial defense mechanism. Another pertinent perspective was the early optimistic notion that a deficit in sensitivity in one sensory system could be counterbalanced by a gain in sensitivity in an intact modality (e.g., Hartmann, 1933; Hayes, 1933; Rönnberg, 1995). Although the empirical evidence in the early cases of compensation was somewhat mixed, the concept spread and proliferated. Among the reasons for the resilience and power of the concept of compensation are the related facts that (a) it

possesses potential theoretical importance of considerable magnitude, and (b) it has immediate and compelling practical implications for several applied areas of research (Dixon & Bäckman, 1995b).

Selected areas of compensation research

In our reviews (Bäckman & Dixon, 1992; Dixon & Bäckman, 1995b, 1999), the concept and empirical deployment of compensation were surveyed in a wide range of literatures. The goal was to develop a comprehensive model of compensation, one that was derived from research in several domains. In the present review, we focus on the following principal literatures, each presented with sample citations and an illustrative compensatory idea.

(1) *Cognitive neurosciences* (e.g., Bäckman *et al.*, 1997; Cabeza *et al.*, 2002; Grady *et al.*, 2003; Horn *et al.*, 1996; Kolb & Gibb, 1999; Reuter-Lorenz & Lustig, 2005; Stern *et al.*, 2005; Teasell *et al.*, 2005) in which behavioral, electrophysiological, neuroimaging, and morphological evidence suggests that the human brain may display plasticity, including reorganization and substitution of function, as a response to impairment, damage and fallibility (errors).

(2) *Neurorehabilitation* (e.g., Bayona *et al.*, 2005b; Becker *et al.*, 1996a, 1996b; Buckner *et al.*, 1996; Craik *et al.*, 2007; Dixon *et al.*, 2003; Glisky & Glisky, 1999; Grady *et al.*, 2003; Mateer, 1996, 1999; Stuss *et al.*, 2007; Turner & Levine, 2004; Wilson, 1997; 1999; Wilson & Watson, 1996) in which deficits associated with either organic diseases (e.g., Alzheimer's disease) or other neurological injuries (e.g., traumatic brain injury, executive disorders) may be compensated by a variety of behavioral strategies for improving cognitive performance (e.g., utilization of preserved skills).

(3) *Acquired speech and language disorders* (e.g., Ahlsén, 1991; Buckner *et al.*, 1996; Crosson *et al.*, 2005; Gonzalez Rothi, 1995; Heiss & Thiel, 2006; Rothi & Horner, 1983; Schaefer *et al.*, 2006; Towne, 1994) in which deficits

resulting from an injury or stroke may be compensated through the use of alternative communication mechanisms or through physiological restitution.

(4) *Sensory injuries or deficits* (e.g., Amedi *et al.*, 2003; Liotti *et al.*, 1998; Neville, 1990; Ohlsson, 1986; Rönnberg, 1995; Smith & Curthoys, 1989; Stevens *et al.*, 1996; Szlyk *et al.*, 1995; Yabe & Kaga, 2005) in which impairment in one sensory modality could be compensated by increased sensitivity in an alternative system.

(5) *Anxiety disorders/phobias* (e.g., Paquette *et al.*, 2003; Straube *et al.*, 2006) in which successful cognitive–behavioral therapy may modify dysfunctional neural networks associated with phobic responses.

(6) *Cognitive aging and decline* (e.g., Bäckman, 1985, 1989; de Frias & Dixon, 2005; Dixon *et al.*, 2001; Jennings & Jacoby, 2003; Kliegl & Philipp, 2007; Marsiske *et al.*, 1995; Salthouse, 1984, 1987, 1990, 1995; Stern *et al.*, 2000) in which aging-related declines in one cognitive component or skill (e.g., speed of processing, memory encoding and retrieval) may be compensated by the development/use of supplemental or alternative mechanisms, and measured with multiple techniques.

(7) *Individual differences in reserve or capacity* (e.g., Bayona *et al.*, 2005a; Springer *et al.*, 2005; Stern, 2002; Stern *et al.*, 2005; Tuokko *et al.*, 2003) in which the probability of compensating for deficits and decline varies across individuals, despite similar pathologies or conditions (e.g., aging; cognitive impairment; Alzheimer's disease (AD)).

Overview

These literatures are too extensive to review in this context (see Dixon & Bäckman, 1995a), but they support a set of principles, definitions, and implications for both theoretical (e.g., cognitive neuroscience) and applied (e.g., rehabilitation and clinical neuropsychology) work. These implications are discussed in the following sections.

Working definition

Our analysis of the concept and principles of compensation has benefited substantially from many scholars contributing to the domains listed above. Several reviews covering different substantive areas, as well as our continuing effort to clarify the concept of compensation, have led to the following working definition. This definition is designed to cut across the selected literatures and stimulate integrative empirical and theoretical activities. Little previous cross-fertilization has occurred in research on compensation despite the fact that, across disciplines, there is both common ground and unique perspectives.

Compensation is a process of overcoming losses or deficits through one of several mechanisms. These compensatory mechanisms vary by level of analysis, technique employed, and degree of automaticity. They include: (a) investing more time and effort through training, practice or trying harder in performing a task reflective of the loss or deficit (remediation); (b) substituting a latent skill for a declining or defective one (substitution with latent process); (c) developing a new skill to take over the performance of an absent, lost, or declining skill (substitution with novel process); (d) adjusting one's goals, expectations, priorities, and criteria to be more concordant with the match between the demands of one's current context and the skills one currently possesses (accommodation); (e) modifying the environment or adjusting the expectations of others (assimilation); and (f) at the neural level, relatively automatic reorganization and substitution of function as a result of injury or accumulated damage. These mechanisms are elaborated below.

Principal features of the process of compensation

- Compensation refers to the moderation of deficits or losses (e.g., sensory, cognitive, neurological).
- Literatures in which compensation has been a prominent concern include cognitive neuroscience,

neurological disorders, acquired speech and language disorders, sensory injuries or deficits, normal and impaired cognitive aging and neurodegenerative diseases.

- Several mechanisms of compensation have been identified from a broad review of the literature. These include remediation, substitution with latent process, substitution with novel process, accommodation, assimilation and neural reorganisation.
- The four principal issues in the process of compensation are origins, mechanisms, awareness and consequences.

We have identified four leading issues in compensation, each of which is relevant to one or more specific literatures. The four principles identified are origins, mechanisms, awareness and consequences. In one sense these may be viewed as phases in the process of compensation, for they roughly represent the chronological progress of compensatory "behavior" from the moment a need or opportunity is presented. That is, compensation originates in a deficit, which provides an opportunity (although not an automatic necessity) for restitution. A variety of mechanisms may be available, depending on the nature and extent of the deficit, as well as on the resources of the individual. In addition, it is often important to consider the role that awareness of the deficit or of compensatory opportunities and efforts may play, as well as the impact compensatory efforts and results may have. These principles are elaborated in the following sections.

Origins

Generally, compensation will have its origin in a mismatch between an individual's aptitude, skills, or neurological integrity, and the actual demands of a cognitive problem, task or environment (Dixon & Bäckman, 1995b). Conceivably, however, when cognitive skills decline as a function of normal or neuropathological changes in the brain, automatic neural mechanisms could activate in the absence of mismatch in a manner consistent with an

interpretation of compensation. In such cases direct or automatic mechanisms of compensatory neural changes (e.g., increased dendritic arborization, collateral sprouting), which may occur across myriad conditions following insult or accumulated damage (e.g., stroke; traumatic brain injury; AD), are required. Such insults or accumulated damage may result in degraded skills (e.g., impaired episodic memory in AD) with no necessary relation to environmental demands or expected performance. Overall, when (a) there is no present cognitive demand or (b) one's skills match the demands of the environment, there is no need or rationale for compensation, except in cases where skills decline and automatic mechanisms (i.e., neural compensation) of compensation become active. In the common cases in which a mismatch does occur (e.g., reduced skill level relative to environmental demands and expected performance), automatic mechanisms may be available in combination with remediation, substitution, accommodation and assimilation.

Reduced skill level relative to environmental demands and expected performance is of most interest in the context of applied sciences such as neurorehabilitation. Deficits (e.g., head injury, progressive diseases, neurological aging) are manifest in a mismatch between the skills individuals possess and the extent to which they are able to adapt to or perform in specific contexts. In such situations, this key premise of compensation is fulfilled. The general purpose of cognitive and other behavioral compensation is to close the gap between expected or required performance and actual level of skill. The challenge is to identify effective strategies, mechanisms, accommodations, or prostheses that can render the deficit less problematic, acute, comprehensive or debilitating. Notably, behavioral compensation does not always occur for every mismatch (Bäckman & Dixon, 1992). From both theoretical and clinical perspectives, there are two important reasons for this. First, if there is a high degree of performance support in the individual's environment – such as caregivers taking over the cognitive load – there may be no need for the affected individual to develop new compensatory skills, whether as a result of self-initiated effort or other-trained experience (as in a rehabilitation setting). Second, if the deficit is too severe, compensation may not be possible at all, or at least not until after some delay. For example, the profound cognitive deficits associated with late stages of AD may be difficult, if not impossible, to behaviorally compensate (Herlitz *et al.*, 1991; Herlitz *et al.*, 1992). On the other hand, severe language deficits associated with stroke may be subject to both self-initiated and other-trained compensation following a delay (Ahlsén, 1991), potentially leading to neural reorganization after training (Crosson *et al.*, 2005).

Mechanisms

Compensatory mechanisms refer to the means through which an alleviation, remediation or attenuation of the mismatch is effected. The mechanisms identified above include remediation (increasing time, effort or training to maintain or recover the affected skill), substitution of latent skill (from the individual's present repertoire of skills), substitution of new skill (developed such that it replaces a declining or defective skill), accommodation (adjusting priorities or criteria, selecting new goals), assimilation (adjusting the expectations of others, constructing forgiving environments), and neural compensation (changes in neural function as a result of injury or accumulated damage). The typical mechanisms of compensation in cognitive neurorehabilitation are the development of new or latent skills to substitute for those affected by the injury or disease; neural compensation is likely also to occur. However, the other mechanisms may be useful in specific instances (e.g., accommodation and assimilation; Wilson & Watson, 1996). Although the mechanisms of compensation are conceptually different, they can be portrayed as contributing to a unified conceptual meaning of compensation, and they may occur in parallel for a given individual. Each mechanism works to accomplish the goal of reducing the gap

between skill level, on the one hand, and expected performance or environmental demands, on the other. Notably, compensatory neural change may also operate in the context of declining skills irrespective of environmental demand and expected performance.

Awareness and self-regulation

To what extent is awareness of the deficit and of mechanisms for overcoming the mismatch a requirement for an inference of compensation? This is a theoretical question about which there has been active discussion (e.g., Dixon & Bäckman, 1995b; Salthouse, 1995). Our position is that compensatory mechanisms may be enacted and effective along a continuum of awareness. This is consistent with a broad range of literature, in which one can locate examples of compensation that occur with full awareness of the deficit and deliberate compensatory efforts (e.g., substitution of novel skills in the face of declining memory with age; Hawley & Cherry, 2004; Jennings & Jacoby, 2003), as well as examples in which little or no awareness is displayed (e.g., neural reorganization; Cabeza *et al.*, 2002; Grady *et al.*, 2003; Kolb & Gibb, 1999). Awareness of compensatory efforts may be measured by standardized verbal techniques, such as structured interviews or questionnaires. One example of the latter is the Memory Compensation Questionnaire (MCQ). The MCQ has been used to evaluate the extent and variety of memory compensation techniques used in everyday life by normal older adults, memory-impaired adults, AD patients, and brain-injured adults (e.g., de Frias & Dixon, 2005; Dixon *et al.*, 2001; Prigatano & Kime, 2003). Results appear to support the notion that healthy and memory-challenged adults are aware both of their memory impairment and their efforts to compensate for their deficits. Two examples will illustrate. First, AD patients reported recruiting other individuals for memory assistance increasingly more over a 6-month period than did an older adult control group (Dixon *et al.*, 2003). Second, memory-impaired older adults were higher in their reported compensatory use of external memory aids and investment of effort than were cognitively healthy older adults (Dixon & de Frias, 2007). Interestingly, over a 6-year period, the initially intact older adults increased their everyday compensatory efforts whereas initially impaired adults decreased their efforts. Such results demonstrate that awareness is dynamic and potentially pegged to changing cognitive status.

In addition, changes in awareness may occur during the process of compensation. Like expert skills, compensatory efforts may become relatively automatised and less effortful to execute across time (Ohlsson, 1986). As one learns and practices mnemonic skills, applying them to suitable memory tasks becomes less effortful and more automatic (Kliegl & Philipp, 2007). This gradual transition from effortful to automatic processing occurs whether an individual is shifting from normal towards expert memory (e.g., Kliegl & Baltes; 1987) or from impaired memory towards normal memory (Wilson & Watson, 1996). Indeed, it may be that one indicator of improvement is a diminishment of effortful requirements.

In recovery from brain injury or accumulated neural damage, automatic and effortful processes may complement one another sequentially. This may happen if relatively automatic neural compensation (e.g., morphological changes, recruitment of alternate neural regions) occurs early and is followed by deliberate efforts on the part of the recovering individual (Bach-y-Rita, 1990; Bach-y-Rita & Bach-y-Rita, 1990; Kolb & Whishaw, 1996). They may also complement one another in a more overlapping or even opposite sequence (e.g., Ahlsén, 1991; Erickson *et al.*, 2007). Overall, if the nature and severity of the injury – and the prognosis for recovery – is such that the principal source of compensation is automatic, organic or pharmacological, then initially awareness may not play a role. However, if behavioral training, monitoring or rehabilitation is involved, awareness may very well play a crucial role in recovery from the effects of decline or injury.

Consequences

The implicit expectation of most scholars has been that compensation results in an improvement in functioning, a restoration of some level of performance in an impaired domain. That compensation may lead to negative consequences has been surprising to some observers, with some even suggesting that a positive outcome should be incorporated into the very definition of compensation. The pertinent literature and arguments for including both positive and negative consequences are described in some detail elsewhere (Dixon & Bäckman, 1995b). One basis of the argument can be found in an Emerson (1900) observation: it is not only that there is a balancing gain for every loss, there is also a balancing loss for every gain. This principle has found empirical and theoretical support in some areas of cognitive and social aging. Given aging-related diminishing resources, compounded by injuries or other losses, maintaining specific resource-demanding skills may result in losses in other skills or domains (Brandtstädter & Wentura, 1995). Maintaining and managing a highly valued skill (skill X) may become ever more difficult as basic resources (e.g., sensory, speed, neurological) decline with aging. Downward pressure on skill X may be relieved, if only temporarily, by relaxing the requirement of simultaneously maintaining (at a high level) skills Y and Z. Thus, there are losses involved (in skills Y and Z) in compensating for declines in a more valued skill (skill X). Alternatively, once efforts to maintain skill X become more automatized over time, skills Y and Z may recover.

Concrete examples of negative consequences of compensation are rare, but several illustrations are available. First, Masterton & Biederman (1983) noted that some behaviors of autistic children (such as reliance on proximal sensory input) were initially viewed as compensatory but, from a long-term perspective, were recognized as limiting adaptation, if not being actually maladaptive. Second, in reading, children with select inefficient skills can compensate in a manner that preserves comprehension but also detracts from higher level processes (such as monitoring) because reserves are taken from the latter and applied to the former (Walczyk *et al.*, 2004). Thus, compensation works to enhance literal understanding of words and text, but comes at the cost of the crucial higher-level reading skill of monitoring overall comprehension. Third, occasionally, well-meaning parents of children with injuries or losses may attempt to buffer or substitute for the child's behavioral deficit. Although this may have the transitory desired effect of helping the child navigate selected daily activities or tasks, the long-term effect may be one of hindering the child's development of his or her own compensatory mechanisms (Wasserman *et al.*, 1985). In fact, Wilson & Watson (1996) noted that this phenomenon could occur for parents of brain-injured adult children, as the following poignant vignette illustrates.

The father of one head-injured young woman with memory problems became very protective after the accident. He had already lost a son in another accident and felt he had to do everything for his daughter. He tried to anticipate her every wish and meet her every need. She, in turn, relied on her father to tell her what to do, when to do it, and how to do it. It is likely that without such intense supervision from her father, the young woman would have learned to use her own compensatory strategies and become more independent (Wilson & Watson, 1996, p. 475).

Fourth, a "hidden cost" of compensation at the neural level was recently explained by Reuter-Lorenz & Lustig (2005). If greater brain activation for older than for younger adults could reflect aging-related compensation, older adults might more quickly reach the limits of the cognitive and neural resources available for responding to further and more difficult tasks.

Research may not focus on or identify circumstances in which compensation is not associated with favorable outcomes. Nevertheless, compensation could result in (a) initial gains but overall long-term losses, (b) losses in overall potential for recovery, (c) gains in one process while losses in another or (d) gains for the individual but losses

for others in the context. For this reason, researchers and rehabilitation specialists may wish to consider the consequences dimension in theory development or clinical pursuits.

Compensation in cognitive neurorehabilitation

- The principles of compensation were derived from the neurosciences, neuropsychology and neurorehabilitation.
- Models of compensation have been linked to issues of rehabilitation for memory impairment resulting from brain injury.
- Prominent strategic or behavioral mechanisms of compensation include substitution, remediation and accommodation.
- Neuroimaging methods have vast potential for unlocking the mysteries of compensation occurring at the neuroanatomical level.
- New examples of compensation via the activation of latent or novel mechanisms or regions in the brain include distribution or recruitment of alternative pathways or activation sites. Research includes mild Alzheimer's disease, aphasia and normal older adults.
- Because automatic neuroanatomical compensation can be boosted or initiated through deliberate behavioral compensation, it deserves further attention in cognitive neurorehabilitation.

Thus far, the main purpose in this chapter has been to present the principles of compensation that can be derived from a broad spectrum of literature. Featuring prominently in this review have been the neighboring research areas of cognitive neurosciences and cognitive development. In addition to the theoretical analysis, our own research in compensation has been in the area of cognitive aging and dementia (Bäckman, 1992; Dixon *et al.*, 2004). We turn now to selected brief illustrations of recent work in compensation and neurorehabilitation. The goal is not to review this literature comprehensively, but rather to illustrate how the principles of compensation – some of which were derived from seemingly disparate literatures – may find a voice and an application in cognitive neurorehabilitation. Therefore, only selected projects are briefly addressed.

Behavioral compensation for organic cognitive impairment

Several reviews of cognitive rehabilitation strategies for adult brain injury have attended to issues and principles of compensation. Wilson (1995; Wilson & Watson, 1996) evaluated a comprehensive model of compensation and its application to issues of rehabilitation for memory impairment resulting from brain injury. For example, Wilson & Watson (1996) reviewed three principles of compensation as they apply to rehabilitation for organic memory impairment. With respect to *origins*, they confirm that the principal origin of interest in this field is that of a decrease in skill as a function of brain injury. Furthermore, although the resultant mismatch is the occasion for compensation, there are circumstances in which compensatory behaviors are not developed. These include circumstances in which a high degree of contextual support (or environmental adaptations) obviates the need for compensatory mechanisms operating through the recovering individual. In addition, Wilson & Watson consider the important role of severity of deficit (Bäckman & Dixon, 1992). They report that, for brain injuries, an expected inverse relationship between the severity of the deficit and the probability of self-initiated behavioral compensation is likely to depend in part on whether executive functioning is implicated. Specifically, when executive deficits are prominent, even people who are only mildly impaired in the criterion skill may not readily or effectively initiate compensatory behavior. Conversely, people with less impaired executive functioning may develop compensatory strategies even though they show more pronounced deficits in the criterion skill.

Wilson & Watson (1996) reported that, not only are *remediation* and *substitution* employed as mechanisms of compensating for organic memory impairment, but so is *accommodation*. They reported examples of injured patients investing more effort in the cognitively demanding tasks of their everyday lives (Wilson, 1995). They also reported that substitutable strategies, such as teaching the use of external aids, may be effective (see Dixon *et al.*, 2001). Wilson (1995) described the case of a young adult law student who, following a cerebral hemorrhage and period of rehabilitation, accommodated to his residual cognitive deficit by rearranging his priorities, devaluing blocked goals, and possibly constructing palliative meanings. Finally, as noted above, Wilson & Watson reported several examples of negative consequences of compensatory behavior in organic memory impairment. The one of most concern to the rehabilitation specialist may well be when a brain-injured person engages in compensatory behavior that is successful in overcoming at least some of the deficit (i.e., positive consequences) but this same behavior has negative consequences for others in close proximity. Their example is as follows: "the amnesic patient who is constantly interrupting to record something on a tape recorder or in a diary is acting sensibly on the one hand, but disruptively on the other" (Wilson & Watson, 1996, p. 475). In being overly focused on the process of compensation, the patient may be "over-compensating," producing negative consequences.

Compensatory brain changes

Another body of research indicates that compensation may occur also at the neuroanatomical level. The notion of neural compensation has a long history (Lashley, 1924; Luria, 1963, 1966; Munk, 1881). In particular, Kolb & Gibb (1999) argue that the mechanisms of cortical plasticity are most likely related to dendritic change (increased arborization and density, potentially resulting in a greater number of synaptic connections). Notably, Kolb & Whishaw's (1996) taxonomy lists a dozen other neural mechanisms that may follow neural damage, such as collateral sprouting and regeneration. In Chapter 1 in this volume, Kolb and Gibb outline several basic principles of brain plasticity, including the notion that the mechanisms and manifestations of neural plasticity may vary greatly. For example, Szot *et al.* (2006) demonstrated that upon loss of noradrenergic (NA) neurons in the locus ceruleus and hippocampus both in AD and Lewy body dementia, remaining NA neurons appeared to compensate through dendritic arborization, collateral sprouting, and increased (as compared with healthy controls) enzymatic activity important for memory functioning. Further, Durany *et al.* (2000) found that neurodegeneration in AD patients resulted in the over-expression of brain-derived neurotrophic factor (BDNF; a protein critical for memory and general neuronal integrity in the adult brain) in the hippocampus and parietal cortex. This observation is consistent with the interpretation that BDNF over-expression may serve a compensatory role. In a related vein, de Kosky *et al.* (2002) found an elevation of a presynaptic marker of cholinergic neurotransmission in the hippocampus and frontal cortex among persons classified with mild cognitive impairment. This elevation was interpreted to reflect a compensatory response to entorhinal cell loss. Consistent with the view that disease severity may constrain brain compensation, this increase of cholinergic activity was not seen in clinically diagnosed AD patients. Neurogenesis (a process through which the brain can generate new neurons) also contributes to brain plasticity (see Kolb and Gibb, Chapter 1, this volume; Wojtowicz, Chapter 20, this volume). Wojtowicz notes that learning, enriched environments, and physical activity can be associated with neurogenesis. Overall, these neuroanatomical and neurobiochemical findings complement other observers' analyses of behavioral compensation, as well as those instances in which behavioral and neural mechanisms may operate serially or interactively (e.g., Ahlsén, 1991; Bach-y-Rita & Bach-y-Rita, 1990; Bäckman & Dixon, 1992; Crosson *et al.*, 2005; Erickson *et al.*, 2007; Paquette *et al.*, 2003; Straube *et al.*, 2006; Wilson & Watson, 1996).

Research on compensatory brain activation has also burgeoned, with rapid advancements due to a surge in neuroimaging research (e.g., Cabeza *et al.*, 2002; Crosson *et al.*, 2005; Grady *et al.*, 2003; Levine *et al.*, 2002; Springer *et al.*, 2005; Stern *et al.*, 2005). The following are some brief examples of this recent work, especially as it is pertinent to compensation theory in the fields of aging, brain injury and Alzheimer's disease. Other perspectives and detailed reviews of this growing area are becoming available elsewhere (Daselaar & Cabeza, 2005; Persson *et al.*, 2006; Reuter-Lorenz & Lustig, 2005).

Cabeza *et al.* (2002) examined the effects of general memory ability in older and young adults on subsequent brain activation during recognition and source memory tasks. All participants were initially screened for overall memory performance. Older adults were then divided into low-performing and high-performing groups. As expected, young and high-performing older adults were significantly more accurate on the source memory task. Positron emission tomography (PET) results demonstrated that young adults and low-performing older adults recruited similar right hemisphere dorsal-lateral and anterior prefrontal (PFC) areas at retrieval on the source memory task, although low-performing older adults recruited anterior PFC to a greater extent. However, high-performing older adults recruited anterior prefrontal regions in both hemispheres on a source memory task, suggesting evidence for compensatory brain activation and a reduction in retrieval-based hemispheric asymmetry seen normally in younger adults. The low-performing older group's greater use of typical PFC regions (i.e., the same as utilized by the young group) was ineffective at compensating for memory deficits. This suggests that although greater activation of a typical neural region may be considered a form of neural reorganization (Prvulovic *et al.*, 2005), it may not always aid performance.

In another study, Levine and colleagues (2002) examined the effects of moderate and severe traumatic brain injury (TBI) on PET-based activation during a cued-recall task. On average, TBI was sustained 4 years prior to testing; all TBI patients had recovered functionally and were free of medical and psychological disorders. Results revealed that the TBI group activated many similar task-related regions as controls, but that the TBI group also activated opposite-hemisphere homologues, and several other regions not activated by the control group. As noted for the Cabeza *et al.* (2002) study, these results provide evidence for hemispheric asymmetry reduction in the frontal lobe during mnemonic tasks, indicating that such neural reorganization may serve a similar compensatory role in those who have functionally recovered from moderate or severe TBI. However, the authors note that whether altered patterns of neural activation result solely as a response to neural damage, or whether changes in strategic approach to cognitive tasks also play a role, cannot be determined from these data. Interpretations regarding the primary causal factors of neural activation change should be made with caution.

Although several studies suggest that altered neural recruitment in specific regions represents a compensatory reallocation of neural resources, only limited evidence demonstrates compensatory activation within neural networks. In an attempt to analyse direct links between potential compensatory activation and task performance, Grady and colleagues (2003) examined PET-based activation during semantic and episodic memory tasks in mild AD and healthy elderly controls. Using a technique known as partial least squares (i.e., where latent variables are calculated that represent distributed regions covarying during a task; McIntosh *et al.*, 1996) the authors were able to investigate the typical role of the PFC in "compensatory" activation, as well as its functional connectivity with other task-related neural regions. Results revealed that, relative to controls, AD patients activated a more elaborate network of bilateral prefrontal and temporoparietal regions, and those patients with greater levels of activation in this distributed bilateral network showed more accurate memory. Notably, the compensatory activation was not limited to typical prefrontal cortices, but involved also temporal and parietal regions found previously to subserve semantic and episodic memory in AD

(e.g., Desgranges *et al.*, 1998; Grossman *et al.*, 1997). Further studies investigating the presence of neural reorganization may benefit from connectivity approaches (such as partial least squares) which allow experimenters to relate directly the phenomenon of neural network-based reorganization to cognitive performance.

A caveat

It is important to note, however, that additional neural recruitment (e.g., bilateral frontal) among cognitively impaired persons is not always associated with better performance. For example, in some conditions greater regional activity among older adults may indicate lack of specificity of neural processing, possibly reflecting deficits in transcallosal inhibitory mechanisms (Bäckman *et al.*, 2006; Li *et al.*, 2001). Direct evidence for this view comes from a study by Persson *et al.* (2006). Using a semantic classification task, these investigators reported that persons who had exhibited 10-year cognitive decline showed a bilateral frontal activation pattern, whereas stable cognitive performers showed the typical left frontal activation pattern. Importantly, degree of bilateral recruitment was strongly linked to a diffusion tensor imaging measure of anterior white-matter integrity. Thus, hemispheric "leakage" because of alterations in white-matter microstructure may have resulted among the decliners. In other research, greater regional activity, for comparable performance levels, has been observed during working memory (i.e., n-back) performance in schizophrenics (Egan *et al.*, 2001) as well as in val carriers of the COMT gene, who have reduced dopamine levels in prefrontal cortex (Mattay *et al.*, 2003). Such findings are typically interpreted in terms of neural inefficiency, that is, less cognitive fuel is obtained per unit of neural investment. Disentangling the conditions under which increased regional activity is associated with favorable versus disadvantageous outcomes remains an intriguing avenue for future investigation (Bäckman & Dixon, 1992; Dixon & Bäckman, 1995a, 1999).

Interactions between neural and behavioral compensation

The two forms of compensation discussed in this section occur at different levels of analysis and involve different compensatory mechanisms. Nevertheless, the concept of compensation occurring in both literatures may be incorporated into the model sketched in this chapter. Accordingly, this section closes with reference to a feature of the model that indicates that, under some conditions, neural and behavioral compensatory mechanisms may be profitably linked, and linked on the basis of the principles of compensation.

Conceivably, the degree of awareness of active compensatory mechanisms is less (and low) in the case of neural compensation than it is (or could be) in the case of behavioral compensation for organic cognitive impairment. That is, as compared to some behavioral mechanisms, neurological mechanisms are less likely to be the product of self-initiated and deliberate effort. Indeed, they may not even be available to awareness, monitoring, or management. In contrast, as noted earlier, with training and deliberate effort adults are able to initiate and effect some strategic compensatory behaviors. For example, in the process of compensation following brain injury, at the neuroanatomical level, it is likely that the initial compensation is automatic. Following this, with guidance in neurorehabilitation or self-initiation, it is possible that some patients will boost the overall functional effectiveness of their compensation through deliberate behavioral efforts. Furthermore, it is possible that the two compensatory processes can continue simultaneously, resulting eventually in even greater levels of recovery of function. Evidence for direct links between behavioral and neural compensation has mounted since the first version of this chapter (Dixon & Bäckman, 1999). We briefly outline two studies that demonstrate the direct impact of behavioral intervention on neural reorganization.

First, Paquette *et al.* (2003) examined the effects of cognitive–behavioral therapy (CBT) on the neural correlates of spider phobia using functional magnetic resonance imaging (fMRI). Spider phobia is classified as an anxiety disorder characterized by persistent and intense fear of spiders, and avoidance of spider-related contexts. Cognitive-behavioral therapy was administered over a 4-week period, where spider phobics were given weekly intensive exposure to spider-related materials (e.g., color pictures, films, exposure to live spiders, physically touching a tarantula). Participants were scanned before and after CBT, and were shown film excerpts of spiders (experimental condition) and butterflies (control condition). Prior to CBT, the transient state of fear exhibited by phobics during the experimental condition activated the right dorsolateral prefrontal cortex (possibly reflecting the use of metacognitive strategies for fear regulation), and bilateral parahippocampal gyri (related potentially to the reactivation of contextual fear memory). Following CBT, participants reported no fear reactions to spider-related materials. Neither the right dorsolateral prefrontal cortex or the bilateral parahippocampal gyri were activated, suggesting that CBT reduces contextual fear through behavioral deconditioning of phobic responses (at the parahippocampal level), and through decreasing catastrophic thinking and cognitive misattributions (at the prefrontal level). These findings support a direct link between behavioral and neural compensation (see also Kolb & Gibb, Chapter 1, this volume). As Paquette *et al.* (2003) note, it is possible that if you "change the mind . . . you change the brain" (p. 408).

Second, Crosson and colleagues (2005) investigated the effects of behavioral treatment for "intention" on neural reorganization in two patients with post-stroke nonfluent aphasia. Intention refers to the selection of one of many possible actions, and may facilitate language through word selection and speech initiation. Nonfluent aphasia is characterised as a "disorder of intention," with common symptoms including word-search difficulties and problems initiating and maintaining language output. Typically, left hemisphere pre-supplementary motor area and lateral frontal areas are critical for intention in language (Heilman *et al.*, 2003). Given that ischemic stroke damaged these areas for both patients (resulting in nonfluent aphasia), Crosson *et al.* attempted to shift intention activation to the intact right hemisphere by combining word-finding trials with complex left-hand movements in the patients' left hemispace. By doing so, the right pre-supplementary motor area (adjacent to the region important for complex left-hand movements; Picard & Strick, 1996) may functionally activate the right lateral prefrontal cortex, resulting in a functional form of intention subserved by the intact right hemisphere. Results indicated that the treatment was successful in improving intention for both patients. Post-treatment fMRI demonstrated a successful shift in activity to right pre-supplementary and lateral frontal areas for the patient with the most extensive stroke-related damage. These results provide further evidence for links between behavioral and neural compensation. Notably, however, the efficacy of behavioral treatment on neural compensation in the context of cognitive neurorehabilitation may be limited to specific conditions.

Conclusions

Compensation is a process that is: (a) surprisingly common and frequently studied as it operates on several levels of analysis in a wide range of literatures; (b) elegantly simple in its basic premise and function but manifestly complex in its applications and generalizability across domains; and (c) scientifically intriguing and practically useful to experimental, theoretical and applied researchers in cognitive neuroscience and neurorehabilitation. This chapter began with the focus on the concept of compensation, and presentation of a sketch of the authors' working definition and model. An underlying premise is that whatever the mechanism, compensation involves gains (mostly), but also losses. Whether as a result of injury, disease, or neurodegeneration, compensation originates in a deficit that may first appear in neurobiological or cognitive–behavioral domains. Through the various mechanisms of substitution, remediation, accommodation, assimilation, or reorganization, compensation

involves closing one or more gaps between skills, expectations and demands, except in cases where neural compensation occurs in the context of impaired or declining skills irrespective of expectations and demands.

There are several principles through which observers may evaluate and categorize exemplars of compensation. These include origins, mechanisms, awareness, and consequences (for more details, see Dixon & Bäckman, 1995b, 1999). In the field of cognitive neurorehabilitation, compensation is an important and evolving concept. The chapter illustrates the application of the concept of compensation to two general areas of research, namely: (a) behavioral compensation for organic cognitive impairment, and (b) neural compensation. Although different in several respects, including level of analysis, compensation is an integrative concept in these two areas. In the first, the emphasis is at the behavioral or strategic level: compensation is often the product of self-initiated or other-initiated behavior. Such compensatory behavior may be deliberate, automatic, or both (whether sequentially or interactively). In the second, compensation may be examined in terms of reorganization or plasticity at the neuroanatomical level. In most cases, compensation is likely to incorporate both automatic biological (e.g., collateral sprouting) and effortful behavioral (e.g., strategic) processes. Further empirical linkages between these levels of analysis should be pursued. Stitching these levels together – using perhaps the thread of compensation – may serve to advance both theoretical and practical goals.

ACKNOWLEDGMENTS

RAD acknowledges grant support from both the US National Institute on Aging (R37 AG08235) and the Canada Research Chairs program. DG acknowledges scholarship support from the Natural Sciences and Engineering Research Council of Canada, and from the Kirshenblatt Award in Gerontology from the Toronto Rehabilitation Institute. LB acknowledges support from both the Swedish Research Council and the Swedish Council for Working Life and Social Research. We thank Gordon Winocur for very helpful comments on an earlier version of this chapter.

REFERENCES

Adler, A. A. (1927; Original published in 1920). *Practice and Theory of Individual Psychology*. New York, NY: Harcourt, Brace.

Ahlsén, E. (1991). Body communication as compensation for speech in a Wernicke's aphasic: a longitudinal study. *Journal of Communication Disorders*, **24**, 1–12.

Amedi, A., Raz, N., Pianka, P., Malach, R., & Zohary, E. (2003). Early "visual" cortex activation correlates with superior verbal memory performance in the blind. *Nature Neuroscience*, **6**, 758–766.

Bach-y-Rita, P. (1990). Brain plasticity as a basis for recovery of function in humans. *Neuropsychologia*, **28**, 547–554.

Bach-y-Rita, P., & Bach-y-Rita, E. W. (1990). Biological and psychosocial factors in recovery from brain damage in humans. *Canadian Journal of Psychology*, **44**, 148–165.

Bäckman, L. (1985). Compensation and recoding: A framework for ageing and memory research. *Scandinavian Journal of Psychology*, **26**, 193–207.

Bäckman, L. (1989). Varieties of memory compensation by older adults in episodic remembering. In L. W. Poon, D. C. Rubin, & B. A. Wilson (Eds.), *Everyday Cognition in Adulthood and Late Life* (pp. 509–544). Cambridge, UK: Cambridge University Press.

Bäckman, L. (1992). *Memory Functioning in Dementia*. Amsterdam, NL: North-Holland.

Bäckman, L., & Dixon, R. A. (1992). Psychological compensation: a theoretical framework. *Psychological Bulletin*, **112**, 259–283.

Bäckman, L., Almkvist, O., Andersson, J., Nordberg, A., Reineck, R., Winblad, B., & Långström, B. (1997). Brain activation in young and older adults during implicit and explicit retrieval. *Journal of Cognitive Neuroscience*, **9**, 378–391.

Bäckman, L., Nyberg, L., Lindenberger, U., Li, S.-C., & Farde, L. (2006). The correlative triad among aging, dopamine, and cognition: current status and future prospects. *Neuroscience and Biobehavioral Reviews*, **30**, 791–807.

Bayona, N. A., Bitensky, J., Foley, N., & Teasell, R. (2005a). Intrinsic factors influencing post stroke brain reorganization. *Topics in Stroke Rehabilitation*, **12**, 27–36.

Bayona, N. A., Bitensky, J., Salter, K., & Teasell, R. (2005b). The role of task-specific training in rehabilitation therapies. *Topics in Stroke Rehabilitation*, **12**, 58–65.

Becker, J. T., Mintun, M. A., Aleva, K., Wiseman, M. B., Nichols, T., & DeKosky, S. T. (1996a). Alterations in functional neuroanatomical connectivity in Alzheimer's disease: positron emission tomography of auditory verbal short-term memory. *Annals of the New York Academy of Sciences*, **777**, 239–242.

Becker, J. T., Mintun, M. A., Aleva, K., Wiseman, M. B., Nichols, T., & DeKosky, S. T. (1996b). Compensatory reallocation of brain resources supporting verbal episodic memory in Alzheimer's disease. *Neurology*, **16**, 692–700.

Brandtstädter, J., & Wentura, D. (1995). Adjustment to shifting possibility frontiers in later life: complementary adaptive modes. In R. A. Dixon & L. Bäckman (Eds.), *Compensating for Psychological Deficits and Declines: Managing Losses and Promoting Gains* (pp. 83–106). Mahwah, NJ: Lawrence Erlbaum.

Buckner, R. L., Corbetta, M., Schatz, J., Raichle, M. E., & Petersen, S. E. (1996). Preserved speech abilities and compensation following prefrontal damage. *Proceedings of the National Academy of Sciences of the United States of America*, **93**, 1249–1253.

Cabeza, R., Anderson, N. D., Locantore, J. K., & McIntosh, A. R. (2002). Aging gracefully: compensatory brain activity in high-performing older adults. *NeuroImage*, **17**, 1394–1402.

Craik, F. I. M., Winocur, G., Palmer, H., Binns, M. A., Edwards, M., Bridges, K., Glazer, P., Chavannes, R., & Stuss, D. T. (2007). Cognitive rehabilitation in the elderly: effects on memory. *Journal of the International Neuropsychological Society*, **13**, 132–142.

Crosson, B., Moore, A. B., Gopinath, K., White, K. D., Wierenga, C. E., Gaiefsky, M. E., Fabrizio, K. S., Peck, K. K., Soltysik, D., Milsted, C., Briggs, R. W., Conway, T. W., & Rothi, L. J. G. (2005). Role of the right and left hemispheres in recovery of function during treatment of intention in aphasia. *Journal of Cognitive Neuroscience*, **17**, 392–406.

Daselaar, S., & Cabeza, R. (2005). Age-related changes in hemispheric organization. In R. Cabeza, L. Nyberg, & D. Park (Eds.), *Cognitive Neuroscience of Aging: Linking Cognitive and Cerebral Aging* (pp. 325–353). Oxford, UK: Oxford University Press.

de Frias, C. M., & Dixon, R. A. (2005). Confirmatory factor structure and measurement invariance of the Memory Compensation Questionnaire. *Psychological Assessment*, **17**, 168–178.

de Kosky, S. T., Ikonomovic, M. D., Styren, S. D., Beckett, L., Wisniewski, S., Bennett, D. A., Cochran, E. J., Kordower, J. H., & Mufson, E. J. (2002). Upregulation of choline acetyltransferase in hippocampus and frontal cortex of elderly subjects with mild cognitive impairment. *Annals of Neurology*, **51**, 145–155.

Desgranges, B., Baron, J.-C., de la Sayette, V., Petit-Taboué, M.-C., Benali, K., Landeau, B., Lechevalier, B., & Eustache, F. (1998). The neural substrates of memory systems impairment in Alzheimer's disease: a PET study of resting brain glucose utilization. *Brain*, **121**, 611–631.

Dixon, R. A., & Bäckman, L. (1995a). *Compensating for Psychological Deficits and Declines: Managing Losses and Promoting Gains*. Mahwah, NJ: Lawrence Erlbaum.

Dixon, R. A., & Bäckman, L. (1995b). Concepts of compensation: Integrated, differentiated, and Janus-faced. In R. A. Dixon & L. Bäckman (Eds.), *Compensating for Psychological Deficits and Declines: Managing Losses and Promoting Gains* (pp. 3–20). Mahwah, NJ: Lawrence Erlbaum.

Dixon, R. A., & Bäckman, L. (1999). Principles of compensation in cognitive neurorehabilitation. In D. T. Stuss, G. Winocur, & I. H. Robertson (Eds.), *Cognitive Neurorehabilitation* (pp. 59–72). New York, NY: Cambridge University Press.

Dixon, R. A., & de Frias, C. M. (2007). Mild memory deficits differentially affect six-year changes in compensatory strategy use. *Psychology and Aging*, **22**, 632–638.

Dixon, R. A., de Frias, C. M., & Bäckman, L. (2001). Characteristics of self-reported memory compensation in older adults. *Journal of Clinical and Experimental Neuropsychology*, **23**, 630–661.

Dixon, R. A., Hopp, G. A., Cohen, A.-L., de Frias, C. M., & Bäckman, L. (2003). Self-reported memory compensation: similar patterns in Alzheimer's disease and very old adult samples. *Journal of Clinical and Experimental Neuropsychology*, **25**, 382–390.

Dixon, R. A., Bäckman, L., & Nilsson, L.-G. (2004). *New Frontiers in Cognitive Aging*. Oxford, UK: Oxford University Press.

Durany, N., Michel, T., Kurt, J., Cruz-Sánchez, F. F., Cervós-Navarro, J., & Riederer, P. (2000). Brain-derived neurotrophic factor and neurotrophin-3 levels in Alzheimer's disease brains. *International Journal of Developmental Neuroscience*, **18**, 807–813.

Egan, M. F., Goldberg, T. E., Kolachana, B. S., Callicott, J. H., Mazzanti, C. M., Straub, R. E., Goldman, D., & Weinberger, D. R. (2001). Effect of COMT Val108/158Met genotype on frontal lobe function and risk for schizophrenia. *Proceedings of the National Academy of Sciences of the United States of America*, **98**, 6917–6922.

Emerson, R. W. (1900). *Compensation*. New York, NY: Caldwell.

Erickson, K. I., Colcombe, S. J., Wadhwa, R., Bherer, L., Peterson, M. S., Scalf, P. E., Kim, J. S., Alvarado, M., & Kramer, A. F. (2007). Training-induced plasticity in older adults: effects of training on hemispheric asymmetry. *Neurobiology of Aging*, **28**, 272–283.

Glisky, E. L., & Glisky, M. L. (1999). Memory rehabilitation in the elderly. In D. T. Stuss, G. Winocur, & I. H. Robertson (Eds.), *Cognitive Neurorehabilitation* (pp. 347–361). New York, NY: Cambridge University Press.

Gonzalez Rothi, L. J. (1995). Behavioral compensation in the case of treatment of acquired language disorders resulting from brain damage. In R. A. Dixon, & L. Bäckman (Eds.), *Compensating for Psychological Deficits and Declines: Managing Losses and Promoting Gains* (pp. 219–230). Mahwah, NJ: Lawrence Erlbaum.

Grady, C. L., McIntosh, A. R., Beig, S., Keightley, M. L., Burian, H., & Black, S. E. (2003). Evidence from functional neuroimaging of a compensatory prefrontal network in Alzheimer's disease. *Journal of Neuroscience*, **23**, 986–993.

Grossman, M., Payer, F., Onishi, K., White-Devine, T., Morrison, D., D'Esposito, M., Robinson, K., & Alavi, A. (1997). Constraints on the cerebral basis for semantic processing from neuroimaging studies of Alzheimer's disease. *Journal of Neurology, Neurosurgery and Psychiatry*, **63**, 152–158.

Hartmann, G. W. (1933). Changes in visual acuity through simultaneous stimulation of other sense organs. *Journal of Experimental Psychology*, **16**, 393–407.

Hawley, K. S., & Cherry, K. E. (2004). Spaced-retrieval effects on name-face recognition in older adults with probable Alzheimer's disease. *Behavior Modification*, **28**, 276–296.

Hayes, S. P. (1933). New experimental data on the old problem of sensory compensation. *Teachers Forum*, **5**, 22–26.

Heilman, K. M., Watson, R. T., & Valenstein, E. (2003). Neglect and related disorders. In K. M. Heilman, & E. Valenstein (Eds.), *Clinical Neuropsychology, 4th Edition* (pp. 296–346). New York, NY: Oxford University Press.

Heiss, W. D., & Thiel, A. (2006). A proposed regional hierarchy in recovery of post-stroke aphasia. *Brain and Language*, **98**, 118–123.

Herlitz, A., Adolfsson, R., Bäckman, L., & Nilsson, L.-G. (1991). Cue utilization following different forms of encoding in mildly, moderately, and severely demented patients with Alzheimer's disease. *Brain and Cognition*, **15**, 119–130.

Herlitz, A., Lipsinska, B., & Bäckman, L. (1992). Utilization of cognitive support for episodic remembering in Alzheimer's disease. In L. Bäckman (Eds.), *Memory Functioning in Dementia* (pp. 73–96). Amsterdam, NL: North-Holland.

Horn, D., Levy, N., & Ruppin, E. (1996). Neuronal-based synaptic compensation: a computational study in Alzheimer's disease. *Neural Computation*, **8**, 1227–1243.

Jennings, J. M., & Jacoby, L. L. (2003). Improving memory in older adults: training recollection. *Neuropsychological Rehabilitation*, **13**, 417–440.

Kliegl, R., & Baltes, P. B. (1987). Theory-guided analysis of development and aging mechanisms through testing-the-limits and research on expertise. In C. Schooler & K. W. Schaie (Eds.), *Cognitive Functioning and Social Structure over the Life Course* (pp. 95–119). Norwood, NJ: Lawrence Erlbaum.

Kliegl, R., & Philipp, D. (2007). Become a demosthenes! Compensating age-related memory deficits with expert strategies. In P. C. Kyllonen, R. D. Roberts, & L. Stankov (Eds.), *Extending Intelligence: Enhancements and New Constructs*. Mahwah, NJ: Lawrence Erlbaum.

Kolb, B., & Gibb, R. (1999). Neuroplasticity and recovery of function after brain injury. In D. T. Stuss, G. Winocur, & I. H. Robertson (Eds.), *Cognitive Neurorehabilitation* (pp. 9–25). New York, NY: Cambridge University Press.

Kolb, B., & Whishaw, I. Q. (1996). *Fundamentals of Human Neuropsychology, 4th Edition*. New York, NY: Freeman.

Lashley, K. S. (1924). Studies of cerebral functioning in learning: V. The retention of motor habits after destruction of the so called motor areas in primates. *Archives of Neurology and Psychiatry*, **12**, 249–276.

Levine, B., Cabeza, R., McIntosh, A. R., Black, S. E., Grady, C. L., & Stuss, D. T. (2002). Functional reorganisation of memory after traumatic brain injury: A study with H2I5O positron emission tomography. *Journal of Neurology, Neurosurgery and Psychiatry*, **73**, 173–181.

Li, S.-C., Lindenberger, U., & Sikstrom, S. (2001). Aging cognition: from neuromodulation to representation. *Trends in Cognitive Sciences*, **5**, 479–486.

Liotti, M., Ryder, K., & Woldorff, M. G. (1998). Auditory attention in the congenitally blind: where, when and what gets organized. *NeuroReport*, **9**, 1007–1012.

Luria, A. R. (1963). *Restoration of Function after Brain Injury*. New York, NY: MacMillan.

Luria, A. R. (1966). *Higher Cortical Functions in Man*. New York, NY: Basic Books.

Marsiske, M., Lang, F. R., Baltes, P. B., & Baltes, M. M. (1995). Selective optimization with compensation: life-span perspectives on successful human development. In R. A. Dixon & L. Bäckman (Eds.), *Compensating for Psychological Deficits and Declines: Managing Losses and Promoting Gains* (pp. 35–79). Mahwah, NJ: Lawrence Erlbaum.

Masterton, B. A., & Biederman, G. B. (1983). Proprioceptive versus visual control in autistic children. *Journal of Autism and Developmental Disorders*, **13**, 141–152.

Mateer, C. A. (1996). Rehabilitation of individuals with frontal lobe impairment. In J. Leon-Carrion (Eds.), *Neuropsychological Rehabilitation and Treatment of Brain Injury* (pp. 285–300). Delory Beach, FL: St Lucie Press.

Mateer, C. A. (1999). The rehabilitation of executive disorders. In D. T. Stuss, G. Winocur, & I. H. Robertson (Eds.), *Cognitive Neurorehabilitation* (pp. 314–332). New York, NY: Cambridge University Press.

Mattay, V. S., Goldberg, T. E., Fara, F., Hariri, A. R., Tessitore, A., Egan, M. F., Kolachana, B., Callicott, J. H., & Weinberger, D. R. (2003). Catechol O-methyltransferase val158-met genotype and individual variation in the brain response to amphetamine. *Proceedings of the National Academy of Sciences of the United States of America.*, **106**, 186–191.

McIntosh, A. R., Bookstein, F. L., Haxby, J. V., & Grady, C. L. (1996). Spatial pattern analysis of functional brain images using partial least squares. *NeuroImage*, **3**, 143–157.

Munk, H. M. (1881). *Über die Funktion der Grosshirnrinde: Gesammelte Mittheilungen aus den Jahren 1877–80 [On the function of the cerebral cortex: collected works from the years 1877–80]*. Berlin, De: Hirschwald.

Neville, H. J. (1990). Intermodal competition and compensation in development: evidence from studies of the visual system in congenitally deaf adults. In A. Diamond (Eds.), *The Development and Neural Bases of Higher Cognitive Functions* (pp. 71–91). New York, NY: New York Academy of Sciences.

Ohlsson, K. (1986). Compensation as skill. In E. Hjelmquist & L.-G. Nilsson (Eds.), *Communication and Handicap: Aspects of Psychological Compensation and Technical Aids* (pp. 85–101). Amsterdam, NL: North-Holland.

Paquette, V., Lévesque, J., Mensour, B., Leroux, J.-M., Beaudoin, G., Bourgouin, P., & Beauregard, M. (2003). "Change the mind and you change the brain": Effects of cognitive-behavioral therapy on the neural correlates of spider phobia. *NeuroImage*, **18**, 401–409.

Persson, J., Nyberg, L., Lind, J., Larsson, A., Nilsson, L.-G., Ingvar, M., & Buckner, R. L. (2006). Structure-function correlates of cognitive decline in aging. *Cerebral Cortex*, **16**, 907–915.

Picard, N., & Strick, P. L. (1996). Motor areas of the medial wall: a review of their location and functional activation. *Cerebral Cortex*, **6**, 342–353.

Prigatano, G. P., & Kime, S. (2003). What do brain dysfunctional patients report following memory compensation training? *Neurorehabilitation*, **18**, 47–55.

Prvulovic, D., Van de Ven, V., Sack, A. T., Maurer, K., & Linden, D. E. J. (2005). Functional activation imaging in aging and dementia. *Psychiatry Research: Neuroimaging*, **140**, 97–113.

Reuter-Lorenz, P. A., & Lustig, C. (2005). Brain aging: reorganizing discoveries about the aging mind. *Current Opinion in Neurobiology*, **15**, 245–251.

Rönnberg, J. (1995). Perceptual compensation in the deaf and blind: Myth or reality? In R. A. Dixon & L. Bäckman (Eds.), *Compensating for Psychological Deficits and Declines: Managing Losses and Promoting Gains* (pp. 251–274). Mahwah, NJ: Lawrence Erlbaum.

Rothi, L. J., & Horner, J. (1983). Restitution and substitution: two theories of recovery with applications to neurobehavioral treatment. *Journal of Clinical Neuropsychology*, **5**, 73–81.

Salthouse, T. A. (1984). Effects of age and skill in typing. *Journal of Experimental Psychology: General*, **113**, 345–371.

Salthouse, T. A. (1987). Age, experience, and compensation. In C. Schooler & K. W. Schaie (Eds.), *Cognitive Functioning and Social Structure over the Life Course* (pp. 142–150). New York, NY: Ablex.

Salthouse, T. A. (1990). Cognitive competence and expertise in aging. In J. E. Birren, & K. W. Schaie (Eds.), *Handbook of the Psychology of Aging* (pp. 310–319). San Diego, CA: Academic Press.

Salthouse, T. A. (1995). Refining the concept of psychological compensation. In R. A. Dixon, & L. Bäckman (Eds.), *Compensating for Psychological Deficits and Declines: Managing Losses and Promoting Gains* (pp. 21–34). Mahwah, NJ: Lawrence Erlbaum.

Schaefer, S., Murrey, M. A., Magee, W., & Wheeler, B. (2006). Melodic intonation therapy with brain-injured patients. In G. J. Murrey (Eds.), *Alternative Therapies in the Treatment of Brain Injury and Neurobehavioral Disorders* (pp. 75–88). New York, NY: Haworth Press.

Smith, P. F., & Curthoys, I. S. (1989). Mechanisms of recovery following unilateral labyrinthectomy: a review. *Brain Research Reviews*, **14**, 155–180.

Springer, M. V., McIntosh, A. R., Winocur, G., & Grady, C. L. (2005). The relation between brain activity during memory tasks and years of education in young and older adults. *Neuropsychology*, **19**, 181–192.

Stern, Y. (2002). What is cognitive reserve? Theory and research application of the reserve concept. *Journal of the International Neuropsychological Society*, **8**, 448–460.

Stern, Y., Moeller, J. R., Anderson, K. E., Luber, B., Zubin, N. R., DiMauro, A. A., Park, A., Campbell, C. E., Marder, K., Bell, K., van Heertum, R., & Sackeim, H. A. (2000). Different brain networks mediate task performance in normal aging and AD: Defining compensation. *Neurology*, **55**, 1291–1297.

Stern, Y., Habeck, C., Moeller, J., Scarmeas, N., Anderson, K. E., Hilton, H. J., Flynn, J., Sackeim, H., & van Heertum, R. (2005). Brain networks associated with cognitive reserve in healthy young and old adults. *Cerebral Cortex*, **15**, 394–402.

Stevens, J. C., Foulke, E., & Patterson, M. Q. (1996). Tactile acuity, ageing and Braille reading in long-term blindness. *Journal of Experimental Psychology*, **2**, 91–106.

Straube, T., Glauer, M., Dilger, S., Mentzel, H.-J., & Miltner, W. H. R. (2006). Effects of cognitive-behavioral therapy on brain activation in specific phobia. *NeuroImage*, **29**, 125–135.

Stuss, D. T., Robertson, I. H., Craik, F. I. M., Levine, B., Alexander, M. P., Black, S., Dawson, D., Binns, M. A., Palmer, H., Downey-Lamb, M., & Winocur, G. (2007). Cognitive rehabilitation in the elderly: a randomized trial to evaluate a new protocol. *Journal of the International Neuropsychological Society*, **13**, 120–131.

Szlyk, J. E., Seiple, W., & Viana, M. (1995). Relative effects of age and compromised vision on driving performance. *Human Factors*, **37**, 430–436.

Szot, P., White, S. S., Greenup, J. L., Leverenz, J. B., Peskind, E. R., & Raskind, M. A. (2006). Compensatory changes in the noradrenergic nervous system in the locus ceruleus and hippocampus of postmortem subjects with Alzheimer's disease and dementia with lewy bodies. *Journal of Neuroscience*, **26**, 467–478.

Teasell, R., Bitensky, J., Salter, K., & Bayona, N. A. (2005). The role of timing and intensity of rehabilitation therapies. *Topics in Stroke Rehabilitation*, **12**, 46–57.

Towne, R. L. (1994). Effect of mandibular stabilization on the diadochokinetic performance of children with phonological disorder. *Journal of Phonetics*, **22**, 317–332.

Tuokko, H., Garrett, D. D., McDowell, I., Silverberg, N., & Kristjansson, B. (2003). Cognitive decline in high-functioning older adults: reserve or ascertainment bias? *Aging and Mental Health*, **7**, 259–270.

Turner, G. R., & Levine, B. (2004). Disorders of executive functioning and self-awareness. In J. Ponsford (Eds.), *Cognitive and Behavioral Rehabilitation: From Neurobiology to Clinical Practice. Science and Practice of Neuropsychology* (pp. 224–268). New York, NY: Guilford Press.

Walczyk, J. J., Marsiglia, C. S., Johns, A. K., & Bryan, K. S. (2004). Children's compensations for poorly automated reading skills. *Discourse Processes*, **37**, 47–66.

Wasserman, G. A., Allen, R., & Solomon, C. R. (1985). At-risk toddlers and their mothers: the special case of physical handicaps. *Child Development*, **56**, 73–83.

Wilson, B. A. (1995). Memory rehabilitation: compensating for memory problems. In R. A. Dixon & L. Bäckman (Eds.), *Compensating for Psychological Deficits and Declines: Managing Losses and Promoting Gains* (pp. 171–190). Mahwah, NJ: Lawrence Erlbaum.

Wilson, B. A. (1997). Cognitive rehabilitation: how it is and how it might be. *Journal of the International Neuropsychological Society*, **3**, 487–496.

Wilson, B. A. (1999). Memory rehabilitation in brain-injured people. In D. T. Stuss, G. Winocur, & I. H. Robertson (Eds.), *Cognitive Neurorehabilitation* (pp. 333–346). New York, NY: Cambridge University Press.

Wilson, B. A., & Watson, P. C. (1996). A practical framework for understanding compensatory behaviour in people with organic memory impairment. *Memory*, **4**, 456–486.

Yabe, T. & Kaga, K. (2005). Sound lateralization test in adolescent blind individuals. *Neuroreport: For Rapid Communication of Neuroscience Research*, **16**, 939–942.

3

The patient as a moving target: the importance to rehabilitation of understanding variability

Donald T. Stuss and Malcolm A. Binns

Introduction

- In the history of understanding human behavior, there has been conflict between two different research approaches: the study of group effects versus the examination of individual differences, more generally described as central tendency versus variability in performance.
- Understanding variability may be key to accurate diagnosis and treatment.
- There are five sections to the chapter: Introduction, Definitions and measurements of variability, Factors affecting intra-individual variability, Potential mechanisms underlying variability and Clinical implications.

The efficacy of rehabilitation depends on several issues, not the least of which is the understanding (and by implication measurement) of fundamental principles of human behavior. This in turn would seem to imply a certain level of consistency of such behavior. The history of psychology reflects this premise. Despite observations by early psychologists of "performance oscillations" during the completion of different tasks (e.g., Flugel, 1928; Hull, 1943; Philpott, 1933 – see Barratt, 1963; Jensen, 1992, for a historical background), the goal of cognitive research eventually became focused on central group tendency (Cronbach, 1957; Surwillo, 1975). Variability was viewed as a nuisance, which was managed by testing more subjects and by averaging scores (Cronbach, 1957; Jensen, 1992). Yet central tendency does not provide the full range of information. In reaction time (RT) tasks, for

example, the distribution is often skewed. Maximum speed of response may be physiologically limited, but slowing is not, resulting in a long right tail as slow responses are more broadly distributed (Logan, 1992; Ulrich & Miller, 1994; Wagenmakers et al., 2005). The inability of a patient to perform a task in a stable manner would appear to be a major impediment to the benefit one obtains from rehabilitation, and would influence his/her ability to transform what they might have learned in rehabilitation to the demands of daily life.

Our first encounter with the problem of variability occurred during a study that attempted to answer the question (e.g., van Zomeren, 1981) of whether there was a focused attention deficit after moderate to severe traumatic brain injury (TBI). Patients were tested twice, one week apart, in an effort to demonstrate the replicability of the effect (Stuss et al., 1989, 1994c). The TBI patients were slow, as expected – but a review of the results of the first week unveiled no evidence of a focused attentional deficit. Analysis of the second week's results, on the other hand, indicated the same slowness, but now there was evidence of the expected focused attention impairment. The data were obviously not replicable, and were going to be rejected. Fortuitously, the data from a second study on the recovery from mild concussion (testing patients five times over a 3-month period) completed at the same time showed a similar, albeit milder, inconsistency of performance (see Figure 3.1). A third factor supported the conclusion that variability was not a nuisance but an important observation – the results

Cognitive Neurorehabilitation, Second Edition: Evidence and Application, ed. Donald T. Stuss, Gordon Winocur and Ian H. Robertson. Published by Cambridge University Press. © Cambridge University Press 2008.

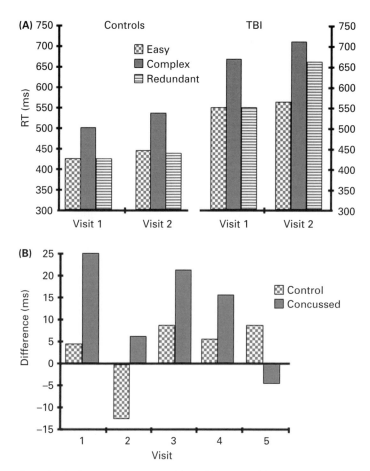

Figure 3.1. Performance on correct trials in all three conditions (Easy, Complex, Redundant) of the Multiple Choice Reaction Time Task: Easy – response to one simple target and three distractors; Complex – target defined by three features (color, form, and shading), with all distractors sharing zero, one, or two features with the target; Redundant – target defined by three features, but the distractors share no features with the target. The target appeared with a probability of 0.25. The Redundant condition was hypothesized to index focused attention since the demands were equivalent to the Easy condition, but the target was visually equivalent to the Complex condition.

(A) The top part of the figure illustrates response time (RT) to correct target responses for all three conditions over two test sessions one week apart. Control participants are on the left, and the patients are on the right. On the first visit, the traumatic brain injured (TBI) patients were slower but the pattern of responses across all three conditions paralleled those of the Control participants. On the second visit, the TBI patients, in addition to slowness, demonstrated a focused attention impairment as shown in their poor performance in the Redundant condition compared with the Easy condition. Reprinted with permission from Stuss *et al.* (1989).

(B) The bottom half of the figure depicts the performance of mildly concussed patients over five visits. The dependent measurement in this figure is the difference in RT between the Redundant and Easy conditions. The Concussed patients were more variable in their focused attention performance across five visits over a 3-month period compared with matched Control participants. Reprinted with permission from Stuss & Gow (1992).

were consonant with clinical experience. Although patients did not indicate a problem with stability of performance, they often complained about their inability to "stay on the job." Thus, although central tendency is important, these observations clearly indicated that individual differences and differences *within* individuals are also important, both theoretically and clinically.

The overall objective of this chapter is to highlight the importance of variability of performance. Specific aims, divided into the major sections of the chapter, are to provide a handy glossary of different types of variability and ways to measure these; to understand what external and internal factors might impact variability; and to examine possible etiological mechanisms, as these might be the key to successful treatment and management of variability. There is little published on actual rehabilitation of variability. We end the chapter with a section on clinical implications, including case studies, that suggest how this knowledge might be implemented in cognitive rehabilitation.

Definitions and measurements of variability

Variability can exist within an individual and between individuals in a group and both play an important role in research trying to understand brain-behavior relations. Minimising group variability is likely a key first step in the study of rehabilitation efficacy. The emphasis in this chapter is on the within- or intra-individual variability, since this type may have a particularly significant impact on clinical rehabilitation, and the outcome of rehabilitation trials.

Central tendency indexes core ability; variability assesses change. It has been claimed that the study of variability within an individual is the best technique to analyse change (Nesselroade, 1991). Changes that influence performance can be long-term or short-term. Longer-term change is more durable and systematic, as seen, for example, in personality traits. The focus in this chapter is on shorter rapid fluctuations that are more or less reversible. For each type of variability, an operational definition is presented, followed by methods of measurement.

- Measurement of variability is key to assessing change.
- Understanding and minimizing between (inter) individual variability is the first step in assessing brain-behavior relations, including the relation of variability to different brain regions or disorders. This diversity of performance can be measured, for example, by the standard deviation of individuals' scores around the mean of the group.
- There are three general types of within (intra) individual variability which we call dispersion, inconsistency and scatter.
- Dispersion is the intra-individual variation of performance across trials within a single task. Dispersion can be measured, for example, by the standard deviation of a subject's observed values within a single test at a single session.
- Inconsistency is the intra-individual variability of performance across different testing sessions. It can be measured, for example, by the standard deviation of an individual's observed values on a given test across several testing sessions.
- Scatter is the intra-individual variability of performance across different tests. It can be measured, for example, by the standard deviation of an individual's observed scaled scores on several tests which perhaps each cover different cognitive domains.

Inter-individual variability

Background

Group variability is defined as differences between individuals (*inter*-individual) performing the same task. Following Hale *et al.* (1988), this inter-individual (sometimes called "between person") variability is labeled diversity (Stuss *et al.*, 1994c, 2003; see also Hultsch & McDonald, 2004; Hultsch *et al.*, 2002; Williams *et al.*, 2005).

Individual differences are normal, and will naturally result in some group variability. The key question is – how much inter-individual variability is reasonable for a defined group? If the group is inadequately defined as might occur if specific factors are not controlled, we may be inflating diversity. As a consequence, inflated variance may obscure statistical evaluation of differences between groups. Our research into the functions of the frontal lobes highlights the importance of this question. For example, studies of memory dysfunction after frontal lobe damage led initially to the conclusion that frontal lobe damage did not result in a recognition memory deficit (Janowsky et al., 1989). However, upon further specification within the frontal lobes, it was clear that damage to specific regions of the frontal lobes did result in a significant recognition deficit (Alexander et al., 2003; Stuss et al., 1994a). A meta-analysis confirmed that this result was obscured by the way frontal groups were defined (Wheeler et al., 1995). That is, in initial studies, "frontal groups" were too broadly defined. When defined more precisely (e.g., in more refined anatomical subgroups, or by controlling for different factors such as depression), group studies can yield important results in the presence of non inflated inter-individual differences (Drai & Grodzinsky, 2006a, 2006b).

Methods

Various techniques have been used to reduce heterogeneity in a group of individuals by constructing new groups that make anatomical and/or behavioral sense. As a general approach in lesion studies, we have conceptualized performance on a given test as an independent variable and lesion location as a dependent variable. One technique, following this general conceptualization, involves overlapping shadows of lesion-extent of individuals who have impaired performance compared with control subjects (e.g., Shammi & Stuss, 1999). Those areas that show a high degree of overlap are considered to be potentially influential in performance of the task. A confounding factor may occur if a non-task-related brain area is lesioned in all of the patients; then a high degree of overlap will be seen at this location among those patients who are impaired on a task.

A modification of the overlapping lesions approach, with a nod to functional neuroimaging's statistical parametric map, involves statistically quantifying the association between presence or absence of damage within defined architectonic regions (e.g., Petrides & Pandya, 1994) and performance (Alexander et al., 2005; Picton et al., 2006; Rorden & Karnath, 2004; Stuss et al., 2005). By comparing performance of patients with damage in a given location to performance of patients without damage in that area, this architectonic localization (or "hotspot") analysis does not suffer from confounding with frequency of lesion occurrence.

As an alternative to identifying patients with abnormal performance, patients' performance can be classified using a median-split partition (Stuss et al., 1994a). That is, undertaking a performance-based division of a set of patients into two subsets of equal size based on their performance as a first step in examining the anatomical or behavioral factors that are relevant to performance. Then, frequency of abnormality in defined anatomical regions can be investigated with respect to these performance-based subsets (Stuss et al., 2001a).

Identification of more homogenous groups demonstrates that diversity may not be simply realizations of random error, but may be related to a combination of one or more relevant factors. This was demonstrated in a study of the recovery of continuous memory after traumatic head injury. When patients were initially grouped by a standard injury severity measure, considerable heterogeneity in recovery time of post-traumatic amnesia was observed (Stuss et al., 2000a). Using the Classification and Regression Tree method (CART; Brieman et al., 1984) and incorporating multiple variables (e.g., demographic information such as the age of the patient; multiple injury severity measures), we were able to meaningfully reduce variability of observed recovery time intervals (see also Temkin et al., 1995).

The importance of deriving a more finely grained partition of patients has been demonstrated in multiple group studies (e.g., Aron et al., 2003; Bechara et al., 1998; Bigler et al., 1994; Damasio & Damasio,

1989; Fellows & Farah, 2005; Godefroy *et al.*, 1998; Godefroy & Rousseaux, 1996; Hornak *et al.*, 2004; Richer & Boulet, 1999; Simons *et al.*, 2005; Tranel *et al.*, 2002). There is obvious application to rehabilitation. Negative findings in group studies may be secondary to group diversity, resulting from inadequate specification of groups. If all individuals in a defined research group do not respond to a given rehabilitation approach and the statistical comparison is negative, the cause may be group constitution and not the efficacy of the rehabilitation.

Intra-individual variability

Background

Intra-individual variability (IIV) (Barratt, 1963) (also termed within-subject, or within-individual, variability) can be exhibited over a spectrum of time scales. At the relatively short-term end of this spectrum – described as "moment to moment" variability (Rabbitt *et al.*, 2001) – are brief inter-observation time intervals such as those associated with millisecond-level sampling rates of neuroelectric signals and minute-level reaction time trials. At the longer-term end of this spectrum – generalized as "day to day" variability (Rabbitt *et al.*, 2001) – are longer time frames such as daily, monthly, or potentially yearly testing sessions. This spectrum suggests categorization of variability at different temporal resolutions.

From a practical perspective the "moment to moment" end of the IIV spectrum can be defined operationally as variability across trials within a continuous testing session (Rabbitt *et al.*, 2001; Stuss *et al.*, 1994c, 2003). The "day to day" end of the spectrum may be operationally defined as intra-individual variation between different testing occasions (Rabbitt 2001 – "between session" variability; Stuss *et al.* 1994c, 2003). In this chapter, these two types of IIV are referred to as *dispersion* (between trials) and *inconsistency* (between sessions), and are discussed below. Not only is it operationally appealing to separate IIV into between-trial and between-session classifications, but this partition

also appears to characterize distinct behavioral facets (Hultsch *et al.*, 2000; Rabbitt *et al.*, 2001; Shammi *et al.*, 1998; see discussion later in this chapter).

Operational definitions of these terms vary among research groups and care should be taken when comparing different papers. Rabbit and colleagues use the term "within session" variability; we use the term "dispersion." Dispersion has also been defined (Hultsch *et al.*, 2002) as the variability of an individual across different tasks tested at a single session (which we define as scatter). The term inconsistency has elsewhere been used to encompass both dispersion and inconsistency: "within person variability in performance on a single task measured on multiple occasions, either across testing sessions, or across separate trials within the same testing session" (Williams *et al.*, 2005, p. 88).

Differences between an individual's scores across tests assessing different cognitive domains, but with numerically comparable scales, can be a useful measure in the analysis of behavioral status. The term "scatter" has been used to describe this variation of an individual's performance on different tests (Matarazzo *et al.*, 1988; Schretlen *et al.*, 2003). Not yet investigated, but a potential area for future research, is the overlap between scatter and dispersion, since different tests (or subscales) are typically evaluated over a substantive interval of time allowing cumulative short-term fluctuations (dispersion) to be exhibited.

Methods

The distinction between predictable variability based on a set of factors and variability that is generated by chance is relevant theoretically and clinically. While we are not suggesting that the factors implicated in predictable variability are easily identifiable or measurable, it is important to investigate these possible sources of variability (such as practice, fatigue, materials and time-of-day effects) as thoroughly as possible so that they are not aggregated into measures of chance-related variability. In this section we present methods of quantifying IIV. Some of the following subheadings address identification of predictable variability (e.g., serial correlation) while others present summary measures of IIV (e.g., coefficient of variation).

Standard deviation

A reasonable measure of the spread of a set of observations is the expected distance between an observation and the center of the distribution of observations. If we allow the center of the distribution to be represented by the average of the observations, then we can compute the sample variance (s^2) as an average of the squared distances:

$$s^2 = \frac{\sum_{i=1}^{n} (x_i - \bar{x})^2}{n-1}$$

where n is the size of the sample. Note that degrees of freedom $(n-1)$ is used in the denominator instead of the sample size (n) in order to obtain an unbiased estimate of the population variance. The sample standard deviation (s) is the square root of the sample variance and has the same units as the observations. The standard deviation of a sample of observations from an individual person is sometimes referred to as the individual standard deviation (ISD).

Coefficient of variation

There are empirical and theoretical reasons for being alert to the possibility that the variance of a variable may be related to its mean. Response time studies, for example, have reported a relationship between location and spread of latency performance (e.g., Jensen, 1992) and many of the distributions that provide a good description of response time data yoke mean and variance together (more on this in the discussion of response time distributions, below). One statistic that attempts to accommodate a relationship between mean and variance in a straightforward manner is the coefficient of variation. The coefficient of variation is defined as the standard deviation divided by the mean. This statistic assumes a constant unitary relationship between mean and standard deviation.

Serial correlation

Given a series of observations on a given individual, it is often expected that there will be an association between consecutive observations and even perhaps between observations that are separated by a given lag. Slifkin & Newell (1998) highlight a couple of methods for describing serial correlation: empirical autocorrelation as a function of lag and approximate entropy which measures the degree of predictability between two sections of a series of observations – see Pincus (1991).

A simple way to visually inspect lag–1 autocorrelation in an observed series is with a scatterplot of the value of each observation (t + 1) versus the value of the immediately preceding observation (t). The sample lag–1 autocorrelation coefficient may be calculated as follows (Wei, 1990):

$$r_{\text{lag}-1} = \frac{\sum_{t=1}^{n-1} (x_t - \bar{x})(x_{t+1} - \bar{x})}{\sum_{t=1}^{n} (x_t - \bar{x})^2}$$

Note that the standard correlation coefficient calculated between two variables in which one is the same as the first but with the observations shifted by one position is not exactly the same as the sample lag–1 autocorrelation for a finite sample size. Lag–1 autocorrelation provides an index of the predictability of the value of the subsequent observation based on the current observation.

Non-stationarity

A (covariance) stationary series of observations has constant mean and variance across time (Wei, 1990). For series which are not stationary in this sense, it is important to accommodate sources of non-stationarity prior to evaluating measures of IIV. Sources of non-stationarity in a series of trial-to-trial observations might include fatigue and practice effects.

If a subject's performance changes (or drifts) linearly over time, for example, then the series is not stationary. Linear regression might be used to accommodate consistently changing performance over time. This change in performance could be seen as theoretically separable from random moment to moment variability and should be excluded from the determination of finer resolution variability.

Outlying observations

Examination of observations with extremely small or large values can be a useful step in verifying that erroneous observations are not being included in the statistical analysis of observed data. While it may seem appealing to simply adhere to a rule of thumb such as rejecting values that fall more than three standard deviations away from the mean, there are various arguments against its application. First, although such an observation may be uncommon, it is not necessarily erroneous. It is expected that about 1 in 526 observations on a random variable with a symmetric normal distribution would exceed the mean by three standard deviations or more. To put this ratio into a context, 1 in 529 people in Canada were 93 years of age or older in 2001. While it may be uncommon to run across someone who is 93 years old or more, you would not want to exclude them from a summary of the population's age distribution.

It is also possible that an observation falling three standard deviations away from the mean is not even uncommon. Consider, for example, a variable with skewed distribution. About 1 in 55 observations on a random variable with an exponential distribution would be expected to exceed the mean by more than three standard deviations. Rather than excluding such an observation it would be more sensible to identify a more appropriate distribution upon which to base characterization of the observed values. The ex-Gaussian distribution, for example, has been used successfully to model long tails often found in response time data (see below).

A method for identifying a threshold below which response time observations might be considered to be generated by a process other than the one under study was described by Ratcliff & Tuerlinckx (2002). This method examines fast trials and sets a threshold at the response latency for which accuracy crosses chance performance. Identifying contaminant observations is described as a critical step since they could inappropriately influence estimation of parameters used to describe the process of interest. In general, this is the important criteria. Observations should not be identified as outlying based on statistics alone but must incorporate information regarding the processes involved in generating the observation.

Response time distributions

Response time tasks are a popular way to study intra-individual variability. Much has been written about statistical distributions which may be motivated by models of mechanisms underlying task performance, or may simply fit observed response time data well. Pertinent to the discussion of variability, these distributions provide an intrinsic association between the mean and variance of the random variable. Both the lognormal (Ulrich & Miller, 1994) and the Weibull (Logan, 1992) distributions, for example, have been found to fit empirical response time data well and can be motivated by models of response time task performance. Both lognormal and Weibull distributions are specified by shape and scale parameters and their means and variances are functions of both parameters. Changing either of these parameters affects both mean and the variance. Wagenmakers and Brown review commonly used response time distributions and examine empirical evidence regarding the relationship between the mean and standard deviation of response time (Wagenmakers & Brown, 2007).

Ex-Gaussian distribution

The ex-Gaussian distribution is the convolution of the one-parameter exponential distribution and the two-parameter normal (or Gaussian) distribution. Specific aspects of the shape of the distribution may be summarized by each of the three ex-Gaussian parameters which index the location (μ) and scale (σ) of the normal distribution and the scale of the exponential distribution (τ). This distribution has been used to model response time data (e.g., Heathcote *et al.*, 1991; Ratcliff & Murdock 1976; West *et al.*, 2002). Estimates of the parameter values may be obtained by various techniques. Van Zandt (2000) assessed six of the more commonly used estimation techniques and found that maximum likelihood estimation on the whole sample recovered parameters with least bias and variability. From a technical perspective, it should be noted that the range of the ex-Gaussian distribution extends into negative numbers which is not generally the case for response time observations – a discrepancy which is typically overlooked in practice.

While the variance of an ex-Gaussian random variable is a function of two scale parameters, σ and τ, it has been argued that analysis of estimates of these separate parameters can be more appropriate than analysis of the sample variance since the effect of manipulated factors on the variance of a distribution of observations could be exhibited either through the general spread of the distribution or by specific changes in the right hand tail (Heathcote *et al.*, 1991). For example, Hultsch and colleagues (2002) found age differences in IIV to be larger for the slowest 20% of an individual's responses.

Scatter

Three indices of scatter were suggested by Matarazzo *et al.* (1988) and were applied to scaled scores for the 11 subscales of the WAIS-R. For an individual's set of observed values on different tests, the range (maximum value minus minimum value) and the standard deviation (both standard measures of spread) may be calculated as indices of scatter. The third proposed index was the number of observed values for a given individual that exceed subject-specific upper and lower thresholds. Thresholds were defined as those beyond which observed values were significantly different from the subject's mean scaled scores. Maximum deviation (Schretlen *et al.*, 2003) is another statistic that has been used to measure scatter.

Mahalanobis distance is a measure of distance of a multivariate observation from the center of a population. This measure has been described as a useful measure of scatter for measures such as the Wechsler Intelligence Scales (Burgess, 1991) because it is more sensitive to discrepancy between strongly correlated subscales than between weakly correlated subscales.

Factors affecting intra-individual variability

Exogenous and endogenous factors may affect IIV. These include task demands, situational factors, normal population factors, neurological conditions and neuropsychiatric disorders.

- Assessment of IIV, and awareness of IIV in rehabilitation, necessitates the awareness of the context during the assessment.
- Task factors, such as difficulty and type, play an important role.
- Situational factors can significantly affect IIV. Factors to consider are fatigue, diurnal rhythms, sleep loss, psychosocial factors, test practice and method of administration.
- Population factors may have substantial impact on IIV, with level of intelligence and age having been most commonly investigated.
- Many neurological disorders have been associated with greater intra-individual variability: mild cognitive impairment, dementia of various types (Alzheimer's, Parkinson's, frontal-temporal lobar degeneration), traumatic brain injury and focal brain damage.
- Severity of disease and type of neurological disorder appear to impact IIV.
- Research on focal brain damage suggests that the frontal lobes and cerebellum are two key areas in a system related to consistency of performance. The role of the basal ganglia in this circuit is still controversial and recent evidence suggests that this region does not play a direct role in temporal processing.
- Different regions of the frontal lobes are related to IIV (see control mechanisms in "Neurological disorders" later in this chapter).
- Schizophrenia causes increased IIV.
- Different factors affecting IIV can interact.

Task factors

Change must be understood in "context;" i.e., those factors which influence change (Cronbach, 1957; Parasuraman, 1976). Task difficulty is an important factor which increases variability. This appears to be true for most populations, but may be particularly relevant in vulnerable populations. This vulnerability has been demonstrated in the elderly (Bunce et al., 2004; Cerella, 1985; Salthouse, 1985, 1992; Shammi et al., 1998; West et al., 2002) and patients with Parkinson's disease (Perbal et al., 2005). The type of task is also relevant, although this factor may well be difficult to dissociate from task difficulty. Increased variability was found in reproduction of timed intervals by Parkinson patients, but not in production of timed intervals (Perbal et al., 2005). Different tasks may elicit IIV differently. For example, three different types of tasks (reasoning, memory, and perceptual speed) were administered to older adults twice a day over 60 consecutive days (Allaire & Marsiske, 2005). Intra-individual variation was not strongly correlated among task pairs but was among pairs of days within task.

It may not be task difficulty or the superficial task characteristics per se that impact IIV as much as the fact that different tasks affect separate timing systems in the brain (Lewis & Miall, 2003). In such cases, the different timing systems may stress brain regions that are less efficient in a particular population. Lewis & Miall (2003) argue that there are at least two systems, one more automatic and related to motor and premotor circuits, and perhaps involved with the cerebellum; there is also a cognitively controlled system, more dependent on prefrontal and parietal cortices.

Situational factors

As might be imagined, there are many situational factors that influence variability of performance: extended work periods and excessive fatigue (Bunce et al., 2004; Henning et al., 1989; Hockey, 1983; Sanders, 1998; see Grady, Chapter 9, this volume); sleep loss (Maruff et al., 2005); psychosocial

factors and related physiological measures such as blood pressure (Ong & Allaire, 2005); and alcohol use (Maruff et al., 2005).

Several situational factors deserve more attention because of the direct clinical application. Diurnal rhythms appear to impact variability (Hockey, 1983; optimal time of day – Murphy et al., 2007), although Rabbitt and colleagues (2001) have argued that both within-session variability (dispersion) and between-session variability (inconsistency) are independent of circadian variability unless you do not take into account IQ differences. Both types of IIV have been observed to be separable from practice effects (Rabbitt et al., 2001), although some tasks show that IIV can be reduced with extended practice (Hofland et al., 1981; Ram et al., 2005). The way a test is administered is also important. In the elderly, power (untimed) testing reduces IIV (Hofland et al., 1981). In patient studies, medication has been found to influence performance (Perbal et al., 2005).

Population factors

Population factors might be considered more endogenous and not driven by exogenous factors. Intelligence and level of education (Christensen et al., 2005; Ram et al., 2005) have been associated with greater variability; lower IQ and less education associated with greater IIV. This has been reported in mentally retarded individuals (Baumeister & Kellas, 1968), the general population (Larson & Alderton, 1990), and in older adults between ages 60 and 80 years, although the effect of intelligence held regardless of age (Rabbitt et al., 2001). Personality variables themselves appear to contribute to variability, at least at the level of neuroticism (Moskowitz & Zuroff, 2005; Robinson & Tamir, 2005).

Perhaps the population variable that most commonly affects both dispersion and inconsistency is age. In general, older adults are more variable than younger adults (Bunce et al., 2004; Fozard et al., 1994; Friedman, 2003; Hultsch et al., 2002; Li & Lindenberger, 1999; Li et al., 2000; Nesselroade & Salthouse, 2004; Rakitin et al., 2005; Salthouse, 1993;

see Morse, 1993, for a meta-analysis comparing the effects of age on IIV across a number of tasks), although task demands may well play a role in demonstrating this (Anstey *et al.*, 2005; Shammi *et al.*, 1998; West *et al.*, 2002;). Not all tasks result in increased IIV with age (Foster *et al.*, 1995). Although mean speed of response is often associated with IIV (Fozard *et al.*, 1994), it is not necessarily so (Hetherington *et al.*, 1996; Segalowitz *et al.*, 1997; Shammi *et al.*, 1998; Stuss *et al.*, 2003).

Neurological disorders

Increased IIV has been reported in children with different disorders (Rovet & Hepworth, 2001; Zahn *et al.*, 1991). Children with attention deficit hyperactivity disorder (ADHD) have higher IIV than control participants, even though there may be no significant differences in average speed of response (Castellanos *et al.*, 2005; Douglas, 1999; Leth-Steensen *et al.*, 2000; Ridderinkhof *et al.*, 2005).

Studies of IIV in adults with neurological disorders can be divided into studies of progressive neurodegenerative disease and acquired focal brain damage. As a general observation in progressive neurodegenerative disease, even mild dementia results in higher IIV than in healthy adults or even those with arthritis, suggesting that this increased IIV is neurological in etiology, and not secondary to general health problems (Hultsch *et al.*, 2000; Strauss *et al.*, 2002). This is true (for at least some abilities) even for mild cognitive impairment (Christensen *et al.*, 2005). In centenarians, inconsistency (between-session variability) was a better predictor of eventual cognitive decline than measures at a single assessment (Kliegel & Sliwinski, 2004).

As might be expected, patients with Alzheimer's disease also exhibit greater IIV than controls (Burton *et al.*, 2006; Duchek *et al.*, 1994). Severity and type of disease have to be considered separately. In a comparison of patients with Alzheimer's and patients with Parkinson's disease (Burton *et al.*, 2006), IIV was related to the severity of the disease process independently of the type of disease. The nature of the disorder also played a role, with

Alzheimer's patients exhibiting more IIV than those with Parkinson's disease. The effect of the type of neurodegenerative disorder, likely reflecting the anatomical systems affected and the clinical symptomatology, is also seen in other comparisons. Ballard *et al.* (2001) found that patients with Alzheimer's disease or Lewy body disease were both more variable than normal elderly individuals, but the IIV was more marked in those with Lewy body disease. A more extended comparison was conducted with the addition of patients who had vascular dementia (Walker *et al.*, 2000). They examined levels of fluctuating consciousness, and found it greatest in Lewy body disease, second largest with vascular dementia, and smallest in those with Alzheimer's disease. In a comparison of patients with Alzheimer's disease and those with frontal-temporal lobar degeneration (Murtha *et al.*, 2002), the latter were more variable, explained by the fact that there was more frontal lobe pathology in frontal temporal lobar degeneration (see below for focal lesion research).

Research on IIV in Parkinson's disease has been relatively plentiful because of the suggestion that these patients have impaired temporal processing. Several studies reported greater variability of performance in Parkinson patients (Artieda *et al.*, 1992; Harrington *et al.*, 1998a; O'Boyle *et al.*, 1996; Perbal *et al.*, 2005; Rammsayer & Classen, 1997). In other studies, there was no such evidence of increased IIV associated with the disease (Duchek *et al.*, 1994; Spencer & Ivry, 2005). Task factors may play a role, as might the question of medication (Perbal *et al.*, 2005). These data suggest caution in interpreting the relationship of diseases that have more widespread anatomical and neurochemical involvement to IIV. Focal lesion studies may be required to help address the controversy.

Traumatic brain injury (TBI) is an excellent example of the importance of understanding and applying knowledge of the different types of variability. As already noted, multiple factors might determine the nature of particular TBI groups, and using this information for clinical purposes such as prediction requires minimizing group variability (Stuss *et al.*,

2000a). Traumatic brain injury is now known to cause both dispersion (Benton & Blackburn, 1957; Bruhn & Parsons, 1971, 1977; Goldstein, 1942; Segalowitz *et al.*, 1997; Spikman *et al.*, 1996; Stuss *et al.*, 1994c; Whyte *et al.*, 1995; Zahn & Mirsky, 1999) and inconsistency (Stuss *et al.*, 1989, 1994a). Intra-individual variability is observed after both more severe and mild TBI, with some proportional relation to the severity of the injury (Bleiberg *et al.*, 1998; Collins & Long, 1996; Stuss *et al.*, 1994c).

A prominent position about IIV, derived to a great degree from functional imaging research, argues for a cortico striatal network involved in timing and variability (Coull *et al.*, 2004; Macar *et al.*, 2002) Studies in patients with focal brain damage, in particular stroke, are therefore key in investigating which nodes in such a network are necessarily involved in consistent behavior. The example of Parkinson's disease is most telling. As noted, damage of various types that involve the basal ganglia have been reported as resulting in impairment in temporal processing, often associated with IIV (Harrington & Haaland, 1999; Harrington *et al.*, 1998a, 1998b; Macar *et al.*, 2002; Rammsayer & Classen, 1997). However, if only patients with unilateral stroke were examined, deficits were found in motor force control but not increased variability in timing for central or motor implementation (Aparicio *et al.*, 2005). The problems may be more related to changes in other regions or systems, or the interaction of these, with the basal ganglia.

In our first studies on TBI and variability, we had hypothesized that a top-down control mechanism was impaired, with the result that an individual could perform any task well, but could not do it consistently (Stuss, 1987; Stuss *et al.*, 1989, 1994c – see also West & Alain, 2000a, 2000b, for the role of prefrontal cortex in maintaining optimal level of control in healthy young adults). We postulated that such a top-down control would involve the frontal lobes, but could not investigate this possibility with TBI patients because of the more diffuse nature of the disorder. To examine this hypothesis a study of IIV in patients with focal frontal and posterior brain damage was completed (Stuss *et al.*, 1999, 2003). The results only partially confirmed the hypothesis. The frontal lobes were involved in a general top-down manner. However, it was not "frontal lobes" in a global sense. Three different regions were involved, each related to a different mechanism of control. Moreover, the posterior regions were also related to control, but only in one condition, which depended to a greater degree on a particular mode of cognitive processing – visual-spatial integration. The focal lesion study therefore suggested that there were different kinds of control of variability, some related to the specific content of the task (domain specific), perhaps more related to the posterior regions, and others more domain general, related to different regions within the frontal lobes.

The cerebellum has also been closely connected with IIV. If one accepts that temporal processing tasks are about variability, then the evidence is consistent that cerebellar damage affects temporal processing (Ivry & Keele, 1989; Ivry *et al.*, 1988). However, the type of task might again be relevant, with impairment on event-based timing tasks, but not on a continuously produced task (Spencer *et al.*, 2003).

Neuropsychiatric disorders

Individuals with schizophrenia demonstrate greater IIV (Brown *et al.*, 2005; Schwartz *et al.*, 1989; Vinogradov *et al.*, 1998). It appears that IIV is independent of psychoticism, and primarily found in those with schizophrenia, and not in affective disorders (Schwartz *et al.*, 1989). There is an important situational factor which might be having a significant impact – medication (Meck, 1996).

Research in depression suggests that individual variability may occur not just in cognitive functions, but in personality variables (Monk *et al.*, 1991). Following the temporal characterization, variations can be seasonal (Reid *et al.*, 2000) or day-to-day (Nezlek *et al.*, 2001). The latter study showed that such variability can be specific; empathy varied daily in depressed individuals, and did not covary with other measures such as daily depressogenic thinking, and self-esteem.

Potential mechanisms underlying variability

What is not known is whether the symptoms of variability should be rehabilitated, or whether it is essential to address the specific impaired mechanisms that cause variable performance. In this section, the postulated mechanisms underlying different types of variability are reviewed. Specific mechanisms underlying group variability are not discussed. Although the underlying cause of scatter can only be speculated in a global sense, the clinical importance of profile analysis recommends review. The emphasis will be on mechanisms of dispersion and inconsistency.

- Cognitive abilities within an individual are not equivalent in terms of performance levels. This "scatter" amongst different measures and abilities is often normal and not necessarily reflective of abnormalities.
- Intra-individual variability is most often interpreted as a disorder of top-down control. In cognitive psychology terminology, phrases such as attentional lapses are used. In neuropsychology, this control is related to the frontal lobes.
- There are different mechanisms of control within the frontal lobes: task setting (left lateral); monitoring and checking (right lateral); energisation (superior medial). Each results in IIV; the importance of uncovering the mechanism relates to the potential specificity of rehabilitation.
- Control mechanisms within the frontal lobes are domain general; that is, they apply to any cognitive function mediated by this region of the brain.
- There are also domain-specific functions, such that impairment of a particular posterior cognitive domain can result in increased IIV for that particular function.

Scatter

Scatter of scores in an individual's profile has been a valuable measure for analyzing the relationships among test scores (Lezak, 1995). If there is a substantial difference between two test scores, the implication has been made that the lower score reflects some abnormal condition. This, however, assumes that individuals have equivalent abilities across different cognitive domains.

In reality, however, individuals have very different abilities across different domains. Matarazzo and colleagues (Matarazzo & Herman, 1985; Matarazzo et al., 1988; Matarazzo & Prifitera, 1989) examined the WAIS III and WAIS-R standardization sample. Over 85% of the sample had differences equaling or exceeding 5 scaled score points between highest and lowest scores; over 15% had differences over 9 scaled score points (3 SD). Schretlen and colleagues (2003) examined scatter over 32 measures derived from 15 neuropsychological tests. Not one individual in the sample of 197 healthy adults aged 20 to 92 years showed "consistent" performance across the different measures, when consistency was defined by a Maximum Discrepancy score (MD) of 1 SD or less. The MD ranged from 1.6 to 6.1. When the neuropsychological measures were compared with IQ estimated by the National Adult Reading Test, the average person's lowest score fell 1.9 MD below his/her IQ. Age affected the MD measure by only 5%; age-correcting the scores did not reduce the scatter. Importantly, the differences did not appear to be due to a small number of tests with unusual psychometric properties. Cognitive abilities within an individual are not equivalent.

Dispersion and inconsistency

Intra-individual variability is commonly seen as a reflection of a disorder of control. In studies of normal populations, the prevailing theory is that IIV is related to attentional oscillations, attentional lapses or mental blocks (Bertelson & Joffe, 1963; Foley & Humphries, 1962; Obersteiner, 1879). This could be influenced by mental fatigue, since IIV is often related to task demand durations, and shown primarily (at least in older adults) in the tail end of the distribution (Hockey, 1983; Lorist et al., 2002; Williams et al., 2005). General slowing is not necessarily directly related to increased IIV (Stuss et al., 2003). The notion that some type of attentional control process is the major factor is supported by other data: distractors affect IIV (Jensen, 1992; Ulrich & Miller, 1994; Stuss *et al.*, 2003); older adults often reveal IIV under conditions of a more difficult task, interpreted as inefficiency of executive control processes (West *et al.*, 2002). The biological mechanism in normal adults is uncertain (see MacDonald *et al.*, 2006, for a review). Catecholamines have been shown to play a role in modulating signal to noise ratio of neurons. Thus, age-related variability may be related to catecholamine changes, with greater neural noise and consequently higher IIV (Li & Lindenberger, 1999).

Lesion data present the most compelling evidence that the frontal lobes, in particular specific areas within the frontal lobes, are significantly involved in mediating consistent behavior. Damage to the frontal lobes does result in increased IIV across a variety of tasks. This type of control is therefore considered to be domain general (Stuss, 2006), in that the processes are superordinate to any number of functional domains. The precise control mechanism depends on which brain region is damaged. That is, there are different control processes within the frontal regions, all of which might impact IIV (Stuss *et al.*, 2002): left lateral – task setting; right lateral – monitoring and checking; superior medial – energization (see also Macar *et al.*, 2002). Although the overt symptom may be increased IIV, the mechanisms resulting in increased IIV vary depending on lesion location (Stuss *et al.*, 2003). In rehabilitation, one probably needs to address the damaged mechanism, and not the symptom of increased IIV.

There are, in addition to the frontal lobe domain-general control processes, domain-specific control mechanisms. These are related to the brain regions involved with that specific cognitive function. As a consequence, likely under conditions of task complexity, damage to a particular non frontal region can result in increased IIV for that particular function. In a complex feature integration reaction time task (but not in simple single feature detection or simple RT), increased IIV was noted in posterior regions as well as frontal (damage to the frontal lobes increased IIV in many tasks) (Stuss *et al.*,

2003). In a similar manner, increased IIV has been reported in patients with right hemisphere lesions and neglect, and was a function of spatial position and not just a general increase in variability (Anderson *et al.*, 2000). Milberg and colleagues (2003) reported variability in lexical decision tasks after left brain injury.

Clinical implications

This overview of variability has shown that there are different kinds of variability, and all may negatively influence rehabilitation efficacy. Although performance fluctuation is almost totally ignored in rehabilitation research, we outline some potential avenues of research and clinical application, and present representative case studies as examples. Analysis of performance variability adds new information above and beyond the general level of performance, and is different from "noise" (Lecerf *et al.*, 2004). Importantly, these individual differences are stable, and therefore amenable to investigation (Hultsch *et al.*, 2000; Rabbitt *et al.*, 2001; Stuss *et al.*, 2003). The impact may be at the level of knowledge, in that being aware of both group constitution and IIV may help in evaluating research on rehabilitation, and the efficacy of clinical interventions. There is a final possibility – perhaps the minimization of IIV should be the specific goal of rehabilitation.

- The clinician must be aware of the different types of variability.
- Scatter should not be over-interpreted for individual diagnostic purposes. At the same time, finding consistent patterns of scatter in specific populations can be very useful.
- There is some evidence that pharmacological or behavioral methods can minimize IIV. However, much research is required to investigate whether specific approaches need to be used for different control mechanisms.
- Intra-individual variability observed in malingering is likely dissociable from that found in neurological conditions.
- Not all variability is maladaptive.

Group variability and scatter

Excessive variability between individuals within a group suggests that the group composition may not be appropriate. Even if significant *rehabilitation efficacy* is found there may be limitations to the generalizablity of results.

Precipitous analysis of individual scatter of performance might lead to over-diagnosis. It would be inappropriate to make diagnostic inferences based only on scatter on psychometric variability (e.g., MD measurement) without clinical context, since in many cases rather large quantitative differences among abilities are normal (Schretlen *et al.*, 2003). The clinical context should consider many factors, including patient complaints, educational and work background (historical strengths and weaknesses), the situational context (e.g., depression), and test interactions. Knowledge of scatter can be used to establish hypotheses, which can be tested. For example, does the profile follow known syndromes, and does this make sense in light of the total history? At the same time, finding the consistency of profile across individuals can be used to great benefit, as in the example of what has been achieved in the learning disability field (e.g., Rourke, 1985).

Assessment

Individual performance fluctuation is an important psychological phenomenon, which has to be considered in both assessment and treatment. Since IIV is virtually never examined clinically, it can be considered a "silent" disorder, which may be reasonably frequent considering all the potential factors affecting stability of performance. Being aware of, and assessing, IIV gives one insight into the processing capabilities of an individual. By varying conditions, insight might be obtained about the potential for learning capacity. In the elderly for example, retesting (practice) and comparing standard (speeded) vs. power (unspeeded) testing, showed that practice and power improved overall correct performance, although the power condition resulted in a different error pattern (Hofland *et al.*, 1981).

Another very significant implication of IIV is that one assessment of a patient may not be representative of their actual level of performance. What you see may not be what you get (Stuss, 1987). Assessing different measures of intra-subject variability provides knowledge that may be crucial to the patient's ability to successfully return to work, and will help guide healthcare providers, caregivers and employers. Performing a task in a less stable manner than the majority of other individuals would have a direct impact on an employee's evaluation.

Case study

The following case study illustrates two important points: intra-individual variability may be the most important index of impairment, against a background of apparently normal functioning; interpreting the IIV against the functional performance of the patient provided the clinical context for interpretation.

The patient was a young male who had been thrown out of a car as a result of an accident on a steep and winding road, hit a tree near the edge of a sharp ravine, and was not found for several days. The traumatic brain injury was considered severe based on biological markers, with a documented loss of consciousness of 2 days and an estimated post-traumatic amnesia of 6 weeks. The patient was seen as a litigant in a medical-legal case some 2 years post-injury. On examination, the patient had mild left facial droop and left-sided weakness. History was remarkable, in that there were few complaints. In fact, post-injury, the young man had done better in school than prior to the injury. He had developed a serious relationship and had returned to work. However, employment positions did not last very long, and the patient had no explanation for this employment failure. In most regards his neuropsychological examination was normal, particularly in light of the severity of his injury. There was no measurable or observed evidence of malingering. What was observed, however, was significant variability of performance. For example, after performing the WCST successfully according to at least one method of scoring (7 categories correct, during a full 128-card presentation), he began to lose set, and for an extended period of time was unable to perform the task correctly

(Stuss *et al.*, 2000b). Had the administration of the WCST been terminated at the end of six consecutive responses, the set loss would not have been demonstrated. He also exhibited IIV on our (at that time unpublished) RT paradigms (Stuss *et al.*, 1989, 2003). There was also inconsistency in performance from session to session. The one striking clinical finding, then, was abnormal IIV, but the awareness of that fact was uncommon in the 1980s. His parents were interviewed. They essentially denied all deficits, saying all that was needed was more effort on his part. In their opinion, the purpose of the neuropsychological examination was to find out where the effort was needed. They did wish that he would close his mouth (left side facial droop) when he ate, but that could be taught. Finally, the appropriate question was felicitously asked. The family owned a business that used machinery. When asked when the son would take over the business, they stated emphatically (paraphrased): "Are you crazy? We don't know from one moment to the next what he might do."

The son had done well post-injury because of the external formal structure of the family. As when the son was young, the parents had in essence again "become the frontal lobes" of their son, enabling him to use maximally whatever abilities he had. Their fears related to what they observed in the less controlled environment. The son's IIV was also the reason he could not maintain consistent employment (see the title for Stuss *et al.*, 2003).

Intra-individual variability and rehabilitation/treatment

Can IIV be treated? Time itself appears to be a healing factor, suggesting some brain plasticity. In a cross-sectional study of severe TBI comparing mean response times (RT) and IIV in patients 5 and 10 years post-injury, there was no change in mean RT (significantly slow), but IIV had notably diminished (Hetherington *et al.*, 1996). Wegesin & Stern (2004) found that estrogen use, but *not* estrogen plus progestin, reduced age-related increase in IIV for at least one form of variability. Bleiberg and colleagues (1993) administered dextroamphetamine in a single subject placebo crossover design to an individual with TBI. With pharmacological treatment

only, variability decreased. However, since only the standard deviation was reported, it is uncertain what the relationship to RT speed was.

There is some suggestion that behavioral interventions may have a beneficial effect. Intra-individual variability can be reduced with practice (Ram *et al.*, 2005), although it may be that there are both adaptive (practice) and maladaptive IIV in the same individuals over time (Allaire & Marsiske, 2005). It is likely that practice alone is not the best intervention.

What may be required is practice combined with cognitive rehabilitation of the specific impaired mechanism. Different control mechanisms within the frontal lobes have been postulated (Stuss *et al.*, 2003). Rather than generic rehabilitation to assist individuals with specific disturbances, knowledge of the lesion location and isolation of the specific deficits through appropriate assessment may provide at least a base for rehabilitation research efforts in rehabilitation targeted at the deficit.

Case study

This case illustrates the potential value of Luria's verbal self-regulation in minimizing IIV, at least in a patient with focal right hemisphere pathology.

A middle-aged gentleman was seen in investigation prior to surgical removal of a large hypodense lesion in the right frontal lobe with extension to the right parietal region (Stuss *et al.*, 1987). The most striking disorder exhibited was motor impersistence, a disorder most commonly found after right frontal pathology when damage is focal. He could initiate tasks successfully (e.g., close your eyes, hold your breath), but could not sustain them. He was also variable in other simple tasks, such as continuous tapping. We used verbal self-regulation (Luria, 1973; Meichenbaum, 1974) to reduce the motor impersistence. If a specific command was repeated within a relatively brief period of time, the patient could sustain the task as long as the command was repeated. The patient then was able to internalize this procedure and repeated the command himself. In anatomical terms, it is likely that his intact left frontal task-setting mechanism could assist the impaired right frontal monitoring and checking mechanism to sustain behavior. However, this patient's use of self-regulation was fragile, in that it was easily disrupted by distractions.

With certain patients, it may be necessary to externalize the control of the patient (see case study above) (Stuss, 1987; Stuss *et al.*, 1994b); i.e., establish a sufficiently rigid external environment that acts to minimize the necessity of top-down control, allowing responses to be more automatic. In such instances, the employer or care-provider has to be a partner, and indeed the leader, in rehabilitation.

Case study

A young man who had suffered a severe TBI returned to work as an autobody mechanic. His performance at work was normal in most aspects. However, if unable to complete a specific task adequately, he would become volatile and destroy what had already been successfully accomplished. His employer, who had suffered a severe TBI himself and had been our patient, over time had learned that external control would help him with his problems. He became aware of the signs preceding such eruptions in his employee, and intervened by telling the young man to take a 5-minute break. The young man would then come back and finish the job without any difficulty. The employer recognized the cause of the variable and erratic performance, and provided external prosthetic time outs to help stabilize performance.

Intra-individual variability and malingering

How might the concept of intra-individual variability relate to the observation of inconsistent performance in malingerers? That is, might variability be a reflection of trying less hard? Cullum *et al.* (1991) proposed that it would be difficult to have the same levels of poor effort over multiple tests; that is, it is difficult to fake consistently. Reitan & Wolfson (1997) compared two traumatic brain-injured groups, one in litigation and the other not, in a 1-year test-retest, and reported that the group in litigation had less consistent scores. Strauss and colleagues (2000) repeated testing on three

occasions with undergraduate students who were asked to pretend to have real impairment to win a lawsuit (malingerers) or do their best. The "malingering" group had less consistent mean scores across the test sessions. What then is the difference between the dispersion and inconsistency caused by brain damage or malingering?

A possible answer can be found in the nature and extent of intra-individual variability as expressed in patients. The principle of "making sense" (Stuss, 1995) can be invoked here. That is, IIV as noted does follow certain principles. It is primarily expected in more complex tasks. IIV is itself consistent. Moreover, in many instances the mean performance of our focal lesion groups was not abnormal, in contrast to many malingerers who present as very significantly impaired. Just as caution is required in interpreting scatter, dispersion and inconsistency must be considered clinically as information that must be interpreted scientifically – by establishing hypotheses and further testing.

General conclusions

The tone of this chapter might suggest that IIV is maladaptive. In fact, our position is that variability of performance is a normal, constant presence in all individuals, and can be either maladaptive or adaptive. The nature of control processes is not just to make processes automatic and uniform, unless this is for the benefit of the organism. Control at some level also requires flexibility in examining options of behavioral responses, and such flexibility will of necessity lead to variability in behavior. Moreover, there are likely levels of control and variability, and the interaction of these need to be studied in greater detail (see Stuss *et al.*, 2001b, for a discussion of levels of control in self-awareness). The brain is a highly distributed super-system, with control at different processing levels (Adi-Japha & Freeman, 2000). This is very aptly illustrated in a study by Miller and colleagues (1996). Patients with Parkinson's disease were treated for gait disturbances. As gait improved, with reduced variability, there was increased variability in muscle and brain measurements. The ultimate goal is to understand and harness both adaptive and maladaptive variability, not to create automatic robotic behaviors.

ACKNOWLEDGMENTS

Research of the senior author related to variability has been supported by grants MT-12853 and GR-14974 from the Canadian Institutes of Health Research; the JSF McDonnell Foundation; the Ontario Mental Health Foundation; the Ontario Heart and Stroke Foundation Centre for Stroke Recovery; and the Posluns Centre for Stroke and Cognition at Baycrest. DTS is supported by the University of Toronto/ Baycrest Reva James Leeds Chair in Neuroscience and Research Leadership. We are grateful to all the co-authors on our previous papers referenced in this chapter. S. Gillingham is thanked for all her assistance in preparing the manuscript.

REFERENCES

Adi-Japha, E., & Freeman, N. H. (2000). Regulation of division of labour between cognitive systems controlling action. *Cognition*, **76**, 1–11.

Alexander, M. P., Stuss, D. T., & Fansabedian, N. (2003). California Verbal Learning Test: Performance by patients with focal frontal and non-frontal lesions. *Brain*, **126**, 1493–1503.

Alexander, M. P., Stuss, D. T., Shallice, T., Picton, T. W., & Gillingham, S. (2005). Impaired concentration due to frontal lobe damage from two distinct lesion sites. *Neurology*, **65**, 572–579.

Allaire, J. C., & Marsiske, M. (2005). Intraindividual variability may not always indicate vulnerability in elders' cognitive performance. *Psychology and Aging*, **20**, 390–401.

Anderson, B., Mennemeier, M., & Chatterjee, A. (2000). Variability not ability: another basis for performance decrements in neglect. *Neuropsychologia*, **38**, 785–796.

Anstey, K. J., Dear, K., Christensen, H., & Jorm, A. F. (2005). Biomarkers, health, lifestyle, and demographic variables as correlates of reaction time performance in early, middle, and late adulthood. *Quarterly Journal of Experimental Psychology: Section A*, **58**, 5–21.

Aparicio, P., Diedrichsen, J., & Ivry, R. B. (2005). Effects of focal basal ganglia lesions on timing and force control. *Brain and Cognition*, **58**, 62–74.

Aron, A. R., Fletcher, P. C., Bullmore, E. T., Sahakian, B. J., & Robbins, T. W. (2003). Stop-signal inhibition disrupted by damage to right inferior frontal gyrus in humans. *Nature Neuroscience*, **6**, 115–116.

Artieda, J., Pastor, M. A., Lacruz, F., & Obesa, J. A. (1992). Temporal discrimination is abnormal in Parkinson's disease. *Brain*, **115**, 199–210.

Ballard, C., O'Brien, J., Gray, A. *et al.* (2001). Attention and fluctuating attention in patients with dementia with Lewy bodies and Alzheimer disease. *Archives of Neurology*, **58**, 977–982.

Barratt, E. S. (1963). Intra-individual variability of performance: ANS and psychometric correlates. *Texas Reports on Biology and Medicine*, **21**, 496–504.

Baumeister, A. A., & Kellas, G. (1968). Distribution of reaction times of retardates and normals. *American Journal of Mental Deficiency*, **72**, 715–718.

Bechara, A., Damasio, H., Tranel, D., & Anderson, S. W. (1998). Dissociation of working memory from decision making within the human prefrontal cortex. *Journal of Neuroscience*, **18**, 428–437.

Benton, A. L., & Blackburn, H. L. (1957). Practice effects in reaction-time tasks in brain-injured patients. *Journal of Abnormal and Social Psychology*, **54**, 109–113.

Bertelson, G., & Joffe, R. (1963). Blockings in prolonged serial responding. *Ergonomics*, **6**, 109–116.

Bigler, E. D., Burr, R., Gale, S. *et al.* (1994). Day of injury CT scan as an index to pre-injury brain morphology. *Brain Injury*, **8**, 231–238.

Bleiberg, J., Garmoe, W., Cederquist, J., Reeves, D., & Lux, W. (1993). Effects of dexedrine on performance consistency following brain injury. *Neuropsychiatry, Neuropsychology, and Behavioral Neurology*, **6**, 245–248.

Bleiberg, J., Halpern, E. L., Reeves, D., & Daniel, J. C. (1998). Future directions for the neuropsychological assessment of sports concussion. *Journal of Head Trauma Rehabilitation*, **13**, 36–44.

Brieman, L., Friedman, J. H., Olshen, R. A., & Stone, C. J. (1984). *Classification and Regression Trees*. Belmont, CA: Wadsworth International Group.

Brown, S. M., Kieffaber, P. D., Carroll, C. A. *et al.* (2005). Eyeblink conditioning deficits indicate timing and cerebellar abnormalities in schizophrenia. *Brain and Cognition*, **58**, 94–108.

Bruhn, P., & Parsons, O. A. (1971). Continuous reaction time in brain damage. *Cortex*, **7**, 278–291.

Bruhn, P., & Parsons, O. A. (1977). Reaction time variability in epileptic and brain-injured patients. *Cortex*, **13**, 373–384.

Bunce, D., MacDonald, S. W. S., & Hultsch, D. F. (2004). Inconsistency in serial choice decision and motor reaction times dissociate in younger and older adults. *Brain and Cognition*, **56**, 320–327.

Burgess, A. (1991). Profile analysis of the Wechsler intelligence scales: A new index of subtest scatter. *British Journal of Clinical Psychology*, **30**, 257–263.

Burton, C., Strauss, E., Hultsch, D., Moll, A., & Hunter, M. (2006). Intraindividual variability as a marker of neurological dysfunction: a comparison of Alzheimer's disease and Parkinson's disease. *Journal of Clinical and Experimental Neuropsychology*, **28**, 67–83.

Castellanos, F. X., Sonuga-Barke, E. J. S., Scheres, A., Di Martino, A., Hyde, C., & Walters, J. R. (2005). Varieties of attention-deficit/hyperactivity disorder-related intra-individual variability. *Biological Psychiatry*, **57**, 1416–1423.

Cerella, J. (1985). Information processing rates in the elderly. *Psychological Bulletin*, **98**, 67–83.

Christensen, H., Dear, K. B. G., Anstey, K. J., Parslow, R. A., Sachdev, P., & Jorm, A. F. (2005). Within-occasion intra-individual variability and preclinical diagnostic status: Is intraindividual variability an indicator of mild cognitive impairment? *Neuropsychology*, **19**, 309–317.

Collins, L. F., & Long, C. J. (1996). Visual reaction time and its relationship to neurological test performance. *Archives of Clinical Neuropsychology*, **11**, 613–623.

Coull, J. T., Vidal, F., Nazarian, B., & Macar, F. (2004). Functional anatomy of the attentional modulation of time estimation. *Science*, **303**, 1506–1508.

Cronbach, L. J. (1957). The two disciplines of scientific psychology. *American Psychologist*, **12**, 671–684.

Cullum, C. M., Heaton, R. K., & Grant, I. (1991). Psychogenic factors influencing neuropsychological performance: Somatoform disorders, factitious disorders, and malingering. In H. O. Doerr & A. S. Carlin (Eds.), *Forensic Neuropsychology: Legal and Scientific Bases* (pp. 141–171). New York, NY: Guilford Press.

Damasio, H., & Damasio, A. R. (1989). *Lesion Analysis in Neuropsychology*. New York, NY: Oxford University Press.

Douglas, V. (1999). Cognitive control processes in attention-deficit/hyperactivity disorder. In H. C. Quay & A. E. Hogan (Eds.), *Handbook of Disruptive Behavior Disorders* (pp. 105–138). New York, NY: Kluwer Academic/Plenum Publishers.

Drai, D., & Grodzinsky, Y. (2006a). A new empirical angle on the variability debate: quantitative neurosyntactic analyses of a large data set from Broca's aphasia. *Brain and Language*, **96**, 117–128.

Drai, D., & Grodzinsky, Y. (2006b). The variability debate: more statistics, more linguistics. *Brain and Language*, **96**, 157–170.

Duchek, J. M., Balota, D. A., & Ferraro, F. R. (1994). Component analysis of a rhythmic finger tapping task in individuals with senile dementia of the Alzheimer type and in individuals with Parkinson's disease. *Neuropsychology*, **8**, 218–226.

Fellows, L. K., & Farah, M. J. (2005). Different underlying impairments in decision-making following ventromedial and dorsolateral frontal lobe damage in humans. *Cerebral Cortex*, **15**, 58–63.

Flugel, J. C. (1928). Practice, fatigue and oscillation. *British Journal of Psychology Monographs, Supplement* **4**, 1–92.

Foley, P. J., & Humphries, M. (1962). Blocking in serial simple reaction tasks. *Canadian Journal of Psychology*, **16**, 128–137.

Foster, J. K., Behrmann, M., & Stuss, D. T. (1995). Aging and visual search: generalized cognitive slowing or selective deficit in attention? *Aging and Cognition*, **2**, 279–299.

Fozard, J. L., Vercruyssen, M., Reynolds, S. L., Hancock, P. A., & Quilter, R. E. (1994). Age differences and changes in reaction time: the Baltimore Longitudinal Study of Aging. *Journals of Gerontology: Series B; Psychological Sciences and Social Sciences*, **49**, 179–189.

Friedman, D. (2003). Cognition and aging: a highly selective overview of event-related potential (ERP) data. *Journal of Clinical and Experimental Neuropsychology*, **25**, 702–720.

Godefroy, O., & Rousseaux, M. (1996). Binary choice in patients with prefrontal or posterior brain damage. A relative judgement theory analysis. *Neuropsychologia*, **34**, 1029–1038.

Godefroy, O., Duhamel, A., Leclerc, X., Saint Michel, T., Henon, H., & Leys, D. (1998). Brain-behaviour relationships. Some models and related statistical procedures for the study of brain-damaged patients. *Brain*, **121**, 1545–1556.

Goldstein, K. (1942). *After Effects of Brain Injuries in War*. New York, NY: Grune and Stratton.

Hale, S., Myerson, J., Smith, G. A., & Poon, L. W. (1988). Age, variability, and speed: between-subjects diversity. *Psychology and Aging*, **3**, 407–410.

Harrington, D. L., & Haaland, K. Y. (1999). Neural under-pinnings of temporal processing: a review of focal lesion, pharmacological, and functional imaging research. *Reviews in the Neurosciences*, **10**, 91–116.

Harrington, D. L., Haaland, K. Y., & Hermanowicz, N. (1998a). Temporal processing in the basal ganglia. *Neuropsychology*, **12**, 3–12.

Harrington, D. L., Haaland, K. Y., & Knight, R. T. (1998b). Cortical networks underlying mechanisms of time perception. *Journal of Neuroscience*, **18**, 1085–1095.

Heathcote, A., Popiel, S. J., & Mewhort, D. J. K. (1991). Analysis of response time distributions: an example using the Stroop task. *Psychological Bulletin*, **109**, 340–347.

Henning, R. A., Sauter, S. L., Salvendy, G., & Krieg, E. F., Jr. (1989). Microbreak length, performance, and stress in a data entry task. *Ergonomics*, **32**, 855–864.

Hetherington, C. R., Stuss, D. T., & Finlayson, M. A. J. (1996). Reaction time and variability 5 and 10 years after traumatic brain injury. *Brain Injury*, **10**, 473–486.

Hockey, G. R. J. (1983). *Stress and Fatigue in Human Performance*. New York, NY: Wiley.

Hofland, B. F., Willis, S. L., & Baltes, P. G. (1981). Fluid intelligence performance in the elderly: intraindividual variability and conditions of assessment. *Journal of Educational Psychology*, **73**, 573–586.

Hornak, J., O'Doherty, J., Bramham, J. *et al.* (2004). Reward-related reversal learning after surgical excisions in orbito-frontal or dorsolateral prefrontal cortex in humans. *Journal of Cognitive Neuroscience*, **16**, 463–478.

Hull, C. L. (1943). The problem of intervening variables in molar behavior theory. *Psychological Review*, **50**, 273–291.

Hultsch, D. F., & MacDonald, S. W. S. (2004). Intraindividual variability in performance as a theoretical window onto cognitive aging. In R. A. Dixon, L. Bäckman, & L.-G. Nilsson (Eds.), *New Frontiers in Cognitive Aging* (pp. 65–88). New York, NY: Oxford University Press.

Hultsch, D. F., MacDonald, S. W. S., Hunter, M. A., Levy-Bencheton, J., & Strauss, E. (2000). Intraindividual variability in cognitive performance in older adults: comparison of adults with mild dementia, adults with arthritis, and healthy adults. *Neuropsychology*, **14**, 588–598.

Hultsch, D. F., MacDonald, S. W. S., & Dixon, R. A. (2002). Variability in reaction time performance of younger and older adults. *Journal of Gerontology: Psychological Sciences*, **57**B, 101–115.

Ivry, R. B., & Keele, S. W. (1989). Timing functions of the cerebellum. *Journal of Cognitive Neuroscience*, **1**, 136–152.

Ivry, R. B., Keele, S. W., & Deiner, H. C. (1988). Dissociation of the lateral and medial cerebellum in movement timing and movement execution. *Experimental Brain Research*, **73**, 167–180.

Janowsky, J. S., Shimamura, A. P., Kritchevsky, M., & Squire, L. R. (1989). Cognitive impairment following frontal lobe damage and its relevance to human amnesia. *Behavioral Neuroscience*, **103**, 548–560.

Jensen, A. R. (1992). The importance of intraindividual variation in reaction time. *Personality and Individual Differences*, **13**, 869–881.

Kliegel, M., & Sliwinski, M. (2004). MMSE cross-domain variability predicts cognitive decline in Centenarians. *Gerontology*, **50**, 39–43.

Larson, G. E., & Alderton, D. L. (1990). Reaction time variability and intelligence: A "worst performance" analysis of individual differences. *Intelligence*, **14**, 309–325.

Lecerf, T., Ghisletta, P., & Jouffray, C. (2004). Intraindividual variability and level of performance in four visuo-spatial working memory tasks. *Swiss Journal of Psychology*, **63**, 261–272.

Leth-Steensen, C., Elbaz, Z. K., & Douglas, V. I. (2000). Mean response times, variability, and skew in the responding of ADHD children: a response time distributional approach. *Acta Psychologica*, **104**, 167–190.

Lewis, P. A., & Miall, R. C. (2003). Distinct systems for automatic and cognitively controlled time measurement: evidence from neuroimaging. *Current Opinion in Neurobiology*, **13**, 250–255.

Lezak, M. D. (1995). *Neuropsychological Assessment (3rd Edition)*. New York, NY: Oxford University Press.

Li, S.-C., & Lindenberger, U. (1999). Cross-level unification: A computational exploration of the link between deterioration of neurotransmitter systems and dedifferentiation of cognitive abilities in old age. In L.-G. Nilsson & H. J. Markowitsch (Eds.), *Cognitive Neuroscience of Memory* (pp. 103–146). Toronto, ON: Hogrefe & Huber.

Li, S.-C., Lindenberger, U., & Frensch, P. A. (2000). Unifying cognitive aging: from neuromodulation to representation to cognition. *Neurocomputing*, 32–33, 879–890.

Logan, G. D. (1992). Shapes of reaction-time distributions and shapes of learning curves: a test of the instance theory of automaticity. *Journal of Experimental Psychology: Learning, Memory, and Cognition*, **18**, 883–914.

Lorist, M. M., Kernell, D., Meijman, T. F., & Zijdewind, I. (2002). Motor fatigue and cognitive task performance in humans. *Journal of Physiology*, **545**, 313–319.

Luria, A. R. (1973). *The Working Brain. An Introduction to Neuropsychology*. New York, NY: Basic Books.

Macar, F., Lejeune, H., Bonnet, M. *et al.* (2002). Activation of the supplementary motor area and of attentional networks during temporal processing. *Experimental Brain Research*, **142**, 475–485.

MacDonald, S. W. S., Nyberg, L., & Bäckman, L. (2006). Intra-individual variability in behavior: links to brain structure, neurotransmission and neuronal activity. *Trends in Neurosciences*, **29**, 474–480.

Maruff, P., Falleti, M. G., Collie, A., Darby, D., & McStephen, M. (2005). Fatigue-related impairment in the speed, accuracy and variability of psychomotor performance: comparison with blood alcohol levels. *Journal of Sleep Research*, **14**, 21–27.

Matarazzo, J. D., & Herman, D. O. (1985). Clinical uses of the WAIS-R: Base rates of differences between VIQ and PIQ in the WAIS-R standardization sample. In B. B. Wolman (Ed.), *Handbook of Intelligence* (pp. 899–932). New York, NY: Wiley & Sons.

Matarazzo, J. D., & Prifitera, A. (1989). Subtest scatter and premorbid intelligence: lessons from the WAIS-R standardization sample. *Psychological Assessment*, **1**, 186–191.

Matarazzo, J. D., Daniel, M. J., Prifitera, A., & Herman, D. O. (1988). Inter-test subtest scatter in the WAIS-R standardization sample. *Journal of Clinical Psychology*, **44**, 940–950.

Meck, W. H. (1996). Neuropharmacology of timing and time perception. *Cognitive Brain Research*, **3**, 227–242.

Meichenbaum, D. (1974). Self-instructional strategy training: a cognitive prosthesis for the aged. *Human Development*, **17**, 273–280.

Milberg, W., Blumstein, S., Giovanello, K. S., & Misiurski, C. (2003). Summation priming in aphasia: evidence for alterations in semantic integration and activation. *Brain and Cognition*, **51**, 31–47.

Miller, R. A., Thaut, M. H., McIntosh, G. C., & Rice, R. R. (1996). Components of EMG symmetry and variability in parkinsonian and healthy elderly gait. *Electroencephalography and Clinical Neurophysiology*, **101**, 1–7.

Monk, T. H., Kupfer, D. J., Frank, E., & Ritenour, A. M. (1991). The social rhythm metric (SRM): measuring daily social rhythms over 12 weeks. *Psychiatry Research*, **36**, 195–207.

Morse, C. K. (1993). Does variability increase with age? An archival study of cognitive measures. *Psychology and Aging*, **8**, 156–164.

Moskowitz, D. S., & Zuroff, D. C. (2005). Robust predictors of flux, pulse, and spin. *Journal of Research in Personality*, **39**, 130–147.

Murphy, K. J., West, R., Armilio, M. L., Craik, F. I. M., & Stuss, D. T. (2007). Word list learning performance in younger and older adults: intra-individual performance variability and false memory. *Aging, Neuropsychology, and Cognition*, **14**, 70–94.

Murtha, S., Cismaru, R., Waechter, R., & Chertkow, H. (2002). Increased variability accompanies frontal lobe damage in dementia. *Journal of the International Neuropsychological Society*, **8**, 360–372.

Nesselroade, J. R. (1991). Interindividual differences in intraindividual change. In L. M. Collins & J. L. Horn (Eds.), *Best Methods for the Analysis of Change* (pp. 92–105). Washington, DC: American Psychological Association.

Nesselroade, J. R., & Salthouse, T. A. (2004). Methodological and theoretical implications of intraindividual variability in perceptual-motor performance. *Journals of Gerontology: Series B; Psychological Sciences and Social Sciences*, **59**, 49–55.

Nezlek, J. B., Feist, G. J., Wilson, F. C., & Plesko, R. M. (2001). Day-to-day variability in empathy as a function of daily events and mood. *Journal of Research in Personality*, **35**, 401–423.

Obersteiner, H. (1879). Experimental researches on attention. *Brain*, **1**, 439–453.

O'Boyle, D. J., Freeman, J. S., & Cody, F. W. J. (1996). The accuracy and precision of timing of self-paced, repetitive movements in subjects with Parkinson's disease. *Brain*, **119**, 51–70.

Ong, A. D., & Allaire, J. C. (2005). Cardiovascular intraindividual variability in later life: the influence of social connectedness and positive emotions. *Psychology and Aging*, **20**, 476–485.

Parasuraman, R. (1976). Consistency of individual-differences in human vigilance performance: abilities classification analysis. *Journal of Applied Psychology*, **61**, 486–492.

Perbal, S., Deweer, B. Pillon, B. *et al.* (2005). Effects of internal clock and memory disorders on duration reproductions and duration productions in patients with Parkinson's disease. *Brain and Cognition*, **58**, 35–48.

Petrides, M., & Pandya, D. N. (1994). Comparative architectonic analysis of the human and macaque frontal cortex. In F. Boller & J. Grafman (Eds.), *Handbook of Neuropsychology: Volume 9* (pp. 17–57). Amsterdam: Elsevier.

Philpott, S. J. F. (1933). Fluctuations in human output. *British Journal of Psychology Monographs, Supplement* **17**, 6.

Picton, T. W., Stuss, D. T., Shallice, T., Alexander, M. P., & Gillingham, S. (2006). Keeping time: effects of focal frontal lesions. *Neuropsychologia*, **44**, 1195–1209.

Pincus, S. M. (1991). Approximate entropy as a measure of system complexity. *Proceedings of the National Academy of Sciences of the United States of America*, **88**, 2297–2301.

Rabbitt, P., Osman, P., Moore, B., & Stollery, B. (2001). There are stable individual differences in performance variability, both from moment to moment and from day to day. *Quarterly Journal of Experimental Psychology: Section A*, **54**, 981–1003.

Rakitin, B. C., Stern, Y., & Malapani, C. (2005). The effects of aging on time reproduction in delayed free-recall. *Brain and Cognition*, **58**, 17–34.

Ram, N., Rabbitt, P., Stollery, B., & Nesselroade, J. R. (2005). Cognitive performance inconsistency: intraindividual change and variability. *Psychology and Aging*, **20**, 623–633.

Rammsayer, T., & Classen, W. (1997). Impaired temporal discrimination in Parkinson's disease: temporal processing of brief durations as an indicator of degeneration of dopaminergic neurons in the basal ganglia. *International Journal of Neuroscience*, **91**, 45–55.

Ratcliff, R., & Murdock, B. B. (1976). Retrieval processes in recognition memory. *Psychological Review*, **83**, 190–214.

Ratcliff, R., & Tuerlinckx, F. (2002). Estimating parameters of the diffusion model: approaches to dealing with contaminant reaction times and parameter variability. *Psychonomic Bulletin and Review*, **9**, 438–481.

Reid, S., Towell, A. D., & Golding, J. F. (2000). Seasonality, social zeitgebers and mood variability in entrainment of mood: implications for seasonal affective disorder. *Journal of Affective Disorders*, **59**, 47–54.

Reitan, R. M., & Wolfson, D. (1997). Consistency of neuropsychological test scores of head-injured subjects involved in litigation compared with head-injured subjects not involved in litigation: development of the retest consistency index. *Clinical Neuropsychologist*, **11**, 69–76.

Richer, F., & Boulet, C. (1999). Frontal lesions and fluctuations in response preparation. *Brain and Cognition*, **40**, 234–238.

Ridderinkhof, K. R., Scheres, A., Oosterlaan, J., & Sergeant, J. A. (2005). Delta plots in the study of individual differences: new tools reveal response inhibition deficits in AD/HD that are eliminated by methylphenidate treatment. *Journal of Abnormal Psychology*, **114**, 197–215.

Robinson, M. D., & Tamir, M. (2005). Neuroticism as mental noise: a relation between neuroticism and reaction time standard deviations. *Journal of Personality and Social Psychology*, **89**, 107–114.

Rorden, C., & Karnath, H. O. (2004). Using human brain lesions to infer function: a relic from a past era in the fMRI age? *Nature Reviews Neuroscience*, **5**, 813–819.

Rourke, B. P. (1985). *Neuropsychology of Learning Disabilities. Essentials of Subtype Analysis.* New York, NY: Guilford Press.

Rovet, J. F., & Hepworth, S. L. (2001). Dissociating attention deficits in children with ADHD and congenital hypothyroidism using multiple CPTs. *Journal of Child Psychology and Psychiatry*, **8**, 1049–1056.

Salthouse, T. A. (1985). Speed of behavior and its implications for cognition. In J. M. Birren & K. W. Schaie (Eds.), *Handbook of the Psychology of Aging* (pp. 400–426). New York: Van Norstrand Reinhold.

Salthouse, T. A. (1992). Why do adult age differences increase with task complexity? *Developmental Psychology*, **28**, 905–918.

Salthouse, T. A. (1993). Attentional blocks are not responsible for age-related slowing. *Journals of Gerontology: Series B; Psychological Sciences and Social Sciences*, **48**, 263–270.

Sanders, A. F. (1998). *Elements of Human Performance: Reaction Time Processes and Attention in Human Skill.* London, UK: Lawrence Erlbaum.

Schretlen, D. J., Munro, C. A., Anthony, J. C., & Pearlson, G. D. (2003). Examining the range of normal intraindividual variability in neuropsychological test performance. *Journal of the International Neuropsychological Society*, **9**, 864–870.

Schwartz, F., Carr, A. C., Munich, R. L. *et al.* (1989). Reaction time impairment in schizophrenia and affective illness: the role of attention. *Biological Psychiatry*, **25**, 540–548.

Segalowitz, S. J., Dywan, J., & Unsal, A. (1997). Attentional factors in response time variability after traumatic brain injury: an ERP study. *Journal of the International Neuropsychological Society*, **3**, 95–107.

Shammi, P., & Stuss, D. T. (1999). Humour appreciation: a role of the right frontal lobe. *Brain*, **122**, 657–666.

Shammi, P., Bosman, E., & Stuss, D. T. (1998). Aging and variability in performance. *Aging, Neuropsychology, and Cognition*, **5**, 1–13.

Simons, J. S., Gilbert, S. J., Owen, A. M., Fletcher, P. C., & Burgess, P. W. (2005). Distinct roles for lateral and medial anterior prefrontal cortex in contextual recollection. *Journal of Neurophysiology*, **94**, 813–820.

Slifkin, A. B., & Newell, K. M. (1998). Is variability in human performance a reflection of system noise? *Current Directions in Psychological Science*, **7**, 165–196.

Spencer, R. M. C., & Ivry, R. B. (2005). Comparison of patients with Parkinson's disease or cerebellar lesions in the production of periodic movements involving event-based or emergent timing. *Brain and Cognition*, **58**, 84–93.

Spencer, R. M. C., Zelaznik, H. N., Diedrichsen, J., & Ivry, R. B. (2003). Disrupted timing of discontinuous but not continuous movements by cerebellar lesions. *Science*, **300**, 1437–1439.

Spikman, J. M., van Zomeren, A. H., & Deelman, B. G. (1996). Deficits of attention after closed-head injury: slowness only? *Journal of Clinical and Experimental Neuropsychology*, **18**, 755–767.

Strauss, E., Hultsch, D. F., Hunter, M., Slick, D. J., Patry, B., & Levy-Bencheton, J. (2000). Using intraindividual variability to detect malingering in cognitive performance. *Clinical Neuropsychologist*, **14**, 420–432.

Strauss, E., MacDonald, S. W. S., Hunter, M., Moll, A., & Hultsch, D. F. (2002). Intraindividual variability in cognitive performance in three groups of older adults: cross-domain links to physical status and self-perceived affect and beliefs. *Journal of the International Neuropsychological Society*, **8**, 893–906.

Stuss, D. T. (1987). Contribution of frontal lobe injury to cognitive impairment after closed head injury: methods of assessment and recent findings. In H. S. Levin, H. M. Eisenberg & J. Grafman (Eds.), *Neurobehavioural Recovery after Head Injury* (pp. 166–177). New York, NY: Oxford University Press.

Stuss, D. T. (1995). A sensible approach to mild traumatic brain injury. *Neurology*, **45**, 1251–1252.

Stuss, D. T. (2006). Frontal lobes and attention: Processes and networks, fractionation and integration. *Journal of the International Neuropsychological Society*, **12**, 261–271.

Stuss, D. T., & Gow, C. A. (1992). "Frontal Dysfunction" after traumatic brain injury. *Neuropsychiatry, Neuropsychology and Behavioural Neurology*, **5**, 272–282.

Stuss, D. T., Delgado, M., & Guzman, D. A. (1987). Verbal regulation in the control of motor impersistence: a proposed rehabilitation procedure. *Journal of Neurologic Rehabilitation*, **1**, 19–24.

Stuss, D. T., Stethem, L. L., Hugenholtz, H. *et al.* (1989). Reaction time after head injury: fatigue, divided and focused attention, and consistency of performance. *Journal of Neurology, Neurosurgery, and Psychiatry*, **52**, 742–748.

Stuss, D. T., Alexander, M. P., Palumbo, C. L. *et al.* (1994a). Organizational strategies of patients with unilateral or bilateral frontal lobe injury in word list learning tasks. *Neuropsychology*, **8**, 355–373.

Stuss, D. T., Mateer, C. A., & Sohlberg, M. M. (1994b). Innovative approaches to frontal lobe deficits. In M. A. J. Finlayson & S. H. Garner (Eds.), *Brain Injury Rehabilitation: Clinical Considerations* (pp. 212–237). Baltimore, MD: Williams & Wilkins.

Stuss, D. T., Pogue, J., Buckle, L., & Bondar, J. (1994c). Characterization of stability of performance in patients with traumatic brain injury: variability and consistency on reaction time tests. *Neuropsychology*, **8**, 316–324.

Stuss, D. T., Murphy, K. J., & Binns, M. A. (1999). The frontal lobes and performance variability: evidence from reaction time. *Journal of the International Neuropsychological Society*, **5**, 123.

Stuss, D. T., Binns, M. A., Carruth, F. G. *et al.* (2000a). Prediction of recovery of continuous memory after traumatic brain injury. *Neurology*, **54**, 1337–1344.

Stuss, D. T., Levine, B., Alexander, M. P. *et al.* (2000b). Wisconsin Card Sorting Test performance in patients with focal frontal and posterior brain damage: effects of lesion location and test structure on separable cognitive processes. *Neuropsychologia*, **38**, 388–402.

Stuss, D. T., Picton, T. W., & Alexander, M. P. (2001b). Consciousness, self-awareness and the frontal lobes. In S. P. Salloway, P. F. Malloy, & J. D. Duffy (Eds.), *The Frontal Lobes and Neuropsychiatric Illness* (pp. 101–109). Washington, DC: American Psychiatric Publishing, Inc.

Stuss, D. T., Floden, D., Alexander, M. P., Levine, B., & Katz, D. (2001a). Stroop performance in focal lesion patient: dissociation of processes and frontal lobe lesion location. *Neuropsychologia*, **39**, 771–786.

Stuss, D. T., Binns, M. A., Murphy, K. J., & Alexander, M. P. (2002). Dissociations within the anterior attentional system: effects of task complexity and irrelevant information on reaction time speed and accuracy. *Neuropsychology*, **16**, 500–513.

Stuss, D. T., Murphy, K. J., Binns, M. A., & Alexander, M. P. (2003). Staying on the job: the frontal lobes control individual performance variability. *Brain*, **126**, 2363–2380.

Stuss, D. T., Alexander, M. P., Shallice, T. *et al.* (2005). Multiple frontal systems controlling response speed. *Neuropsychologia*, **43**, 396–417.

Surwillo, W. W. (1975). Reaction-time variability, periodicities in reaction-time distributions, and the

EEG gating-signal hypothesis. *Biological Psychology*, **3**, 247–261.

Temkin, N. R., Holubkov, R., MacHamer, J. E., Winn, H. R., & Dikmen, S. S. (1995). Classification and regression trees (CART) for prediction of function at 1 year following head trauma. *Journal of Neurosurgery*, **82**, 764–771.

Tranel, D., Bechara, A., & Denburg, N. L. (2002). Asymmetric functional roles of right and left ventromedial prefrontal cortices in social conduct, decision making and emotional processing. *Cortex*, **38**, 589–612.

Ulrich, R., & Miller, J. (1994). Effects of truncation on reaction time analysis. *Journal of Experimental Psychology: General*, **123**, 34–80.

van Zandt, T. (2000). How to fit a response time distribution. *Psychonomic Bulletin and Review*, **7**, 424–465.

van Zomeren, A. H. (1981). *Reaction Time and Attention After Closed Head Injury*. Lisse: Swets & Zeitlinger, BV.

Vinogradov, S., Poole, J. H., Willis-Shore, J., Ober, B. A., & Shenaut, G. K. (1998). Slower and more variable reaction times in schizophrenia: what do they signify? *Schizophrenia Research*, **32**, 183–190.

Wagenmakers, E.-J., & Brown, S. (2007). On the linear relation between the mean and the standard deviation of a response time distribution. *Psychological Review*, **114**, 830–841.

Wagenmakers, E.-J., Grasman, R. P. P. P., & Molenaar, P. C. M. (2005). On the relation between the mean and the variance of a diffusion model response time distribution. *Journal of Mathematical Psychology*, **49**, 195–204.

Walker, M. P., Ayre, G. A., Cummings, J. L. *et al.* (2000). Quantifying fluctuation in dementia with Lewy bodies, Alzheimer's disease, and vascular dementia. *Neurology*, **54**, 1616–1625.

Wegesin, D. J., & Stern, Y. (2004). Inter- and intraindividual variability in recognition memory: effects of aging and estrogen use. *Neuropsychology*, **18**, 646–657.

Wei, W. W. S. (1990). *Time Series Analysis*. New York, NY: Addison-Wesley Publishing Company, Inc.

West, R., & Alain, C. (2000a). Effects of task context and fluctuations of attention on neural activity supporting performance of the Stroop task. *Brain Research*, **873**, 102–111.

West, R., & Alain, C. (2000b). Evidence for the transient nature of a neural system supporting goal-directed action. *Cerebral Cortex*, **10**, 748–752.

West, R., Murphy, K. J., Armilio, M. L., Craik, F. I. M., & Stuss, D. T. (2002). Lapses of intention and performance variability reveal age-related increase in fluctuations of executive control. *Brain and Cognition*, **49**, 402–419.

Wheeler, M. A., Stuss, D. T., & Tulving, E. (1995). Frontal lobe damage produces episodic memory impairment. *Journal of the International Neuropsychological Society*, **1**, 525–536.

Whyte, J., Polansky, M., Fleming, M., Coslett, H. B., & Cavallucci, C. (1995). Sustained arousal and attention after traumatic brain injury. *Neuropsychologia*, **33**, 797–813.

Williams, B. R., Hultsch, D. F., Strauss, E. H., Hunter, M. A., & Tannock, R. (2005). Inconsistency in reaction time across the life span. *Neuropsychology*, **19**, 88–96.

Zahn, T. P., & Mirsky, A. F. (1999). Reaction time indicators of attention deficits in closed head injury. *Journal of Clinical and Experimental Neuropsychology*, **21**, 352–367.

Zahn, T. P., Kruesi, M. J. P., & Rapoport, J. L. (1991). Reaction time indices of attention deficits in boys with disruptive behavior disorders. *Journal of Abnormal Child Psychology*, **19**, 233–252.

4

Hormones and allostasis in brain disease and repair

Richard G. Hunter and Bruce S. McEwen

Introduction

- Hormones are involved in the maintenance of homeostasis.
- The concept of allostasis is allowing us to better understand how hormones and environment interact to modify brain function.

Hormones influence many aspects of behavior as well as cognitive function. When the various steroid hormones were first identified in the 1930s, they were noted for their effects on peripheral physiology, particularly with regard to homeostasis and reproduction. However, the identification of receptor sites in the brain (McEwen *et al.*, 1968; McGuire & Lisk, 1968; Pfaff & Keiner, 1973) led to the realization that the brain, as a master controller of physiological processes throughout the body, is implicated, through hormonal feedback, in the maintenance of homeostasis. It follows that an understanding of the actions of hormones within the brain may provide insight into how the brain copes with various insults.

The concept of homeostasis is central to modern physiology. Within the conceptual field of homeostasis, stress is an example of an experience or state which pushes an organism away from homeostasis. In common usage, "stress" can mean a number of things. In the stress literature the concept of allostasis has been proposed to describe states of adaptation to change, and "allostatic load or overload" has been proposed to describe the burden placed upon an animal by responding to changing circumstances (McEwen, 1998; McEwen & Wingfield, 2003).

Some aspects of homeostasis, such as plasma electrolytes, are too tightly regulated to be subject to allostatic changes, as changes of even a few percent can be deadly. Others, like energy balance, can vary more substantially without impairing health in the short to medium term, though the long-term consequences of the allostatic load of obesity, for example, are well known. Energy balance is nowhere more important than in the brain, which utilises 20% of the body's energy budget while constituting only 2% of its mass (Clark & Sokoloff, 1998). The major portion of that 20% goes to the maintenance of intrinsic neuronal activity, most of which involves neurons using glutamate as a transmitter (Magistretti, 2006) and as we shall see below, glutamatergic transmission is a major substrate of the changes wrought in the brain by allostasis.

Still other aspects of homeostasis involve mediators, such as stress and metabolic hormones, that act to maintain or restore homeostasis. These are the mediators of allostasis that maintain stability through change (McEwen, 1998; McEwen & Wingfield, 2003).

Allostatic load has two defined subtypes. Type 1 allostatic load, where energy demand may exceed supply, can occur, for example, as a result of exhaustion after or during a narrow escape from life-threatening circumstances. Type 2 allostatic loads are found even when energy reserves are high but when the source of the overload is of long duration, such as during chronic psychosocial stress. Type 2 allostatic load is a significant contributor to many, if not most, of the common diseases of affluent societies, where the levels of morbidity and mortality from the traditional killers of mankind (e.g., infectious disease, famine) have dropped to levels inconceivable even a few generations ago.

Since most organisms find life to be more complex than merely maintaining a positive energy balance, the idea of life history stage has been added to the basic concept of allostasis in acknowledgement of the fact that the homeostatic and energy demands vary across the organism's lifetime. A life history stage can be developmental, such as childhood or adolescence, or situational (e.g., an emergency life history stage such as when an animal's life is at stake (McEwen & Wingfield, 2003). Energy demands vary circannually (e.g., reproduction or hibernation) on shorter time scales, and, of course, in an "emergency life history stage" where survival is at stake, the response is immediate (McEwen & Wingfield, 2003). The interaction between hormones and life history stage is readily apparent when one is speaking of puberty or menopause, but less so when one is talking about maintenance of cognitive function during aging.

Life history is particularly important when discussing many of the diseases which are common in developed countries, as many of these disorders, notably obesity, type 2 diabetes, depression and cardiovascular disease, have a substantial contribution of lifestyle to their etiology. In addition, these pathologies contribute to increased cognitive decline in aging humans (Gorelick, 2005; Hendrickx et al., 2005; Messier & Teutenberg, 2005; O'Brien et al., 2004) and in both aging and chronic diseases the health of the neuroendocrine axis is important. Concepts like allostasis and life history stages provide a framework within which the "Darwinian concept of stress" (Korte et al., 2005) is beginning to allow us to understand the diverse roles of steroid and other hormones in an integrated way.

The steroid hormones are important mediators of many functions, including the stress response. They are not the only mediators, nor are they even the most important actors at the level of energy balance.

In fact, recent work points to complex interactions involving steroids and a medley of other hormones, such as insulin, leptin, as well as a host of other peptides, such as Cocaine-Amphetamine Regulated Transcript (CART), in the regulation of brain structure and behavior. Our understanding of how many of these hormones impact cognition and brain physiology is still in its infancy, as is our understanding of how behavioral interventions, such as better diet and exercise regimes, contribute to improved brain health, though there is little doubt that they do (Cotman & Berchtold, 2002; Barbour & Blumenthal, 2005; Hendrickx et al., 2005; Dishman et al., 2006; Morgan et al., 2007).

In this chapter we will examine the influence of the most extensively studied steroid hormones, the adrenal steroids and the gonadal steroids, upon brain plasticity and cognition. We have chosen to focus on the hippocampus as it is one of only two sites in the adult mammalian brain where neurogenesis has been conclusively demonstrated to occur (Lledo et al., 2006) and because it is particularly sensitive to damage and remodeling in a variety of disorders, such as depression and stroke. At the end of the chapter we will explain how our understanding of plasticity in the hippocampus is expanding to include a number of peptide hormones associated with metabolic regulation and how this knowledge is being integrated with our understanding of steroid action in health and disease.

Adrenal steroids

- The two types of adrenal steroids, mineralocorticoids and glucocorticoids, have different effects upon the brain.
- High levels of glucocorticoids result in gross changes in the structure of the hippocampus as well as alterations in memory and behavior.
- Disorders such as major depression and Cushing's disease can result in hippocampal atrophy and drugs, such as SSRI antidepressants, can stop or reverse these changes.

Classification of adrenal steroids and their receptors

Corticosteroids belong to two subclasses, the glucocorticoids and the mineralocorticoids. The former are so called due to their impact on carbohydrate metabolism and the latter for their role in regulating salt metabolism. In addition to their role in normal physiology, the corticosteroids, particularly the glucocorticoids, play a significant role in the stress response and in the biology of a number of disorders. Most significantly in terms of this discussion, excess glucocorticoids have been demonstrated to produce atrophy of the hippocampus, and associated cognitive deficits, in animals and humans (Bourdeau et al., 2002; Sapolsky, 2000; Sapolsky et al., 1986, 1990; Starkman et al., 1999, 2003). Corticosteroids have two receptors, the high affinity type I or mineralocorticoid receptor (MR), at which aldosterone and cortisol/corticosterone are agonists and type II or glucocorticoid receptor (GR), which has a 10-fold lower affinity for corticosterone and little affinity for aldosterone (de Kloet et al., 1990). Both of these receptors are expressed in the brain, particularly within the hypothalamus and hippocampus, and in the latter region, they are implicated in expressions of brain plasticity, ranging from memory consolidation to neurogenesis (de Kloet et al., 1998). Corticosteroids are also thought to act through membrane receptors to produce rapid effects, but these receptors are as yet poorly characterized (Stellato, 2004).

Corticosteroid effects on neural structure and cognitive function

Corticosteroids, principally cortisol or corticosterone, have significant effects on cognitive function and brain structure. A number of disorders exhibiting hypercortisolemia have been shown to produce brain atrophy, particularly of the hippocampus. These include Cushing's disease, major depression, and post-traumatic stress disorder (Bremner et al., 1995; Gurvits et al., 1996; Sapolsky, 2000; Sheline et al., 1996; Starkman et al., 1999). The structural changes correlate with the ability to recall specific experiences (declarative memory) and are at least partially reversible (Bremner, 2006; Starkman et al., 2003). Cortisol levels at the circadian nadir also correlate with dementia in the elderly (Magri et al., 2006). These effects appear to be mediated by the capacity of corticosteroids to sculpt the hippocampus through their effects on dendritic structure, glia and neurogenesis.

Chronic stress and glucocorticoid treatment induce shrinkage of the apical dendritic trees of CA3 pyramidal neurons (Magariños & McEwen, 1995; Magariños et al., 1996; Watanabe et al., 1992a,1992b,1992c; Woolley et al., 1990). This effect appears to be transient as it resolves within 10 days following removal of the stressor (Conrad et al., 1999), but it may contribute to vulnerability to other insults or disease processes such as excitotoxicity (Conrad et al., 2004), depression (Sheline et al., 1996) or obesity (Raber, 1998). Glucocorticoids are implicated because chronic administration of corticosterone in the rat reproduces the stress effect (Woolley et al., 1990) and blockade of corticosterone production with a synthesis inhibitor, cyanoketone, blocks it (Magariños & McEwen, 1995).

The functional purpose of dendritic retraction in response to stress is not yet clear. One hypothesis is that stress-induced dendritic remodeling may protect against excitotoxicity. For example, restraint stress, which leads to dendritic remodeling, raises both glutamate release (Gilad et al., 1990; Lowy et al., 1993) and glutamate transporter expression (Reagan et al., 2004) in the hippocampus, and inhibiting excitatory transmission with phenytoin blocks dendritic remodeling in the CA3 region of hippocampus (Magariños et al., 1996; Watanabe et al., 1992a). Conrad, however, recently demonstrated that chronic stress renders the CA3 of male rats more vulnerable to an excitotoxic lesion than unstressed controls (Conrad et al., 2004), while stressed females, that did not show remodeling in the CA3, did not show increased vulnerability. The latter findings suggest that stress-induced remodeling in the CA3 is not protective, but pathological, though the question remains open until the consequences of blocking the remodeling process for excitotoxicity are fully determined. Glucocorticoids also influence the morphology and function of other regions of the brain including the CA1, amygdala, and prefrontal cortex (Arbel *et al.*, 1994; Cerqueira *et al.*, 2007; Cook & Wellman, 2004; de Kloet *et al.*, 1998; Radley *et al.*, 2004; Vyas *et al.*, 2002). In the amygdala dendritic arborization actually appears to increase following chronic stress, suggesting different processes govern dendritic plasticity there than those in the hippocampus.

Neurons are not the only targets of corticosteroid action in the brain. Glial cells, particularly astrocytes also express corticosteroid receptors. Glial proteins, such as GFAP, Ndrg2, and TGF-β1, are regulated by adrenalectomy and corticosteroid administration (Nichols *et al.*, 2005). Chronic high doses of corticosterone elevate the fraction of hippocampal volume occupied by astrocytes (Tata *et al.*, 2006), as well as acutely interfering with their ability to clear excitatory amino acids (Chou, 1998), which may contribute to excitotoxicity. Corticosterone also appears to negatively impact astrocytic ATP levels during a hypoxic stressor (Tombaugh *et al.*, 1992). Further, evidence suggests that neurons and glia are metabolically coupled, particularly with regard to glutamate transmission, and that metabolic plasticity in hippocampal memory tasks may parallel synaptic plasticity (Magistretti, 2006).

Neurogenesis, or the birth of new neurons, has only recently begun to be studied in earnest in the adult mammalian brain. Neurogenesis is addressed in more detail in other chapters of the present volume (see Chapter 20 by Wojtowicz, Chapter 21 by Vinters and Carmichael, and Chapter 22 by Stickland, Weiss and Kolb) but it is important to note that stress and corticosteroids also affect neurogenesis in the dentate gyrus of the hippocampus (Gould *et al.*, 1999). Chronic stress reduces levels of neurogenesis and produces atrophy in the hippocampus (Duman, 2004a; McEwen, 1999; Sapolsky, 2001). Administration of high doses of corticosterone, acting via the GR, reduces neurogenesis (Cameron & Gould, 1994; Gould *et al.*,

1992). Adrenalectomy, which removes circulating corticosteroids, increases neurogenesis in this region, while increasing neurodegeneration, the latter effect being rescued by MR agonism (Woolley *et al.*, 1991). The presence of a functional MR appears necessary to maintain normal levels of neurogenesis (Gass *et al.*, 2000). The reduction of neurogenesis in response to stress or high corticosterone can be blocked by antagonists of the NMDA glutamate receptor subtype (Gould & Cameron, 1996), which provides a further link between the glutamate system and steroid induced plasticity. Serotonin is also implicated as stress increases its levels in the hippocampus and reduces serotonin transporter binding (McKittrick *et al.*, 1995, 2000).

Treatment with the antidepressant, tianeptine, blocks the effects of stress on dendritic structure and behavior (Conrad *et al.*, 1996; Magariños *et al.*, 1999; Watanabe *et al.*, 1992b). Corticosterone also reduces levels of the neurotrophic factor Brain Derived Neurotrophic Factor (BDNF), which helps promote the survival of new neurons. Treatment with antidepressants, including electroconvulsive therapy and exercise, increases both BDNF and neurogenesis. Blockade of neurogenesis by irradiation or deletion of the 5-HT1A receptor blocks behavioral responses to antidepressant treatment (Santarelli *et al.*, 2003). These findings have led to the neurotrophic and neurogenic hypothesis of depression outlined by Duman (Duman, 2004a, 2004b; Warner-Schmidt & Duman, 2006).

Corticosteroid effects on memory and anxiety

Behaviorally, chronic stress and glucocorticoids influence the ability of animals to perform hippocampus-dependent memory tasks (de Kloet *et al.*, 1998). These effects are time and dose dependent. Acute administration of corticosterone typically elevates the performance of animals in memory tasks provided the glucocorticoid is administered in close temporal proximity to the learning event (Lupien & McEwen, 1997; McEwen *et al.*, 1986). However, stress experienced 30 minutes prior to testing tends to disrupt memory (de Quervain *et al.*, 2000).

Conversely, reduction of corticosterone levels during recall improves memory performance (Wright *et al.*, 2006). Adrenalectomy generally impairs perform-ance and corticosterone restores normal behavior, an effect which appears to depend upon its activity at both MR and GR receptors, as specific agonists either partially restore or antagonize corticoster-one's effects (de Kloet *et al.*, 1998). The two recep-tors seem to affect different aspects of behavior as well, since MR activation influences response selection and response to novelty and GR to alter consolidation. Interestingly, chronic continuous GR antagonism seems to improve spatial learning and memory, whereas phasic antagonism of glu-cocorticoid actions impairs it (Oitzl *et al.*, 1998a,1998b).

In humans, chronic elevation of cortisol, as seen in Cushing's disease, also impairs memory (Lupien *et al.*, 1998). Studies of animals with reduced levels of GR expression show that reduction of brain GR expression impairs spatial learning strategy (Kellendonk *et al.*, 2002). These animals also show an increase in depression-like behaviors, while ani-mals over-expressing GR show a depression-resistant phenotype (Boyle *et al.*, 2005; Ridder *et al.*, 2005) which fits well with findings of hippo-campal and HPA axis abnormalities in depression (de Kloet *et al.*, 1998; McEwen, 2005). Glucocorticoid receptor is also linked to anxiety, as mice over- and under-expressing the receptor show increased and reduced anxiety levels, respectively (Howell & Muglia, 2006). Animals with brain-specific MR knock-outs do not show alterations in anxiety, but they do show deficits in learning and working memory, as well as perseverance and increased exploratory activity toward novel objects (Berger *et al.*, 2006).

Summary

Corticosteroids represent some of the most impor-tant modulators of brain plasticity. They have important impacts on gross and cellular morphol-ogy, as well as cognition and behavior in both ani-mals and humans.

Gonadal steroids

- Androgens and estrogens have been demonstra-ted to have a positive impact on neuronal plasti-city in the hippocampus.
- On balance, estrogen seems to improve cognitive function in both animal models and human trials.

The gonadal steroids, androgens and estrogens, are responsible for the maintenance and expression of reproductive behavior and sexual differentiation in mammals. In terms of neural development, a peri-natal androgen surge organizes different nuclei of the limbic system and hypothalamus to induce a male brain phenotype. A female phenotype occurs in the absence of this surge (de Vries & Simerly, 2002). The gonadal steroids are the major inducers of reproductive life history stages. Starting with puberty and throughout adulthood, gonadal ster-oids drive further changes in behavior, brain struc-ture and function (Arnold & Breedlove, 1985; MacLusky *et al.*, 2006; McEwen & Alves, 1999; Romeo *et al.*, 2002).

Estrogens

Estrogens activate mating behaviors and reproduc-tive endocrine functions in the hypothalamo-pituitary-gonadal (HPG) axis via receptors in the hypothalamus (Pfaff, 1980). It was not until the dis-covery of estrogen receptors (ER) in the hippocam-pus (Loy *et al.*, 1988) that the possibility was considered that estrogen might alter cognition and alter neural processes beyond the HPG axis. A key discovery was the finding that estradiol promotes the formation of new dendritic spines and glutama-tergic synapses in the adult hippocampus (Gould *et al.*, 1990; Rudick & Woolley, 2001; Woolley & McEwen, 1992; Woolley *et al.*, 1997). Further, it has been shown that estrogen enhances hippocampal neurogenesis (Tanapat *et al.*, 1999), at least acutely and principally via co-involvement of serotonin (Banasr *et al.*, 2001).

It was found that the density of apical dendrites on the pyramidal cells of the CA1 fluctuate by roughly 30% during the course of the estrus cycle in the female rat and that this fluctuation could be modeled with ovariectomy (OVX) and estrogen replacement. Progesterone was shown to initially augment the effect of estrogen in the OVX model and then rapidly decrease spine density. Subsequent investigation showed that the changes observed in spine density correlated with changes in glutamate receptor binding (Weiland, 1992) and immunoreactivity (Gazzaley *et al.*, 1996), which led to studies demonstrating that estrogen acted upon NMDA receptors to increase CA1 LTP (Foy *et al.*, 1999) in a fashion which parallels the changes observed in spine density.

CA1 pyramidal neurons do not express many, if any, nuclear estrogen receptors, but abundant cell nuclear ERα is found in some interneurons (Hart *et al.*, 2001; Weiland *et al.*, 1997), and so the morphologic and physiologic changes seen in hippocampal pyramidal neurons during the estrus cycle or following estrogen treatment are not thought to occur via direct nuclear receptor activation. Rather the effects are thought to result from estrogen-regulated signaling in dendrites of CA1 neurons via non-nuclear forms of ERα and ERβ, coordinated by estrogen dependent reduction in GABA tone via the aforementioned interneurons (Blurton-Jones & Tuszynski, 2006; Murphy *et al.*, 1998; Rudick & Woolley, 2001; Rudick *et al.*, 2003; Steffensen *et al.*, 2006). Trans-synaptic influences from afferents to the hippocampus appear to be involved (Leranth *et al.*, 2000), because estrogen induction of spine synapses was absent when the fimbria/fornix was transected.

The estrogen effects on synapse formation in hippocampus led to the demonstration that ovarian hormones influence hippocampus-dependent functions. The most robust effects have been observed in tests of spatial working memory. The Morris water maze (MWM) is a behavioral test in which animals must remember the location of a concealed platform in a pool of water; performance in this test is linked to the function of the dorsal hippocampus (Morris *et al.*, 1982). Using the MWM, Sandstrom & Williams (2001) tested animals over 10 days following estrogen treatment. They observed that memory for platform location was substantially improved during the period (1–4 days) when estrogen has its greatest impact upon spine density, but not before or after this period when spine densities are lower. Another research group observed similar effects in the radial arm maze test of spatial memory (Daniel & Dohanich, 2001).

Estrogen also has been shown to have acute effects on memory retention, presumably independent of its more long-term impact on spine densities. Local injection of estradiol hydroxypropyl-β-cyclodextrin into the dorsal hippocampus of both male and female rats immediately after MWM training improved performance the next day (Packard *et al.*, 1996; Packard & Teather, 1997). If injections were delayed by 2 hours, however, this effect was not observed. Similarly, systemic 17-β estradiol improved performance in an inhibitory avoidance task if given immediately after training, but not when given 2 hours later (Rhodes & Frye, 2006). Luine and colleagues found that injection of various estrogens either 30 minutes before, or immediately after, training in object recognition or place memory improved performance when animals were retested 4 hours later (Luine *et al.*, 2003).

Thus, in animals, estrogens can have both acute and chronic effects on cognition, and these effects are generally beneficial. In human studies the effects of estrogens are somewhat more ambiguous. As far back as the early 1950s, there was evidence of a positive effect of estrogen upon cognition in older women (Caldwell & Watson, 1952), whereas other studies showed no benefit. Notably in the case of the recent Women's Health Initiative Memory Study, a slight increase in the probability of dementia was reported (Shumaker *et al.*, 2003). The reasons for these disparities are discussed at length in a recent review by Sherwin (2006) and may be related to the length of time that elapsed between menopause and initiation of hormone therapy, as well as the fact that the preponderance of hormone therapy involved concurrent administration of an estrogen plus a synthetic progestin. Nonetheless, many human studies support the thesis that estrogen improves and conserves cognitive function, at least in younger women.

Androgens

The effects of androgenic steroids on brain plasticity and cognition are similar, if somewhat less well described than those of estrogens. Androgens have been demonstrated to influence plasticity at the level of synaptic structure and survival of proliferating neurons in the hippocampus (Galea et al., 2006; MacLusky et al., 2006).

With regard to neurogenesis, most studies to date have been correlational. Alvarez-Buylla & Kirn (1997) demonstrated that neuron number in the high vocal center (HVC) of songbirds correlated with seasonal fluctuations in androgens and Galea demonstrated a similar phenomenon in meadow voles (Galea & McEwen, 1999; Galea et al., 1999). Further study in both rodents and birds has shown that androgens such as testosterone and DHT seem to enhance survival of new neurons rather than promoting proliferation (Absil et al., 2003; Ormerod & Galea, 2003; Rasika et al., 1994). Another androgen, DHEA, seems to impact proliferation as well (Karishma & Herbert, 2002; Suzuki et al., 2004). Unlike estrogen, androgen receptors (AR) are present in the hippocampus (Kerr et al., 1995) so these effects may be due to the direct action of androgens upon their receptors.

At the structural level, it has been shown that in some strains of rodents the dentate gyrus is larger in the male than in the female (Roof, 1993; Roof & Havens, 1992; Wimer & Wimer, 1989). Sex differences also exist in the number of spine synapses in the CA1 (Shors et al., 2001) and these appear to depend directly upon androgenic effects as opposed to aromatization of androgens to estrogen (Leranth et al., 2003, 2004b). Interestingly, these studies also demonstrated that estrogen had little effect on spine synapse density in males. This is in contrast to females where androgens do seem to have an effect on synapse density in addition to those produced by estrogen (Leranth et al., 2004a). It is possible that these effects are mediated directly via local androgen receptors. This would appear to be partially true as fimbria/fornix transection reduces, but does not block the effects of androgens upon spine density (Kovacs et al., 2003). Some further difficulty in attributing the changes in synapse density to local androgen receptor activation comes from the observation that the AR antagonist flutamide acts as an agonist with regard to synaptic remodeling (MacLusky et al., 2004). For the time being, the mechanism responsible for these observations remains unknown.

Summary

While the effects of gonadal steroids on the brain are less well studied than those of adrenal steroids, there is no doubt that they have an effect on brain structure and cognition. Future studies will certainly elaborate our understanding of their actions in the nervous system.

Peptides and the metabolic axis

- In addition to the steroid hormones, there are a number of peptide hormones which have important effects on hippocampal function, notably leptin and insulin.

In addition to the steroids, a number of other hormonal mediators of energy balance, life stage and behavior, are worthy of mention with regard to behavioral and brain plasticity. This is especially true of the hippocampus, which in addition to being one of the most plastic regions of the brain, expresses high levels of receptors for insulin, IGF-1, ghrelin, leptin and a number of other transmitters and hormones involved in energy balance. While this area of study is still in its infancy, there is growing evidence that insulin and leptin, as well as a growing number of other peptide signals, such as ghrelin or cocaine-amphetamine regulated transcript (CART), may be involved in the control of brain plasticity.

Leptin is a peptide hormone secreted by adipocytes, and is involved in the maintenance of body weight, feeding and adiposity (Jéquier, 2002). While leptin research has centered on its role in body weight regulation, only recently has it become a focus of attention with regard to its role in brain regions such as the hippocampus. There is evidence that diets high in saturated fats impair hippocampal dependent memory and dendritic structure (Baran et al., 2005; Winocur & Greenwood, 1999). Furthermore, fatty Zucker rats, which are leptin-receptor deficient, show deficits in hippocampal-dependent memory (Winocur et al., 2005). Leptin receptors are present in hippocampus (Mercer et al., 1996) and leptin appears to enhance hippocampal LTP via NMDA receptors (Shanley et al., 2001). Leptin, which is reduced in human depressives and suicides (Eikelis et al., 2006), has been shown to act on the hippocampus as an antidepressant (Lu et al., 2006). There is now preliminary evidence that leptin increases neurogenesis in the hippocampus (Yao et al., 2006), findings which fit well in the context of the neurogenic hypothesis of depression. Interestingly, women have higher circulating levels of leptin than men, even when relative adiposity is controlled for (Saad et al., 1997), a finding which could have relevance to the higher levels of depression in women. All of this strongly suggests that leptin has a role in hippocampal pathologies in a number of disorders.

Insulin, the first protein to be fully sequenced (Sanger, 1959), has been the subject of enormous amounts of research due to its role in diabetes. Its significance in regulating carbohydrate metabolism is well known. Impaired glucose tolerance and diabetes in humans are associated with cognitive deficits (Hendrickx et al., 2005) and reduced glycemic control is associated with hippocampal volume changes in human aging as well (Convit et al., 2003). In the hippocampus both insulin and IGF-1 receptors are present (Doré et al., 1997). In the hypothalamus, insulin acts via the same PI3 kinase pathway that leptin does (Niswender & Schwartz, 2003). Insulin is responsible for the translocation of certain glucose transporters to the neuronal membrane (Reagan, 2005) and the transport of one of these, GLUT4, is impaired in the Zucker rat model

of obesity (Winocur et al., 2005). There is some evidence insulin can produce changes in synaptic plasticity in the hippocampus (Wan et al., 1997) and an animal model of type 1 diabetes shows an increased rate of dendritic remodeling (McEwen et al., 2002). IGF-1 also has an impact on neurogenesis (Aberg et al., 2000) and synaptic number as over-expression of it increases both in transgenic mice (O'Kusky et al., 2000). Of particular interest is the finding that IGF-1 appears to mediate some of the effects of exercise on neurogenesis (Carro et al., 2000), as exercise is an antidepressant (Ernst et al., 2006) in addition to its recognized benefits for physical health.

A number of gut-brain peptides appear to have a role in brain plasticity as well. Ghrelin increases memory retention and anxiety (Carlini et al., 2004) as well as spine synapse density (Diano et al., 2006) in the hippocampus. Cocaine-amphetamine regulated transcript (CART) is expressed in the dentate gyrus (Koylu et al., 1998). It also promotes the survival of cultured hippocampal neurons (Wu et al., 2006) and mediates the neuroprotective properties of estrogen in cerebral ischemia (Xu et al., 2006). Interestingly, CART appears to be regulated by corticosterone (Balkan et al., 2001; Hunter et al., 2005; Vrang et al., 2003), as well as leptin (Kristensen et al., 1998), suggesting it may act to integrate the actions of these hormones. Recently it has been shown that CART levels rise in the hippocampus and amygdala after chronic and acute stress respectively (Balkan et al., 2006; Hunter et al., 2007); thus it would appear that CART has a role in the hippocampal response to stress.

Summary

Besides those discussed above, other peptides are known to be or are likely to be involved in brain plasticity, and much future research will focus on determining not only the roles of individual hormones and transmitters but how they interact with one another and with the steroid hormones. Ultimately, it is hoped that a clear picture of the mechanisms of plasticity will emerge.

Methods of intervention

- Treatment of hormonal disorders is complicated by their chronic and complex nature.
- In addition to pharmacotherapy, clinicians should also include exercise and social support in their approach to treatment.

There are many ways to treat the pathologies associated with chronic dysregulation of the stress and metabolic axes. Some are straightforward while others are less so. Iatrogenic Cushing's disease can be treated merely by terminating chronic steroid treatment or removing the endogenous source of excess cortisol, whereas treatment and prevention of chronic diseases such as diabetes and depression is more complex.

Pharmaceutical interventions are generally the most desirable in our culture, since compliance with a treatment regime is simple and they do not require any major change in behavior. For example, antidepressants reverse or stop the progression of structural changes in the hippocampus, while statins improve cholesterol profiles. In the case of depression, at our present state of understanding it would seem imperative that antidepressant drugs be used as early as possible in every case of major depression in order to stop progressive loss of cognitive function. Yet drugs often have side effects, and this is particularly true when one is treating a disorder resulting from the primary distortion of mediators of allostasis that results in allostatic load, which is in itself a "side effect" of coping with external or internal demands. The potential costs and benefits of chronic treatment with corticosteroids is the most obvious illustration of this issue. That is, while it may be possible to treat a dangerous inflammatory condition with corticosteroids, there is the potential risk of adversely affecting cognition and brain structure. Furthermore, the use of drugs over the course of decades as a preventative for diseases, which may or may not present in late life, is medically and ethically dubious, given the potential for adverse outcomes and side effects. While drugs will remain an important part of the medical armamentarium, it is important, particularly when

we are speaking of what have been termed "lifestyle" diseases, that we look further afield for means of therapeutic intervention.

Humans living in affluent societies enjoy many advantages over their early ancestors, and one of these is not having to go much further than the refrigerator to find something to eat. One of the most important health consequences of our wealth of easily accessible food is a highly sedentary lifestyle which predisposes us to many diseases, ranging from diabetes to dementia and depression. A number of recent studies have demonstrated a protective and preventative role for even moderate physical activity, such as a daily walk (Barbour & Blumenthal, 2005; Bernadet, 1995; Dishman *et al.*, 2006; Kramer *et al.*, 2003; Perseghin *et al.*, 1996; Rovio *et al.*, 2005). In the brain, exercise increases neurogenesis in the dentate gyrus of aging animals (van Praag *et al.*, 2005) as well as the levels of neurotrophins in the hippocampus and cortex (Cotman & Berchtold, 2002). That dietary restriction seems to have similar effects on neurogenesis, and expression of the neurotrophin BDNF (Lee *et al.*, 2002) suggests that diet and exercise act via a convergent pathway to improve the health of the brain, most likely via pathways involved in energy balance. Thus exercise fits with the neurogenic definition of an antidepressant mentioned above. In humans, exercise is an effective antidepressant (Lawlor & Hopker, 2001) in addition to its ability to improve cognition in the aged (Colcombe & Kramer, 2003; van Gelder *et al.*, 2004).

Social support, which is addressed in more detail elsewhere in this volume, is both a predictor of allostatic load and a likely means of intervention. Social support and social status are important predictors of risk for chronic diseases (Adler & Ostrove, 1999; Ahern & Hendryx, 2005). Social support reduces allostatic load scores (Seeman *et al.*, 2002) and improves both physical and mental health (Adams *et al.*, 2006; Leskela *et al.*, 2006; Saxena *et al.*, 2006; Silver *et al.*, 2006). Obviously, it is more difficult for many people to adhere to an exercise program than to a pill taken once a day and even more difficult to increase social support.

Nonetheless, research is advancing our knowledge of those elements of social support which are vital to health and which are amenable to intervention. It is important that recommendations about exercise, diet, and social stimulation are made in the course of interactions between doctors and patients. It is imperative that these ideas make their way into the broader culture, where there is little awareness of the fact that diseases like diabetes and depression take a physical toll on the brain, and that these can be prevented or slowed by regular exercise, appropriate diet and an effective social network.

Conclusions

A variety of hormones, including the steroids, interact to maintain healthy cognitive function in the mammalian brain. The hippocampus is a particularly sensitive region to the perturbations in these hormones produced by stress and metabolic disease and it is evident that both can alter hippocampal structure and function, as well as cognition and memory in both humans and animals. The hippocampus, while not the only site of steroid action in the brain, is particularly susceptible to the effects of steroids, particularly corticosteroids, due to high levels of steroid receptors and its sensitivity to excitotoxic and metabolic insult. Recent research has shown that the steroid hormones are not the only players in hippocampal plasticity and that an increasing number of peptide hormones, particularly those with a role in maintaining energy balance, have an influence on plasticity as well.

The conceptual framework of allostasis and allostatic load provides a framework for thinking about both the purpose of brain plasticity as well as a means to understand the relations between different hormones and other mediators in the maintenance of healthy brain structure and function. At present the number of available pharmaceutical interventions includes antioxidants, anti-inflammatory agents, anxiolytics and antidepressants, but future research holds out the likelihood of other potential pharmacological approaches as more is learned about

the interactions of the peptide metabolic hormones with the brain. However, low technology and low-cost interventions, such as physical exercise have much to recommend them, and should be encouraged wherever possible, especially due to the fact that those with the least access to expensive healthcare are most likely to suffer from chronic diseases related to stress and metabolic dysfunction.

REFERENCES

Åberg, M. A. I., Åberg, N. D., Hedbäcker, H., Oscarsson, J., & Eriksson, P. S. (2000). Peripheral infusion of IGF-1 selectivity induces neurogenesis in the adult rat hippocampus. *Journal of Neuroscience*, **20**, 2896–2903.

Absil, P., Pinxten, R., Balthazart, J., & Eens, M. (2003). Effect of age and testosterone on autumnal neurogenesis in male European starlings (*Sturnus vulgaris*). *Behavioural Brain Research*, **143**, 15–30.

Adams, R. E., Boscarino, J. A., & Galea, S. (2006). Social and psychological resources and health outcomes after the World Trade Center disaster. *Social Science and Medicine*, **62**, 176–188.

Adler, N. E., & Ostrove, J. M. (1999). Socioeconomic status and health: what we know and what we don't. *Annals of the New York Academy of Sciences*, **896**, 3–15.

Ahern, M. M., & Hendryx, M. S. (2005). Social capital and risk for chronic illnesses. *Chronic Illness*, **1**, 183–190.

Alvarez-Buylla, A., & Kirn, J. R. (1997). Birth, migration, incorporation, and death of vocal control neurons in adult songbirds. *Journal of Neurobiology*, **33**, 585–601.

Arbel, I., Kadar, T., Silbermann, M., & Levy, A. (1994). The effects of long-term corticosterone administration on hippocampal morphology and cognitive performance of middle-aged rats. *Brain Research*, **657**, 227–235.

Arnold, A. P., & Breedlove, S. M. (1985). Organizational and activational effects of sex steroids on brain and behavior: a reanalysis. *Hormones and Behavior*, **19**, 469–498.

Balkan, B., Koylu, E. O., Kuhar, M. J., & Pogun, S. (2001). The effect of adrenalectomy on cocaine and amphetamine-regulated transcript (CART) expression in the hypothalamic nuclei of the rat. *Brain Research*, **917**, 15–20.

Balkan, B., Gozen, O., Yararbas, G. *et al.* (2006). CART expression in limbic regions of rat brain following forced swim stress: sex differences. *Neuropeptides*, **40**, 185–193.

Banasr, M., Hery, M., Brezun, M., & Daszuta, A. (2001). Serotonin mediates oestrogen stimulation of cell proliferation in the adult dentate gyrus. *European Journal of Neuroscience*, **14**, 1417–1424.

Baran, S. E., Campbell, A. M., Kleen, J. K. *et al.* (2005). Combination of high fat diet and chronic stress retracts hippocampal dendrites. *NeuroReport*, **16**, 39–43.

Barbour, K. A., & Blumenthal, J. A. (2005). Exercise training and depression in older adults. *Neurobiology of Aging*, **26**, *Suppl. 1*, S119–S123.

Berger, S., Wolfer, D. P., Selbach, O. *et al.* (2006). Loss of the limbic mineralocorticoid receptor impairs behavioral plasticity. *Proceedings of the National Academy of Sciences of the United States of America*, **103**, 195–200.

Bernadet, P. (1995). Benefits of physical activity in the prevention of cardiovascular diseases. *Journal of Cardiovascular Pharmacology*, **25**, *Suppl. 1*, S3–S8.

Blurton-Jones, M., & Tuszynski, M. H. (2006). Estradiol-induced modulation of estrogen receptor-β and GABA within the adult neocortex: a potential transsynaptic mechanism for estrogen modulation of BDNF. *Journal of Comparative Neurology*, **499**, 603–612.

Bourdeau, I., Bard, C., Noël, B. *et al.* (2002). Loss of brain volume in endogenous Cushing's syndrome and its reversibility after correction of hypercortisolism. *Journal of Clinical Endocrinology and Metabolism*, **87**, 1949–1954.

Boyle, M. P., Brewer, J. A., Funatsu, M. *et al.* (2005). Acquired deficit of forebrain glucocorticoid receptor produces depression-like changes in adrenal axis regulation and behavior. *Proceedings of the National Academy of Sciences of the United States of America*, **102**, 473–478.

Bremner, J. D. (2006). The relationship between cognitive and brain changes in posttraumatic stress disorder. *Annals of the New York Academy of Sciences*, **1071**, 80–86.

Bremner, J. D., Randall, P., Scott, T. M. *et al.* (1995). MRI-based measurement of hippocampal volume in patients with combat-related posttraumatic stress disorder. *American Journal of Psychiatry*, **152**, 973–981.

Caldwell, B. M., & Watson, R. I. (1952). An evaluation of psychologic effects of sex hormone administration in aged women. 1. Results of therapy after 6 months. *Journals of Gerontology*, **7**, 228–244.

Cameron, H. A., & Gould, E. (1994). Adult neurogenesis is regulated by adrenal steroids in the dentate gyrus. *Neuroscience*, **61**, 203–209.

Carlini, V. P., Varas, M. M., Cragnolini, A. B. *et al.* (2004). Differential role of the hippocampus, amygdala, and dorsal raphe nucleus in regulating feeding, memory, and anxiety-like behavioral responses to ghrelin. *Biochemical and Biophysical Research Communications*, **313**, 635–641.

Carro, E., Nuñez, A., Busiguina, S., & Torres-Aleman, I. (2000). Circulating insulin-like growth factor I mediates effects of exercise on the brain. *Journal of Neuroscience*, **20**, 2926–2933.

Cerqueira, J. J., Taipa, R., Uylings, H. B. M., Almeida, O. F., & Sousa, N. (2007). Specific configuration of dendritic degeneration in pyramidal neurons of the medial prefrontal cortex induced by differing corticosteroid regimens. *Cerebral Cortex*, **17**, 1998–2006.

Chou, Y.-C. (1998). Corticosterone exacerbates cyanide-induced cell death in hippocampal cultures: role of astrocytes. *Neurochemistry International*, **32**, 219–226.

Clark, D. D., & Sokoloff, L. (1998). Circulation and energy metabolism of the brain. In G. J. Siegal, B. W. Agranoff, R. W. Albers, S. K. Fisher, & M. D. Uhler (Eds.), *Basic Neurochemistry: Molecular, Cellular and Medical Aspects* (pp. 637–670). Philadelphia, PA: Lippencott-Raven.

Colcombe, S., & Kramer, A. F. (2003). Fitness effects on the cognitive function of older adults: a meta-analytic study. *Psychological Science*, **14**, 125–130.

Conrad, C. D., Galea, L. A. M., Kuroda, Y., & McEwen, B. S. (1996). Chronic stress impairs rat spatial memory on the Y maze and this effect is blocked by tianeptine pretreatment. *Behavioral Neuroscience*, **110**, 1321–1334.

Conrad, C. D., Magariños, A. M., LeDoux, J. E., & McEwen, B. S. (1999). Repeated restraint stress facilitates fear conditioning independently of causing hippocampal CA3 dendritic atrophy. *Behavioral Neuroscience*, **113**, 902–913.

Conrad, C. D., Jackson, J. L., & Wise, L. S. (2004). Chronic stress enhances ibotenic acid-induced damage selectively within the hippocampal CA3 region of male, but not female rats. *Neuroscience*, **125**, 759–767.

Convit, A., Wolf, O. T., Tarshish, C., & de Leon, M. J. (2003). Reduced glucose tolerance is associated with poor memory performance and hippocampal atrophy among normal elderly. *Proceedings of the National Academy of Sciences of the United States of America*, **100**, 2019–2022.

Cook, S. C., & Wellman, C. L. (2004). Chronic stress alters dendritic morphology in rat medial prefrontal cortex. *Journal of Neurobiology*, **60**, 236–248.

Cotman, C. W., & Berchtold, N. C. (2002). Exercise: a behavioral intervention to enhance brain health and plasticity. *Trends in Neurosciences*, **25**, 295–301.

Daniel, J. M., & Dohanich, G. P. (2001). Acetylcholine mediates the estrogen-induced increase in NMDA receptor binding in CA1 of the hippocampus and the associated improvement in working memory. *Journal of Neuroscience*, **21**, 6949–6956.

de Kloet, E. R., Reul, J. M. H. M., & Sutanto, W. (1990). Corticosteroids and the brain. *Journal of Steroid Biochemistry and Molecular Biology*, **37**, 387–394.

de Kloet, E. R., Vreugdenhil, E., Oitzl, M. S., & Joëls, M. (1998). Brain corticosteroid receptor balance in health and disease. *Endocrine Reviews*, **19**, 269–301.

de Quervain, D. J.-F., Roozendaal, B., Nitsch, R. M., McGaugh, J. L., & Hock, C. (2000). Acute cortisone administration impairs retrieval of long-term declarative memory in humans. *Nature Neuroscience*, **3**, 313–314.

de Vries, G. J., & Simerly, R. B. (2002). Anatomy, development, and function of sexually dimorphic neural circuits in the mammalian brain. In D. W. Pfaff, A. P. Arnold, A. M. Etgen, S. E. Fahrback, & R. T. Rubin (Eds.), *Hormones, Brain and Behavior* (pp. 137–191). San Diego: Academic Press.

Diano, S., Farr, S. A., Benoit, S. C. *et al.* (2006). Ghrelin controls hippocampal spine synapse density and memory performance. *Nature Neuroscience*, **9**, 381–388.

Dishman, R. K., Berthoud, H. R., Booth, F. W. *et al.* (2006). Neurobiology of exercise. *Obesity (Silver Spring)*, **14**, 345–356.

Doré, S., Kar, S., Rowe, W., & Quirion, R. (1997). Distribution and levels of [^{125}I]IGF-I, [^{125}I]IGF-II and [^{125}I]Insulin receptor binding sites in the hippocampus of aged memory-unimpaired and -impaired rats. *Neuroscience*, **80**, 1033–1040.

Duman, R. S. (2004a). Depression: A case of neuronal life and death? *Biological Psychiatry*, **56**, 140–145.

Duman, R. S. (2004b). Role of neurotrophic factors in the etiology and treatment of mood disorders. *Neuromolecular Medicine*, **5**, 11–25.

Eikelis, N., Esler, M., Barton, D. *et al.* (2006). Reduced brain leptin in patients with major depressive disorder and in suicide victims. *Molecular Psychiatry*, **11**, 800–801.

Ernst, C., Olson, A. K., Pinel, J. P. J., Lam, R. W., & Christie, B. R. (2006). Antidepressant effects of exercise: evidence for an adult-neurogenesis hypothesis? *Journal of Psychiatry and Neuroscience*, **31**, 84–92.

Foy, M. R., Xu, J., Xie, X., Brinton, R. D., Thompson, R. F., & Berger, T. W. (1999). 17beta-estradiol enhances NMDA receptor-mediated EPSPs and long-term potentiation. *Journal of Neurophysiology*, **81**, 925–929.

Galea, L. A. M., & McEwen, B. S. (1999). Sex and seasonal differences in the rate of cell proliferation in the dentate gyrus of adult wild meadow voles. *Neuroscience*, **89**, 955–964.

Galea, L. A. M., Perrot-Sinal, T. S., Kavaliers, M., & Ossenkopp, K.-P. (1999). Relations of hippocampal volume and dentate gyrus width to gonadal hormone levels in male and female meadow voles. *Brain Research*, **821**, 383–391.

Galea, L. A. M., Spritzer, M. D., Barker, J. M., & Pawluski, J. L. (2006). Gonadal hormone modulation of hippocampal neurogenesis in the adult. *Hippocampus*, **16**, 225–232.

Gass, P., Kretz, O., Wolfer, D. P. *et al.* (2000). Genetic disruption of mineralocorticoid receptor leads to impaired neurogenesis and granule cell degeneration in the hippocampus of adult mice. *EMBO Reports*, **1**, 447–451.

Gazzaley, A. H., Weiland, N. G., McEwen, B. S., & Morrison, J. H. (1996). Differential regulation of NMDAR1 mRNA and protein by estradiol in the rat hippocampus. *Journal of Neuroscience*, **16**, 6830–6838.

Gilad, G. M., Gilad, V. H., Wyatt, R. J., & Tizabi, Y. (1990). Region-selective stress-induced increase of glutamate uptake and release in rat forebrain. *Brain Research*, **525**, 335–338.

Gorelick, P. B. (2005). William M. Feinberg Lecture: cognitive vitality and the role of stroke and cardiovascular disease risk factors. *Stroke*, **36**, 875–879.

Gould, E., & Cameron, H. A. (1996). Regulation of neuronal birth, migration and death in the rat dentate gyrus. *Developmental Neuroscience*, **18**, 22–35.

Gould, E., Woolley, C. S., Frankfurt, M., & McEwen, B. S. (1990). Gonadal steroids regulate dendritic spine density in hippocampal pyramidal cells in adulthood. *Journal of Neuroscience*, **10**, 1286–1291.

Gould, E., Cameron, H. A., Daniels, D. C., Woolley, C. S., & McEwen, B. S. (1992). Adrenal hormones suppress cell division in the adult rat dentate gyrus. *Journal of Neuroscience*, **12**, 3642–3650.

Gould, E., Tanapat, P., Hastings, N. B., & Shors, T. J. (1999). Neurogenesis in adulthood: a possible role in learning. *Trends in Cognitive Sciences*, **3**, 186–192.

Gurvits, T. V., Shenton, M. E., Hokama, H. *et al.* (1996). Magnetic resonance imaging study of hippocampal volume in chronic, combat-related posttraumatic stress disorder. *Biological Psychiatry*, **40**, 1091–1099.

Hart, S. A., Patton, J. D., & Woolley, C. S. (2001). Quantitative analysis of ERα and GAD colocalization in the hippocampus of the adult female rat. *Journal of Comparative Neurology*, **440**, 144–155.

Hendrickx, H., McEwen, B. S., & van der Ouderaa, F. (2005). Metabolism, mood and cognition in aging: the importance of lifestyle and dietary intervention. *Neurobiology of Aging*, **26**, *Suppl. 1*, S1–S5.

Howell, M. P., & Muglia, L. J. (2006). Effects of genetically altered brain glucocorticoid receptor action on behavior and adrenal axis regulation in mice. *Frontiers in Neuroendocrinology*, **27**, 275–284.

Hunter, R. G., Vicentic, A., Rogge, G., & Kuhar, M. J. (2005). The effects of cocaine on CART expression in the rat nucleus accumbens: a possible role for corticosterone. *European Journal of Pharmacology*, **517**, 45–50.

Hunter, R. G., Bellani, R., Bloss, E. *et al.* (2007). Regulation of CART mRNA by stress and corticosteroids in the hippocampus and amygdala. *Brain Research*, **1152**, 234–240.

Jéquier, E. (2002). Leptin signaling, adiposity, and energy balance. *Annals of the New York Academy of Sciences*, **967**, 379–388.

Karishma, K. K., & Herbert, J. (2002). Dehydroepiandrosterone (DHEA) stimulates neurogenesis in the hippocampus of the rat, promotes survival of newly formed neurons and prevents corticosterone-induced suppression. *European Journal of Neuroscience*, **16**, 445–453.

Kellendonk, C., Gass, P., Kretz, O., Schütz, G., & Tronche, F. (2002). Corticosteroid receptors in the brain: Gene targeting studies. *Brain Research Bulletin*, **57**, 73–83.

Kerr, J. E., Allore, R. J., Beck, S. G., & Handa, R. J. (1995). Distribution and hormonal regulation of androgen receptor (AR) and AR messenger ribonucleic acid in the rat hippocampus. *Endocrinology*, **136**, 3213–3221.

Korte, S. M., Koolhaas, J. M., Wingfield, J. C., & McEwen, B. S. (2005). The Darwinian concept of stress: benefits of allostasis and costs of allostatic load and the trade-offs in health and disease. *Neuroscience and Biobehavioral Reviews*, **29**, 3–38.

Kovacs, E. G., MacLusky, N. J., & Leranth, C. (2003). Effects of testosterone on hippocampal CA1 spine synaptic density in the male rat are inhibited by fimbria/fornix transection. *Neuroscience*, **122**, 807–810.

Koylu, E. O., Couceyro, P. R., Lambert, P. D., & Kuhar, M. J. (1998). Cocaine- and amphetamine-regulated transcript peptide immunohistochemical localization in the rat brain. *Journal of Comparative Neurology*, **391**, 115–132.

Kramer, A. F., Colcombe, S. J., McAuley, E. *et al.* (2003). Enhancing brain and cognitive function of older adults through fitness training. *Journal of Molecular Neuroscience*, **20**, 213–221.

Kristensen, P., Judge, M. E., Thim, L. *et al.* (1998). Hypothalamic CART is a new anorectic peptide regulated by leptin. *Nature*, **393**, 72–76.

Lawlor, D. A., & Hopker, S. W. (2001). The effectiveness of exercise as an intervention in the management of depression: systematic review and meta-regression analysis of randomised controlled trials. *British Medical Journal*, **322**, 763–767.

Lee, J., Seroogy, K. B., & Mattson, M. P. (2002). Dietary restriction enhances neurotrophin expression and neurogenesis in the hippocampus of adult mice. *Journal of Neurochemistry*, **80**, 539–547.

Leranth, C., Shanabrough, M., & Horvath, T. L. (2000). Hormonal regulation of hippocampal spine synapse density involves subcortical mediation. *Neuroscience*, **101**, 349–356.

Leranth, C., Petnehazy, O., & MacLusky, N. J. (2003). Gonadal hormones affect spine synaptic density in the CA1 hippocampal subfield of male rats. *Journal of Neuroscience*, **23**, 1588–1592.

Leranth, C., Hajszan, T., & MacLusky, N. J. (2004a). Androgens increase spine synapse density in the CA1 hippocampal subfield of ovariectomized female rats. *Journal of Neuroscience*, **24**, 495–499.

Leranth, C., Prange-Kiel, J., Frick, K. M., & Horvath, T. L. (2004b). Low CA1 spine synapse density is further reduced by castration in male non-human primates. *Cerebral Cortex*, **14**, 503–510.

Leskelä, U., Rytsälä, H., Komulainen, E. *et al.* (2006). The influence of adversity and perceived social support on the outcome of major depressive disorder in subjects with different levels of depressive symptoms. *Psychological Medicine*, **36**, 779–788.

Lledo, P.-M., Alonso, M., & Grubb, M. S. (2006). Adult neurogenesis and functional plasticity in neuronal circuits. *Nature Reviews Neuroscience*, **7**, 179–193.

Lowy, M. T., Gault, L., & Yamamoto, B. K. (1993). Adrenalectomy attenuates stress-induced elevations in extracellular glutamate concentrations in the hippocampus. *Journal of Neurochemistry*, **61**, 1957–1960.

Loy, R., Gerlach, J. L., & McEwen, B. S. (1988). Autoradiographic localization of estradiol-binding neurons in the rat hippocampal formation and entorhinal cortex. *Developmental Brain Research*, **39**, 245–251.

Lu, X.-Y., Kim, C. S., Frazer, A., & Zhang, W. (2006). Leptin: a potential novel antidepressant. *Proceedings of the National Academy of Sciences of the United States of America*, **103**, 1593–1598.

Luine, V. N., Jacome, L. F., & MacLusky, N. J. (2003). Rapid enhancement of visual and place memory by estrogens in rats. *Endocrinology*, **144**, 2836–2844.

Lupien, S. J., de Leon, M., de Santi, S. *et al.* (1998). Cortisol levels during human aging predict hippocampal atrophy and memory deficits. *Nature Neuroscience*, **1**, 69–73.

Lupien, S. J., & McEwen, B. S. (1997). The acute effects of corticosteroids on cognition: integration of animal and human model studies. *Brain Research Reviews*, **24**, 1–27.

MacLusky, N. J., Hajszan, T., & Leranth, C. (2004). Effects of dehydroepiandrosterone and flutamide on hippocampal CA1 spine synapse density in male and female rats: implications for the role of androgens in maintenance of hippocampal structure. *Endocrinology*, **145**, 4154–4161.

MacLusky, N. J., Hajszan, T., Prange-Kiel, J., & Leranth, C. (2006). Androgen modulation of hippocampal synaptic plasticity. *Neuroscience*, **138**, 957–965.

Magariños, A. M., & McEwen, B. S. (1995). Stress-induced atrophy of apical dendrites of hippocampal CA3c neurons: involvement of glucocorticoid secretion and excitatory amino acid receptors. *Neuroscience*, **69**, 89–98.

Magariños, A. M., McEwen, B. S., Flügge, G., & Fuchs, E. (1996). Chronic psychosocial stress causes apical dendritic atrophy of hippocampal CA3 pyramidal neurons in subordinate tree shrews. *Journal of Neuroscience*, **16**, 3534–3540.

Magariños, A. M., Deslandes, A., & McEwen, B. S. (1999). Effects of antidepressants and benzodiazepine treatments on the dendritic structure of CA3 pyramidal neurons after chronic stress. *European Journal of Pharmacology*, **371**, 113–122.

Magistretti, P. J. (2006). Neuron-glia metabolic coupling and plasticity. *Journal of Experimental Biology*, **209**, 2304–2311.

Magri, F., Cravello, L., Barili, L. *et al.* (2006). Stress and dementia: the role of the hypothalamic-pituitary-adrenal axis. *Aging Clinical and Experimental Research*, **18**, 167–170.

McEwen, B. S. (1998). Stress, adaptation, and disease: allostasis and allostatic load. *Annals of the New York Academy of Sciences*, **840**, 33–44.

McEwen, B. S. (1999). Stress and hippocampal plasticity. *Annual Review of Neuroscience*, **22**, 105–122.

McEwen, B. S. (2005). Glucocorticoids, depression, and mood disorders: structural remodeling in the brain. *Metabolism*, **54**, *Suppl 1.*, 20–23.

McEwen, B. S., & Alves, S. E. (1999). Estrogen actions in the central nervous system. *Endocrine Reviews*, **20**, 279–307.

McEwen, B. S., & Wingfield, J. C. (2003). The concept of allostasis in biology and biomedicine. *Hormones and Behavior*, **43**, 2–15.

McEwen, B. S., Weiss, J. M., & Schwartz, L. S. (1968). Selective retention of corticosterone by limbic structures in rat brain. *Nature*, **220**, 911–912.

McEwen, B. S., de Kloet, E. R., & Rostene, W. (1986). Adrenal steroid receptors and actions in the nervous system. *Physiological Reviews*, **66**, 1121–1188.

McEwen, B. S., Magariños, A. M., & Reagan, L. P. (2002). Studies of hormone action in the hippocampal formation: possible relevance to depression and diabetes. *Journal of Psychosomatic Research*, **53**, 883–890.

McGuire, J. L., & Lisk, R. D. (1968). Estrogen receptors in the intact rat. *Proceedings of the National Academy of Sciences of the United States of America*, **61**, 497–503.

McKittrick, C. R., Blanchard, D. C., Blanchard, R. J., McEwen, B. S., & Sakai, R. R. (1995). Serotonin receptor binding in a colony model of chronic social stress. *Biological Psychiatry*, **37**, 383–393.

McKittrick, C. R., Magariños, A. M., Blanchard, D. C. *et al.* (2000). Chronic social stress reduces dendritic arbors in CA3 of hippocampus and decreases binding to serotonin transporter sites. *Synapse*, **36**, 85–94.

Mercer, J. G., Hoggard, N., Williams, L. M. *et al.* (1996). Localization of leptin receptor mRNA and the long form splice variant (Ob-Rb) in mouse hypothalamus and adjacent brain regions by in situ hybridization. *FEBS Letters*, **387**, 113–116.

Messier, C., & Teutenberg, K. (2005). The role of insulin, insulin growth-factor, and insulin-degrading enzyme in brain aging and Alzheimer's disease. *Neural Plasticity*, **12**, 311–328.

Morgan, T. E., Wong, A. M., & Finch, C. E. (2007). Anti-inflammatory mechanisms of dietary restriction in slowing aging processes. *Interdisciplinary Topics in Gerontology*, **35**, 83–97.

Morris, R. G. M., Garrud, P., Rawlins, J. N. P., & O'Keefe, J. (1982). Place navigation impaired in rats with hippocampal lesions. *Nature*, **297**, 681–683.

Murphy, D. D., Cole, N. B., Greenberger, V., & Segal, M. (1998). Estradiol increases dendritic spine density by reducing GABA neurotransmission in hippocampal neurons. *Journal of Neuroscience*, **18**, 2550–2559.

Nichols, N. R., Agolley, D., Zieba, M., & Bye, N. (2005). Glucocorticoid regulation of glial responses during hippocampal neurodegeneration and regeneration. *Brain Research Reviews*, **48**, 287–301.

Niswender, K. D., & Schwartz, M. W. (2003). Insulin and leptin revisited: adiposity signals with overlapping physiological and intracellular signaling capabilities. *Frontiers in Neuroendocrinology*, **24**, 1–10.

O'Brien, J. T., Lloyd, A., McKeith, I., Gholkar, A., & Ferrier, N. (2004). A longitudinal study of hippocampal volume, cortisol levels, and cognition in older depressed subjects. *American Journal of Psychiatry*, **161**, 2081–2090.

Oitzl, M. S., Fluttert, M., & de Kloet, E. R. (1998a). Acute blockade of hippocampal glucocorticoid receptors facilitates spatial learning in rats. *Brain Research*, **797**, 159–162.

Oitzl, M. S., Fluttert, M., Sutanto, W., & de Kloet, E. R. (1998b). Continuous blockade of brain glucocorticoid receptors facilitates spatial learning and memory in rats. *European Journal of Neuroscience*, **10**, 3759–3766.

O'Kusky, J. R., Ye, P., & D'Ercole, A. J. (2000). Insulin-like growth factor-I promotes neurogenesis and synaptogenesis in the hippocampal dentate gyrus during postnatal development. *Journal of Neuroscience*, **20**, 8435–8442.

Ormerod, B. K., & Galea, L. A. M. (2003). Reproductive status influences the survival of new cells in the dentate gyrus of adult male meadow voles. *Neuroscience Letters*, **346**, 25–28.

Packard, M. G., & Teather, L. A. (1997). Intra-hippocampal estradiol infusion enhances memory in ovariectomized rats. *Neuroreport*, **8**, 3009–3013.

Packard, M. G., Kohlmaier, J. R., & Alexander, G. M. (1996). Posttraining intrahippocampal estradiol injections enhance spatial memory in male rats: interaction with cholinergic systems. *Behavioral Neuroscience*, **110**, 626–632.

Perseghin, G., Price, T. B., Petersen, K. F. *et al.* (1996). Increased glucose transport-phosphorylation and muscle glycogen synthesis after exercise training in insulin-resistant subjects. *New England Journal of Medicine*, **335**, 1357–1362.

Pfaff, D. W. (1980). *Estrogens and Brain Function: Neural Analysis of a Hormone-Controlled Mammalian Reproductive Behavior*. New York, NY: Springer-Verlag.

Pfaff, D., & Keiner, M. (1973). Atlas of estradiol-concentrating cells in the central nervous system of the female rat. *Journal of Comparative Neurology*, **151**, 121–157.

Raber, J. (1998). Detrimental effects of chronic hypothalamic-pituitary-adrenal axis activation: from obesity to memory deficits. *Molecular Neurobiology*, **18**, 1–22.

Radley, J. J., Sisti, H. M., Hao, J. *et al.* (2004). Chronic behavioral stress induces apical dendritic reorganization in pyramidal neurons of the medial prefrontal cortex. *Neuroscience*, **125**, 1–6.

Rasika, S., Nottebohm, F., & Alvarez-Buylla, A. (1994). Testosterone increases the recruitment and/or survival of new high vocal center neurons in adult female canaries. *Proceedings of the National Academy of Sciences of the United States of America*, **91**, 7854–7858.

Reagan, L. P. (2005). Neuronal insulin signal transduction mechanisms in diabetes phenotypes. *Neurobiology of Aging*, **26**S, S56–S59.

Reagan, L. P., Rosell, D. R., Wood, G. E. *et al.* (2004). Chronic restraint up-regulates GLT-1 mRNA and protein expression in the rat hippocampus: reversal by tianeptine. *Proceedings of the National Academy of Sciences of the United States of America*, **101**, 2179–2184.

Rhodes, M. E., & Frye, C. A. (2006). ERβ-selective SERMs produce mnemonic-enhancing effects in the inhibitory avoidance and water maze tasks. *Neurobiology of Learning and Memory*, **85**, 183–191.

Ridder, S., Chourbaji, S., Hellweg, R. *et al.* (2005). Mice with genetically altered glucocorticoid receptor expression show altered sensitivity for stress-induced depressive reactions. *Journal of Neuroscience*, **25**, 6243–6250.

Romeo, R. D., Richardson, H. N., & Sisk, C. L. (2002). Puberty and the maturation of the male brain and sexual behavior: recasting a behavioral potential. *Neuroscience and Biobehavioral Reviews*, **26**, 381–391.

Roof, R. L. (1993). The dentate gyrus is sexually dimorphic in prepubescent rats: testosterone plays a significant role. *Brain Research*, **610**, 148–151.

Roof, R. L., & Havens, M. D. (1992). Testosterone improves maze performance and induces development of a male hippocampus in females. *Brain Research*, **572**, 310–313.

Rovio, S., Kåreholt, I., Helkala, E.-L. *et al.* (2005). Leisure-time physical activity at midlife and the risk of dementia and Alzheimer's disease. *Lancet Neurology*, **4**, 705–711.

Rudick, C. N., & Woolley, C. S. (2001). Estrogen regulates functional inhibition of hippocampal CA1 pyramidal cells in the adult female rat. *Journal of Neuroscience*, **21**, 6532–6543.

Rudick, C. N., Gibbs, R. B., & Woolley, C. S. (2003). A role for the basal forebrain cholinergic system in estrogen-induced disinhibition of hippocampal pyramidal cells. *Journal of Neuroscience*, **23**, 4479–4490.

Saad, M. F., Damani, S., Gingerich, R. L. *et al.* (1997). Sexual dimorphism in plasma leptin concentration. *Journal of Clinical Endocrinology and Metabolism*, **82**, 579–584.

Sandstrom, N. J., & Williams, C. L. (2001). Memory retention is modulated by acute estradiol and progesterone replacement. *Behavioral Neuroscience*, **115**, 384–393.

Sanger, F. (1959). Chemistry of insulin. *Science*, **129**, 1340–1344.

Santarelli, L., Saxe, M., Gross, C. *et al.* (2003). Requirement of hippocampal neurogenesis for the behavioral effects of antidepressants. *Science*, **301**, 805–809.

Sapolsky, R. M. (2000). Glucocorticoids and hippocampal atrophy in neuropsychiatric disorders. *Archives of General Psychiatry*, **57**, 925–935.

Sapolsky, R. M. (2001). Depression, antidepressants, and the shrinking hippocampus. *Proceedings of the National Academy of Sciences of the United States of America*, **98**, 12320–12322.

Sapolsky, R. M., Krey, L. C., & McEwen, B. S. (1986). The neuroendocrinology of stress and aging: the glucocorticoid cascade hypothesis. *Endocrine Reviews*, **7**, 284–301.

Sapolsky, R. M., Uno, H., Rebert, C. S., & Finch, C. E. (1990). Hippocampal damage associated with prolonged glucocorticoid exposure in primates. *Journal of Neuroscience*, **10**, 2897–2902.

Saxena, S., Jané-Llopis, E., & Hosman, C. (2006). Prevention on mental and behavioral disorders: implications for policy and practice. *World Psychiatry*, **5**, 5–14.

Seeman, T. E., Singer, B. H., Ryff, C. D., Love, G. D., & Levy-Storms, L. (2002). Social relationships, gender, and allostatic load across two age cohorts. *Psychosomatic Medicine*, **64**, 395–406.

Shanley, L. J., Irving, A. J., & Harvey, J. (2001). Leptin enhances NMDA receptor function and modulates hippocampal synaptic plasticity. *Journal of Neuroscience*, **21**, RC186.

Sheline, Y. I., Wang, P. W., Gado, M. H., Csernansky, J. G., & Vannier, M. W. (1996). Hippocampal atrophy in recurrent major depression. *Proceedings of the National Academy of Sciences of the United States of America*, **93**, 3908–3913.

Sherwin, B. B. (2006). Estrogen and cognitive aging in women. *Neuroscience*, **138**, 1021–1026.

Shors, T. J., Chua, C., & Falduto, J. (2001). Sex differences and opposite effects of stress on dendritic spine density in the male versus female hippocampus. *Journal of Neuroscience*, **21**, 6292–6297.

Shumaker, S. A., Legault, C., Rapp, S. R. *et al.* (2003). Estrogen plus progestin and the incidence of dementia and mild cognitive impairment in postmenopausal women. The Women's Health Initiative Memory Study: a randomized controlled trial. *Journal of the American Medical Association*, **289**, 2651–2662.

Silver, E. J., Heneghan, A. M., Bauman, L. J., & Stein, R. E. K. (2006). The relationship of depressive symptoms to parenting competence and social support in inner-city mothers of young children. *Maternal and Child Health Journal*, **10**, 105–112.

Starkman, M. N., Giordani, B., Gebarski, S. S. *et al.* (1999). Decrease in cortisol reverses human hippocampal atrophy following treatment of Cushing's disease. *Biological Psychiatry*, **46**, 1595–1602.

Starkman, M. N., Giordani, B., Gebarski, S. S., & Schteingart, D. E. (2003). Improvement in learning associated with increase in hippocampal formation volume. *Biological Psychiatry*, **53**, 233–238.

Steffensen, S. C., Jones, M. D., Hales, K., & Allison, D. W. (2006). Dehydroepiandrosterone sulfate and estrone sulfate reduce GABA-recurrent inhibition in the hippocampus via muscarinic acetylcholine receptors. *Hippocampus*, **16**, 1080–1090.

Stellato, C. (2004). Post-transcriptional and nongenomic effects of glucocorticoids. *Proceedings of the American Thoracic Society*, **1**, 255–263.

Suzuki, M., Wright, L. S., Marwah, P., Lardy, H. A., & Svendsen, C. N. (2004). Mitotic and neurogenic effects of dehydroepiandrosterone (DHEA) on human neural stem cell cultures derived from the fetal cortex. *Proceedings of the National Academy of Sciences of the United States of America*, **101**, 3202–3207.

Tanapat, P., Hastings, N. B., Reeves, A. J., & Gould, E. (1999). Estrogen stimulates a transient increase in the number of new neurons in the dentate gyrus of the adult female rat. *Journal of Neuroscience*, **19**, 5792–5801.

Tata, D. A., Marciano, V. A., & Anderson, B. J. (2006). Synapse loss from chronically elevated glucocorticoids: relationship to neuropil volume and cell number in hippocampal area CA3. *Journal of Comparative Neurology*, **498**, 363–374.

Tombaugh, G. C., Yang, S. H., Swanson, R. A., & Sapolsky, R. M. (1992). Glucocorticoids exacerbate hypoxic and hypoglycemic hippocampal injury in vitro: biochemical correlates and a role for astrocytes. *Journal of Neurochemistry*, **59**, 137–146.

van Gelder, B. M., Tijhuis, M. A. R., Kalmijn, S. *et al.* (2004). Physical activity in relation to cognitive decline in elderly men: the FINE Study. *Neurology*, **63**, 2316–2321.

van Praag, H., Shubert, T., Zhao, C., & Gage, F. H. (2005). Exercise enhances learning and hippocampal neurogenesis in aged mice. *Journal of Neuroscience*, **25**, 8680–8685.

Vrang, N., Larsen, P. J., Tang-Christensen, M., Larsen, L. K., & Kristensen, P. (2003). Hypothalamic cocaine-amphetamine regulated transcript (CART) is regulated by glucocorticoids. *Brain Research*, **965**, 45–50.

Vyas, A., Mitra, R., Shankaranarayana, R., & Chattarji, S. (2002). Chronic stress induces contracting patterns of dendritic remodeling in hippocampal and amygdaloid neurons. *Journal of Neuroscience*, **22**, 6810–6818.

Wan, Q., Xiong, Z. G., Man, H. Y. *et al.* (1997). Recruitment of functional GABA$_A$ receptors to postsynaptic domains by insulin. *Nature*, **388**, 686–690.

Warner-Schmidt, J. L., & Duman, R. S. (2006). Hippocampal neurogenesis: opposing effects of stress and antidepressant treatment. *Hippocampus*, **16**, 239–249.

Watanabe, Y., Gould, E., Cameron, H. A., Daniels, D. C., & McEwen, B. S. (1992a). Phenytoin prevents stress- and corticosterone-induced atrophy of CA3 pyramidal neurons. *Hippocampus*, **2**, 431–436.

Watanabe, Y., Gould, E., Daniels, D. C., Cameron, H., & McEwen, B. S. (1992b). Tianeptine attenuates stress-induced morphological changes in the hippocampus. *European Journal of Pharmacology*, **222**, 157–162.

Watanabe, Y., Gould, E., & McEwen, B. S. (1992c). Stress induces atrophy of apical dendrites of hippocampal CA3 pyramidal neurons. *Brain Research*, **588**, 341–345.

Weiland, N. G. (1992). Estradiol selectively regulates agonist binding sites on the *N*-methyl-D-aspartate receptor complex in the CA1 region of the hippocampus. *Endocrinology*, **131**, 662–668.

Weiland, N. G., Orikasa, C., Hayashi, S., & McEwen, B. S. (1997). Distribution and hormone regulation of estrogen receptor immunoreactive cells in the hippocampus of male and female rats. *Journal of Comparative Neurology*, **388**, 603–612.

Wimer, C. C., & Wimer, R. E. (1989). On the sources of strain and sex differences in granule cell number in the dentate area of house mice. *Developmental Brain Research*, **48**, 167–176.

Winocur, G., & Greenwood, C. E. (1999). The effects of high fat diets and environmental influences on cognitive performance in rats. *Behavioural Brain Research*, **101**, 153–161.

Winocur, G., Greenwood, C. E., Piroli, G. G. *et al.* (2005). Memory impairment in obese Zucker rats: an investigation of cognitive function in an animal model of insulin resistance and obesity. *Behavioral Neuroscience*, **119**, 1389–1395.

Woolley, C. S., & McEwen, B. S. (1992). Estradiol mediates fluctuation in hippocampal synapse density during the estrous cycle in the adult rat. *Journal of Neuroscience*, **12**, 2549–2554.

Woolley, C. S., Gould, E., & McEwen, B. S. (1990). Exposure to excess glucocorticoids alters dendritic morphology of adult hippocampal pyramidal neurons. *Brain Research*, **531**, 225–231.

Woolley, C. S., Gould, E., Sakai, R. R., Spencer, R. L., & McEwen, B. S. (1991). Effects of aldosterone or RU28362 treatment on adrenalectomy-induced cell death in the dentate gyrus of the adult rat. *Brain Research*, **554**, 312–315.

Woolley, C. S., Weiland, N. G., McEwen, B. S., & Schwartzkroin, P. A. (1997). Estradiol increases the sensitivity of hippocampal CA1 pyramidal cells to NMDA receptor-mediated synaptic input: correlation with dendritic spine density. *Journal of Neuroscience*, **17**, 1848–1859.

Wright, R. L., Lightner, E. N., Harman, J. S., Meijer, O. C., & Conrad, C. D. (2006). Attenuating corticosterone levels on the day of memory assessment prevents chronic stress-induced impairment in spatial memory. *European Journal of Neuroscience*, **24**, 595–605.

Wu, B., Hu, S., Yang, M., Pan, H., & Zhu, S. (2006). CART peptide promotes the survival of hippocampal neurons by upregulating brain-derived neurotrophic factor. *Biochemical and Biophysical Research Communications*, **347**, 656–661.

Xu, Y., Zhang, W., Klaus, J. *et al.* (2006). Role of cocaine- and amphetamine-regulated transcript in estradiol-mediated neuroprotection. *Proceedings of the National Academy of Sciences of the United States of America*, **103**, 14489–14494.

Yao, H., Garza, J., Kim, C., Olson, C. L., & Lu, X. (2006). Leptin reverses chronic stress-induced suppression of hippocampal neurogenesis and behavioral deficits in an animal model of depression. *Society for Neuroscience*. Atlanta, Georgia.

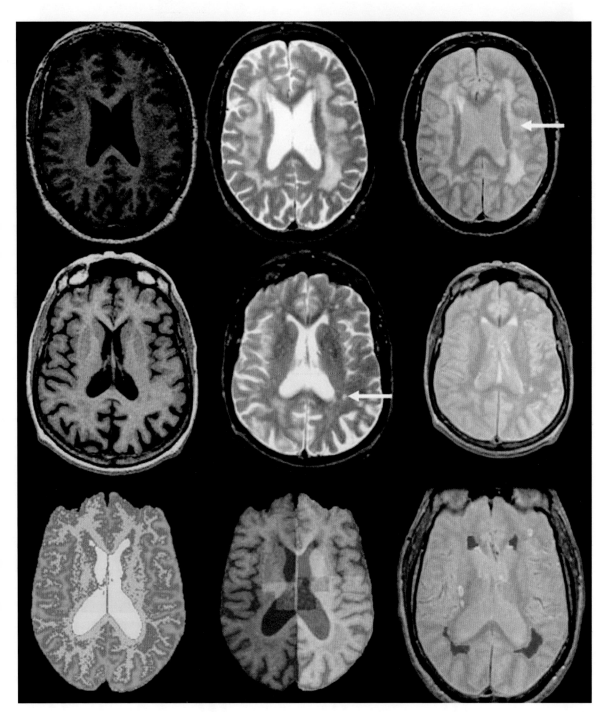

Fig 8.4

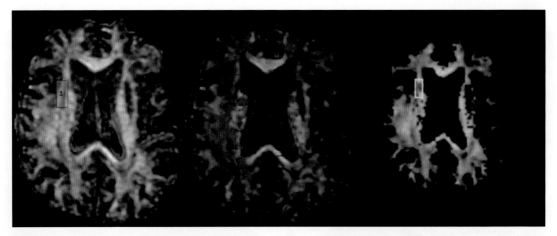

Fig 8.8 (above)

Fig 8.16 (below)

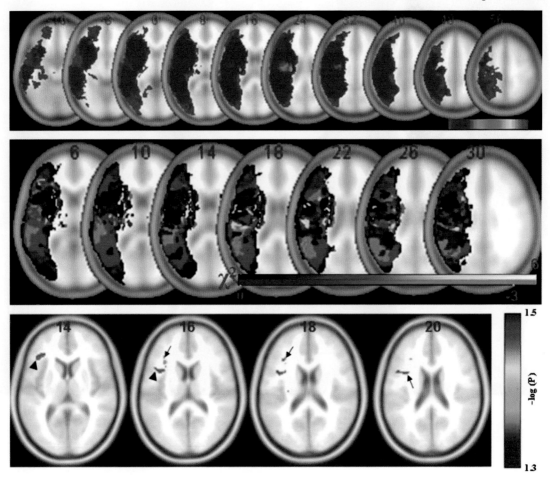

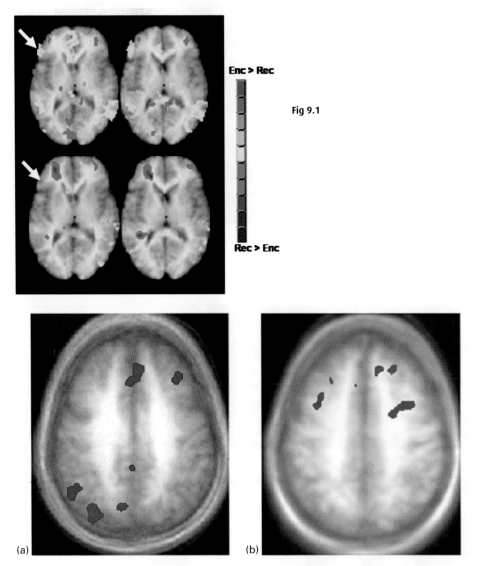

Fig 9.1

(a)

(b)

Fig 9.2

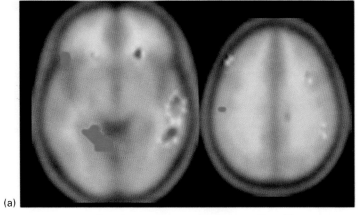

(a)

Fig 9.4

Z = –8   Z = +32

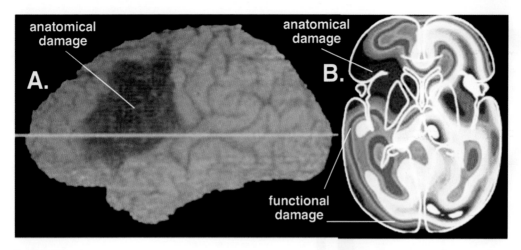

Fig 10.2 (above)

Fig 10.3 (below)

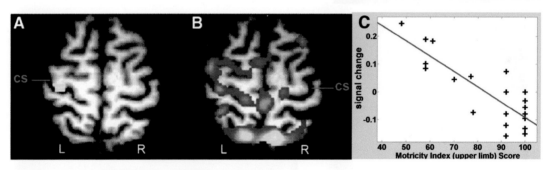

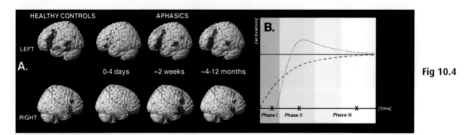

Fig 10.4

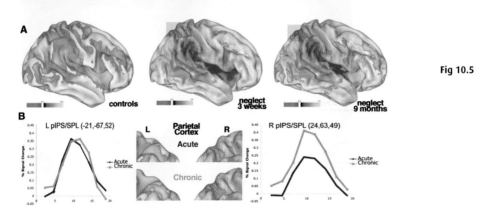

Fig 10.5

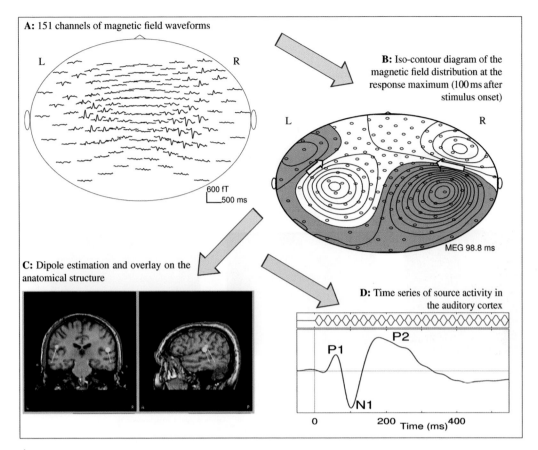

A: 151 channels of magnetic field waveforms

L R

600 fT
500 ms

B: Iso-contour diagram of the magnetic field distribution at the response maximum (100 ms after stimulus onset)

L R

MEG 98.8 ms

C: Dipole estimation and overlay on the anatomical structure

D: Time series of source activity in the auditory cortex

P1
P2
N1

0 200 Time (ms) 400

Fig 11.1

B)

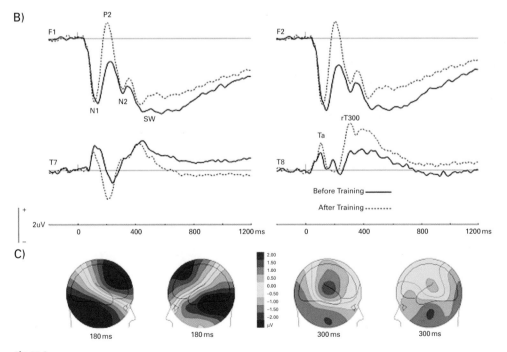

F1
P2
N1 N2
SW

F2
rT300
Ta

T7

T8

Before Training ———
After Training ·········

2uV

0 400 800 1200 ms

0 400 800 1200 ms

C)

2.00
1.50
1.00
0.50
0.00
−0.50
−1.00
−1.50
−2.00
µV

180 ms 180 ms 300 ms 300 ms

Fig 11.2

Time line of neurogenesis

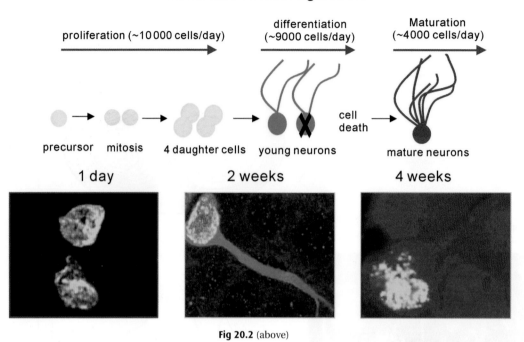

Fig 20.2 (above)

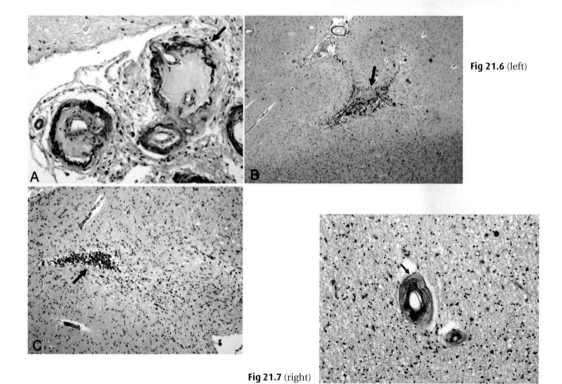

Fig 21.6 (left)

Fig 21.7 (right)

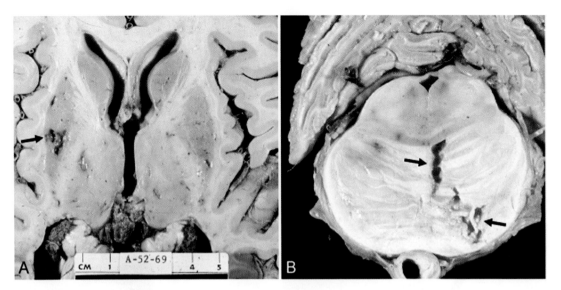

Fig 21.1 (above)

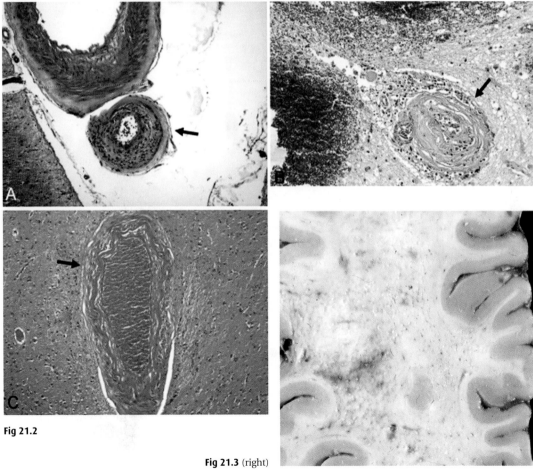

Fig 21.2

Fig 21.3 (right)

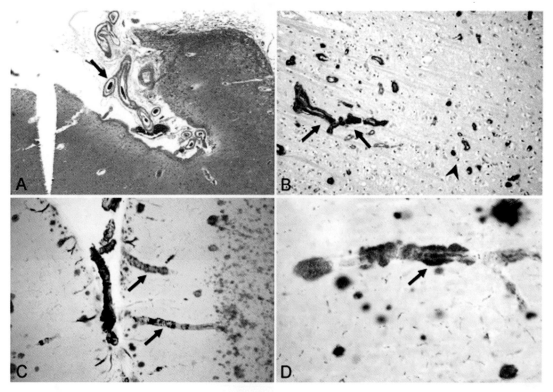

Fig 21.4 (above)

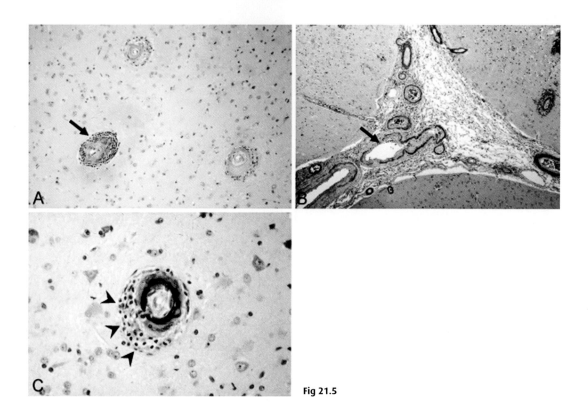

Fig 21.5

5

Principles in conducting rehabilitation research

Amy D. Rodriguez and Leslie J. Gonzalez Rothi

Introduction

- The concept of the maturational process of research is introduced.
- History and current state of rehabilitation are reviewed.
- Barriers to conducting rehabilitation research are identified.

Future research should move beyond the simple question of whether cognitive rehabilitation is effective, and examine the therapy factors and patient characteristics that optimize the clinical outcomes of cognitive rehabilitation. (Cicerone *et al.*, 2005)

All practical solutions to biomedical conditions such as cognitive disorders resulting from neurologic disease or injury begin with discovery yielded by basic research. Evolution of this basic knowledge toward its practical application requires a series of steps along a continuum referred to as clinical trials, stages or phases. Sufficient research within each stage is required to confirm methodological adequacy or to allow resolution of necessary modifications before moving along the stream toward more evolved stages of clinical evidence. The process of moving from one phase to the next is referred to as "translational" with each transition posing its own set of challenges unique to the maturity of the treatment.

Points of translation in research are particularly inefficient and these impediments have limited progress in delivering the biomedical discovery to clinical practice in general. In the case of cognitive rehabilitation, scientists face additional challenges at every level of investigation beginning with concept development. One difficulty at this most early stage is the inherently complex nature of the human behaviors that serve as the targets of cognitive rehabilitation. Throughout the continuum of a clinical trial evolution, there are difficulties unique to participating in rehabilitation research that include, in the earliest stages, the process of recruiting select participants who meet constrained subject criteria. The simple act of participation (whatever level of clinical trial) requires endurance and compliance due to the protracted nature of the process of cognitive rehabilitation. An additional impediment is found in the dearth of adequate outcome measures for appropriately measuring the impact of various forms of cognitive rehabilitation. Finally, it is difficult to obtain funding for early clinical trials in rehabilitation and journals appear reluctant to publish the results of such trials, reflecting perhaps a lack of appreciation for the value of early phase trials (Rothi, 2006). The result of these and other challenges is that cognitive rehabilitation research lags well behind other forms of rehabilitation research and remains in its infancy with much ahead to be achieved. The purpose of this chapter is to review some issues related to these impediments in hopes of encouraging/enabling the successful translation of good ideas into effective and efficient clinical practices for those that we seek to serve and who need/ deserve our best efforts.

Cognitive Neurorehabilitation, Second Edition: Evidence and Application, ed. Donald T. Stuss, Gordon Winocur and Ian H. Robertson. Published by Cambridge University Press. © Cambridge University Press 2008.

The evolution of neurorehabilitation: from optimism to nihilism and back again

Early reports of the use of "mechanism targeted" techniques to rehabilitate functional deficits resulting from neural injury or disease can be dated back to 2500 BC when the early Egyptians used charms and potions in medicine and in particular in the case of stroke. The assumption was that the functional deficits resulted from demonic possession and thus they developed treatments they felt would make the body unwelcoming to their presence (Finger, 1994). On through history, mechanism-based treatments further evolved when, in 400 BC, attempts were made to treat neurobehavioral deficits by using phlebotomy to realign the four humors within the body, assumed to be out of balance and thus creating the behavioral consequences of stroke (Rothi, 2006).

Even in modern day we continue to evolve our view of rehabilitation (Rothi, 2001). For example, through advances in basic science we have moved past the longstanding notion put forth by Cajal (1928) that a damaged central nervous system (CNS) is unchangeable after puberty and irreparable following injury. Rehabilitation scientists now embrace the notion of plasticity as it relates to the mature CNS, recognizing also that structural and functional change can be seen well after acute stages of injury (Rothi, 2001, 2006) and are particularly sensitive to experience. In this volume, Chapter 1 by Kolb and Gibb, Chapter 2 by Dixon, Garrett and Bäckman, and Chapter 20 by Wojtowicz, review evidence supporting this plastic view of the chronically compromised, mature nervous system and reveal the potential that neurorehabilitation efforts undoubtedly will play in the future. However, we have not yet realized the promise of a plastic mature CNS through rehabilitation efforts.

The promise that lies ahead for neurorehabilitation has prompted a critical desire and value placed upon communication and collaboration between basic scientists and rehabilitation scientists that until now has been lacking. The union of the sciences has developed into what is known as translational research. Through translational research, innovative treatments based on basic science discoveries are applied to humans. During this process, basic science informs clinical practice and, in turn, clinical practice informs basic science. In other words, research moves from bench to bedside and back to the bench. While the National Institutes of Health (NIH) Roadmap endorses the value of translational research by establishing institutional funding mechanisms and pilot programs that support clinical and translational research programs, the actualization of these kinds of partnerships continue to be difficult to accomplish for a number of reasons, beginning with a lack of a commonly shared vocabulary. Additionally, Kleim (2006) believes that barriers also include pervasive communication problems (basic scientists fail to understand/pose clinically relevant questions while clinicians fail to understand basic science findings), a lack of appropriate animal models for cognition, and few standard methods for assessing functional outcome within various cognitive domains with none that are comparable across animal and human models.

Neurorehabilitation clinical trials

The popular belief that only randomised, controlled trials produce trustworthy results and that all observational studies are misleading does a disservice to ... clinical investigation . . . . (Concato *et al.*, 2000)

A major fault with evidence-based medicine is its emphasis on randomised controlled trials. (Iggo, 1995)

The role of rehabilitation science in the evolutionary process is to develop treatments based on the principles of neuroplasticity and apply them to individuals with neurologic injury in a series of systematically conducted clinical trials. While we are beginning to embrace our role in this translation, we as yet do not fully appreciate the evolutionary nature of the process itself. Research is a process, and unfortunately there appears to be a lack of respect for the evolution involved in the development and maturation of the process. In part, this has been brought on by the call for evidence-based medicine in clinical practice. Evidence-based medicine is defined as "the conscientious, explicit, and judicious use of current best evidence in making decisions about the care of individual patients" (Sackett *et al.*, 1996). The notion that randomized clinical trials (RCTs) are the "gold standard" for guidance in clinical practice is widely held. Unfortunately, this has been erroneously extended to the belief that RCTs are also the gold standard in clinical research (Frattali, 1998; Robey & Schultz, 1998). Consequently, reviewers' perspectives are often clouded by this belief and there has been an increasingly strong bias for funding and publishing RCTs, with little regard shown for exploratory studies and their critical role in evolving experimental treatment methods.

Evidenced-based care has the potential to rescue us from sinking in a sea of papers . . . however, proponents of the movement threaten to swamp us in a tidal wave of enthusiasm . . . Categorizing interventions by evidence makes an implicit value judgment. It is a short step from "without substantial evidence" to "without substantial value". (Bradley & Field, 1995)

The result of pre-empting early phases and jumping directly to late phase trials is that the research is undermined by a lack of what should have been accomplished in earlier phases. As an example, beginning with an RCT means that a large number of people are subjected to a treatment that has not been shown to be reasonably tolerable (rehabilitation's version of "safety"), has not been demonstrated as having potency (i.e., a therapeutic effect), has not had the opportunity to "tweak the methods" based upon experience to refine procedures to efficiently deliver and maximally effect change, and finally to take advantage of the opportunity to select outcome measures that adequately measure the targeted behaviors at multiple functional levels (World Health Organization (WHO) ICF models). With all that is necessary to achieve the best structured RCT, it is not only discouraging but disconcerting that funding for early phase studies is rarely granted, and that even when these studies are conducted

reviewers are reluctant to publish the results. If our interest is conducting research that informs clinical practice, we must value early phase treatment studies. While they involve small numbers, targeted unidimensional outcome measures, and within-subject designs rather than comparison control groups, we must appreciate their role in the maturational process of research, realizing that they lay the foundation for later phases of research (i.e., RCTs). Although treatment studies may be costly and time consuming, if they are not conducted systematically, the cost (human and financial) of not treating may be far greater in the long run. This chapter describes essential principles in conducting rehabilitation research, providing a new phase model to guide research development and a framework that guides selection of appropriate outcome measures.

Phase models in rehabilitation research

- Introduction to the use of phase models in rehabilitation research is provided.
- The concepts of therapeutic effect, efficacy and effectiveness are reviewed.
- Barriers to progressing through stages of research are addressed.

Rehabilitation scientists are faced with the challenge of establishing the efficacy and effectiveness of treatments for a number of reasons, not the least of which is providing evidence for clinical practice. While the push for evidence-based medicine has effected positive changes in clinical practice, the application of its standards to rehabilitation research has had negative consequences on the process of conducting systematic research. Phase models originated in pharmaceutical research but are not well suited for use in clinical outcomes research because of inconsistencies with behavioral rehabilitation. Despite its shortcomings, the concept of using a "phase" model for clinical outcomes research was initially proposed by the WHO in 1975 and subsequently adopted in behavioral research (Robey & Schultz, 1998). Over time, models have undergone a number of iterations, including fluctuation in the number of phases and creation of subphases. One consistency, however, is that according to these models the only justification for advancing from one phase to the next is a positive outcome in the previous phase. That is, the research process must begin at the beginning and undergo a maturational process before reaching the end. Currently, the most widely accepted standard for clinical outcomes research is the five-phase model put forth by the National Cancer Institute (NCI). This model guides research from infancy to maturity by first generating evidence for a treatment's therapeutic effect, and then systematically determining its efficacy and effectiveness. As stated by Robey & Schultz (1998), who adapted the NCI model for use in aphasiology, the requirements for each of the elements are as follows:

Therapeutic effect: Develop hypotheses, protocols, methods; establish safety and activity; determine best outcome measure; determine responders vs. nonresponders; determine optimal intensity/duration; determine why treatment is producing an effect.

Efficacy: Determine probability of benefit to individuals in a defined population under ideal conditions; determine if any unexpected consequences, benefits and applications exist; conduct follow-up tests of efficacy in specified subpopulations.

Effectiveness: Determine probability of benefit to individuals in a defined population under average (typical) conditions; determine unexpected side effects; compare magnitude of effect under ideal conditions and average (typical) conditions; determine how to minimize waste; determine cost-effectiveness and cost–benefit.

Each of the above elements occurs during a certain phase of research, and thus, each phase has a specific purpose, design and methodology. For example, early phases are conducted to determine therapeutic effect and typically require small numbers of subjects and experimental control is managed within-subject rather than by group comparison. The requirement of an RCT emerges later when the *efficacy* of a treatment is being investigated. Thus, according to phase models, RCTs are not considered until early phase studies have successfully demonstrated a therapeutic effect. Thus, rehabilitation scientists must advocate adherence to phase models and maintain respect for the maturational process of research in order to maximize treatment outcomes and advance the science of rehabilitation.

Our model for rehabilitation research development

- A model describing the maturational process of rehabilitation research from basic science to health services research is described.
- Examples of two lines of research that originated in basic science and systematically progressed through the phases of research are provided.

In a recent article, Rothi (2006) proposed a model that summarizes the maturational process of rehabilitation research (see Table 5.1). The benefit of this model over other phase models is that it includes the purpose, design and methodology of rehabilitation research from basic science to health services research. The addition of basic science and translational research to the continuum of currently accepted standards for clinical outcomes research captures the union between basic science and clinical research in rehabilitation science. This is an important addition because the relationship between these disciplines is critical for rehabilitation research development to thrive. Since the model proposed by Rothi (2006) is actually an extension of Robey's five-phase model, comparisons between the two will be made where appropriate. Examples relevant to each stage of research will also be provided and shall hereafter simply be referred to as the Rothi's Revision of the Robey Model.

According to Rothi's Revision of the Robey Model, rehabilitation research begins with the Basic Science stage. The purpose of this stage is to initiate the evolutional process of research through *Discovery*. During *Discovery*, scientists conduct research at the basic elemental (behavioral and/or

Table 5.1. Maturational process of rehabilitation research.

	Basic Science	Translational Research	Exploratory Clinical Study	Phase I Clinical Trial	Phase II Clinical Trial	Phase III Clinical Trial	Health Services Research
Purpose	Basic discovery	Translation from animal to human application; normal human to pathology	Treatment innovation	Treatment evolution/ formalisation	Treatment efficacy	Treatment effectiveness	Delivery Method/ Societal Impact
Participant model	Animal or human	Animal to human, normal to pathology	Human individuals	Human individuals from defined population	Human individuals from defined population (ideal conditions) and specified sub-populations	Human individuals from defined population (average of typical conditions)	Human individuals and institutions
Research methodology	Within-subject and small group designs	Within-subject and small group designs	Within-subject and small group designs	Small group designs, case studies, within-subject with replication across subjects	Parallel group designs with large sample sizes	Multi-site randomized clinical trials with large samples and within-subject with replication across subjects	Large group designs. Within-subject with multiple replication across subjects, and meta-analysis

physiologic) level. This involves investigation of neural mechanisms in animals and/or humans using within-subject designs or group comparisons. One example of *Discovery* in the literature was the finding of Merzenich & Jenkins (1995), when studying experience-dependent plasticity in auditory cortex, that neurons responsible for mapping sensory events in the brains of adult monkeys are highly adaptive. They found that functional representations in regions of auditory cortex reorganized after intensive exposures to complex auditory stimuli. Additionally, basic science involving humans has also contributed to rehabilitation strategies as well. One example can be found in the studies confirming two distinctive pathways within the human visual system (ventral and dorsal) that are known to be organized hierarchically and to have specialized functions. The ventral stream is concerned with "what," or the perceptual identification of objects. The dorsal stream is concerned with "where," or the spatial location of objects and the sensorimotor transformation needed for visually guided action (Goodale & Milner, 1992; Ungerleider & Haxby, 1994). The basic science *Discovery* regarding the functions of these two pathways provokes us to consider that failures to process visual information may result from mechanisms that warrant distinctions in treatment approaches.

The second phase of Rothi's Revision of the Robey Model is Translational Research. Accordingly, its purpose is *Translation* of a basic science *Discovery* to a human condition. Using similar design methodologies as the basic science phase, research conducted with animals is translated to human application. Or, if previous research was conducted in a normal human population, it is extended to humans with a defined pathological state. Continuing down the prior thread of Merzenich & Jenkins' basic findings that the auditory cortex of monkeys could be "tuned" by exposures to a range of acoustic stimuli, Tallal & Piercy (1973a, 1973b) found that children with language learning impairment (LLI) required more time between acoustic events than age- and intelligence-matched cohorts, and that extending the duration of elements in

acoustic wave forms of speech syllables significantly improved acoustic discrimination in children with LLI (Tallal & Piercy, 1975). Furthermore, they found that temporal integration threshold highly correlated with severity of receptive language deficits and difficulty with phonological encoding necessary for reading (Tallal, 1980a, 1980b; Tallal *et al.*, 1985). Armed with this knowledge, and Merzenich & Jenkins' basic science discovery, Merzenich and colleagues hypothesized that training exercises used in monkeys may remediate auditory temporal integration deficits of children with LLI (Merzenich *et al.*, 1996).

Similarly, the discoveries made by Ungerleider and colleagues about the functional distinctions of the dorsal and ventral streams in the visual system have been translated from basic psychological discovery to individuals with brain damage. For example, a number of studies found that brain damage could result in the inability to discriminate perceptual (ventral stream) features but preserved ability to make appropriate (dorsal stream) motoric responses to those features (Goodale, 1996; Milner & Goodale, 1995). Again, this is an example of communication between basic scientist and rehabilitation scientist that provided an opportunity for *Translation* of a basic science discovery to a certain clinical population. This type of *Translation* research leads to the next stage in Rothi's Revision of Robey's Model called Exploratory Clinical Study.

Exploratory Clinical Study is a time of *Innovation*. During this stage, clinical studies are developed using the principles previously established in the Basic Science and Translational Research stages. In our example of Tallal & Merzenich's work with children with LLI, a treatment was developed for remediation of their auditory temporal integration deficits using adaptive computer games that changed acoustic cues in speech and non-speech stimuli (Merzenich *et al.*, 1996) and listening exercises that used acoustically modified speech to train phonological discrimination and language comprehension (Nagarajan *et al.*, 1998). These stimuli and methods were designed consistent with principles emanating from Merzenich's early phase work in experience dependent adaptations of the monkey auditory cortex.

Regarding our thread of the tale of the dorsal and ventral visual systems, Robertson and colleagues began to develop ideas about treatment for individuals with unilateral spatial neglect by developing distinctive methods that respected "what" vs. "where" information. For example, in a 1995 study, Robertson *et al.* proposed that changing responses to spatially extended objects may modify their deficits. The results of two experiments involving reaching for and pointing to the center of objects, and another set of experiments involving pointing and grasping which were replicated (Edwards & Humphreys, 1999), suggested that some spatial information is lost when motor responses are initiated. That is, activation of the dorsal stream affects the ventral stream. Thus, *Innovation* is a time of translating theories into novel approaches for rehabilitation. Since *Innovation* is a time of exploration, within-subject and small group designs are typically utilized. Following this stage, a treatment is ready for the first formal phase of a human clinical trial.

Rothi's Revision of Robey's Model proposes that the purpose of a phase I clinical trial is *Evolution/Formalization*, or what was previously defined in this chapter as therapeutic effect. This stage is similar to phase I/II of Robey's five-phase model. Thus, the design methodologies are similar. During *Evolution/Formalization*, studies include participants who are chosen based upon highly constrained inclusion criteria in order to maximize the possibility of being able to detect any activity related to the intervention. Therefore they do not represent well the general population to which this treatment may eventually be applied. Multiple baseline within-subject experimental designs with replication across subjects and/or behaviors are utilized to enforce strict experimental control. Thus, the use of a comparison control group is not necessary. Within our example of treatments being developed for children with LLI is the further evolution of the treatment described in the study by Merzenich *et al.* (1996) in which treatment methods involving the

computer games and listening exercises were further formalized and applied to a series of children. This study resulted in findings of a significant effect of improvement in speech and language performance, providing justification for further investigation in the form of the next clinical trial phase.

Using our example of visual processing rehabilitation, Robertson *et al.* (1997) continued their research of unilateral neglect in a study that required individuals to lift the center of a rod placed horizontally in front of them. The nature of this procedure allowed proprioceptive and visual feedback when the rod was not lifted in the center. This rehabilitation technique resulted in the temporary improvement of neglect; thus a treatment effect was presumed to have occurred, at least transiently. When a positive outcome is attained during the *Evolution/Formalization* stage progression to the next stage is warranted.

A phase II clinical trial in Rothi's Revision of Robey's Model has one distinct purpose, establishing treatment *Efficacy*, as defined in the previous section. Thus, Rothi's Revision of Robey's Model phase II is akin to phase III/IV of Robey's model. At this stage, parallel group experiments with larger samples (the size of which are suggested by effect sizes established in phase I) are utilized. During *Efficacy* studies the size of the group may be large enough to consider multi-site data collection. The success of this is limited by the fact that reliability of providers varies and the protracted term of treatment research is already ripe for drift. However this threat would be greatly mitigated by the investment in the phase 1 period in the strict honing of the protocol and refinement into a formal structure. Thus again, we see the value of each phase to the success of each subsequent phase.

Again, Tallal and colleagues conducted a number of studies of *Efficacy* of their treatment approach as it was refined in early phase trials. In Tallal *et al.* (1996) the evolved formal protocol was utilized but a treatment control group was added. The results of this study replicated those of the Merzenich *et al.* (1996) study. Subsequently, a study of 500 participants across 35 sites was conducted to extend the population spectrum further. The training program was expanded and the duration/intensity revised. In addition, the treatment was applied to individuals with LLI and other comorbid language disorders. Results replicated the 1996 studies, showing improvement in auditory processing and speech-language skills in a larger, less constrained subset of children (Tallal *et al.*, 1997).

A phase III clinical trial, according to Rothi's Revision of Robey's Model, is a time for establishing treatment *Effectiveness*. Though considered part of phase IV/V of Robey's model, the methodology is much the same in that large, multi-site RCTs are appropriate. The goal is to establish that the treatment is applicable to as broad a spectrum of exemplars (people with the problem targeted) as possible. Miller *et al.* (1997) extended their research into *Effectiveness* by conducting a study using the established treatment in children with LLI who also had comorbidities including attention deficit disorder, dyslexia, autism and central auditory processing disorder. Similar positive outcomes were obtained in this population, suggesting that the treatment was appropriate for other developmental disabilities as well. This type of positive outcome in phase III leads to the final stage in the process of research development, Health Services Research.

Finally, the purpose of Health Services Research is *Delivery* and *Impact*, which encompasses research regarding the structure, process and outcome of applying an effective rehabilitation technique or method to persons suffering the consequences of a medical condition. *Delivery* is concerned with how a system (healthcare, social services, educational and so on) delivers an intervention and *Impact* addresses the effect an individual's participation in this rehabilitation program has on society in general. *Delivery* and *Impact* in Rothi's Revision of Robey's Model are synonymous with the concept of cost-effectiveness and cost–benefit in Robey's model. Since the efficacy of a treatment has already been established by this phase of study, the design requirements differ from previous phases. Large group or multiple-replication single subject studies

with large sample sizes and no external controls are appropriate. Meta-analyses may also be utilized to determine effectiveness (Robey & Schultz, 1998).

Cost-effectiveness compares the functional outcome of treatment (i.e., return to work) with the cost of providing that treatment (i.e., clinic costs). In regard to our examples of the evolution of the treatment of auditory temporal integration in children with LLI, no studies are yet available. However, a different example of this level of study is offered by Boysen & Wertz (1996) who provide a thoughtful account of the importance of determining cost-effectiveness of aphasia rehabilitation, asking the question "How much is a word worth?". According to these researchers, the estimated cost of efficacious aphasia treatment ranged from $2512 to $8500, depending on the medical setting and the location of the individual within the medical setting.

Impact can also be measured by the cost–benefit, or comparing the cost of a treatment to the financial contribution of the effect of that treatment to the economy. That is, if an individual participates in a treatment that costs approximately $8500 and is consequently able to return to work, what is the economic gain associated with this functional outcome? Other important aspects of cost–benefit include consumer satisfaction and quality of life, which are also included in phase V of Robey's model.

The influence of *Delivery* and *Impact* on public policy and legislation may also be addressed. For example, if a treatment is found to be effective at high intensity and short duration, how is that treatment delivered within a healthcare system that is set up to provide services at a low intensity and short duration? Should other methods of treatment delivery, such as robotics, artificial intelligence, telehealth or computers, be considered? The only way to answer these questions and accomplish successful service delivery is to conduct research that goes beyond establishing a treatment's efficacy to provide evidence that supports change in current systems of delivery and care policy.

Selecting outcome measures
in rehabilitation research

- A model of rehabilitation research is described.
- Selection of outcome measures are discussed in terms of the model and the phases of research.
- Barriers created by selecting inappropriate outcomes are discussed.

The practice of rehabilitation has long realized that those suffering chronic conditions associated with stroke and the like are best considered not only in the context of their health status, but most importantly in the context of their social and psychological circumstance. The science of rehabilitation is more recently moving toward a more integrated approach that includes not only an understanding of the symptoms of disease or injury but also the importance of performance, context of performance, and psychosocial issues based on conceptual models of health state such as the *International Classification of Function, Disability and Health* (ICF) model put forth by the World Health Organization (2001). The ICF is a model which allows rehabilitation practitioners and scientists to understand and measure outcomes by classifying functioning and disability associated with health conditions in ways that account for multiple perspectives. That is, the ICF differs from other approaches to healthcare in that it seeks to integrate aspects of both the medical model and social model. It proposes that disability is the result of (1) a problem with the individual due to a disease state, trauma or health condition (medical perspective) as well as (2) a problem created by society that is not directly linked to an individual attribute (social perspective). Additionally, the ICF model recognizes contextual factors that may positively or negatively influence health state.

The three domains of the ICF include body function and structures, activity and participation. Body function is defined as the physiological or psychological functions of body systems. Body structure refers to anatomical parts of the body. Deficits of body structure and function due to deviation or loss are called impairments. Methods for measurement

in this domain have become increasingly sophisticated and allow rehabilitation scientists to capture changes that occur at the physiologic level. Activity refers to execution of a task or action by the individual. Measurement in this domain is strictly associated with capacity to perform a task, such as ability to read a word. Participation refers to the ability to execute a task when performing life roles, such as reading words on a menu. Careful measurement is important because ability to execute a task (e.g., reading single words aloud) does not necessarily mean an individual will successfully execute that task while fulfilling life roles (e.g., comprehending the words indicating gender on public bathrooms and using this information to correctly distinguish their target), a distinction which is critical when considering the outcome of a treatment. Finally, contextual factors, such as environmental and personal factors, may influence an individual's performance either positively or negatively. For example, if an individual is motivated and seeks to engage in positive social behaviors but lives in a community that does not embrace his or her culture, that individual's health state is positively influenced by personal factors and negatively influenced by environmental factors. While contextual factors are often difficult to measure, they are an important part of rehabilitation and as such have gained more attention in recent years.

The ICF conceptualizes domains of functioning and disability at multiple levels simultaneously. Understanding these domains can aid rehabilitationists in selecting appropriate outcome measures, the importance of which is attested to in studies that have demonstrated that improvement in one domain does not predict improvement in another (Brandt & Pope, 1997; Jette, 2003). For example, a measure of impairment will not predict whether or not an individual will be able to participate in life roles, which is the ultimate outcome of rehabilitation (Cardol *et al.*, 2002; Perenboom & Chorus, 2003).

Interestingly, one of the greatest challenges in rehabilitation research is evaluating treatment outcomes. While we are overwhelmed with impairment level measures in cognitive research, there is a lack of options for measuring outcomes at other levels. Additionally, one should ask how we can effectively apply these multilevel medical/social perspectives with the distinctive questions being asked in each phase of clinical trial evolution. For example, would it be appropriate to ask the question of phase I (safety, feasibility and activity of treatment) yet use outcome measures at a participation level perspective? In this instance, the information provided by the outcome level and the question being asked are not compatible. Few have addressed the need to align outcome perspective with the experimental question and problems with outcome measures remain a major challenge to rehabilitation research. Utilization of inappropriate outcome measures may lead to invalid assumptions about treatment results. Thus, rehabilitation scientists must charge themselves with developing outcome measures that provide information to answer the questions posed in each stage of research.

Conclusion

We have experienced the dawning of a new era in rehabilitation research. The union of basic scientists and rehabilitation scientists has paved the way for translational research that brings new hope to cognitive rehabilitation. But we must be patient in our endeavors, keeping in mind that rehabilitation research is an evolutionary process. As rehabilitation scientists, we must remember that rehabilitation research progresses through a sequence of studies with unique questions that build upon each other. We must respect what each phase of research contributes to this maturational process. We must also remember that vigilance in our adherence to this process involves being careful to utilize the methods and outcome measures appropriate to each phase of research. And, finally, we must be advocates for a process of clinical trials rehabilitation research that endorses that each phase is valuable and necessary in order to realize the promise of what lies ahead.

Postscript: wisdom from a participant to those who perform rehabilitation research

I'm here to share some thoughts from the perspective of my personal experience as a subject/consumer of rehabilitation research. In this respect I thought I would share with you who I am as a "research subject" . . . (My) injury has a profound impact on my life, and on the lives of my family, friends and colleagues . . . If I did not suffer from such a condition, you would have little purpose or passion for devoting your efforts to alleviating suffering. I am a research subject . . . the sine qua non of your research, your funding, your resources, and your students. I am a researcher . . . my personal commitment, participation and effort is essential to the implementation of your intervention protocol. I am a teacher . . . I use feedback from my unique perspective as the individual experiencing both the medical condition and your intervention to inform and instruct students, nurses, technicians and yes . . . principal investigators . . . on my subjective experience of the intervention protocol. I am a collaborator . . . an essential member of the research team. I'm invested in the outcome of your research and the knowledge it generates . . . not only for the benefits I experience directly, but for the welfare of individuals suffering from my condition who may experience future benefits as a consequence of our collaboration . . . On behalf of all the subjects . . . and future beneficiaries . . . of your research efforts, I offer my deepest gratitude. Whether you are a funding agent, an administrator, a principal investigator or project staff . . . you each play an essential role in moving forward our ability to promote healing and alleviate suffering. I thank you for your involvement in this noble cause. (Schauble, 2004, participant in a study funded by NIH grant #K01HD01348-01 – A. Behrman, PI, VA BRRC and University of Florida.)

REFERENCES

Boysen, A. E., & Wertz, R. T. (1996). Clinical costs in aphasia treatment: how much is a word worth? In M. L. Lemme (Ed.), *Clinical Aphasiology*, **24**, 207–213. Austin, TX: PRO-ED.

Bradley, F., & Field, J. (1995). Evidence-based medicine: a response. *Lancet*, **346**, 838–839.

Brandt, E. N., Jr., & Pope, A. M. (1997). Models of disability and rehabilitation. In E. N. Brandt, & A. M. Pope (Eds.),

Enabling America: Assessing the Role of Rehabilitation Science and Engineering (pp. 24–39). Washington, DC: National Academy Press.

Cajal, R. Y. (1928). *Degeneration and Regeneration of the Nervous System*. Oxford, UK: Oxford University Press.

Cardol, M., de Jong, B. A., van den Bos, G. A. M. *et al.* (2002). Beyond disability: perceived participation in people with a chronic disabling condition. *Clinical Rehabilitation*, **16**, 27–35.

Cicerone, K. D., Dahlberg, C., Malec, J. F. *et al.* (2005). Evidence-based cognitive rehabilitation: updated review of the literature from 1998 through 2002. *Archives of Physical Medicine and Rehabilitation*, **86**, 1681–1692.

Concato, J., Shah, N., & Horwitz, R. I. (2000). Randomized, controlled trials, observational studies, and the hierarchy of research designs. *New England Journal of Medicine*, **342**, 1887–1892.

Edwards, M. G., & Humphreys, G. W. (1999). Pointing and grasping in unilateral visual neglect: effect of on-line visual feedback in grasping. *Neuropsychologia*, **37**, 959–973.

Finger, S. (1994). *Origins of Neuroscience: A History of Explorations into Brain Function*. New York, NY: Oxford University Press.

Frattali, C. M. (1998). Outcomes measurement: definitions, dimensions, and perspectives. In C. M. Frattali (Ed.), *Measuring Outcomes in Speech-Language Pathology* (pp. 1–27). New York, NY: Theime.

Goodale, M. A. (1996). One visual experience, many visual systems. In T. Inui & J. L. McClelland (Eds.), *Attention and Performance: Information Integration in Perception and Communication* (pp. 369–394). Cambridge, MA: MIT Press.

Goodale, M. A., & Milner, A. D. (1992). Separate visual pathways for perception and action. *Trends in Neurosciences*, **15**, 20–25.

Iggo, N. (1995). Evidence-based medicine: A response. *Lancet*, **346**, 839.

Jette, A. M. (2003). Assessing disability in studies on physical activity. *American Journal of Preventive Medicine*, **25**, Suppl. 2, 122–128.

Kleim, J. A. (2006). Can understanding basic principles of neural plasticity improve rehabilitation? *Academy of Neurologic Communications Sciences and Disorders*. ANCDS Annual Meeting, 15 November, Miami, FL.

Merzenich, M. M., & Jenkins, W. M. (1995). Cortical plasticity, learning, and learning dysfunction. In B. Julesz & I. Kovacs (Eds.), *Maturational Windows and Adult Cortical Plasticity, SFI Studies in the Sciences of Complexity (Vol. XXIII)* (pp. 247–272). Boston, MA: Addison-Wesley.

Merzenich, M. M., Jenkins, W. M., Johnston, P. *et al.* (1996). Temporal processing deficits of language-learning impaired children ameliorated by training. *Science*, **271**, 77–81.

Miller, S., Merzenich, M. M., Saunders, G. H., Jenkins, W. M., & Tallal, P. (1997). Language improvements with training of children with both attentional and language impairments. *Society for Neuroscience Abstracts*, **23**, 490.

Milner, A. D., & Goodale, M. A. (1995). *The Visual Brain in Action*. Oxford, UK: Oxford University Press.

Nagarajan, S. S., Wang, X., Merzenich, M. M. *et al.* (1998). Speech modifications algorithms used for training language learning-impaired children. *IEEE Transactions on Rehabilitation Engineering*, **6**, 257–268.

Perenboom, R. J. M., & Chorus, A. M. J. (2003). Measuring participation according to the International Classification of Functioning, Disability and Health. *Disability and Rehabilitation*, **25**, 577–587.

Robertson, I. H., Nico, D., & Hood, B. M. (1995). The intention to act improves unilateral left neglect: two demonstrations. *Neuroreport*, **7**, 246–248.

Robertson, I. H., Nico, D., & Hood, B. M. (1997). Believing what you feel: using proprioceptive feedback to reduce unilateral neglect. *Neuropsychology*, **11**, 53–58.

Robey, R. R., & Schultz, M. C. (1998). A model for conducting clinical-outcome research: an adaptation of the standard protocol for use in aphasiology. *Aphasiology*, **12**, 787–810.

Rothi, L. J. G. (2001). Neurophysiologic basis of rehabilitation. *Journal of Medical Speech-Language Pathology*, **9**, 117–127.

Rothi, L. J. G. (2006). Cognitive rehabilitation: the role of theoretical rationales and respect for the maturational process needed for our evidence. *Journal of Head Trauma Rehabilitation*, **21**, 194–197.

Sackett, D. L., Rosenberg, W. M. C., Gray, J. A. M., Haynes, R. B., & Richardson, W. S. (1996). Evidence-based medicine: what it is and what it isn't. *British Medical Journal*, **312**, 71–72.

Schauble, P. (2004). An invited keynote presentation at UF-VA Rehabilitation Research Day. *UF-VA Rehabilitation Research Day*. Gainesville, FL.

Tallal, P. (1980a). Auditory temporal perception, phonics, and reading disabilities in children. *Brain and Language*, **9**, 182–198.

Tallal, P. (1980b). Language and reading: some perceptual prerequisites. *Bulletin of the Orton Society*, **30**, 170–178.

Tallal, P., & Piercy, M. (1973a). Defects of non-verbal auditory perception in children with developmental aphasia. *Nature*, **241**, 468–469.

Tallal, P., & Piercy, M. (1973b). Developmental aphasia: impaired rate of non-verbal processing as a function of sensory modality. *Neuropsychologia*, **11**, 389–398.

Tallal, P., & Piercy, M. (1975). Developmental aphasia: the perception of brief vowels and extended stop consonants. *Neuropsychologia*, **13**, 69–74.

Tallal, P., Stark, R. E., & Mellits, D. (1985). The relationship between auditory temporal analysis and receptive language development: evidence from studies of developmental language disorder. *Neuropsychologia*, **23**, 527–534.

Tallal, P., Miller, S. L., Bedi, G. *et al.* (1996). Language comprehension in language-learning children improved with acoustically modified speech. *Science*, **271**, 81–84.

Tallal, P., Saunders, G. H., Miller, S. *et al.* (1997). Rapid training-driven improvement in language ability in autistic and PPD-NOS children. *Society for Neuroscience Abstracts*, **23**, 490.

Ungerleider, L. G., & Haxby, J. V. (1994). 'What' and 'where' in the human brain. *Current Opinion in Neurobiology*, **4**, 157–165.

World Health Organization (2001). *International Classification of Function, Disability and Health*. Geneva: WHO.

6

Outcome measurement in cognitive neurorehabilitation

Nadina Lincoln and Roshan das Nair

Introduction

The aim of this chapter is to consider the criteria for selecting outcome measures for evaluating the effects of cognitive neurorehabilitation. The *International Classification of Function, Disability and Health* (ICF) (World Health Organization, 2001) is used as a framework for deciding what to measure. The properties of the ideal outcome measure are discussed. Examples of outcome measures commonly used in clinical studies are provided and their strengths and limitations considered. The focus is on self-report measures rather than neuropsychological tests as these reflect the effect of cognitive rehabilitation on daily life.

Outcome

- Outcomes may be assessed at the levels of impairment, activity or participation.
- Activity measures are the most important outcomes for cognitive rehabilitation.
- Quality of life is best assessed as component domains rather than a single measure.

Rehabilitation may be considered in terms of process, structure and outcome (Donabedian, 1966). Process consists of the activities which are designed to improve the functioning of the individual, such as the treatment techniques used by members of the multidisciplinary team to foster recovery or adaptation. Structure refers to the facilities provided to enable the treatments to be administered, such as the environment, staff and equipment. Outcome refers to the result of the rehabilitation endeavor. It is the endpoint against which the effectiveness of rehabilitation is judged. In cognitive rehabilitation, the aim is to help the patient to function to the maximum level of ability possible within the constraints of deficits resulting from brain damage. In addition, that individual should be as contented and satisfied with his or her condition as is possible, and so should the relatives. The assessment of outcome is the means by which we determine whether rehabilitation has achieved these aims.

Measurement of outcome

The ICF (World Health Organization, 2001) is recognized as providing a useful framework for the selection of appropriate outcome measures (Heinemann, 2005; Jette & Haley, 2005; Mermis, 2005; Wade, 2003). The concepts are as follows.

(a) Body functions and deficits: these are impairments or the loss or abnormality of psychological, physiological or anatomical structure or function. They include cognitive deficits such as disorders of memory, attention and language.

(b) Activity limitation is the difficulties an individual may have in executing activities, including learning and applying knowledge; self-care; domestic life; interpersonal interactions; and community, social and civic life. It includes the effects of cognitive impairments on daily life, such as difficulties in telling the time and losing

Cognitive Neurorehabilitation, Second Edition: Evidence and Application, ed. Donald T. Stuss, Gordon Winocur and Ian H. Robertson. Published by Cambridge University Press. © Cambridge University Press 2008.

items around the home, and the disruption to interpersonal relationships that may occur following a head injury.

(c) Participation is the involvement in life situations at a societal level. It includes the social, cultural, economic and environmental effects of activity limitation.

An impairment, such as visual inattention, usually will give rise to an activity limitation, such as the inability to dress independently, which in turn may affect participation, through loss of personal independence. An effective rehabilitation program would reduce the impairments and the activity limitations which are consequent upon those impairments. In many instances, it is not possible to ameliorate the impairment, but nevertheless significant gains may be made by attempting directly to increase activity. Although it would be desirable to improve participation, this can rarely be achieved directly and may not entirely be within the remit of the rehabilitation service. Provided the activity limitation has been reduced, the assumption is that there will be a beneficial effect on participation.

Quality of life is an elusive outcome which relates to participation. Most assessments of quality of life incorporate several domains, which include both activities and participation. It is beyond the scope of assessment procedures to assess adequately all domains which contribute to quality of life and produce a satisfactory single quality-of-life measure. For this reason it does not seem practical even to attempt to assess general quality of life, but rather only the specific domains, even though improving the quality of life must be the ultimate goal of rehabilitation.

Selection of measures

- The psychometric properties of measures need to be considered.
- Measures of motor, sensory and cognitive impairment provide standardized descriptions of patients.
- Cognitive tests measure cognitive impairment and not the effect in daily life.

In order to choose an outcome measure it is important to know that the measure meets the requirements of a measurement tool. These requirements are:

(a) Validity: any measure must measure what it purports to measure. For example, measures of activities of daily living should include those activities people would consider to be essential for independence in daily life. Measures should relate to other measures of the same underlying ability and include all the relevant aspects of the attributes they measure. Hypotheses generated based on the measure should be upheld. For example, one would predict that head-injured people will do less well on a measure of memory than normal participants, and if this is supported it indicates that the measure has construct validity.

(b) Reliability: any outcome measure should provide the same information if used by different assessors (inter-rater reliability) or by the same assessor on different occasions (intra-rater reliability). If the assessment is to be used to monitor change it needs to have minimal practice effects and to show no variation simply as a result of repeating the assessment (test-retest reliability).

(c) Sensitivity: outcome measures in rehabilitation need to be sensitive to change, i.e., able to detect change in ability when change has occurred, and responsive to differences between rehabilitation programs.

(d) Practicality: the selection of outcome measures is dominated by practical constraints. An outcome measure must be short, easy to administer and acceptable to patients. Those measures which are tiring, detailed, intrusive or repetitive will not be tolerated. It must also be easy to communicate the findings to others.

Many studies evaluating the effects of rehabilitation have used single-case experimental designs. Measures are repeated frequently and therefore need to be very short, in order not to induce fatigue and not to interfere with the treatment program. They also need to have minimal practice effects so that stable baselines can be achieved. Alternative versions of tests may be used but few standardized tests have sufficient alternative versions available to be suitable for monitoring progress in single-case experimental designs. When using a randomized controlled trial to evaluate an intervention, it is necessary to use measures which have been used in other studies, so that comparisons between trials are possible. It is also important to include sufficient patients to be sure that a small difference in outcome has not been missed, yet from a patient's perspective even a small gain in function may be worthwhile. A common strategy to resolve this is to conduct a meta-analysis of several trials, which is facilitated by the use of a common outcome measure.

Measures of impairment

Cognitive rehabilitation is designed to improve cognitive abilities. Most cognitive impairments can be assessed by a range of measures but few have been designed as measures of outcome. Some cognitive assessments are intended as screening devices, to identify cognitive impairments which require further evaluation. Others are diagnostic tools, to detect cognitive impairment and differentiate particular impairments from each other. Assessments for screening or diagnostic purposes may not be suitable measures of outcome. Their validity will be based on their ability to classify and therefore those which give clear cut-off points will be most robust. In contrast outcome measures need to have continuous scales such that they are sensitive to changes in ability rather than whether a patient fits a particular category. Measures of specific cognitive impairments can be found in later chapters and therefore are not reviewed in detail here. However, impairments other than cognitive deficits may affect a patient's response to a cognitive rehabilitation program, and it is therefore appropriate to assess these. They will not be used as outcome assessments, as few cognitive rehabilitation techniques would be expected to decrease, for example,

motor impairments. However, the treatment of visual inattention could be predicted to reduce sensory inattention or visual field deficits. For this reason, such assessments are considered.

Motor function may be assessed using summed indices, such as the Rivermead Motor Assessment (Lincoln & Leadbitter, 1979) and the Motor Assessment Scale (Carr et al., 1985), to indicate the level of motor impairment. The Rivermead Mobility Index (Collen et al., 1991) is a comprehensive assessment which includes sitting, transfers, walking and getting up stairs. It has been used as an outcome measure in rehabilitation studies on stroke (Wade et al., 1992) and is sensitive to change in people with multiple sclerosis (Vaney et al., 1996). The Expanded Disability Status Scale (Kurtzke, 1983) and Guys Neurological Disability Scale (Sharrack & Hughes, 1999), despite their names, are predominantly measures of impairments in multiple sclerosis and include aspects of motor function.

Sensory impairment is assessed as part of a clinical examination but there are only a few standardized scales available (Lincoln et al., 1998, Winward et al., 2002). Tactile inattention, proprioception and stereognosis may affect the outcome of cognitive rehabilitation, so it is important that they are assessed. Visual impairment will affect patients' ability to participate in cognitive rehabilitation but conventional acuity measurement techniques require language skills, and visual field assessment may be confounded by the presence of inattention (Walker et al., 1991).

Cognitive impairments are assessed by a wide range of psychological tests. Assessments are available to determine the severity of deficits in language, perception, memory, reasoning, attention, movement disorders and other cognitive functions. Standardized cognitive tests may assess "pure" levels of impairment specific to one cognitive domain. For example, memory can be assessed in terms of encoding ability or working memory capacity. However, such tests may not be of much value as outcome measures. In order for a cognitive assessment to be used as an outcome measure, it must be sensitive to changes over time but have minimal practice effects. For example, although recognition memory tests are sensitive to differences between individuals, they are not appropriate for evaluating change unless there are parallel versions available. Many cognitive tests, while reliable over time, will show sufficient improvement simply as a result of practice to make them insensitive to small differences between interventions.

Activities

The main aim of cognitive rehabilitation is an increase in activity, which includes functional, cognitive, emotional and social activities.

- The most important outcomes for cognitive rehabilitation are cognitive activities, yet the measurement of these is poorly developed.
- Independence in activities of daily living and mood measures provide proxy measures for the outcome of cognitive rehabilitation.
- The Extended Activities of Daily Living (EADL) and Functional Independence Measure (FIM) are the most suitable measures of independence in activities of daily living.
- Mood should be assessed on questionnaires designed to detect change.

Limitations in functional activities

The ability to perform functional activities in everyday life may be assessed by scales of activities of daily living (ADL), including basic personal self-care skills and instrumental activities of daily living. The choice of scale is governed by practical considerations and there is little consensus on the "best" measures (Jette & Haley, 2005). Most ADL scales consist of summed indices, but concerns have been expressed about treating such scales as ordinal, though some have been demonstrated to be acceptable using Guttman scaling, e.g., EADL and Barthel, or a Rasch model, e.g., Barthel and FIM.

The Barthel Index (Mahoney & Barthel, 1965) is a widely used measure of personal activities of daily living which has almost become the gold standard for stroke rehabilitation studies. It is sensitive to differences between rehabilitation interventions (Indredavik et al., 1991) and reliable when administered verbally or by post. It is sensitive in the inpatient phase of rehabilitation (Houlden et al., 2006) but less sensitive to change in community-based patients. The original index was scored on a 0–100 scale, but this implies a spurious degree of accuracy, and the revised 20-point version (Collin et al., 1988) has become the standard. The main limitation is its ceiling effect; therefore, rehabilitation studies may include a measure of instrumental activities of daily living in addition to the Barthel Index.

Two widely used measures of instrumental activities of daily living are the Nottingham Extended Activities of Daily Living (EADL) scale (Nouri & Lincoln, 1987) and the Frenchay Activities Index (Holbrook & Skilbeck, 1983). Each includes domestic activities such as preparing meals and washing up, mobility outside the home, leisure and social activities. Both scales have been found to be sensitive to differences between rehabilitation interventions (Forster & Young, 1996; Fuller et al., 1996). The EADL is suitable for multi-center studies as it has been validated for postal administration. Cognitive rehabilitation programs are more likely to have an effect on instrumental activities of daily living than on personal self-care skills. Therefore, these scales may be appropriate for assessing the generalization of cognitive retraining to daily life skills.

The main measure of personal ADL used with a wide range of patients is the Functional Independence Measure (FIM) (Granger et al., 1986). This covers personal self-care and motor activities and has cognitive items on comprehension, expression, social interaction, problem solving and memory. Inter-rater reliability has been found to be higher for physical disability than communication and social cognition sections (Brosseau & Wolfson, 1994; Kidd et al., 1995; Pollak et al., 1996). Because the effect of a cognitive rehabilitation program is most relevant to these items, further improvement to the reliability is needed. Rasch analysis has indicated that the motor and cognitive items form two distinct scales, though this has been questioned by Dickson & Kohler (1996), who identified six factors from a factor analysis of the FIM. Differential item functioning has also been identified in different patient groups (Dallmeijer *et al.*, 2005), particularly in the motor domain and disordered thresholds, leading to the suggestion that the number of response categories should be reduced (Dallmeijer *et al.*, 2005; Nilsson *et al.*, 2005). The cognitive scale has shown ceiling effects in people with multiple sclerosis (van der Putten *et al.*, 1999) and administration requires prolonged observation of the patient, which means the scale would be difficult to administer in the context of a randomized controlled trial by an independent assessor. Houlden *et al.* (2006) demonstrated comparable responsiveness between the Barthel and the FIM.

The Functional Assessment Measure (FAM), which was developed to assess the specific problems of brain-injured patients (Hall *et al.*, 1993), contains additional items emphasizing cognitive, communicative and psychosocial function. McPherson *et al.* (1996) found high inter-rater reliability, but greatest discrepancies occurred on cognitive, communication and behavioral items. Hobart *et al.* (2001b) compared the psychometric properties of the Barthel, FIM and FIM+FAM and found them similar, and highlighted that the FIM and FIM+FAM have significant redundancy of items and confer few advantages over the shorter simpler Barthel for patients receiving inpatient rehabilitation. For the FIM+FAM to be used to evaluate the outcome of cognitive rehabilitation, further work is needed to check the reliability and sensitivity.

The Rivermead Head Injury Follow-Up Questionnaire (Crawford *et al.*, 1996) was developed as an outcome measure for patients with mild to moderate head injury. It is short, simple and can be administered by post or at interview. It was found to have good inter-rater reliability, to be sensitive to changes over time and to detect differences in outcome in a randomized controlled trial (Wade *et al.*, 1997). The Brain Injury Community Rehabilitation Outcome 39 (BICRO39) (Powell *et al.*, 1998) covers aspects of personal and social functioning for brain

injury patients living in the community. It has good test-retest and inter-rater reliability and has also been found to be sensitive to the effects of intervention (Powell *et al.*, 2002).

Measures of activity for people with multiple sclerosis seem to be few. The FIM (Brosseau & Wolfson, 1994) and Assessment of Motor and Process Skills (AMPS) (Doble *et al.*, 1994) and Functional Assessment of MS (Cella *et al.*, 1996) have been used, but there are few data to indicate the most appropriate measure for this group. The AMPS requires patients to perform tasks and so takes longer, but it covers instrumental activities of daily living, which may be more important to assess than personal activities of daily living, when the effects of cognitive rehabilitation are being evaluated and has adequate reliability (Doble *et al.*, 1999).

In addition there are general rehabilitation outcome measures, which are predominantly measures of activity limitation. The Sickness Impact Profile (Bergner *et al.*, 1981), the British version of which is the Functional Limitations Profile (Charlton *et al.*, 1983), assesses the impact of sickness on daily activities and behavior. It provides subscales in 12 areas, including ambulation, body care and household management. It is lengthy and complex to administer.

Mood

Although mood disorders might be considered either as an impairment, i.e., a direct consequence of some underlying pathology, or as a consequence of impairments, in the context of cognitive rehabilitation they are probably best considered as emotional disabilities. Many mood scales are available but few have been validated for patients with neurological disorders. Those which have items affected by physical disability are likely to be insensitive to mood changes. Many mood questionnaires were developed as screening devices to detect significant levels of depression or anxiety. To evaluate the outcome of cognitive neurorehabilitation, measures need to be sensitive to change and therefore not all screening questionnaires will be suitable for this purpose.

The Hospital Anxiety and Depression Scale (Zigmund & Snaith, 1983) is a short, easy to complete measure which provides separate scores for both anxiety and depression. Although it was designed for hospitalized medically ill patients, several items reflect physical disability. It is probably more suitable as a screening measure than for assessing outcome. In contrast, other scales, such as the Beck Depression Inventory II (Beck *et al.*, 1996) and Center for Epidemiologic Studies Depression Scale (Radloff, 1977), were designed as measures of the severity of depressive symptoms. They are likely to be more sensitive to the effects of intervention than measures designed for screening purposes (Turner-Stokes & Hassan, 2002).

Cognitive rehabilitation would be expected to improve mood. If patients' cognitive performance improves following treatment, they will probably suffer from less depression, be less anxious and suffer less general distress. The most widely used measure of general psychological distress is the General Health Questionnaire (Goldberg & Williams, 1988). The GHQ28 and GHQ30 have been found to be sensitive to the effects of psychological interventions in randomized controlled trials (Juby *et al.*, 1996, Watkins *et al.*, 2007); the GHQ12 is shorter but its sensitivity to the effects of intervention in neurological patients has not been established.

One problem in assessing mood in neurological patients is that many have communication difficulties. The Stroke Aphasic Depression Questionnaire (Lincoln *et al.*, 2000; Sutcliffe & Lincoln, 1998) was developed to assess mood in aphasic patients. Items that could be observed by relatives or nursing staff were taken from mood questionnaires and rephrased in terms of observable behaviors. The Visual Analog Mood Scales (Stern, 1997) provide a pictorial method of assessing mood. The Neuropsychiatric Inventory (Cummings *et al.*, 1994) was developed to assess mood disorders in people with dementia and has been used as an outcome measure for pharmacological treatments in dementia (Ringman & Cummings, Chapter 19, this

volume). These scales have good validity and reliability, but their sensitivity to change in response to cognitive rehabilitation has not been established.

Limitations in cognitive activities

Limitations in cognitive activities are a major concern for patients and carers and are primary targets for cognitive rehabilitation programs. (For further discussion see Cicerone, Chapter 7, this volume.) Outcome is assessed in several ways, including semi-structured interviews, questionnaires or patient observation. The most common strategy has been to employ a questionnaire that includes items on the behavioral manifestations of cognitive impairments. These may be completed by patients or carers, to determine the subjective effects of cognitive impairment on daily life. These are important indicators of the outcome of cognitive neurorehabilitation, but there are few scales available and not all possible cognitive deficits are included. Another problem is the reliability of eliciting this kind of information from individuals who may not be able to judge their functioning accurately due to their cognitive deficits. For example, frontal lobe damage after brain injury results in impaired metacognitive processing (Hanten *et al.*, 2000), patients with MS underestimate their memory problems on questionnaires (Beatty & Monson, 1991) and patients with memory problems and epilepsy, tended to overstate memory problems on questionnaires, compared with "objective" tests of memory (Piazzini *et al.*, 2001). Semi-structured interviews may provide valuable information regarding the patients' experience of cognitive rehabilitation, but may not be accurate measures of outcome.

Ecological validity

Cognitive assessments can use ecologically valid tests that assess cognitive functions in the context of everyday tasks. For example, the Rivermead Behavioral Memory Test (RBMT) (Wilson *et al.*, 1985) has tasks, such as remembering where an object was placed in a room or remembering to do things at appointed times. This task-based performance is related to a number of cognitive functions, and not a specific one, but provides a clinical assessment which approximates the patient's functioning in everyday life. Two approaches to ecological validity (Franzen & Wilhelm, 1996) have been adopted. One is developing tests with high face validity which simulate daily tasks (requiring the underlying cognitive functions to complete these tasks to be intact). The other relates performance on pre-existing (traditional) tests to daily functioning (Chaytor & Schmitter-Edgecombe, 2003). Assessments of cognitive function which are designed to reflect the cognitive skills needed in everyday life, such as the RBMT (Wilson *et al.*, 1985), Behavioral Inattention Test (BIT) (Wilson *et al.*, 1987), Behavioral Assessment of the Dysexecutive Syndrome (Wilson *et al.*, 1996) and Test of Everyday Attention (TEA) (Robertson *et al.*, 1994), may be considered to measure limitations to cognitive activities rather than impairment. They include items which are likely to be predictive of everyday performance rather than assessing everyday performance itself. Although they have the advantage of ecological validity, unlike many assessments of cognitive impairment, they are probably not true measures of activity limitation, because they comprise artificial activities and not those which people necessarily perform on a daily basis. Ecologically valid tests of memory and attention (e.g., RBMT and TEA) have been found to be better at predicting functional disability than memory questionnaires (Higginson *et al.*, 2000). However, there is a trade-off when developing ecologically valid tests: the more they approximate real-world scenarios, the less structured they are; and consequently have poor psychometric properties (Van Zomeren & Spikman, 2003). Assessments in the main cognitive domains will be considered.

Memory

Subjective memory impairment has been investigated using the Everyday Memory Questionnaire (EMQ) (Sunderland *et al.*, 1983) in studies of stroke (Tinson & Lincoln, 1987), head injury (Sunderland *et al.*, 1984) and MS (Taylor, 1990). The questionnaire has been used both for patients to assess their own problems and for relatives. Five factors, reflecting the underlying memory processes, have been identified in healthy individuals: retrieval, task monitoring, conversational monitoring, spatial memory and memory for activities (Cornish, 2000). The EMQ has validity in that it correlates moderately with tests of memory, and its reliability is acceptable, though not good. The Subjective Memory Assessment Questionnaire (Davis *et al.*, 1995) is short and has been validated for stroke patients. The Memory Failures Questionnaire (Gilewski *et al.*, 1990) contains more items in four subscales, including one on the use of mnemonics. There is conflicting evidence on the extent to which it correlates with prospective memory (Kinsella *et al.*, 1996; Zelinski *et al.*, 1990).

In general, memory questionnaires appear to have adequate reliability, but low validity, particularly when completed by patients (Ruisel, 1991). To complement memory questionnaires, and to compensate for some of their limitations, memory "performance" tests are frequently used. Such tests, which approximate real-life scenarios, may be more valid measures of rehabilitation outcome than traditional memory tests. The Rivermead Behavioral Memory Test (RBMT) (Wilson *et al.*, 1985) was developed to assess everyday memory problems in individuals with acquired brain damage. The extended version (RBMT-E) (Wilson *et al.*, 1998), with two parallel forms, is sensitive to milder memory deficits. It has age norms (years 11–95), and has been translated into many languages.

Visual neglect

The behavioral manifestations of visual neglect have also been assessed by questionnaires. Towle & Lincoln (1991) developed the Problems in Everyday Living Questionnaire as a subjective measure of visual neglect. The patient has to report how often problems, such as bumping into door frames and making errors when dialling the telephone, have occurred. The Catherine Bergego Scale (Azouvi *et al.*, 1996) contains ten items which the patient has to rate according to their severity. It has been found to have good inter-rater reliability and validity. Test-retest reliability and sensitivity to change need to be checked. Neither scale has been demonstrated to be sensitive to differences between interventions. An alternative approach has been to ask patients to carry out practical tasks and to observe their performance. Zoccolotti *et al.* (1992) described a scale which differentiated tasks involving the exploration of external space, dealing cards and serving tea, from those which related to one's own body, using a comb or razor. The scales were found to have high inter-rater reliability and internal consistency, and concurrent validity in relation to conventional impairment measures.

An ecologically valid test of unilateral visual neglect that reflects patients' daily life is the Behavioral Inattention Test (BIT) (Wilson *et al.*, 1987). This short, easy to administer test has six conventional tests (such as line cancellation) and nine behavioral tests (such as telephone dialling). Hartman-Maeir & Katz (1995) found construct and predictive validity of most of the behavioral subtests as functional measures of neglect. To assess the effects of domain-specific interventions, tests of neglect for body space, peripersonal space and locomotor space may be used. Robertson *et al.* (1998) used a variant of the Hair Combing Task (Zoccolotti & Judica, 1992) to measure neglect of body space, the Baking Tray Task (Tham & Tegnér, 1996) to assess peripersonal space and a tailor-made navigation task to assess locomotor neglect. The Shapes Task (Maddicks *et al.*, 2003), in which the patient has to name 20 shapes on a wall three meters away, has also been used for this purpose. Although some neglect tests have been designed for diagnosis, imaginative adaptations can render them suitable outcome measures.

Attention

van Zomeren & Spikman (2003) discussed impairments of attention in terms of hemi-neglect, mental slowness, lack of control (focused and divided attention) and poor sustained attention. Some traditional tests, e.g., the Stroop Color Word and Trail Making, have been used to assess these, but as tests of impairment, they can only be used as proxy measures of rehabilitation outcome. An alternative has been to use questionnaires.

Changes associated with attention training have been assessed with the Attention Questionnaire (Sohlberg *et al.*, 2000), the Dysexecutive Questionnaire (Wilson *et al.*, 1996) and the Attention Rating and Monitoring Scale (ARMS) (Cicerone, 2002). The latter consists of 15 items measuring concentration, mental effort, and cognitive symptoms associated with attentional difficulties. An observational rating scale, the Moss Attention Rating Scale (MARS) (Whyte *et al.*, 2003) is completed by occupational and physical therapists. The inter-rater reliability is good but further evaluation of reliability and validity is needed.

The Rating Scale of Attentional Behavior (Ponsford & Kinsella, 1991) showed moderate correlations with neuropsychological measures of attention, good internal consistency and intrarater reliability but agreement between raters working in different contexts was less satisfactory. Scores showed change over time with treatment but the correspondence to neuropsychological measures of attention was low. Discrepancies seemed to occur as a result of emotional factors and expectations of the therapists. This highlights the difficulty of validating such scales, and Ponsford & Kinsella (1991) suggested that more concrete descriptions of scale items might reduce this subjectivity.

The Test of Everyday Attention (TEA) (Robertson *et al.*, 1994) is an ecologically valid test of selective attention, sustained attention and attentional switching. It consists of eight subtests that approximate attentional tasks carried out by people in daily life, such as listening to winning numbers in a lottery, searching telephone directories and scanning maps. It takes about 60 minutes to complete and normative data exists for ages 18–80. It has three parallel forms and high test-retest reliability. Discriminative validity has been established in brain injury (Chan, 2000).

Executive functions

People with impairment of executive function display problems in initiating and stopping behaviors, shifting set, paying attention and being aware of themselves and others. Cognitive rehabilitation of executive dysfunctions has aimed to reduce the barriers to participation and activity limitations. Worthington (2005) recommended that outcomes be measurable as "socially meaningful (as opposed to statistically significant) change" (p. 259). A rating scale for problem-solving behaviors was developed by Von Cramon et al. (1991) to evaluate the behavioral effects of treatment. Aspects of problem-solving behavior were rated according to the frequency of their occurrence. The scale was found to be reliable and sensitive to improvements.

The Behavioral Assessment of the Dysexecutive Syndrome (BADS) (Wilson et al., 1996) assesses problems related to planning, organizing, initiating, monitoring and adapting behavior. It comprises six tests which simulate real-life scenarios. The Dysexecutive Questionnaire (DEX) has 20 items on a Likert scale that describe behaviors related to the dysexecutive syndrome. Patient and carer versions exist. Reliability has been evaluated by the authors, and validity by other small studies (Norris & Tate, 2000). Significant correlations have been reported between executive tests, such as Wisconsin Card Sorting (0.37) and phonemic fluency (0.35), and ratings on the DEX (Burgess et al., 1998), and with the Disability Rating Scale (0.52) (Hanks et al., 1999).

Language

The effects of language problems on everyday life have been investigated in detail. The Communicative Activities for Daily Living (Holland et al., 1999) presents language tasks through role play. This is more sensitive to communication strengths than traditional testing but is not a naturalistic observation. The Functional Communication Profile (Sarno, 1969) and Edinburgh Functional Communication Profile (Skinner et al., 1984) provide ratings of everyday language behavior but are very subjective. The Profile of Functional Impairment in Communication (Linscott et al., 1996) contains a detailed analysis of communication skills but requires an experienced assessor. Aphasia batteries have been employed as measures of change over time, but these are not sensitive (Weniger, 1990), with some subtests being sensitive but having few stimuli, and overall scores being too generic (Nickels, 2005).

Assessment of general cognitive functions

In addition there are scales which do not attempt to assess specific cognitive domains but consider cognitive ability in general.

The Level of Cognitive Functioning Scale (LCFS) (Hagen et al., 1972) (also referred to as Rancho Los Amigo Scale) has been used to assess cognitive functioning in post-coma patients. This scale has an 8-level classification of functioning, ranging from "no response" to "purposeful-appropriate." It has good test-retest and inter-rater reliability and concurrent and predictive validity (Gouvier et al., 1987). However, the categories are broad, making detection of small changes difficult.

The Cognitive Failures Questionnaire (CFQ) (Broadbent et al., 1982) is a 5-point self-rating scale that determines the frequency with which cognitive slips (arising from failures in perception, memory, and motor functions) have occurred, with versions for both patients and significant others. It is less specific to memory and includes the behavioral consequences of other cognitive deficits. It has been used as a measure of outcome of treatment, including light therapy for neuropsychological functions in seasonal affective disorder (Michalon et al., 1997) and cognitive assessment in stroke rehabilitation (McKinney et al., 2002). A similar scale, the Cognitive Log (Cog-Log) (Alderson & Novack, 2003), is suitable for assessing recovery of higher neuropsychological processes with inpatients. The Log assesses verbal recall, attention, working memory, motor sequencing and response inhibition, and is reported to have good inter-rater reliability and high internal consistency (Alderson & Novack, 2003).

Limitation in social and occupational activities

Behavioral and psychosocial problems are common consequences of traumatic brain injury and need to be assessed, particularly in the later stages of rehabilitation (see Dawson & Winocur, Chapter 14, this volume). Assessment procedures have been criticised for their lack of rigorous evaluation (Hall, 1992). The Neurobehavioral Rating Scale (Levin et al., 1987) is based on behavior, symptoms and skills measured in a structured clinical setting. The Neurobehavioral Functioning Inventory can be used with informants to record their perceptions of everyday problems (Kreutzer et al., 1996). Neither scale has well-established reliability or validity nor shown to be a sensitive indicator of rehabilitation outcome. However, the scales would seem to be worth developing further as they tap the activity limitation associated with cognitive impairment.

Participation

- There are few measures of participation.
- The best developed measures are the London Handicap Scale and Short Form 36.
- Global measures which include impairment, activity and participation are unlikely to be sensitive to the effects of cognitive rehabilitation.

Although it is unlikely that cognitive rehabilitation will have a direct effect on participation, because multiple factors will determine participation and cognitive problems are only one of many, it may be useful to assess participation as an effect of an overall rehabilitation package. Several measures have recently been developed (Heinemann, 2005) and some overlap with indicators of quality of life. Participation is subjective and inherently more difficult to measure than activity limitation, particularly in people with cognitive impairments.

The London Handicap Scale (Harwood et al., 1994) generates a profile of handicaps in the six survival roles: orientation, physical independence, mobility, occupation of time, social integration and economic self-sufficiency and an overall severity score. Other potential measures include the Community Integration measure (McColl et al., 2001), Craig Handicap Assessment and Reporting Technique (Whiteneck et al., 1992) and MS Impact Scale (Hobart et al., 2001a).

Generic measures of quality of life may also be used as indicators of participation. The Short Form 36 (Stewart & Ware, 1992) is a short questionnaire with good construct validity (Ware et al., 1993). However, there are doubts about its applicability with the elderly (Hill & Harries, 1994) and it has floor effects in physically disabled groups (Freeman et al., 1996). Wade (2003) questioned whether measurement of quality of life was appropriate in the context of rehabilitation.

Future developments

- The psychometric properties of most measures need further evaluation.
- Activity measures are needed for the evaluation of outcome in single case experimental design studies.
- Researchers conducting randomized controled trials should attempt to reach consensus on a few standard activity measures in order to facilitate meta-analyses.

For each of the measures mentioned, further work is needed to establish the validity and reliability of the scale. In particular, the validity is often only established with one diagnostic group. Validation studies should be carried out in several groups of patients to confirm the underlying construct. The reliability needs to be checked in a variety of situations (inpatient, outpatient, hospital, community), conditions and over a variety of time intervals. For most scales this task has hardly yet begun. Sensitivity to the effects of intervention will not be established until there are far more efficacy studies. Most single case experimental design studies use measures of impairment to assess the effect of intervention. However, it is the effect on daily life that is of most concern to patients and their families. Therefore, activity measures need to be developed for use in this context. Few of the measures described above are sensitive to the small changes in ability that need to be detected and many are too long to be administered with the frequency that is necessary in single case experimental design studies. The alternative approach to treatment evaluation is the randomized controlled trial. Several measures described above have been found to be sensitive to differences between rehabilitation procedures in randomized controlled trials. However, there have been few well-designed, methodologically sound trials of cognitive rehabilitation (see Cicerone, Chapter 7, this volume; Lincoln & Bowen 2006). It is hard to recruit sufficient patients within a single center; therefore multi-center trials of cognitive rehabilitation are needed. This requires consensus about which outcome measure to use. In addition, consistency of outcome measures is important for meta-analysis. The main way forward, therefore, seems to be to agree on a group of outcome measures suitable for trials of cognitive neurorehabilitation. These measures need to be refined in terms of their psychometric properties. If this is achieved in the context of research, it will also then be possible to use the measures for the audit of clinical services and the evaluation of the progress of an individual patient in a rehabilitation setting.

Conclusions

Standardized measures are available for evaluating the outcome of cognitive neurorehabilitation. These include measures at the levels of impairment, activity and participation. At each level, the measures chosen should be reliable, valid, sensitive to the effects of intervention and consistent with those used by other researchers. There is a particular need for the development of measures of limitations in cognitive activities.

REFERENCES

Alderson, A. L., & Novack, T. A. (2003). Reliable serial measurement of cognitive processes in rehabilitation: the cognitive log. *Archives of Physical Medicine and Rehabilitation*, **84**, 668–672.

Azouvi, P., Marchal, F., Samuel, C. *et al.* (1996). Functional consequences and awareness of unilateral neglect: study of an evaluation scale. *Neuropsychological Rehabilitation*, **6**, 133–150.

Beatty, W. W., & Monson, N. (1991). Metamemory in multiple sclerosis. *Journal of Clinical and Experimental Neuropsychology*, **13**, 309–327.

Beck, A. T., Steer, R. A., & Brown, G. K. (1996). *Beck Depression Inventory Manual (2nd Edition)*. San Antonio, TX: The Psychological Corporation.

Bergner, M., Bobbitt, R. A., Carter, W. B., & Gilson, B. S. (1981). The Sickness Impact Profile: development and final revision of a health status measure. *Medical Care*, **19**, 787–805.

Broadbent, D. E., Cooper, P. F., Fitzgerald, P., & Parkes, K. R. (1982). The Cognitive Failures Questionnaire (CFQ) and its correlates. *British Journal of Clinical Psychology*, **21**, 1–16.

Brosseau, L., & Wolfson, C. (1994). The inter-rater reliability and construct validity of the Functional Independence Measure for multiple sclerosis subjects. *Clinical Rehabilitation*, **8**, 107–115.

Burgess, P. W., Alderman, N., Evans, J., Emslie, H., & Wilson, B. A. (1998). The ecological validity of tests of executive function. *Journal of the International Neuropsychological Society*, **4**, 547–558.

Carr, J. H., Shepherd, R. B., Nordholm, L., & Lynne, D. (1985). Investigation of a new motor assessment scale for stroke patients. *Physical Therapy*, **65**, 175–180.

Cella, D. F., Dineen, K., Arnason, B. *et al.* (1996). Validation of the Functional Assessment of Multiple Sclerosis quality of life instrument. *Neurology*, **47**, 129–139.

Chan, R. C. K. (2000). Attentional deficits in patients with closed head injury: a further study to the discriminative validity of the test of everyday attention. *Brain Injury*, **14**, 227–236.

Charlton, J. R. H., Patrick, D. L., & Peach, H. (1983). Use of multi-variate measures of disability in health surveys. *Journal of Epidemiology and Community Health*, **37**, 296–304.

Chaytor, N., & Schmitter-Edgecombe, M. (2003). The ecological validity of neuropsychological tests: a review of the literature on everyday cognitive skills. *Neuropsychological Review*, **13**, 181–197.

Cicerone, K. D. (2002). Remediation of 'working attention' in mild traumatic brain injury. *Brain Injury,* **16**, 185–195.

Collen, F. M., Wade, D. T., Robb, G. F., & Bradshaw, C. M. (1991). The Rivermead Mobility Index: a further development of the Rivermead Motor Assessment. *International Disability Studies,* **13**, 50–54.

Collin, C., Wade, D. T., Davis, S., & Home, V. (1988). The Barthel Index: a reliability study. *International Disability Studies,* **10**, 61–63.

Cornish, I. M. (2000). Factor structure of the Everyday Memory Questionnaire. *British Journal of Psychology,* **91**, 427–438.

Crawford, S., Wenden, F. J., & Wade, D. T. (1996). The Rivermead Head Injury Follow-up Questionnaire: a study of a new rating scale and other measures to evaluate outcome after head injury. *Journal of Neurology, Neurosurgery, and Psychiatry,* **60**, 510–514.

Cummings, J. L., Mega, M., Gray, K. *et al.* (1994). The Neuropsychiatric Inventory: comprehensive assessment of psychopathology in dementia. *Neurology,* **44**, 2308–2314.

Dallmeijer, A., Dekker, J., Roorda, L. *et al.* (2005). Differential item functioning of the functional independence measure in higher performing neurological patients. *Journal of Rehabilitation Medicine,* **37**, 346–352.

Davis, A. M., Cockburn, J. M., Wade, D. T., & Smith, P. T. (1995). A subjective memory assessment questionnaire for use with elderly people after stroke. *Clinical Rehabilitation,* **9**, 238–244.

Dickson, H. G., & Kohler, F. (1996). The multi-dimensionality of the FIM motor items precludes an interval scaling using Rasch analysis. *Scandinavian Journal of Rehabilitation Medicine,* **26**, 159–162.

Doble, S. E., Fisk, J. D., Fisher, A. G., Ritvo, P. O., & Murray, T. J. (1994). Functional competence of community dwelling persons with multiple sclerosis using the assessment of motor and process skills. *Archives of Physical Medicine and Rehabilitation,* **75**, 843–851.

Doble, S. E., Fisk, J. D., Lewis, M., & Rockwood, K. (1999). Test-retest reliability of the assessment of motor and process skills in elderly adults. *Occupational Therapy Journal of Research,* **19**, 203–215.

Donabedian, A. (1966). Evaluating the quality of medical care. *Evaluating the Quality of Medical Care,* **44**, 166–206.

Forster, A., & Young, J. (1996). Specialist nurse support for patients with stroke in the community: a randomised controlled trial. *British Medical Journal,* **312**, 1642–1646.

Franzen, M. D., & Wilhelm, K. L. (1996). Conceptual foundations of ecological validity in neuropsychology. In R. J. Sbordone & C. J. Long (Eds.), *Ecological Validity of Neuropsychological Testing* (pp. 91–112). Delray Beach, FL: GR Press/St Lucie Press.

Freeman, J. A., Langdon, D. W., & Thompson, A. J. (1996). Health related quality of life in people with multiple sclerosis undergoing in-patient rehabilitation. *Journal of Neurologic Rehabilitation,* **10**, 185–194.

Fuller, K. J., Dawson, K., & Wiles, C. M. (1996). Physiotherapy in chronic multiple sclerosis: a controlled trial. *Clinical Rehabilitation,* **10**, 195–204.

Gilewski, M. J., Zelinski, E. M., & Schaie, K. W. (1990). The Memory Functioning Questionnaire for assessment of memory complaints in adulthood and old age. *Psychology and Aging,* **5**, 482–490.

Goldberg, D., & Williams, P. (1988). *A User's Guide to the General Health Questionnaire.* Windsor, UK: NFER-Nelson.

Gouvier, W. D., Blanton, P. D., LaPorte, K. K., & Nepomuceno, C. (1987). Reliability and validity of the Disability Rating Scale and the Levels of Cognitive Functioning Scale in monitoring recovery from severe head injury. *Archives of Physical Medicine and Rehabilitation,* **68**, 94–97.

Granger, C. V., Hamilton, B. B., & Sherwin, F. S. (1986). *Guide for Use of the Uniform Data Set for Medical Rehabilitation.* Buffalo, NY: Department of Rehabilitation Medicine, Buffalo General Hospital.

Hagen, C., Malkmus, D., & Durham, P. (1972). *Levels of Cognitive Functioning.* Downey, CA: Rancho Los Amigos Hospital.

Hall, K. M. (1992). Overview of functional assessment scales in brain injury rehabilitation. *Neurorehabilitation,* **2**, 98–113.

Hall, K. M., Hamilton, B. B., Gordon, W. A., & Zasler, N. D. (1993). Characteristics and comparisons of functional assessment indices: Disability Rating Scale, Functional Independence Measure and Functional Assessment Measure. *Head Trauma Rehabilitation,* **8**, 60–71.

Hanks, R. A., Rapport, L. J., Millis, S. R., & Deshpande, S. A. (1999). Measures of executive functioning as predictors of functional ability and social integration in a rehabilitation sample. *Archives of Physical Medicine and Rehabilitation,* **80**, 1030–1037.

Hanten, G., Bartha, M., & Levin, H. S. (2000). Metamemory following pediatric traumatic brain injury: a preliminary study. *Developmental Neuropsychology,* **18**, 383–398.

Hartman-Maeir, A., & Katz, N. (1995). Validity of the Behavioural Inattention Test (BIT): relationships with functional tasks. *American Journal of Occupational Therapy,* **49**, 507–516.

Harwood, R. H., Rogers, A., Dickinson, E., & Ebrahim, S. (1994). Measuring handicap: London Handicap Scale, a new outcome measure for chronic disease. *Quality Health Care*, **3**, 11–16.

Heinemann, A. W. (2005). Putting outcome measurement in context: a rehabilitation psychology perspective. *Rehabilitation Psychology*, **50**, 6–14.

Higginson, C. I., Arnett, P. A., & Voss, W. D. (2000). The ecological validity of clinical tests of memory and attention in multiple sclerosis. *Archives of Clinical Neuropsychology*, **15**, 185–204.

Hill, S., & Harries, U. (1994). *Assessing the Outcome of Health Care for the Older Person in Community Settings: Should we use the SF-36?* Leeds, UK: Clearing House on Health Outcomes, Nuffield Institute for Health.

Hobart, J., Lamping, D., Fitzpatrick, R., Riazi, A., & Thompson, A. (2001a). The Multiple Sclerosis Impact Scale (MSIS-29): a new patient-based outcome measure. *Brain*, **124**, 962–973.

Hobart, J. C., Lamping, D. L., Freeman, J. A. *et al.* (2001b). Evidence-based measurement: which disability scale for neurologic rehabilitation? *Neurology*, **57**, 639–644.

Holbrook, M., & Skilbeck, C. E. (1983). An activities index for use with stroke patients. *Age and Ageing*, **12**, 166–170.

Holland, A. L., Frattali, C. M., & Fromm, D. (1999). *Communication Activities for Daily Living (2nd Edition)*. Austin, TX: Pro-E.

Houlden, H., Edwards, M., McNeil, J., & Greenwood, R. (2006). Use of the Barthel Index and the Functional Independence Measure during early inpatient rehabilitation after single incident brain injury. *Clinical Rehabilitation*, **20**, 153–159.

Indredavik, B., Bakke, F., Solberg, R. *et al.* (1991). Benefit of a stroke unit: a randomized controlled trial. *Stroke*, **22**, 1026–1031.

Jette, A., & Haley, S. (2005). Contemporary measurement techniques for rehabilitation outcomes assessment. *Journal of Rehabilitation Medicine*, **37**, 339–345.

Juby, L. C., Lincoln, N. B., Berman, P. *et al.* (1996). The effect of a stroke rehabilitation unit on functional and psychological outcome: a randomised controlled trial. *Cerebrovascular Diseases*, **6**, 106–110.

Kidd, D., Stewart, G., Baldry, J. *et al.* (1995). The functional independence measure: a comparative validity and reliability study. *Disability and Rehabilitation*, **17**, 10–14.

Kinsella, G., Murtagh, D., Landry, A. *et al.* (1996). Everyday memory following traumatic brain injury. *Brain Injury*, **10**, 499–507.

Kreutzer, J. S., Marwitz, J. H., Seel, R., & Serio, C. D. (1996). Validation of a neurobehavioral functioning inventory for adults with traumatic brain injury. *Archives of Physical Medicine and Rehabilitation*, **77**, 116–124.

Kurtzke, J. F. (1983). Rating neurologic impairment in multiple sclerosis: an expanded disability status scale (EDSS). *Neurology*, **33**, 1444–1452.

Levin, H. S., High, W. M., Goethe, K. E. *et al.* (1987). The Neurobehavioral Rating Scale: assessment of the behavioral sequelae of head injury by the clinician. *Journal of Neurology, Neurosurgery, and Psychiatry*, **50**, 183–193.

Lincoln, N. B., & Bowen, A. (2006). The need for randomised treatment studies in neglect research. *Restorative Neurology and Neuroscience*, **24**, 401–408.

Lincoln, N. B., & Leadbitter, D. (1979). Assessment of motor function in stroke patients. *Physiotherapy*, **65**, 48–51.

Lincoln, N. B., Jackson, J. M., & Adams, S. A. (1998). Reliability and revision of the Nottingham Sensory Assessment for stroke patients. *Physiotherapy*, **84**, 358–365.

Lincoln, N. B., Sutcliffe, L. M., & Unsworth, G. (2000). Validation of the Stroke Aphasic Depression Questionnaire (SADQ) for use with patients in hospital. *Clinical Neuropsychological Assessment*, **1**, 88–96.

Linscott, R. J., Knight, R. G., & Godefroy, H. P. D. (1996). The Profile of Functional Impairment in Communication (PFIC): a measure of communication impairment for clinical use. *Brain Injury*, **10**, 397–412.

Maddicks, R., Marzillier, S. L., & Parker, G. (2003). Rehabilitation of unilateral neglect in the acute recovery stage: the efficacy of limb activation therapy. *Neuropsychological Rehabilitation*, **13**, 391–408.

Mahoney, F. I., & Barthel, D. W. (1965). Functional evaluation: Barthel Index. *Maryland State Medical Journal*, **14**, 61–65.

McColl, M. A., Davies, D., Carlson, P., Johnston, J., & Minnes, P. (2001). The community integration measure: development and preliminary validation. *Archives of Physical Medicine and Rehabilitation*, **82**, 429–434.

McKinney, M., Blake, H., Treece, K. A. *et al.* (2002). Evaluation of cognitive assessment in stroke rehabilitation. *Clinical Rehabilitation*, **16**, 129–136.

McPherson, K. M., Pentland, B., Cudmore, S. F., & Prescott, R. J. (1996). An inter-rater reliability study of the Functional Assessment Measure (FIM + FAM). *Disability and Rehabilitation*, **18**, 341–347.

Mermis, B. J. (2005). Developing a taxonomy for rehabilitation outcome measurement. *Rehabilitation Psychology*, **50**, 15–23.

Michalon, M., Eskes, G. A., & Mate-Kole, C. C. (1997). Effects of light therapy on neuropsychological function and mood in seasonal affective disorder. *Journal of Psychiatry and Neuroscience*, **22**, 19–28.

Nickels, L. (2005). Tried, tested and trusted? Language assessment for rehabilitation. In P. W. Halligan & D. Wade (Eds.), *Effectiveness of Rehabilitation for Cognitive Deficits* (pp. 169–184). Oxford, UK: Oxford University Press.

Nilsson, Å. L., Sunnerhagen, K. S., & Grimby, G. (2005). Scoring alternatives for FIM in neurological disorders applying Rasch analysis. *Acta Neurologicalica Scandinavica*, **111**, 264–273.

Norris, G., & Tate, R. L. (2000). The Behavioural Assessment of the Dysexecutive Syndrome (BADS): ecological, concurrent and construct validity. *Neuropsychological Rehabilitation*, **10**, 33–45.

Nouri, F. M., & Lincoln, N. B. (1987). An extended ADL scale for use with stroke patients. *Clinical Rehabilitation*, **1**, 301–305.

Piazzini, A., Canevini, M. P., Maggiori, G., & Canger, R. (2001). The perception of memory failures in patients with epilepsy. *European Journal of Neurology*, **8**, 613–620.

Pollak, N., Rheault, W., & Stoecker, J. L. (1996). Reliability and validity of the FIM for persons aged 80 years and above from a multilevel continuing care retirement community. *Archives of Physical Medicine and Rehabilitation*, **77**, 1056–1061.

Ponsford, J., & Kinsella, G. (1991). The use of a rating scale of attentional behavior. *Neuropsychological Rehabilitation*, **1**, 241–257.

Powell, J. H., Beckers, K., & Greenwood, R. (1998). Measuring progress and outcome in community rehabilitation after brain injury with a new assessment instrument – The BICRO-39 scales. *Archives of Physical Medicine and Rehabilitation*, **79**, 1213–1225.

Powell, J., Heslin, J., & Greenwood, R. (2002). Community based rehabilitation after severe traumatic brain injury: a randomised controlled trial. *Journal of Neurology, Neurosurgery, and Psychiatry*, **72**, 193–202.

Radloff, L. S. (1977). The CES-D Scale: a self-report depression scale for research in the general population. *Applied Psychological Measurement*, **1**, 385–401.

Robertson, I. H., Hogg, K., & McMillan, T. M. (1998). Rehabilitation of unilateral neglect: improving function by contralesional limb activation. *Neuropsychological Rehabilitation*, **8**, 19–29.

Robertson, I. H., Ward, T., Ridgeway, V., & Nimmo-Smith, I. (1994). *The Test of Everyday Attention*. Titchfield: Thames Valley Test Company.

Ruisel, I. (1991). Memory rating. *Studia Psychologica*, **33**, 71–77.

Sarno, M. T. (1969). *The Functional Communication Profile Manual of Directions*. New York, NY: Institute of Rehabilitation Medicine, New York University Medical Center.

Sharrack, B., & Hughes, R. A. C. (1999). The Guy's Neurological Disability Scale (GNDS): a new disability measure for multiple sclerosis. *Multiple Sclerosis*, **5**, 223–233.

Skinner, C., Wirz, S., Thompson, I., & Davidson, J. (1984). *The Edinburgh Functional Communication Profile*. Oxford: Winslow Press.

Sohlberg, M. M., McLaughlin, K. A., Pavese, A., Heidrich, A., & Posner, M. I. (2000). Evaluation of attention process training and brain injury education in persons with acquired brain injury. *Journal of Clinical and Experimental Neuropsychology*, **22**, 656–676.

Stern, R. A. (1997). *Visual Analog Mood Scales*. Odessa, FL: Psychological Assessment Resources, Inc.

Stewart, A. L., & Ware, J. E. (1992). *Measuring Functioning and Well-Being: The Medical Outcomes Study Approach*. Durham, NC: Duke University Press.

Sunderland, A., Harris, J. E., & Baddeley, A. D. (1983). Do laboratory tests predict everyday memory? A neuropsychological study. *Journal of Verbal Learning and Verbal Behavior*, **22**, 341–357.

Sunderland, A., Harris, J. E., & Gleave, J. (1984). Memory failures in everyday life following severe head injury. *Journal of Clinical Neuropsychology*, **6**, 127–142.

Sutcliffe, L., & Lincoln, N. (1998). The assessment of depression in aphasic stroke patients: the development of the Stroke Aphasic Depression Questionnaire. *Clinical Rehabilitation*, **12**, 506–513.

Taylor, R. (1990). Relationships between cognitive test performance and everyday cognitive difficulties in multiple sclerosis. *British Journal of Clinical Psychology*, **29**, 251–253.

Tham, K., & Tegnér, R. (1996). The Baking Tray Task: a test of spatial neglect. *Neuropsychological Rehabilitation*, **6**, 19–25.

Tinson, D. J., & Lincoln, N. B. (1987). Subjective memory impairment after stroke. *International Disability Studies*, **9**, 6–9.

Towle, D., & Lincoln, N. B. (1991). Development of a questionnaire for detecting everyday problems in stroke patients with unilateral visual neglect. *Clinical Rehabilitation*, **5**, 135–140.

Turner-Stokes, L., & Hassan, N. (2002). Depression after stroke: a review of the evidence base to inform the development of an integrated care pathway. Part 1: Diagnosis, frequency and impact. *Clinical Rehabilitation*, **16**, 231–247.

van der Putten, J. J. M. F., Hobart, J. C., Freeman, J. A., & Thompson, A. J. (1999). Measuring change in disability after inpatient rehabilitation: comparison of the responsiveness of the Barthel Index and the Functional Independence Measure. *Journal of Neurology, Neurosurgery, and Psychiatry*, **66**, 480–484.

van Zomeren, A. H., & Spikman, J. M. (2003). Assessment of attention. In P. W. Halligan, U. Kischka, & J. C. Marshall (Eds.), *Handbook of Clinical Neuropsychology* (pp. 73–88). Oxford, UK: Oxford University Press.

Vaney, C., Blaurock, H., Gattlen, B., & Meisels, C. (1996). Assessing mobility in multiple sclerosis using the Rivermead Mobility Index and gait speed. *Clinical Rehabilitation*, **10**, 216–226.

von Cramon, D. Y., Matthes-von Cramon, G., & Mai, N. (1991). Problem solving deficits in brain-injured patients: a therapeutic approach. *Neuropsychological Rehabilitation*, **1**, 45–64.

Wade, D. T. (2003). Outcome measures for clinical rehabilitation trials: impairment, function, quality of life, or value? *American Journal of Physical Medicine and Rehabilitation*, **82**, S26–S31.

Wade, D. T., Collen, F. M., Robb, G. F., & Warlow, C. P. (1992). Physiotherapy intervention late after stroke and mobility. *British Medical Journal*, **304**, 609–613.

Wade, D. T., Crawford, S., Wenden, F. J., King, N. S., & Moss, N. E. G. (1997). Does routine follow up after head injury help? A randomised controlled trial. *Journal of Neurology, Neurosurgery, and Psychiatry*, **62**, 478–484.

Walker, R., Findlay, J. M., Young, A. W., & Welch, J. (1991). Disentangling neglect and hemianopia. *Neuropsychologia*, **29**, 1019–1027.

Ware, J. E., Snow, K. K., Kosinski, M., & Gandek, B. (1993). *SF-36 Health Survey Manual and Interpretation Guide*. Boston, MA: The Health Institute, New England Medical Center.

Watkins, C. L., Auton, M. F., Deans, C. F. *et al.* (2007). Motivational interviewing early after acute stroke: a randomized, controlled trial. *Stroke*, **38**, 1004–1009.

Weniger, D. (1990). Diagnostic tests as tools of assessment and models of information processing: a gap to bridge. *Aphasiology*, **4**, 109–113.

Whiteneck, G., Charlifues, W., Gerhart, K., Overholser, J. D., & Richardson, G. N. (1992). Quantifying handicap: a new measure of long term rehabilitation outcomes. *Archives of Physical Medicine and Rehabilitation*, **73**, 519–526.

Whyte, J., Hart, T., Bode, R. K., & Malec, J. F. (2003). The Moss Attention Rating Scale for traumatic brain injury: Initial psychometric assessment. *Archives of Physical Medicine and Rehabilitation*, **84**, 268–276.

Wilson, B. A., Cockburn, J., & Baddeley, A. (1985). *The Rivermead Behavioural Memory Test*. Bury St Edmunds, UK: Thames Valley Test Company.

Wilson, B. A., Cockburn, J., & Halligan, P. W. (1987). *Behavioural Inattention Test*. Bury St Edmunds, UK: Thames Valley Test Company.

Wilson, B. A., Alderman, N., Burgess, P., Emslie, H., & Evans, J. (1996). *Behavioural Assessment of the Dysexecutive Syndrome*. Bury St Edmunds, UK: Thames Valley Test Company.

Wilson, B. A., Clare, L., Baddeley, A., Watson, P., & Tate, R. (1998). *Rivermead Behavioural Memory Test – Extended Version (RBMT-E)*. Bury St Edmunds, UK: Thames Valley Test Company.

Winward, C. E., Halligan, P. W., & Wade, D. T. (2002). The Rivermead Assessment of Somatosensory Performance (RASP): standardization and reliability data. *Clinical Rehabilitation*, **16**, 523–533.

World Health Organization (2001). *International Classification of Functioning, Disability and Health*. Geneva, Switzerland: WHO.

Worthington, A. (2005). Rehabilitation of executive deficits: Effective treatments of related disabilities. In P. W. Halligan & D. Wade (Eds.), *Effectiveness of Rehabilitation for Cognitive Deficits* (pp. 257–267) Oxford: Oxford University Press.

Zelinski, E. M., Gilewski, M. J., & Anthony-Bergstone, C. R. (1990). Memory Functioning Questionnaire: concurrent validity with memory performance and self-reported memory failures. *Psychology and Aging*, **5**, 388–399.

Zigmund, A. S., & Snaith, R. P. (1983). The Hospital Anxiety and Depression Scale. *Acta Psychiatrica Scandinavia*, **67**, 361–370.

Zoccolotti, P., & Judica, A. (1992). Functional evaluation of hemineglect by means of a semi-structured scale: personal extrapersonal differentiation. *Neuropsychological Rehabilitation*, **2**, 33–44.

Zoccolotti, P., Antonucci, G., & Judica, A. (1992). Psychometric characteristics of two semi-structured scales for the functional evaluation of hemi-inattention in extrapersonal and personal space. *Neuropsychological Rehabilitation*, **2**, 179–191.

7

Principles in evaluating cognitive rehabilitation research

Keith D. Cicerone

Introduction

- Judgments about the clinical effectiveness of interventions are complex and subject to biases.

Nothing is so firmly believed as what we least know. (Michel de Montaigne)

The practice of evidence-based rehabilitation is based on the "integration of individual clinical experience with the best available external clinical evidence from systematic research" (Sackett *et al.*, 2000, p. 2). In the absence of scientific evidence, claims for the effectiveness of any medical or rehabilitation practice rely upon clinical "expert opinion," typically reflecting the judgments and beliefs acquired by individual clinicians through their professional experience and clinical practice. Unfortunately, clinical judgments are fraught with potential biases (Elstein & Schwarz, 2002) and these appear to be a fundamental aspect of human reasoning and decision making (Ditto & Lopez, 1992; Kahneman, 2003). The impact of potential bias is greatest and is most apparent in situations that require the integration of complex and incomplete information (Elstein & Schwarz, 2002), which, of course, is characteristic of most aspects of rehabilitation planning and decision making. Within the context of rehabilitation, even judgments about patients' functional status that rely on well-established, standardized instruments are highly susceptible to biases that are difficult to overcome (Wolfson *et al.*, 2000). Clinical experience is generally inadequate to overcome subjective biases, and may even exacerbate

errors in judgment. Practicing clinicians frequently fail to initiate a search for relevant information or suppress the recognition of a need for additional information (Cabana *et al.*, 1999) and are less likely to acknowledge information that is inconsistent with their past experience and practices (Burgers *et al.*, 2003).

The evaluation of rehabilitation research as an aide to effective clinical decision making relies on assumptions regarding the level of evidence based on a hierarchy of research designs and the associated strength of recommendations. Evidence-based evaluation of the available research typically requires the classification of individual studies according to their methodological rigor and quality.

Levels of evidence and the hierarchy of research designs

- Evidence-based reviews of rehabilitation are based on a hierarchy of research design ranging from randomized clinical trials to expert opinion.
- Several systematic reviews of cognitive rehabilitation have been conducted.
- These reviews have reached different conclusions, based on their reliance on randomized trials and subjective interpretation of results.

The movement in evidence-based medicine has been occurring for two decades, although this pursuit has been somewhat slower in rehabilitation

Cognitive Neurorehabilitation, Second Edition: Evidence and Application, ed. Donald T. Stuss, Gordon Winocur and Ian H. Robertson. Published by Cambridge University Press. © Cambridge University Press 2008.

research (DeLisa, 1999). A number of procedures have been developed to systematically review and explicitly characterize the levels of evidence in primary research and relate these to healthcare recommendations. The initial approaches to developing guidelines for clinical practice relied on informal or formal consensus development. This approach represented a form of collective expert opinion, and retained all of the potential limitations and biases of individual expert opinion, as well as introducing additional variance due to group dynamics and politics (Woolf, 1992). In 1990, an explicit process for guideline development was introduced based primarily on the nature of research design employed by the relevant primary studies. According to the guideline, randomized controlled trials (RCTs) represent "good" evidence (level I), observational studies using concurrent controls (cohort or case-control analyses) represent "fair" evidence (level II), and studies using historical controls, uncontrolled case series, single case reports or expert opinion are considered "poor" evidence (level III) (Eddy, 1990). While a large number of systems for grading the evidence have been developed subsequently, these have retained generally the logic of classification based on a hierarchy of research design (Atkins *et al.*, 2004b) and this approach is characteristic of attempts to evaluate the effectiveness of cognitive rehabilitation.

Systematic reviews of cognitive rehabilitation

As part of a consensus conference on interventions for the cognitive and behavioral sequelae of TBI, Carney *et al.* (1999) reviewed 32 studies of cognitive rehabilitation for TBI, including 11 randomized, controlled studies. Their review noted that data on the effectiveness of cognitive rehabilitation programs was limited by the heterogeneity of subjects, interventions and outcomes studied. It was noted specifically that efficacy had been demonstrated for the use of compensatory devices, such as memory books, to improve particular cognitive functions and to compensate for specific deficits. It was also noted that comprehensive, interdisciplinary programs that

included individually tailored interventions for cognitive deficits were commonly used for persons with TBI. Although this personalized approach led to difficulty in the scientific evaluation of effectiveness, several uncontrolled studies and a nonrandomized clinical trial supported the effectiveness of these approaches.

The Brain Injury-Interdisciplinary Special Interest Group (BI-ISIG) of the American Congress of Rehabilitation Medicine reviewed 171 studies of cognitive rehabilitation following TBI or stroke (Cicerone *et al.*, 2000). This review considered 29 RCTs (level I), 35 controlled observational studies (level II), and 107 uncontrolled or single-subject studies (level III). Of the 29 RCTs, 20 provided some evidence to support the effectiveness of cognitive rehabilitation for subjects with traumatic brain injury (TBI) or stroke. Evidence from eight studies supported the use of visuospatial remediation of visual scanning deficits resulting from right hemisphere stroke, and evidence from four studies supported the use of language remediation following left hemisphere stroke. Twelve RCTs evaluated the effectiveness of cognitive remediation for persons with TBI. Eight of these studies provided support for the effectiveness of cognitive remediation for impairments of attention, functional communication, memory and problem solving following TBI. Subsequently, Cicerone *et al.* (2005) reviewed an additional 87 studies, including 17 level I studies, 8 level II studies, and 62 level III studies. This review concluded that there was substantial evidence to support clinical recommendations for cognitive-linguistic therapies for people with language deficits after left hemisphere stroke, and visuospatial rehabilitation for deficits associated with visual neglect after right hemisphere stroke. In addition, there was substantial evidence to support strategy training for people with TBI with mild memory impairment or post-acute attention deficits.

In 2003, a task force under the auspices of the European Federation of Neurological Societies (Cappa *et al.*, 2003) concluded that there is substantial evidence to support attention training in the post-acute phase after TBI (but not during the period of acute recovery) and compensatory memory training for subjects with mild memory impairments. Evidence of effectiveness of pragmatic conversational therapy after TBI was found to be based on a limited number of studies with small samples, and in need of confirmation. Several methods of rehabilitation for spatial neglect were found to be effective, as was the treatment of apraxia with compensatory strategies. As part of a broader effort by the Academy of Neurologic Communication Disorders and Sciences to develop practice guidelines for treating cognitive-communication disorders after TBI, Sohlberg et al. (2003) examined the evidence for the effectiveness of direct attention training following TBI. They concluded that there was evidence of improvement in attention-based skills with direct training, although the interpretation of studies was limited by factors such as subject heterogeneity and the lack of replications.

In contrast to the studies noted above, two Cochrane Reviews found limited evidence for the effectiveness of cognitive rehabilitation for attention deficits (Lincoln et al., 2000) or memory deficits (Majid et al., 2000) after stroke. Only level I studies with 20 or more participants in each condition were considered for inclusion in these analyses. Lincoln et al. (2000) concluded that there was some evidence that training improves alertness and sustained attention but insufficient evidence of improved functional independence after stroke. Majid et al. (2000) identified a single study that met their criteria for inclusion, and found insufficient evidence to support or refute the effectiveness of cognitive rehabilitation for memory problems after stroke.

Several systematic reviews (Bowen & Lincoln, 2007; Jutai et al., 2003; Pierce & Buxbaum, 2002) found evidence that cognitive rehabilitation, including visual scanning training, improves spatial neglect after right hemisphere stroke, but also noted that there is limited or insufficient evidence for the long-term benefits of treatment effects or relevance to everyday functioning. Systematic reviews of treatment for aphasia have reached conflicting conclusions. Robey (1998) conducted a meta-analytic review of 55 studies of clinical outcomes after

aphasia rehabilitation. These were generally observational studies, rather than randomized controlled trials. Outcomes for treated individuals were found to be superior for untreated individuals in all stages of recovery, particularly when treatment was begun in the acute stage of recovery, and the magnitude of treatment effects was positively associated with amount of treatment. There were too few studies to examine the differential effects of treatments for different types of aphasia. Cappa et al. (2003) also found some evidence for the effectiveness of aphasia therapy, again based largely on level II and level III studies. In contrast, a Cochrane Review of aphasia rehabilitation identified only 12 randomized clinical trials suitable for their review, and none of these was considered methodologically adequate quality in terms of description and analysis (Greener et al., 1999). The main conclusion of this last review was that aphasia therapy after stroke has not been shown to be clearly effective within a randomized controlled trial.

It seems clear that the reliance on a classification of research based on the levels of evidence does not guarantee consensus regarding the evaluation of available evidence. Several factors may contribute to these discrepancies, including the degree of reliance on level I evidence (RCTs) to the exclusion of other evidence, subjectivity in the interpretation of study results (McCormack & Greenhalgh, 2000), and inchoate criteria for considering the quality of evidence beyond the level of research design (Moja et al., 2005).

Evaluation of methodological quality in rehabilitation research

- Factors other than research design influence the quality of rehabilitation research.
- Indicators of methodological quality have been applied to the evaluation of rehabilitation research.
- Evaluation of research quality includes consideration of randomization and concealment of treatment allocation, eligibility criteria and subject characteristics, blinding and masked outcome

assessment, adequate description of interventions, relevance of outcome measures, and appropriate statistical analyses.

There is increasing recognition of the need to consider factors beyond the basic study design in evaluating treatment effectiveness. For example, a recent paper from the GRADE working group (Atkins et al., 2004a) identified four key elements to consider in systematic evaluations of evidence: study design, study quality, the consistency of effects across different studies, and directness (the extent to which people, interventions and outcomes are similar to those of interest). Although prospective, randomized trials are generally considered to provide the most rigorous evaluation and best evidence for treatment effectiveness, RCTs and observational studies have been shown to produce remarkably similar magnitudes of effect for equivalent treatments in many, but not all cases (Benson & Hartz, 2000; Concato et al., 2000). When differences due to study design have been detected, these have often reflected worse prognosis and outcomes for controls in observational studies than for control participants in RCTs (with no difference between the treated participants in RCTs and observational studies), suggesting the substantial influence of participant selection factors (Concato et al., 2000). In some cases, participants in RCTs represent a highly selected sample relative to the population of interest, making it difficult to generalize results. Observational studies will be difficult to interpret when the factors influencing treatment selection and outcome are strongly related to prognostic factors, but might be successfully used to evaluate naturally occurring variations in services (Whyte, 2002). Observational studies of similar interventions conducted in different settings may provide the best evidence of clinical utility and generalizability (Bonell et al., 2006). Ideally, these observational studies are conducted within the appropriate context of research development after the efficacy of the intervention(s) has been evaluated.

Randomized trials will not be feasible where the behaviors of interest have a low rate of occurrence, and in these instances observational methods, including single case studies, represent the most feasible and valuable alternative. Small case series or single subject studies are particularly valuable for describing and evaluating innovative treatment approaches, where large observational studies or RCTs are unlikely to be appropriate or possible. The major limitation of single case studies is the potential lack of generalizability. In general, the evaluation of study design should be placed in the appropriate context of research development, as described by Gonzalez Rothi (2006; Chapter 5 by Rodriguez & Gonzalez Rothi, this volume).

The American Academy of Neurology (Edlund et al., 2005) has incorporated several indicators of study quality that go beyond basic study design in its procedure for rating and classifying therapeutic articles (Table 7.1). Within this framework, level I evidence relies on the use of a prospective randomized clinical trial in which the primary outcome(s) are clearly defined and measurement of outcome is masked, exclusion and exclusion criteria are clearly defined, the sample is representative of the population of interest, relevant baseline characteristics are presented and equivalent among treatment groups, and there is adequate accounting for study dropouts. This framework has been applied to the evaluation of rehabilitation research (Gordon et al., 2006; Johnston et al., 2006).

There have been several recent attempts to develop criteria for evaluating the quality of research specifically within the area of rehabilitation effectiveness. Initial efforts to apply a uniform operationalization of specific quality criteria were conducted by van Tulder (van Tulder et al., 1997, 2003) in the area of treatment for neck and back pain. These methods and criteria were subsequently applied to the area of occupational therapy for stroke patients (Steultjens et al., 2003) and multidisciplinary rehabilitation for acquired brain injury (TBI and stroke) (Turner-Stokes et al., 2005). These methods for the assessment of study quality include criteria relating to the internal validity of the study, adequate description of basic elements of the study design, and statistical analyses and appear applicable to the evaluation of cognitive rehabilitation research (Table 7.2).

Table 7.1. Levels of evidence. (Adapted from Edlund *et al.*, 2005.)

Level I	Prospective, randomized, controlled clinical trial with masked outcome assessment, in a representative population, with:
	(a) primary outcome(s) clearly defined;
	(b) exclusion/inclusion criteria clearly defined;
	(c) sufficiently low numbers and adequate accounting for drop-outs and withdrawals;
	(d) relevant baseline characteristics are reported and substantially equivalent among treatment groups.
Level II	Prospective matched group cohort study in a representative population with masked outcome assessment that meets (a–d) above OR an RCT in a representative population that lacks one criterion from (a–d).
Level III	All other controlled trials (including historical controls and patients serving as their own controls) in a representative population, where outcome is independently assessed or derived from objective measurement that is unlikely to be affected by bias.
Level IV	Evidence from uncontrolled studies, case series, case reports or expert opinion.

Table 7.2. Proposed indicators of methodological quality in cognitive rehabilitation research. (Adapted from van Tulder *et al.*, 1997, 2003, and Turner-Stokes *et al.*, 2005.)

Internal validity	Eligibility criteria specified: A list of inclusion and exclusion criteria are explicitly stated.
	Method of randomization: an unpredictable, random sequence is used to assign participants to treatment condition.
	Treatment allocation concealed: assignment of participants to condition is concealed from the investigators.
	Similarity of baseline characteristics: characteristics of both the experimental and control groups should be described, and participants in different treatment conditions should be comparable at baseline (start of treatment) on important characteristics.
	Treatment and control interventions are specifically described.
	Co-interventions are avoided or equivalent.
	Compliance: compliance rates should not be below 80%, or differences between compliance rates in the two groups differ by more than 20%.
	Outcome assessor blinded to intervention: the person conducting the outcome assessment should be unaware of the participant's treatment condition.
	Outcome measures are relevant: for cognitive rehabilitation, relevant outcome measures might include
	(1) assessment of impairment, e.g., neuropsychological test scores, neurobehavioral or psychosocial symptoms,
	(2) assessment of activity limitations, participation, health-related quality of life, and subjective well-being.
	The primary outcomes should be specified.
Descriptive criteria	Withdrawal and drop-out rates are described and acceptable.
	Short-term outcome measurement is conducted (at the end of treatment).
	Long-term outcome measurement is conducted 3 or more months after completion of treatment.
	Timing of outcome assessment(s) should be identical for all intervention groups and for all important outcome assessments.
	Sample size is described for each group.
Statistical criteria	Intention-to-treat analysis: all patients who were randomized should be reported and analyzed.
	Point estimates and measures of variability should be reported.
	Statistical comparison of treatment effect: should include a direct comparison between treatment conditions.

*Randomization and adequate concealment
of treatment allocation*

Randomization requires that participants are
assigned to treatment condition based on an unpredictable sequence in order to ensure that uncontrolled variables (some of which may be known, but
many of which will be unknown) are distributed equi-
tably among treatment groups. While this is a fundamental aspect of research design that is central to the
evaluation of study quality, it has been inconsistently
applied within the research on cognitive rehabilitation. We reviewed 24 planned RCTs for patients with
traumatic brain injury (TBI) that were included in
ongoing evidence-based reviews of cognitive rehabilitation (Cicerone *et al.*, 2000, 2005) for adequate
description and adherence to the principles of randomization. In only three of these studies (12.5%) was
there evidence of adequate randomization. In 13
reports (54%) there was insufficient description of
the process of random assignment of participants,
and eight studies (33%) either broke randomization
or used a quasi-randomized method of subject
assignment, such as alternation according to a fixed
sequence or matching subjects prior to assignment.

The problem with these latter procedures is related
to the need for adequate concealment of the
sequence of randomization from the investigators.
Concealment of treatment allocation is also related
to reduction or elimination of selection biases, and
appears to be equally if not more important than the
use of randomization. There is evidence from the
general medical literature that the inadequate concealment of treatment allocation is associated with
exaggerated magnitude of effects that surpasses the
influence of randomized versus observational study
designs (Kunz & Oxman, 1998; Schulz *et al.*, 1995)
and can be larger than the effect size associated with
the actual interventions (Kunz & Oxman, 1998).
Despite the importance of adequate concealment of
treatment allocation, adequate concealment was
found in only 56% of RCTs published in four of the
most prestigious general medical journals (Hewitt
et al., 2005). A review of 208 randomized trials
addressing interventions for various aspects of head

or brain injury found that the method of concealment of allocation was reported in only 47 (23%) of
the trials, and was judged to be adequate in only 22
(11%) of trials (Dickinson *et al.*, 2000). Among the
studies addressing multidisciplinary treatment for
brain injury (Turner-Stokes *et al.*, 2005) 5 of 14
(36%) studies indicated concealment of allocation.
In reviewing the RCTs of cognitive rehabilitation
after traumatic brain injury, adequate concealment
of treatment allocation was reported and found to be
adequate in only two (8%) studies.

*Specification of eligibility criteria and
comparability of baseline characteristics*

Intervention studies need to report in adequate
detail the inclusion and exclusion criteria used to
select subjects, as restrictiveness of eligibility criteria also makes a significant contribution to the size
of treatment effects (Horwitz *et al.*, 1990). The finding that participants in the control arm of observational studies have poorer outcomes than the
control participants in randomized trials (Concato
et al., 2000; Kunz & Oxman, 1998) may be related to
the tendency to apply more restrictive inclusion
criteria in RCTs in order to evaluate only those
patients most likely to benefit from the intervention.
The specification of eligibility criteria in RCTs can
also represent a selection bias and influence the
conclusions regarding both the effectiveness and
generalizability of interventions. For example,
Salazar *et al.* (2000) conducted a RCT of cognitive
rehabilitation for injured military personnel, compared with a low-intensity home program, and
found no significant differences between groups
on neuropsychological functioning, psychological
adjustment, return to work or fitness for duty at 1
year after treatment. Participants were still in the
acute stage of recovery at the time of treatment,
were generally healthy and well educated prior to
their injuries, and all were in the military healthcare
system. The selective nature of the population represents a potentially important limitation. Glenn
et al. (2001) noted that the patients in this study

were highly atypical of most patients admitted for inpatient rehabilitation with respect to severity and recovery; only 2 of 643 (0.3%) patients enrolled in a national TBI database during the time-frame of the Salazar *et al.* (2000) study were far enough recovered to have met the entrance criteria. The participants in both arms of the Salazar *et al.* (2000) study demonstrated extraordinarily high return to work rates after treatment, suggesting that the good prognosis of patients may have masked any potential differences attributable to different interventions.

There are numerous patient characteristics that might potentially impact the effects of treatment. Unfortunately, little is known about how these factors might influence the response to cognitive rehabilitation, and this is an area of investigation that sorely needs additional research. Both the consistency and generalizability of findings from intervention studies are likely to be affected by differences in eligibility criteria. The determination of relevant and appropriate inclusion and exclusion criteria will depend on the phase of research development and the questions being addressed. For example, during the exploratory phase of research, investigators might elect to employ broad eligibility criteria in order to identify participants who are more or less likely to benefit from a given intervention. On the other hand, preliminary studies of innovative interventions designed to determine whether it is possible to identify a meaningful treatment effect might want to include a relatively restrictive and homogenous sample of participants, to maximize the probability of detecting an effect. However, later stages of treatment reflecting phase 3 clinical trials and health services research would be more likely to employ samples that are representative of the general clinical population, across various settings, to assess the applicability of the intervention in clinical practice (see discussion by Rodriguez and Gonzalez Rothi in Chapter 5, this volume).

Studies of cognitive rehabilitation need to describe the characteristics of participants in all arms of the study, and report on the similarity of baseline characteristics on relevant variables. Although little is currently known regarding which patients are likely to benefit from what interventions, participants should be comparable on basic demographic characteristics, injury-related variables and value(s) of the primary outcome measure(s). The range of relevant patient characteristics is likely to be related to the complexity of the intervention under investigation: treatments with multiple potential active treatment components are more likely to interact with multiple relevant patient characteristics, making the detection of treatment effects complex.

Blinding of participants and therapists and masked outcome assessment

In a double-blind trial, neither the patient nor the therapist is aware of the treatment assignment. While randomization and concealment of treatment allocation are intended largely to prevent or minimize participant selection biases, blinding is intended to minimize the effects of ascertainment bias, e.g., the influence of therapists' and participants' knowledge about treatment conditions on the delivery or response to treatment. In the context of rehabilitation interventions, full blinding is typically not feasible, and may not even be desirable. The relevance and impact of blinding is likely to vary depending on various aspects of the intervention. To the extent that interventions are less narrowly focused, less standardized, allow for greater treatment accommodations, depend on the motivation of participants, and depend on more subjective outcome criteria, the lack of patient or therapist blinding will represent a greater source of potential bias on outcomes.

An additional form of blinding refers to the use of masked outcome assessments, i.e., the degree to which the people measuring the effects of treatment are not involved in the delivery of treatment and are unaware of the assignment of participants to treatment conditions. Even in circumstances in which patient and therapist blinding are not possible, the blind assessment of outcomes is still achievable, although this will depend on the nature of the outcome being assessed. In cases where the outcome is assessed using objective and standardized instruments, such as many neuropsychological tests, it is reasonable to expect the use of masked outcome assessments. Although most studies of cognitive rehabilitation have relied on some aspect of neuropsychological evaluation as a measure of treatment effectiveness, we found that only 5 (21%) of 24 RCTs of cognitive rehabilitation for TBI used masked outcome assessments. When measures of disability are used as the primary outcome, masked outcome assessment was applied in only 26% of medical interventions for brain injury (Dickinson *et al.*, 2000) and 57% of the multidisciplinary interventions for brain injury (Turner-Stokes *et al.*, 2005). Masked outcome assessment is neither possible nor desirable for patient-centered measures such as subjective well-being.

Adequate description of the treatment and control interventions

Although all of the 24 RCTs of cognitive rehabilitation for TBI provided a general description of the interventions, these varied with regard to the degree of detail and few of the studies provided enough information to allow for replication of the intervention. This situation is likely to improve with increasing emphasis on the use of standardized and manualized intervention protocols (Whyte & Hart, 2003). There continues to be significant variation in the extent to which published reports of cognitive rehabilitation specify the exact frequency, intensity, timing and duration of interventions, as well as the characteristics (discipline, training and experience) of the people providing the interventions. This appears to be another aspect of the quality of intervention studies that should be remediable once given adequate attention.

The adequacy of description of treatments will also vary depending on the complexity of the intervention being studied. Complex interventions have been described as those that include several components (Campbell *et al.*, 2000) and it has been noted that "the greater the difficulty in defining precisely what exactly are the 'active ingredients' of an intervention and how they relate to each other, the greater the likelihood that you are dealing with a complex intervention" (Hawe *et al.*, 2004).

Whyte & Hart (2003) have described two approaches to the analysis of treatments that are relevant to the description and specification of complex interventions. One approach is to begin with the investigation of specific, isolated treatment components, and progressively investigate the addition and integration of multiple treatment components. The other approach is to begin with the investigation of less well-specified, global interventions and systematically attempt to isolate and tease apart the contributions of specific aspects of the complex intervention. This approach might be guided by both the availability of empirical information regarding the presumed treatment components in isolation, and theoretical constructs describing the presumed interaction of treatment components. The investigation and validation of complex interventions should be considered within the maturational framework of rehabilitation research development (Campbell *et al.*, 2000; Rothi, 2006). Exploratory studies and phase I clinical trials might be conducted with the intent of identifying the fixed (specific) and variable (nonspecific) aspects of a complex intervention through a qualitative analysis, or determining the feasibility of implementing and replicating the complex intervention within and between participants and settings. Tunis *et al.* (2003) have described the role of *practical clinical trials* (PCTs) that may bridge the gap between efficacy and effectiveness studies, and provide direct value and relevance to clinical decision making. According to Tunis *et al.* (2003), the characteristic features of PCTs are that they (1) compare and evaluate clinically relevant alternative interventions, that (2) include a diverse population of participants (3) referred from representative, heterogenous practice settings and (4) assess the effects of treatment using a broad range of outcome measures. While explanatory clinical trials are designed primarily to understand why and how an intervention might work, practical clinical trials are attempts to formulate hypotheses and study designs based on the information needed to make decisions in clinical practice.

There are several potential indicators of methodological quality that are closely related to the specification of interventions, including assessment of treatment compliance and treatment integrity. Treatment compliance refers to the degree to which the participants' behaviors were actually consistent with the presumed application of the intervention, while treatment integrity refers to the degree to which therapists' behaviors reflected the theoretical and/or procedural prescriptions underlying the intervention.

A major aspect of treatment compliance is the number of participants who drop out or withdraw from treatment following randomization. This is probably again related to prognostic factors, and has the potential to influence estimates of treatment effectiveness since participants remaining in treatment might reflect a bias towards those participants most likely to benefit. Unfortunately, estimates of the impact of withdrawals on the magnitude of treatment effects can be limited by the failure to report this information in clinical trials (Schulz et al., 1995). Only 50% of RCTs in our review of cognitive rehabilitation for TBI reported withdrawal rates, and the inability to determine the withdrawal rates in observational studies may represent a major methodological limitation. Additional aspects of treatment compliance might reflect participants' attendance, participation or engagement in therapy, as well as their actual application of the intended interventions. For example, Dirette et al. (1999) compared the effects of remedial (restorative) versus compensatory interventions for visual information processing deficits after TBI. The compensatory intervention consisted of instruction in the use of three compensatory strategies (verbalization, chunking and pacing). The restorative intervention was designed as remedial computer activities without instruction in the use of compensatory strategies. Both groups improved, with no evidence of a differential treatment effect. Actual use of strategies was examined through self-report and observation. Despite the different intended effects of the interventions, 80% of the patients used compensatory strategies whether or not they

were instructed to do so. On the other hand, within the context of a physical therapy intervention, it has been noted the effectiveness of constraint-induced therapy can be strongly influenced by patients' willingness and ability to comply with the protocol within their treatment setting (Page et al., 2002) and the effectiveness of compensatory memory strategies is influenced by patients' willingness or ability to actually employ memory aids (Evans et al., 2003).

The assessment of treatment integrity involves an evaluation of the extent to which the treatment(s) are provided in accordance with their original intentions. This might include not only the actual delivery of the experimental condition, but the extent to which there was potential for contamination between treatment conditions and the extent to which other potential co-interventions are avoided, or equivalent, between treatment conditions.

Relevance and equivalence of outcome measures

The relevant outcomes of cognitive rehabilitation include those at the level of impairment (symptoms, neuropsychological functioning), activity limitations, participation and quality of life. Most studies of cognitive rehabilitation have assessed the effects on measures of neuropsychological functioning. Rather than relying on a broad range of neuropsychological tests, it is preferable to identify the primary outcome(s) expected to change in relation to the intended effects of the intervention, which Whyte (1997) has termed "congruent outcome measurement." For example, Kaschel et al. (2002) generated specific predictions regarding the expected benefits of training compensations for visual imagery on verbal memory, while predicting less effect on other aspects of memory. A study of memory notebook training (Schmitter-Edgecombe et al., 1995) used a number of outcome measures of memory functioning, including both laboratory-based measures and observations of everyday memory failures. Patients who received the notebook training reported fewer observed everyday memory failures (with the use of the notebook), although there were no significant treatment effects for the laboratory-based tests of memory (which did not allow use of the notebook). Although the intended effects of the intervention were related to use of the memory notebook, a clinically beneficial treatment effect would not have been detected if the investigators had relied solely on laboratory-based memory measures.

There is increasing emphasis on the application of ecologically valid or real world functional outcomes, including measures of participation and quality of life. Although it is generally agreed that the goal of cognitive rehabilitation is improvement on aspects of patients' daily functioning, this has not been reflected in most cognitive rehabilitation research.

The assessment of treatment effect should include both short-term measurement (at the completion of treatment) as well as assessment of the stability of treatment effects at follow-up, typically at least 3 months after the completion of treatment. For example, an RCT of memory training initially demonstrated training in compensatory memory strategies to be superior to pseudo-treatment and no treatment conditions (Berg *et al.*, 1991). When participants were re-evaluated 4 years after training there were no differences between treatment conditions in overall memory performance or subjective memory complaints, which appeared to be related to the continued use (or lack of use) of compensatory memory strategies by participants (Milders *et al.*, 1995). The timing of outcome measurements should be identical for all intervention groups and for all important outcome assessments.

Statistical analyses

The quality of intervention studies is related to the use of appropriate and complete statistical analysis. This should include, at minimum, a complete description of the number of participants that were screened, enrolled and participated in the study. Although a number of systematic reviews of cognitive rehabilitation have imposed a minimum number of subjects as a criterion for study quality,

the logic of this approach has been questioned (van Tulder *et al.*, 1997). It is likely that the absolute number of participants is less important than an adequate analysis of sample size required for detection of the presumed effect size, and the limitations related to studies with small sample sizes could presumably be overcome by replicating the effects of interventions. The reporting of statistical results should include both point estimates of central tendency and measures of variability; measures of effect size are valuable for determining the clinical significance of any observed treatment effects as well as for the planning and development of subsequent research (Guyatt *et al.*, 1998). The analysis of treatment effects should include a direct comparison of treatment conditions using the appropriate multivariate techniques.

While there is obvious value in reporting the effects of treatment for participants who completed treatment, a conservative assessment of treatment effectiveness should include an intent-to-treat analysis in which all participants who were randomized and completed baseline evaluations are included in the reporting of results (following the same logic as that discussed for reporting participants who withdrew from treatment). The use of intent-to-treat analysis represent another area where the quality of cognitive rehabilitation research might be readily improved, since this was completed in only 10 (42%) studies that we evaluated and only 5 of 14 (36%) studies of multidisciplinary rehabilitation (Turner-Stokes *et al.*, 2005).

Conclusions

The goal of clinical research is to improve the quality of care. It is not reasonable to assume that clinicians will be able to integrate the large amounts of information and make the complex judgments to effectively treat patients in all circumstances. For that reason, efforts to systematically review and synthesise the available evidence are worthwhile. The systematic review and evaluation of research has relied on the classification of studies according to a hierarchy of research designs, ranging from randomized controlled trials to expert opinion. This framework is likely to evolve, but the basic tenets and value associated with the various research designs is unlikely to change dramatically. This does not mean that "lower" levels of evidence such as small case series and single case studies are not valuable (particularly for infrequent clinical problems and innovative interventions), any more than it means that these designs are less appropriate methods for conducting research in relation to the appropriate questions and stages of research development. In moving beyond procedures for grading and classifying evidence based solely on the level of research design, it is possible to identify a number of indicators of methodological quality that contribute to the evaluation of the available evidence within the field of rehabilitation, including cognitive rehabilitation. An appreciation of these principles will allow researchers to design more rigorous and sensitive investigations, facilitate the evaluation of existing research and allow clinicians to make decisions that can best guide clinical practice.

REFERENCES

Atkins, D., Best, D., Briss, P. A. *et al.* (2004a). Grading quality of evidence and strength of recommendations. *British Medical Journal*, **328**, 1490–1497.

Atkins, D., Eccles, M., Flottorp, S. *et al.* (2004b). Systems for grading the quality of evidence and the strength of recommendations I: critical appraisal of existing approaches. The GRADE Working Group. *BMC Health Services Research*, **4**, 38–44.

Benson, K., & Hartz, A. J. (2000). A comparison of observational studies and randomized, controlled trials. *New England Journal of Medicine*, **342**, 1878–1886.

Berg, I. J., Koning-Haanstra, M., & Deelman, B. G. (1991). Long-term effects of memory rehabilitation: a controlled study. *Neuropsychological Rehabilitation*, **1**, 97–111.

Bonell, C., Oakley, A., Hargreaves, J., Strange, V., & Rees, R. (2006). Assessment of generalisability in trials of health interventions: suggested framework and systematic review. *British Medical Journal*, **333**, 346–349.

Bowen, A., & Lincoln, N. B. (2007). Cognitive rehabilitation for spatial neglect following stroke (Review). *Cochrane Database of Systematic Reviews*, **2**, 1–43.

Burgers, J. S., Grol, R. P. T. M., Zaat, J. O. M. *et al.* (2003). Characteristics of effective clinical guidelines for general practice. *British Journal of General Practice*, **53**, 15–19.

Cabana, M. D., Rand, C. S., Powe, N. R. *et al.* (1999). Why don't physicians follow clinical practice guidelines? A framework for improvement. *Journal of the American Medical Association*, **282**, 1458–1465.

Campbell, M., Fitzpatrick, R., Haines, A. *et al.* (2000). Framework for design and evaluation of complex interventions to improve health. *British Medical Journal*, **321**, 694–696.

Cappa, S. F., Benke, T., Clarke, S. *et al.* (2003). EFNS guidelines on cognitive rehabilitation: report of an EFNS task force. *European Journal of Neurology*, **10**, 11–23.

Carney, N., Chesnut, R. M., Maynard, H. *et al.* (1999). Effect of cognitive rehabilitation on outcomes for persons with traumatic brain injury: a systematic review. *Journal of Head Trauma Rehabilitation*, **14**, 277–307.

Cicerone, K. D., Dahlberg, C., Kalmar, K. *et al.* (2000). Evidence-based cognitive rehabilitation: recommendations for clinical practice. *Archives of Physical Medicine and Rehabilitation*, **81**, 1596–1615.

Cicerone, K. D., Dahlberg, C., Malec, J. F. *et al.* (2005). Evidence-based cognitive rehabilitation: updated review of the literature from 1998 through 2002. *Archives of Physical Medicine and Rehabilitation*, **86**, 1681–1692.

Concato, J., Shah, N., & Horwitz, R. I. (2000). Randomized, controlled trials, observational studies, and the hierarchy of research designs. *New England Journal of Medicine*, **342**, 1887–1892.

DeLisa, J. A. (1999). Issues and challenges for physiatry in the coming decade. *Archives of Physical Medicine and Rehabilitation*, **80**, 1–12.

Dickinson, K., Bunn, F., Wentz, R., Edwards, P., & Roberts, I. (2000). Size and quality of randomised controlled trials in head injury: review of published studies. *British Medical Journal*, **320**, 1308–1311.

Dirette, D. K., Hinojosa, J., & Carnevale, G. J. (1999). Comparison of remedial and compensatory interventions for adults with acquired brain injuries. *Journal of Head Trauma Rehabilitation*, **14**, 595–601.

Ditto, P. H., & Lopez, D. F. (1992). Motivated skepticism: use of differential decision criteria for preferred and non-preferred conclusions. *Journal of Personality and Social Psychology*, **63**, 568–584.

Eddy, D. M. (1990). Practice policies: guidelines for methods. *Journal of the American Medical Association*, **263**, 1839–1841.

Edlund, W., Gronseth, G., So, Y., & Franklin, G. (2005). *Clinical Practice Guideline Process Manual*. Saint Paul, MN: American Academy of Neurology.

Elstein, A. S., & Schwarz, A. (2002). Clinical problem solving and diagnostic decision making: selective review of the cognitive literature. *British Medical Journal*, **324**, 729–732.

Evans, J. J., Wilson, B. A., Needham, P., & Brentnall, S. (2003). Who makes good use of memory aids? Results of a survey of people with acquired brain injury. *Journal of the International Neuropsychological Society*, **9**, 925–935.

Glenn, M. B., Yablon, S. A., Whyte, J., & Zafonte, R. (2001). Letter to the editor. *Journal of Head Trauma Rehabilitation*, **16**, vii–viii.

Gonzalez Rothi, L. J. (2006). Cognitive rehabilitation: the role of theoretical rationales and respect for the maturational process needed for our evidence. *Journal of Head Trauma Rehabilitation*, **21**, 194–197.

Gordon, W. A., Zafonte, R., Cicerone, K. *et al.* (2006). Traumatic brain injury rehabilitation: state of the science. *American Journal of Physical Medicine and Rehabilitation*, **85**, 343–382.

Greener, J., Enderby, P., & Whurr, R. (1999). Speech and language therapy for aphasia following stroke. *Cochrane Database of Systematic Reviews*, **4**, 1–62.

Guyatt, G. H., Juniper, E. F., Walter, S. D., Griffith, L. E., & Goldstein, R. S. (1998). Interpreting treatment effects in randomised trials. *British Medical Journal*, **316**, 690–693.

Hawe, P., Shiell, A., & Riley, T. (2004). Complex interventions: how "out of control" can a randomised controlled trial be? *British Medical Journal*, **328**, 1561–1563.

Hewitt, C., Hahn, S., Torgerson, D. J., Watson, J., & Bland, J. M. (2005). Adequacy and reporting of allocation concealment: review of recent trials published in four general medical journals. *British Medical Journal*, **330**, 1057–1058.

Horwitz, R. I., Viscoli, C. M., Clemens, J. D., & Sadock, R. T. (1990). Developing improved observational methods for evaluating therapeutic effectiveness. *American Journal of Medicine*, **89**, 630–638.

Johnston, M. V., Sherer, M., & Whyte, J. (2006). Applying evidence standards to rehabilitation research. *American Journal of Physical Medicine and Rehabilitation*, **85**, 292–309.

Jutai, J. W., Bhogal, S. K., Foley, N. C. *et al.* (2003). Treatment of visual perceptual disorders post stroke. *Topics in Stroke Rehabilitation*, **10**, 77–106.

Kahneman, D. (2003). A perspective on judgment and choice: mapping bounded rationality. *American Psychologist*, **58**, 697–720.

Kaschel, R., Della Sala, S., Cantagallo, A., Fahlböck, A., Laaksonen, R., & Kazen, M. (2002). Imagery mnemonics for the rehabilitation of memory: a randomised group controlled trial. *Neuropsychological Rehabilitation*, **12**, 127–153.

Kunz, R., & Oxman, A. D. (1998). The unpredictability paradox: review of empirical comparisons of randomised and non-randomised clinical trials. *British Medical Journal*, **317**, 1185–1190.

Lincoln, N. B., Majid, M. J., & Weyman, N. (2000). Cognitive rehabilitation for attention deficits following stroke (Review). *Cochrane Database of Systematic Reviews*, **4**, 1–9.

Majid, M. J., Lincoln, N. B., & Weyman, N. (2000). Cognitive rehabilitation for memory deficits following stroke (Review). *Cochrane Database of Systematic Reviews*, **3**, 1–9.

McCormack, J., & Greenhalgh, T. (2000). Seeing what you want to see in randomised controlled trials: versions and perversions of UKPDS data. *British Medical Journal*, **320**, 1720–1723.

Milders, M. V., Berg, I. J., & Deelman, B. G. (1995). Four-year follow-up of a controlled memory training study in closed-head injured patients. *Neuropsychological Rehabilitation*, **5**, 223–238.

Moja, L. P., Telaro, E., D'Amico, R. *et al.* (2005). Assessment of methodological quality of primary studies by systematic reviews: results of the metaquality cross sectional study. *British Medical Journal*, **330**, 1053–1057.

Page, S. J., Levine, P., Sisto, S., Bond, Q., & Johnston, M. V. (2002). Stroke patients' and therapists' opinions of constraint-induced movement therapy. *Clinical Rehabilitation*, **16**, 55–60.

Pierce, S. R., & Buxbaum, L. J. (2002). Treatments of unilateral neglect: a review. *Archives of Physical Medicine and Rehabilitation*, **83**, 256–268.

Robey, R. R. (1998). A meta-analysis of clinical outcomes in the treatment of aphasia. *Journal of Speech, Language, and Hearing Research*, **41**, 172–187.

Sackett, D. L., Richardson, W. S., Rosenberg, W., & Haynes, R. B. (2000). *Evidence-based Medicine: How to Practice and Teach EBM*. London, UK: Churchill Livingstone.

Salazar, A. M., Warden, D. L., Schwab, K. *et al.* (2000). Cognitive rehabilitation for traumatic brain injury: a randomized trial. *Journal of the American Medical Association*, **283**, 3075–3081.

Schmitter-Edgecombe, M., Fahy, J. F., Whelan, J. P., & Long, C. J. (1995). Memory remediation after severe closed head injury: notebook training versus supportive therapy. *Journal of Consulting and Clinical Psychology*, **63**, 484–489.

Schulz, K. F., Chalmers, I., Hayes, R. J., & Altman, D. G. (1995). Empirical-evidence of bias: dimensions of methodological quality associated with estimates of treatment effects in controlled trials. *Journal of the American Medical Association*, **273**, 408–412.

Sohlberg, M. M., Avery, J., Kennedy, M., *et al.* (2003). Practice guidelines for direct attention training. *Journal of Medical Speech-Language Pathology*, **11**, xix–xxxix.

Steultjens, E. M. J., Dekker, J., Bouter, L. M. *et al.* (2003). Occupational therapy for stroke patients: a systematic review. *Stroke*, **34**, 676–687.

Tunis, S. R., Stryer, D. B., & Clancy, C. M. (2003). Practical clinical trials: increasing the value of clinical research for decision making in clinical and health policy. *Journal of the American Medical Association*, **290**, 1624–1632.

Turner-Stokes, L., Disler, P. B., Nair, A., & Wade, D. T. (2005). Multi-disciplinary rehabilitation for acquired brain injury in adults of working age (Review). *Cochrane Database of Systematic Reviews*, **3**, 1–30.

van Tulder, M. W., Assendelft, W. J. J., Koes, B. W., & Bouter, L. M. (1997). Method guidelines for systematic reviews in the Cochrane Collaboration Back Review Group for Spinal Disorders. *Spine*, **22**, 2323–2330.

van Tulder, M., Furlan, A., Bombardier, C., & Bouter, L. (2003). Updated method guidelines for systematic reviews in the Cochrane Collaboration Back Review Group. *Spine*, **28**, 1290–1299.

Whyte, J. (1997). Distinctive methodologic challenges. In M. J. Fuhrer (Ed.), *Assessing Medical Rehabilitation Practices: The Promise of Outcome Research* (pp. 43–59). London, UK: Paul H. Brookes.

Whyte, J. (2002). Traumatic brain injury rehabilitation: are there alternatives to randomized clinical trials? *Archives of Physical Medicine and Rehabilitation*, **83**, 1320–1322.

Whyte, J., & Hart, T. (2003). It's more than a black box; It's a Russian Doll: defining rehabilitation treatments. *American Journal of Physical Medicine and Rehabilitation*, **82**, 639–652.

Wolfson, A. M., Doctor, J. N., & Burns, S. P. (2000). Clinician judgments of functional outcomes: how bias and perceived accuracy affect rating. *Archives of Physical Medicine and Rehabilitation*, **81**, 1567–1574.

Woolf, S. H. (1992). Practice guidelines, a new reality in medicine. II. Methods of developing guidelines. *Archives of Internal Medicine*, **152**, 946–952.

Application of imaging technologies

Introduction to Section 2

Donald T. Stuss

How does one measure the efficacy of a cognitive rehabilitation intervention? The science of cognitive neurorehabilitation certainly requires a behavioral level of evidence – do our interventions result in genuine improvement at some level of functioning? In one sense this is all that matters – patients getting better. However, is this by itself sufficient? There are many levels of potential benefit. For example, clinicians have strenuously emphasized that one must examine the type and value of the outcome measure. Not all are of equal value. Improvement in performance after rehabilitation on a memory score may not be as meaningful as positive changes in memory functioning in everyday activities. Both may be relevant, but each may be telling only part of the story. How can one achieve breakthroughs in rehabilitation that are transformative?

There may be other levels of explanation to the story – those addressing underlying mechanisms (e.g., neurochemical, biophysiological), and changes in the neural processes underlying behavior. When the first edition of this book was published in 1999, there were only two chapters that presented the use of imaging in neurorehabilitation, and we decided at that time that these chapters did not deserve an independent section, or a unique focus. In this second edition, we felt that research in neurorehabilitation had advanced so significantly that a section on the use of structural and functional imaging should stand independently. The four chapters in this section are methodologically oriented with other chapters in the book providing direct evidence resulting from the use of imaging

(see Chapters 1, 2, 12, 13, 17, 19, 21, 23, 24, 27, 28, 30 and 31).

The inclusion of a new section on imaging in this second edition on cognitive neurorehabilitation reflects the editors' judgment of the importance of measuring what happens *in* and *to* the brain (see also Robertson and Fitzpatrick, Chapter 32) in relation to behavioral performance. Is it relevant to know where the damage in the brain is before initiating treatment? That is, in rehabilitating memory dysfunction, should one consider if the damage involves the hippocampus, dorsomedial nucleus of the thalamus, frontal regions or connecting white matter? How should these be measured? At a functional level, is it important to be able to evaluate how brain functioning changes after rehabilitation? Two examples illustrate how functional imaging is used to understand what is happening at the biological level following different treatment approaches. In physiotherapeutic approaches to motor dysfunction, a major adaptive strategy was to have the patient use the nonaffected limb. The use of functional imaging evaluating the efficacy of that approach indicated that not only might this not be the best way, to some degree, it may be harmful to the eventual overall successful outcome (Taub *et al.*, 1993, 1998; Wolf *et al.*, 1989). Using functional imaging as an additional measure led to a truly counter-intuitive approach to motor recovery. Imaging can also be used to evaluate the value of specific pharmacotherapeutics (see Chapter 17 by McAllister & Arnsten).

The four chapters in Section 2 emphasize different imaging techniques: structural magnetic resonance

Cognitive Neurorehabilitation, Second Edition: Evidence and Application, ed. Donald T. Stuss, Gordon Winocur and Ian H. Robertson. Published by Cambridge University Press. © Cambridge University Press 2008.

imaging (MRI); functional magnetic resonance imaging (fMRI); and event-related potentials (ERP) and magnetoencephalography (MEG). The title of Chapter 8, by Ramirez, Gao and Black clearly defines the importance of structural imaging: *defining the cerebral context* for cognitive neurorehabilitation. As the authors argue, if one is to understand diagnosis, plan interventions, and design rigorous research studies, it is essential to determine the cause, location, and extent of any acquired brain pathology, and also evaluate the potential presence of pre-existing brain pathology. The chapter focuses on cerebrovascular disease, with the understanding that in older individuals the two often co-exist. There are many strengths in this chapter. There are clear definitions of the disorders; the most important structural imaging approaches are reviewed, including a historical context; the use of the different approaches are brought to life with case studies and examples of research; the figures clearly illustrate the text. This chapter is a necessary read for all those who use structural imaging in their cognitive neurorehabilitation research, or indeed clinically (see Chapters 1, 13, 17, 19, 21, 23, 24, 27, 28 and 30).

In Chapter 9, Grady summarizes how functional imaging, in addition to behavioral memory performance, has led to new insights into the aging process. As Grady notes, it was not surprising to observe that older adults showed less brain activity when performing memory tasks, particularly if the elderly were performing less well. What was surprising was the increased recruitment of task-relevant brain areas, as well as the recruitment of new areas, particularly if the elderly were performing similar to the young. This increased activity is most frequent in the prefrontal regions, perhaps reflecting the use of different strategies to perform the task. Grady also describes the use of a relatively new technique in functional imaging, neural network analysis, which suggests that an important aspect of brain plasticity may be brain network reorganization. The promise of brain plasticity may be at many levels, such as increased activity in brain regions, compensation by another region for damage to one area, and brain network reorganization. The reader is encouraged

to review, in the context of Grady's chapter, other chapters that discuss rehabilitation in aging and related disorders (see Chapters 1, 2, 3, 4, 8, 11, 14, 15, 16, 19, 20, 21, 22, 24, 27, 30 and 31).

Corbetta in Chapter 10 uses the example of stroke to discuss how imaging might be used to "separate the wheat from the chaff," that is, examine whether the changes are natural secondary to the brain injury, or are related to the behavioral recovery. He emphasizes the use of fMRI, since it is a technique that provides a measure of metabolic demands in a region that reflects the integration of information at that region. If one can answer this basic question, then one can develop an algorithm that categorizes patients, predicts outcomes, and measures the value of new methods of interventions. Corbetta rightfully points out that this is an enormous challenge, since it requires understanding the brain at all the interactive levels, from molecules to networks to real functional outcome, including the changes in the course of recovery. This is a critical review, pointing out three main strategies needed for the study of neurological recovery, and highlighting pitfalls in the interpretation of functional imaging data. Corbetta emphasizes that those engaged in rehabilitation must consider that neurological deficits reflect not only focal injury, but the impact on connected networks both close and far. One interesting aspect of this chapter is that three different patient types of deficits are considered: motor, language (aphasia) and visual spatial. The reader is encouraged to cross-reference this chapter by Corbetta with the other imaging chapters, and the chapters on rehabilitation of motor impairments (Chapter 23), aphasia (Chapter 25) and spatial neglect (Chapter 26).

There is an important aspect of brain activity that is often overlooked – the unfolding of processes over rapid time periods. Alain and Ross, in their chapter, highlight two methods that provide measures of millisecond by millisecond timing related to neuroplastic changes in the brain – event-related potentials and magnetoencephalography. The chapter provides a nice summary of the methods for those not knowledgeable about the techniques. A major value of scalp recording of EEG and extra-cranial MEG recordings are that they are noninvasive techniques for investigating neuroplastic changes in humans. Both Alain and Ross have used this approach to correlate brain neuroplasticity with behavioral improvement in perceptual skills, particularly in learning paradigms. They report that extended training results in specific changes in sensory evoked responses, measured in different ways, such as an increase in the size of cortical areas representing the trained attribute, changes in the locus of representation of the trained function, or even increased synchronization within different regions. Their data imply that ERPs and MEG can be used to study cortical remodeling after training and, in particular, add measures that are not available to other functional imaging modalities such as PET and fMRI. An important emphasis in their work is one that is often overlooked – training the perceptual processes that are essential for higher order cognitive functioning. We see great potential in developing the use of functional imaging to evaluate the efficacy of cognitive neurorehabilitation programs – using neural network analysis to examine changes in brain integration across the time span of a process and, indeed, over the longer time span of recovery.

In summary, the chapters in Section 2 underscore one recurring message of this edited volume. For cognitive neurorehabilitation to achieve its potential, the behavioral, functional and psychosocial approaches must be grounded in science and the biology of the brain.

REFERENCES

Taub, E., Miller, N. E., Novack, T. A. *et al.* (1993). Technique to improve chronic motor deficit after stroke. *Archives of Physical Medicine and Rehabilitation*, **74**, 347–354.

Taub, E., Crago, J. E., & Uswatte, G. (1998). Constraint-Induced Movement Therapy: a new approach to treatment in physical rehabilitation. *Rehabilitation Psychology*, **43**, 152–170.

Wolf, S. L., Lecraw, D. E., Barton, L. A., & Jann, B. B. (1989). Forced use of hemiplegic upper extremities to reverse the effect of learned nonuse among chronic stroke and head-injured patients. *Experimental Neurology*, **104**, 104–132.

8

Structural neuroimaging: defining the cerebral context for cognitive rehabilitation

Joel Ramirez, Fu Qiang Gao and Sandra E. Black

Introduction

Recovery from brain injury depends not only on severity and location of damage, but also on many host factors such as age, genetics, concomitant illnesses and the premorbid condition of the brain in the person who has incurred the injury. As our population ages, rehabilitationists are increasingly faced with the restorative challenge posed by older individuals, many of whom have vascular risk factors which have already inflicted chronic injury to an already aging brain. Given that the prevalence of dementia from Alzheimer's disease (AD) increases from 6% at age 65 to 25% by age 85 (Anonymous, 2000), many older individuals with stroke or head injury will be challenging to rehabilitate due to underlying neurodegeneration. This is particularly true for stroke patients whose average age is increasing, because of the interactions between ischemia and AD pathogenesis. Hence structural brain imaging is necessary not only to determine the cause, location and extent of acute brain damage such as stroke, but also to evaluate pre-existing brain disease. This is important not only clinically for understanding prognosis and planning intervention, but also for designing and interpreting research studies.

This chapter outlines how structural neuroimaging measures can be used to assess the baseline state of the brain by applying tissue classification methods, which can provide quantification of regional brain atrophy as well as the volume and location of subcortical cerebrovascular disease

(CVD) in the white matter and deep brain nuclei. In addition, traditional planimetric tracing methods are described enhanced by computational methodology to determine the volume and location of focal injury in group as well as individual case studies. Structural neuroimaging is an extension of the clinical and neurobehavior examination, providing neuroanatomical information needed to develop an informed picture of the individual's baseline injuries, build reasonable expectations for recovery and guide interventions.

To illustrate structural imaging approaches, this chapter draws primarily from injury due to cerebrovascular disease, but the same methodologies can be applied to other brain disorders such as traumatic brain injury, brain tumors, epilepsy and multiple sclerosis. Traditionally, in cognitive neuroscience, human stroke has provided the natural ablation experiments that have allowed us to infer which brain structures are necessary, though often not sufficient, for particular cognitive functions. Cognitive rehabilitation is a relatively new venture, based on fundamental advances in cognitive neuroscience but also dependent on the compassion, skill and dedicated, individualized coaching that has always distinguished the successful rehabilitation therapist. Armed with new knowledge of the injured brain's neuroplastic potential and capacity to change with the right guidance, cognitive rehabilitation aims to push beyond the limits of natural recovery by finding ways to enhance repair and to develop rational compensatory strategies. Careful analysis and inventory of neuroanatomical damage, both acute and chronic, through structural imaging can not only guide assessment and intervention, but also one day may be used to document tissue restoration.

Epidemiological considerations

- Epidemiological and community-based autopsy studies show that Alzheimer's disease (AD) is often combined with cerebrovascular disease (CVD) and the two together cause more injury than either alone.
- The most common cerebrovascular disease is small vessel disease, which should be evaluated in standard clinical practice. Rating scales can be used and quantification utilizing semi-automatic tissue segmentation techniques is desirable in research studies of brain–behavior relationships.
- Prevention of vascular injury could reduce the development and expression of dementia associated with both stroke and Alzheimer's disease.

Cerebrovascular disease

Cerebrovascular disease is a term broadly used to describe pathological changes in the brain parenchyma resulting from abnormalities in the brain's vasculature, such as atherosclerosis or amyloid angiopathy. It is heterogenous and can arise from large and small vessel disease, both on the arterial and venous sides of the circulation, from inflammation of vessels, cardiogenic embolism, hemorrhage and hypoperfusion. In addition to overt strokes that cause paralysis or loss of speech, there are so-called silent strokes which often affect brain networks involved in behavior and cognition.

Cognitive deficits may be masked by more obvious sensorimotor deficits and can initially be overlooked. Stroke occurs when there is a loss of blood supply to brain tissue either through occlusion or bleeding from a blood vessel. When damage is confined to the brain's white matter, brain connectivity is disrupted since the white matter is made up of nerve fibers joining the different brain regions together, as well as various types of supporting cells. Deficits will depend on the size and location of damage, but even small injuries through accumulation and strategic location can disrupt or degrade information transfer and reduce speed and efficiency of information processing. A clinically evident stroke occurs every 45 seconds in North America with approximately 5 million people living with the consequence of their stroke. Silent strokes are estimated to be 10–20 times as prevalent (Longstreth *et al.*, 1996) and on average only 4.4% of the elderly do not have evidence of white matter disease. Overt or covert ischemic brain injury from small vessel disease appears to be the commonest form of cerebrovascular disease (MRC CFAS, 2001). This cerebrovascular epidemic, soon to be exacerbated by the baby boomer bulge, is a sobering reality that will confront cognitive rehabilitation in the coming decades of the twenty-first century.

Dementia

Dementia is defined as a deterioration in memory and at least one other area of cognitive functioning sufficient to impair independence in activities of daily living. Worldwide, the prevalence of dementia is estimated to be 26.6 million. In the USA alone, care for the 4 million affected costs over $100 billion annually. In the absence of new prevention or disease-modifying therapies, given the aging of the human population, dementia constitutes a major challenge for healthcare and social systems around the world. Dementia also poses a particular challenge for cognitive rehabilitation in the elderly, the fastest growing sector of the human population in developed countries.

Recent epidemiological and pathological studies show that Alzheimer's disease (AD) is often combined with cerebrovascular disease, especially in the elderly, and the two together cause more injury than either alone to the aging human brain, leading more readily to the expression of dementia as a clinical syndrome (DeCarli, 2003). Silent stroke and white matter disease can gradually accumulate over time, as does the cell death caused by neurodegenerative disorders. In a prospective autopsy study of Catholic sisters over the age of 75, prevalence of dementia in those with AD pathology was only 57%, but it was 93% for those with small vessel infarcts in the subcortical regions (Snowdon *et al.*, 1997). Community-based autopsy studies suggest that cerebrovascular disease and AD may account for 80% of dementing illnesses; for example, one community-based autopsy series reported that 30% of cases had pure AD alone, 45% had mixed Alzheimer's and vascular lesions with less than 10% attributed to pure vascular pathologies (Lim *et al.*, 1999). A British community autopsy study (average age in the 80s) showed that 78% of cases had vascular pathology and 70% had Alzheimer's disease (MRC CFAS, 2001). In longitudinal population studies such as the Rotterdam study (Schmidt *et al.*, 2004; van Dijk *et al.*, 2004) and the Honolulu study of Japanese men, cerebrovascular risk factors such as hypertension, diabetes and hypercholesterolemia were risk factors not only for stroke but also for Alzheimer's disease (de la Torre, 2002; Launer *et al.*, 2000; Petrovitch *et al.*, 2000). Such findings suggest that prevention of vascular injury could reduce the development and expression of dementia associated with stroke and with Alzheimer's disease (Forette *et al.*, 1998; Snowdon, 2003).

Given the comorbidity of cerebrovascular disease and AD, both of which have detrimental effects on cognition and behavior, standardized methods to acquire scans and quantify both brain atrophy and cerebrovascular disease are advisable. In particular, evaluation of small vessel disease is highly desirable and should become as routine as the application of standard clinical assessment tools. The following section describes techniques to quantify the small vessel disease, with an emphasis on magnetic resonance imaging (MRI) – currently the most sensitive tool for its detection. A brief glossary of terms for MRI signal abnormalities is also provided at the end of this chapter, with Figures 8.1–8.8,

to guide the rehabilitationist through the labyrinth of technical jargon.

Overview of signal abnormalities seen on MRI

- Intensity differences as seen on MRI are used to classify brain tissue into gray matter, white matter, cerebrospinal fluid (CSF), and pathological changes such as cerebrovascular damage, which can appear as hyperintensities on T2-weighted MRI in the deep nuclei and white matter.
- Varying pathologies underlie these subcortical hyperintensities (SH), including occlusive disease (lipohyalinosis) of small vessels, demyelination, ependymal loss and gliosis, amyloid angiopathy, arteriosclerosis and small infarcts, and astrocytic changes.

Brain MRI is typically viewed as grayscale images where intensity differences are used to discriminate different tissue types. Each digital expression of an MRI comprises *voxels* with different intensity values, analogous to *pixels* which make up a picture from a digital camera. Depending on the scanning protocols, the brain's gray matter, white matter, cerebrospinal fluid (CSF), and more importantly, pathological changes, can be identified based on voxel intensity differences. Proton density (PD), T2-weighted (T2), and fluid attenuated inversion recovery (FLAIR) images are routinely used to identify subcortical hyperintensities (SH).

Varying pathologies underlie the SH (Pantoni & Lammie, 2002), including occlusive disease (lipohyalinosis) of small vessels, demyelination, ependymal loss and gliosis, amyloid angiopathy (Chen *et al.*, 2006), arteriosclerosis, small infarcts and astrocytic changes (Sahlas *et al.*, 2002). Subcortical hyperintensity rating, classification, and quantification have posed a challenge to researchers and clinicians to this day and no one method or gold standard has prevailed. The following section discusses approaches used to process an MRI to obtain volumetric and topographic information for different types of SH.

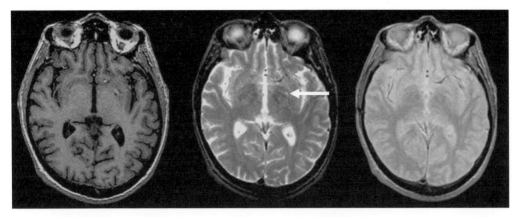

Figure 8.1. Dilated Virchow–Robin spaces appear as subcortical hyperintensities on T2-weighted MRIs and are often seen in the white matter and basal ganglia (i.e., bright on T2, isointense on PD), and occasionally co-exist with gliosis and small areas of infarction (Awad *et al.*, 1986). They appear as dots or lines, isointense relative to CSF, and generally 1 mm or less in diameter. Shown above is an example of a Virchow–Robin space (perivascular space) in the basal ganglia. Each image shows the same axial slice on a T1-weighted, T2-weighted, and Proton Density, magnetic resonance image (MRI). Images courtesy of the LC Campbell Cognitive Neurology Research Unit at Sunnybrook Health Sciences Centre, Toronto, Canada.

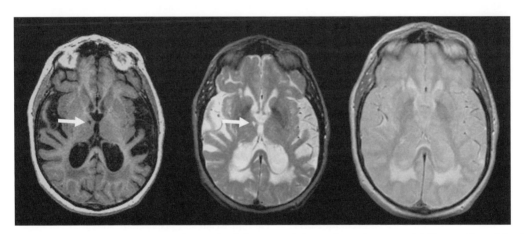

Figure 8.2. An example of a lacunar infarct in the thalamus. Each image shows the same axial slice on a T1-weighted, T2-weighted, and Proton Density (PD), magnetic resonance image (MRI). Images courtesy of the LC Campbell Cognitive Neurology Research Unit at Sunnybrook Health Sciences Centre, Toronto, Canada.

Historical overview of subcortical hyperintensities

- Prior to modern *in vivo* medical imaging techniques, Binswanger and Alzheimer described dementia characterized as "subcortical arteriosclerotic encephalopathy" commonly referred to as Binswanger's disease.
- More recent terms for this white matter disease include leukoaraiosis (rarefaction (araiosis) of white (leuko) matter), leukoencephalopathy, white matter or subcortical hyperintensities, and unidentified bright objects.

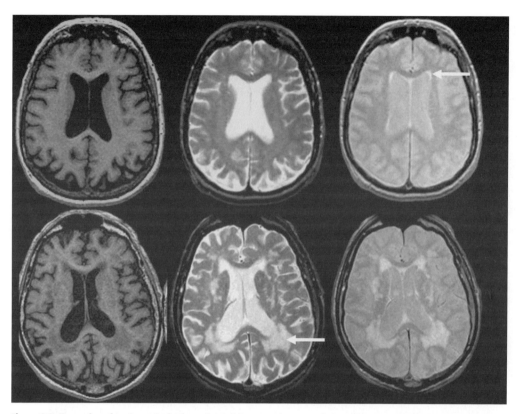

Figure 8.3. Examples of periventricular hyperintensities: anterior smooth cap (Top Row) and posterior irregular shaped (Bottom Row). Each row shows the same axial slice on a T1-weighted, T2-weighted, and Proton Density (PD), magnetic resonance image (MRI). Images courtesy of the LC Campbell Cognitive Neurology Research Unit at Sunnybrook Health Sciences Centre, Toronto, Canada.

In 1894, Otto Binswanger described eight patients with a form of dementia characterized by a progressive decline in various mental and motor functions including speech, memory and weakness in the lower extremities (Blass *et al.*, 1991). Autopsy revealed enlarged ventricles with thickened ependymal lining, atrophy of the subcortical white matter with normal-appearing cerebral cortex and sparing of the U-fibers. In 1902, Aloysius Alzheimer provided a histological report of a similar case confirming Binswanger's suggestion that this was related to ischemia, noting subcortical atherosclerosis and lacunar infarction of the white matter, internal capsule, basal ganglia, thalamus and pons (Schorer, 1992). In a 1962 review of Binswanger and Alzheimer's reports, the term

"subcortical arteriosclerotic encephalopathy" was introduced to characterize this neuropathologic entity (Olszewski, 1962). (For informative reviews, see Pantoni & Garcia, 1995; Roman, 2002.)

The advent of computed tomography (CT) in the early 1970s and of magnetic resonance imaging (MRI) in the early 1980s changed our understanding of the neuropathology first observed by Binswanger and Alzheimer. These imaging techniques, CT measuring tissue density using x-ray and MRI measuring proton density and relaxation properties of water when radio-frequency pulses are applied in a high magnetic field, allowed premortem examination of the human brain and revealed subcortical signal changes interpreted to be observable manifestation of Binswanger's disease

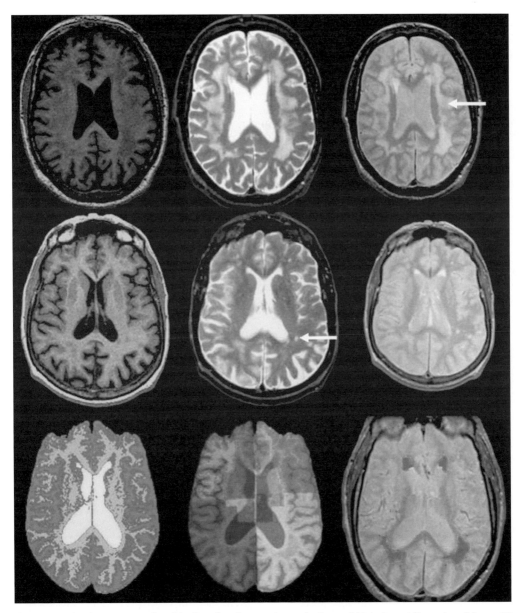

Figure 8.4. (This figure is reproduced in the color plate section at the front of this volume.) Examples of deep white hyperintensities: large confluent (Top Row) and discrete punctate (Middle Row). Each row shows the same axial slice on a T1-weighted, T2-weighted, and Proton Density (PD), magnetic resonance image (MRI). Bottom row from left to right shows post-processed images: a tissue segmented image (dark gray: gray matter, light gray: white matter, blue: CSF, yellow: vCSF); a regionally parcellated image using SABRE (Dade *et al.*, 2004); and a lesion segmentation overlayed on a PD image (red: periventricular, light blue: deep white). Images courtesy of the LC Campbell Cognitive Neurology Research Unit at Sunnybrook Health Sciences Centre, Toronto, Canada. Post-processed images provided courtesy of the Sunnybrook Dementia Study.

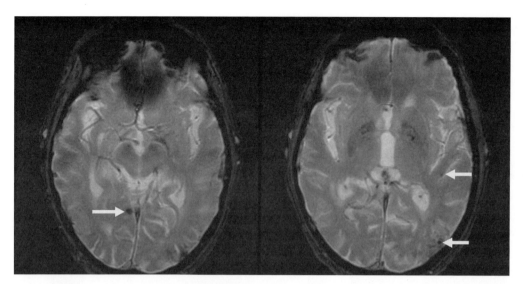

Figure 8.5. Examples of iron deposits corresponding to old hemorrhages as evidence of cerebral amyloid angiopathy. Microbleeds shown appear as hypointense dark spots on gradient echo MRIs. Images courtesy of the LC Campbell Cognitive Neurology Research Unit at Sunnybrook Health Sciences Centre, Toronto, Canada.

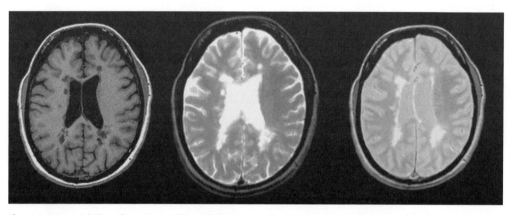

Figure 8.6. An axial slice of a patient with multiple sclerosis. Each image shows the same axial slice on a T1-weighted, T2-weighted, and Proton Density (PD), magnetic resonance image (MRI). Images courtesy of Dr. A. Feinstein, MS Research Group at Sunnybrook Health Sciences Centre, Toronto, Canada.

in vivo. Using gray-scale display, these signal abnormalities were hypodense (dark) regions on CT, hyperintense (white) on T2-weighted and proton density MRI, and isointense or hypointense to gray matter on T1-weighted MRI. It was soon realized that these abnormalities could be present in both clinically demented and nondemented individuals, leading to

a reconsideration of the diagnosis of Binswanger's disease (Babikian & Ropper, 1987; Roman, 2002).

In 1987, Hachinski and colleagues proposed the term *leuko-araiosis*, describing a rarefaction (araiosis) of the cerebral white (leuko) matter (Hachinski *et al.*, 1987). Other studies offer different nomenclatures to describe the same phenomenon, emphasizing

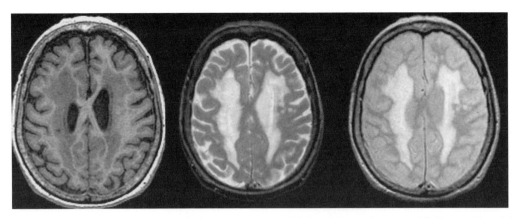

Figure 8.7. An axial slice of a patient with clasmatodendrosis. Each image shows the same axial slice on a T1-weighted, T2-weighted, and Proton Density (PD), magnetic resonance image (MRI). Images courtesy of the LC Campbell Cognitive Neurology Research Unit at Sunnybrook Health Sciences Centre, Toronto, Canada.

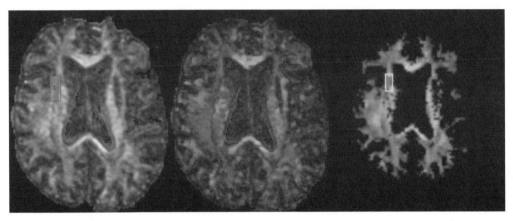

Figure 8.8. (This figure is reproduced in the color plate section at the front of this volume.) Fractional anisotropy (FA), corresponding color map, and FA image masked for white matter with selected region of interest (ROI) (red box) for obtaining mean FA value. Processed from a 12 orientation diffusion tensor image. Images courtesy of the LC Campbell Cognitive Neurology Research Unit at Sunnybrook Health Sciences Centre, Toronto, Canada.

different suggested pathologies, disease characteristics, and/or appearance on different neuroimaging techniques (e.g., unidentified bright objects, leukoencephalopathy, white matter hyperintensities). In the following section, we refer to these signal abnormalities in the most inclusive sense as "subcortical hyperintensities" (SH) to reflect both the "hyperintense appearance" and the general location "under" the cortex in the deep white matter, periventricular white matter and/or in the deep brain nuclei.

Quantifying signal abnormalities

- Rating scales provide quick estimates of the extent and location of SH using a T2-weighted/proton density or FLAIR MRI.
- Microbleeds (e.g., from traumatic injury), hypertension or amyloid angiopathy can also be assessed and counted using susceptibility-weighted gradient-echo MRI.

- Computational methods for full quantification of SH are available, the best of which allow separate regional volumetric analysis of brain parenchyma and hyperintense lesions, permitting simultaneous evaluation of the contribution of different regional compartments.
- Advanced new structural imaging techniques allow interrogation of: (a) myelin status (magnetization transfer ratio); (b) metabolite and neurotransmitter profiles (magnetic resonance spectroscopy); and (c) microstructural integrity (quantitative-T2 and diffusion tensor imaging).

In order to examine possible brain-behavior influences of SH in relation to recovery, a method of quantification is required to analyse their extent and location. Numerous subjective rating scales have been developed to estimate the severity and location of SH (e.g., Bocti et al., 2005; Scheltens et al., 1993; Wahlund et al., 1990). Computational quantification methods have also been developed to more objectively quantify these signal abnormalities. Below is a brief summary of a number of different techniques employed to classify and quantify SH volume on MRI.

A typical approach is to extend the tissue segmentation procedures used for brain parenchyma by adding an additional lesion compartment to the standard tissue classification into gray, white and CSF. Fuzzy clustering models using T1, T2 and PD images can be extended to include a fourth lesion class (e.g., Gosche et al., 1999). Gaussian curve fitting can be adapted to include a lesion intensity cutoff point such as +3 SDs on a Gaussian curve (e.g., DeCarli et al., 2005). Similarly, modal intensity cutoffs applied to slice-by-slice intensity histograms can be used to include a lesion segmentation (Jack et al., 2001). Co-registration to normal templates, such as the SPM99 segmentation, can be used to compare the voxel probabilities from FLAIR images to a white matter probability map using a weighting function (Burton et al., 2004; Wen & Sachdev, 2004). Tri-feature combination (PD, T2 and T1) procedures can be applied to combine a T1-segmentation (e.g., Kovacevic et al., 2002) with a PD/T2 lesion segmentation – allowing for quantification of

periventricular and deep white hyperintensities, T1 infarcts and Virchow–Robin (VR) spaces (Quddus et al., 2004; Ramirez et al., 2005).

Some lesion segmentation procedures have been designed specifically to only separate parenchyma and lesion using PD, T2, and/or FLAIR images that emphasize SH through fuzzy clustering (e.g., Admiraal-Behloul et al., 2005) or through KNN clustering algorithms (e.g., Swartz et al., 2002). These procedures generally provide whole brain quantification volumes without regional or gray-white parcellations. What is important is to use a method that allows separate quantification of both brain parenchyma and hyperintense lesion volumes so that the relative contributions of each can be understood.

Despite numerous clinically based research studies, the clinical relevance of SH remains to be fully elucidated. The most well-documented risk factors for presence of SH are aging, hypertension and other cerebrovascular disease risk factors (Boone et al., 1992; Liao et al., 1996; Manolio et al., 1994; Schmidt, 1992). Subcortical hyperintensities have also been associated with cognitive decline, particularly speed of information processing and executive functions (DeCarli et al., 1995; Gunning-Dixon & Raz, 2000; Longstreth et al., 1996; van Swieten et al., 1991), as well as physical disability, particularly gait disorders and poor motor dexterity (Masdeu et al., 1989; Sachdev et al., 2005; Starr et al., 2003; Whitman et al., 2001). In neuropsychological studies, correlations with poor attention and reduced speed of mental processing have been consistent across many series (Boone et al., 1992; Steingart et al., 1987; Ylikoski et al., 1993). However, when simultaneously considered with measures of gray and white matter atrophy, SH often explain only a small proportion of the variance, usually in relation to executive function measures (Fein et al., 2000; Mungas et al., 2001; Swartz et al., 2008). These correlations seem to hold irrespective of hyperintense lesion location.

In order to study subcortical white matter disease more consistently across many populations and many sites, standardized acquisition of MRI scans is needed. These should include 3D T1-weighted, and either FLAIR or T2-weighted/proton density scans, as well as gradient echo sequences to evaluate microbleeds, as recommended by the recent Harmonization Consensus guidelines for vascular cognitive impairment (Hachinski *et al.*, 2006). Ideally, what is necessary for post-processing are the following: (a) removal of brain from the skull and non-brain soft tissues; (b) a set of tissue segmentation protocols that reliably classify tissue compartments for gray matter, white matter, CSF, ventricular-CSF, subcortical hyperintensities and T1-"black hole" lacunar infarcts; and (c) a parcellation procedure to determine the neuroanatomical regions for the tissue volumes. Larger focal lesions, especially if they involve the cortex, are best traced and analysed separately (see next section).

Advanced neuroimaging techniques that further elucidate structural changes include diffusion tensor imaging (DTI), quantitative T2-weighted imaging and magnetization transfer ratio imaging. Magnetic resonance spectroscopy can give additional information on metabolite and even neurotransmitter profiles. Specifically, quantitative T2 measures intrinsic T2 characteristics of myelin and water. It provides information about changes in relative populations of these compartments (Webb *et al.*, 2003). Magnetization transfer (MT) provides information about interactions between water and macromolecular protons associated with myelin sheath lipids and indirectly measures demyelination and remyelination (Sled *et al.*, 2004; Stanisz *et al.*, 2005; Webb *et al.*, 2003). White matter exhibits the highest MT effect because of the highly structured lipid-rich macromolecular context provided by myelin. Magnetization transfer ratio has become an important metric in multiple sclerosis and has revealed abnormalities in amnestic mild cognitive impairment (Kabani *et al.*, 2002a, 2002b). Alterations in cellular function can be inferred from metabolite ratios using proton magnetic resonance spectroscopy (MRS), typically using creatine concentration as a reference. Commonly used cellular markers

include N-acetylaspartate (NAA), a marker of neuronal axonal integrity and density, myo-inositol, a marker of glial density, choline, a marker of myelin integrity, as well as lactate, a marker of anaerobic metabolism seen in ischemia. Magnetic resonance spectroscopy in the posterior cingulate, for example, can identify early changes in mild cognitive impairment (Kantarci *et al.*, 2002b), may predict conversion to dementia (Kantarci *et al.*, 2002a), and correlates with cognitive measures. Diffusion tensor imaging (DTI) is more sensitive than conventional T1 and T2 to changes in tissue microstructure, such as cellular geometry, extra- and intracellular volume fractions and cell membrane permeability and generates two parameters, mean diffusivity and fractional anisotropy. This will be discussed in more detail as it may elucidate brain–behavior relationships, both in relation to white matter hyperintensities and to large focal areas of brain injury. Importantly, these new structural imaging measures provide novel parameters of brain structure that can be related to cognitive test performance, daily function and behavioral scores based on questionnaires, protein biomarkers, and when possible, neuropathological information from biopsy or autopsy.

It is also important to mention gradient echo imaging, a quick acquisition protocol that is susceptibility-weighted causing blooming of any iron-containing lesions in the brain. Most commonly, this is useful in patients with stroke, dementia and traumatic brain injury. Microbleeds from traumatic diffuse axonal injury, hypertension or amyloid angiopathy can be visualized as dark black areas and can reveal the extent of silent brain bleeding. In the context of head injury, this may be the footprint of diffuse axonal injury, which may explain ongoing cognitive symptoms or difficulties with recovery. In the context of stroke, lobar hemorrhage with or without microbleeds, in the absence of a vascular formation, may be a clue that there is underlying Alzheimer's disease pathology (Cordonnier *et al.*, 2006). All of this may be important in planning treatment and rehabilitation strategies.

Diffusion tensor imaging (DTI)

- Diffusion tensor imaging measures the extent to which free diffusion is constrained (anisotropic diffusion) as occurs within myelinated fiber bundles. Fractional anisotropy is a new parameter reflecting this tissue microstructure, which can map the integrity of white matter tracts.

Diffusion tensor imaging provides an estimate of the 3-dimensional (3D) shape of water diffusion in the brain (Mori & Zhang, 2006). Conditions disrupting the brain's white matter cause increased free diffusion (equal in all directions) of water in and around the white matter fibers. This free diffusion is called isotropic diffusion. In contrast, anisotropic (unidirectional) diffusion represents a healthy condition whereby axon bundles are highly ordered and often myelinated, posing a perpendicular barrier to the free diffusion of water and creating an anisotropic path for water parallel to the orientation of the white matter fibers. Free diffusion of water implies structural damage to the white matter tracts while more constrained and unidirectional measures implies tract integrity. Fractional anisotropy (FA) (ranging from 0–1) is an index of the degree of anisotropic diffusion with a high value indicating high anisotropic diffusion.

Diffusion parameters can be estimated by acquiring diffusion weighted scans at various orientations, with a larger number of orientations generally allowing for higher resolution images. With the assistance of computerized DTI software, a trained operator can semi-automatically identify and trace the large association, projection and commissural tracts of an individual or group, a procedure called tractography.

It has been speculated that deep small subcortical hyperintensities can be more damaging than large ones because they may disrupt association tracts. Along the same lines, quantification of whole brain volumes of SH may be too crude a measure to understand brain–behavior relationships, particularly in specific cognitive domains. The ability to specifically quantify small strategic lesions in the basal ganglia and along the association tracts joining anterior and posterior cortical regions, such as

the superior longitudinal fasciculus, may correlate more specifically to cognitive impairments than measuring whole brain hyperintensity volumes. With DTI, subcortical hyperintensities can be accurately localized within white matter, allowing for recognition of disruption of specific fiber tracts. This technique can bring brain connectivity into direct scrutiny for analysing brain networks. This has potential application not only for better understanding the impact of white matter disease (DeCarli *et al.*, 1995) but also in neurodegenerative conditions (Zhang *et al.*, 2007). It also means that inferences about network disruptions from focal brain injury in stroke or surgical resection can now be tested directly (Thiebaut De Schotten *et al.*, 2007).

Focal brain lesion localization and lesion-behavior analysis

- Focal brain lesion analysis provides more accurate measurement of neuroanatomical location and volume and may aid prognostication and rehabilitation planning as well as help to develop a deeper understanding of structural-functional relationships.

Focal lesions, such as stroke, traumatic brain contusion, brain tumor and neurosurgical resections, can provide a unique window into human brain function through disease-related ablations of brain tissue. Structural neuroimaging (e.g., MRI or CT) enables identification of damaged brain regions in vivo in correlation with the clinical and neurobehavioral findings in individuals and groups of people. For instance, evidence strongly implicating the hippocampus and extra-hippocampal medial temporal lobe (MTL) in declarative memory came from single-case studies such as K.C., who showed dramatic loss of both anterograde and retrograde episodic memory after closed head injury from a motor vehicle accident (Tulving *et al.*, 1988). Tracing medial temporal structures using 3D MRI parallel to the long axis of the hippocampus revealed that K.C.'s hippocampus and some parahippocampal structures were extensively damaged

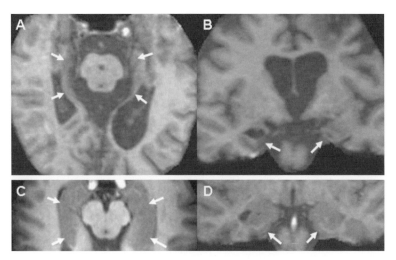

Figure 8.9. All images are 3D-T1 MR images. A (the patient K.C.) and C (healthy control) are the slices parallel to the long axis of the hippocampus (LAH). The hippocampi (double arrows in each side) are severely damaged bilaterally in the patient compared to the control. B (the patient K.C.) and D (healthy control) are scans perpendicular to the LAH. The entorhinal cortices bilateral (arrows) are markedly injured in the patient compared to the control. This patient exhibits anterograde and retrograde amnesia in aspects of recollective and familiarity processes after the brain injury (Rosenbaum *et al.*, 2000 with permission).

bilaterally, in addition to damage to medial occipital cortex and left frontal subcortical white matter (see Figure 8.9).

The results from his MTL damage included impaired acquisition of episodic memory with very poor recognition and no recollection of either episodic or generic/semantic details of his personal life (Gilboa *et al.*, 2006; Rosenbaum *et al.*, 2000, 2005). Animal experiments have suggested that distinct subregions within the MTL have dissociable functions subserving recollection processes and a sense of familiarity (Eichenbaum *et al.*, 1994). The hippocampus and the fornix, which links the hippocampus, thalamus and septal nuclei are critical for normal episodic memory (Gaffan, 1992a, 1992b) and the perirhinal, entorhinal or parahippocampal cortices are important for generic memory or familiarity processes (Aggleton & Brown, 1999). This dissociation is very difficult to demonstrate in humans, but A.D., another amnesic patient, provides further evidence to support this hypothesis (Gilboa *et al.*, 2006). 3D-MRI using multiple angles to track the fornix demonstrated that AD had bilateral fornix disruptions as well as damage to the

septal nuclei caused by a stereotactic probe used for trans-cortical surgery to remove a colloid cyst from the anterior third ventricle (see Figure 8.10). Bilateral damage to the fornix, which is almost equivalent to bilateral hippocampal ablation, induced severe anterograde as well as retrograde episodic amnesia, but left familiarity memory intact.

However, most brain lesions are unlikely to affect only one neural substrate, let alone be restricted to the fornix, and often involve many functional modules. It is not easy to precisely identify the region that is required for a particular function on the basis of the behavior of a single patient. Therefore, parallel case series or group studies are an important approach to identify regions that are commonly damaged in different individuals with the same deficit, but with lesions of different locations and sizes.

Conventionally, standardized focal lesion localizations used two-dimensional (2D) lesion-to-template translation methods, in which lesions from 2D-CT or MRI were manually traced onto a template atlas, such as those provided by Talairach (Talairach & Tournoux, 1988), Damasio (Damasio &

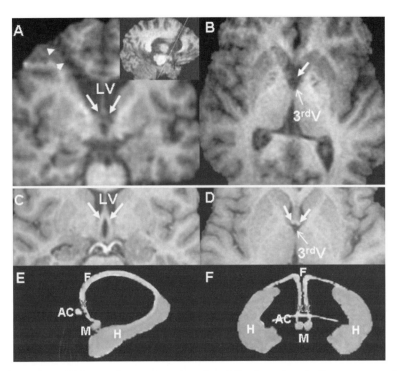

Figure 8.10. A and B are 3D-T1 MR images from an amnesic patient, A.D., after a stereotactic surgery removing a colloid cyst in the anterior 3rd ventricle (3rdV) (thin arrow) (Gilboa *et al.*, 2006 with permission). A is an oblique coronal section oriented at the line inside the inserted sagittal image, passing through the surgical stereotactic pathway (arrowheads). B is an axial image at level of 4 mm above the anterior-posterior commissure plane. A shows the anterior fornix is disrupted bilaterally (thick arrows) and B shows the fornix is not visible (indicating injuries), comparing to the control in C and D respectively. E (lateral view) and F (front-post view) are 3D reconstruction of the hippocampus (H), fornix (F), mammillary body (M) and anterior commissure (AC) from the control with 'x' indicating approximate level of the disrupted fornix in the patient A.D. LV: lateral ventricle. 3rdV: the third ventricle.

Damasio, 1989), or DeArmond (DeArmond *et al.*, 1989) (see an illustration in Figure 8.11). Lesion locations from different patients could then be compared on the template atlas, which contains localisation information on brain coordinates in stereotactic space, on anatomical regions and on Brodmann's areas (BA). If patients with focal damage are grouped by a common cognitive deficit and their lesions are superimposed on the common template, and if there is a common area of overlap which is mostly spared in patients lacking this deficit, it is inferred that this area is related to the cognitive deficit. Using this method, for example, Dronkers found that in stroke patients with verbal apraxia, an

articulatory planning deficit, the common area of lesion overlap was the left precentral gyrus of the insula (Dronkers, 1996). In another series, stroke patients with ideomotor limb apraxia showed the greatest overlap in white matter tracts at the left temporoparietal junction (Roy *et al.*, 1998).

Conventional template tracing methods are limited by the need to translate the position of a lesion from an individual scan to a standard template, as the scan angle, orientation and thickness often vary among subjects (Damasio & Damasio, 1989; Rorden & Brett, 2000). It is also difficult to precisely replicate localization, as different image interpreters use different anatomical

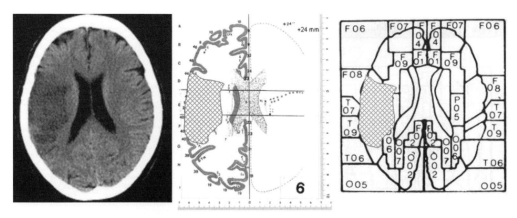

Figure 8.11. The left image is a CT axial section showing a right hemisphere hypodensity in the territory of the middle cerebral artery. The middle and right figures show the infarction has been manually mapped on the corresponding brain slice in the Talairach atlas (shaded area), and in the Damasio template (shaded area) respectively. The coded anatomical cells represent specified brain regions in the Damasio template (Damasio & Damasio, 1989).

landmarks to define lesion locations (Rorden & Brett, 2000).

Using a statistical overlap method to fractionate regional frontal lobe functions in correlation with damage in different frontal subregions, Stuss and colleagues showed that "energization" as measured by slow reaction times and poor response to a warning signal was associated with right superior medial frontal damage (BA24, 32, 9) (Stuss *et al.*, 2005). Failure to use cues to enhance response time was seen with right dorsolateral frontal damage. A follow-up study further implicated right lateral frontal regions in monitoring time intervals and controlling timed behavior, and the superior medial regions in sustaining consistent timed performance over time (Picton *et al.* 2006; Stuss, 2006; Stuss *et al.*, 2005). His group showed that lesions to the left superior frontal cortex (area 6) are associated with deficits in withholding responses, while lesions to the right cingulate area (area 24, 32, 9) cause slowness of response and inconsistency in both timing and accuracy (Picton *et al.*, 2007; Stuss *et al.*, 2005). Such studies demonstrate that careful lesion-behavior correlations continue to expand our understanding of the role played by different brain regions in specific cognitive processes.

With digital technology, computerized lesion analysis using spatial normalization methods has become increasingly popular (Bates *et al.*, 2003; Rorden & Brett, 2000). This approach has the following advantages: (a) spatial coordinates of focal lesions in the normalized brain template are easy to determine; (b) lesion volumes can be made comparable across patients, as overall size of brains are normalized; (c) it is easier to compare lesion location across subjects and across publications; (d) it is automated and therefore more objective (Ashburner & Friston, 1999; Rorden & Brett, 2000; Woods *et al.*, 1992). The major steps of this approach are discussed below.

Imaging acquisition and lesion tracing

- Three-dimensional T1-weighted MRI provides the best images to measure brain necrosis. Two-dimensional images are less ideal but can be converted into 3D images.

Three-dimensional MR images are best for documenting scan normalization, as they give the most accurate view of anatomical landmarks and structures, and need less transformation in the spatial normalization process and in interpolating the extent of the lesion between slices (Rorden & Brett, 2000). Three-dimensional, T1-weighted, 1mm thick images

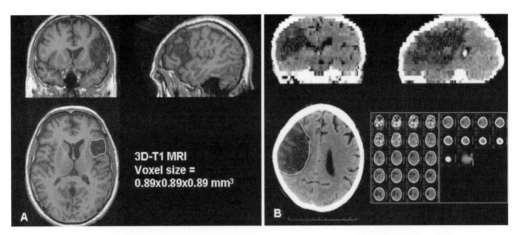

Figure 8.12. (A) is a 3D-T1 MRI from a patient with an infarction in the territory of the left middle cerebral artery (MCA), (B) is a 2D-CT hardcopy (lower/right images) from another patient with right MCA stroke, which has been digitized and transferred to 3D-CT. Lesion tracings using the ANALYZE region of interest module (Robb *et al.*, 1989 with permission) are shown in the axial slices and the actual lesion outline is performed slice-by-slice to obtain entire lesion volume.

also offer the best anatomical definition for lesions causing brain necrosis, which appears hypointense on T1 (see Figure 8.12A), or for hemorrhagic lesions, which cause hyperintense signal change on T1 images in the acute phase. Other MR sequences can help to define the full extent of tissue alteration and extend lesion boundaries. For instance, T2-weighted and Proton Density (PD) images will show greater lesion extent than T1 with gliosis, demyelination, edema and encephalomalacia appearing as hyperintense as described above. Fluid attenuated inversion recovery (FLAIR) may show a necrotic hypointense core, surrounded by a hyperintense border. Gradient echo sequence will cause hemosiderin deposits from microhemorrhages or hemotomas to "bloom" and be more visible as black spots or areas displayed on each slice. Although CT scans do not provide the same anatomical accuracy as MRI, it is still possible, though not ideal, to co-register scans and normalize them to the same brain template using a 2D-to-3D technique, as demonstrated in Figure 8.12B (Davidson *et al.*, 2008).

To obtain acute volume information, focal lesions have to be traced and segmented on each slice of the raw image series in acquisition space (see Figure 8.12). Although some semi-automated methods can help determine lesion boundaries (Kaus *et al.*, 2001), this is still best done manually by a trained observer, due to low contrast between brain tissue and lesion, or to individual topologic variations.

Spatial normalization

- Spatial normalization is the technique for scaling, rotating and warping individual brains (the source images) of different sizes, shapes and orientations to align with a "standard" brain (template image).
- Lesion masking can prevent lesions from being distorted in the spatial normalization process.

Spatial normalization is generally referred to as the technique of scaling, rotating and warping individual brains (source image) of different sizes, shapes and orientations to align with a "standard" brain (template image). It can be implemented using normalization packages, such as Statistical Parametric Mapping (SPM) (Ashburner & Friston, 1999; Friston *et al.*, 1995) (free at: www.fil.ion.ucl.ac.uk.spm). Normalization is an iterative computational process matching two images based on intensity difference between their corresponding regions, using

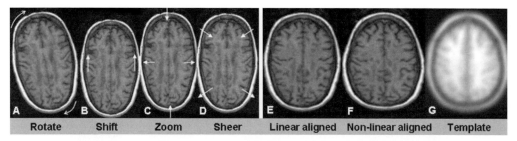

Figure 8.13. Illustrations of linear and nonlinear spatial normalization. (A–D) are MR source images presenting an unusual brain shape with an elongated anterior-to-posterior extent and short width. The directions (arrows) of the linear transformation required to fit the template G are shown globally, including rotating (A), shifting (B), zooming (C) and sheering (D). (E), the same image of (A–D) shown after the linear transformation, has to fit to the template (G) roughly, and (F) is the image after further nonlinear warping, using SPM, which has matched the source images (A–D) to the template. The template (G) is a smoothed average image of a large group of brains created by the Montreal Neurological Institute (Collins *et al.*, 1994) and freely distributed in SPM (www.fil.ion.ucl.ac.uk.spm).

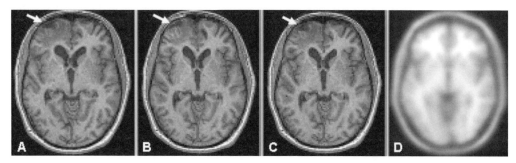

Figure 8.14. Illustrations of using lesion mask in SPM to prevent lesions from being distorted in the nonlinear normalization process. (A) is an image with linear transformation showing a lesion in the right frontal pole (arrow). (B) is the same image after the nonlinear transformation without using a lesion mask, showing that the lesion (arrow) is compressed and becomes smaller than that lesion in (A). (C) is the image using nonlinear normalization while the lesion is masked, illustrating that the lesion (arrows) is well preserved in shape and size compared to the lesion in (A). (D) is the Montreal Neurological Institute template.

linear and nonlinear transformations. Linear transformation (also referred as to affine spatial transformation) matches the source image to the template across the whole brain, using rotating, shifting, zooming and sheering, to make two images in rough alignment globally. Nonlinear transformation (also referred to as warping) can further optimize the matching between the source and template images. The warping process will selectively compress some portions of the image while expanding other regions, and tends to be more sensitive to local differences than affine transforms (Ashburner & Friston, 1999) (see illustrations in Figure 8.13). However, the nonlinear functions can also squash, distort or eliminate the region of a lesion by compressing that region, and cause considerable distortion of the brain, because lesions (such as stroke) usually have a very different intensity in a patient's scan than the corresponding area in the template. This problem can be resolved if the region of lesion is masked during the nonlinear normalization process (Brett *et al.*, 2001), as the masked region (e.g., area of a lesion) does not influence the parameter estimation of nonlinear functions (see Figure 8.14).

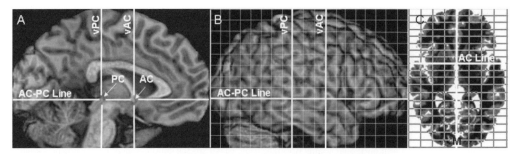

Figure 8.15. Talairach system. (A) (MR T1 inter-hemispheric sagittal plane) shows the three reference lines forming the basis of the Talairach proportional grid system (Talairach & Tournoux, 1988): the anterior commissure–posterior commissure line (AC–PC), the vertical line traversing the AC (vAC), and the midline of inter-hemispheric sagittal plane. (B) (MR T1 lateral view) and (C) (MR T1 axial view at the AC–PC plane) demonstrate the actual proportional grid. M: the midline of the inter-hemispheric fissure. vPC: the vertical line tranversing the PC.

Lesion localization and lesion-behavior analysis

- Lesion-behavior analysis can be done by overlapping lesions in patients dichotomously categorised into groups with and without a specific behavior using chi-square to test for statistical significance.
- Voxel-based lesion symptom-mapping dichotomises voxels into lesion and nonlesion and statistically tests the means for voxels affected and those not affected with t-tests using a continuous behavioral measure.

After the spatial normalization, the lesions in each scan are reconstructed in the template using the transformation. The Talairach stereotactic coordinate system in which the axis is aligned parallel to the baseline joining the anterior and posterior commissure (the so-called AC–PC line) (Talairach & Tournoux, 1988) is typically used to describe spatial location of lesions in the template. It is based on the assumption of proportionality of brain structures (i.e., brain size changes between different subjects, but proportions of brain structures are constant) (see Figure 8.15). Although lesion location also can be defined using standard Brodmann areas and anatomical regions (e.g., Talairach & Tournoux, 1988; or www.MRIcro.com), reporting lesion data in terms of Talairach coordinates is often more appropriate for neuropsychological correlations

than trying to specify the site of the lesion in terms of Brodmann's areas, especially for functional imaging studies with positron emission tomography (PET) or functional MRI. This is because the normalization process described above can reduce fine image details such as the position of small sulci (Rorden & Brett, 2000).

A clear advantage of the spatial normalization is that it allows direct comparison of focal lesions across patients or between groups in a single standard space using the lesion overlapping technique. Two voxelwise lesion-behavior analyses, e.g., the lesion subtraction analysis (Rorden & Brett, 2000) and voxel-based lesion-symptom mapping (VLSM) (Bates *et al.*, 2003) have been developed in recent years to identify regions that are commonly damaged in different individuals with the same cognitive deficit.

The subtraction method uses study subjects dichotomized into groups with and without a specific behavior (Rorden & Brett, 2000). The lesions from each subject in the symptom-present group are added together, creating an overlap image showing the region of mutual involvement. Then, the lesions for the nonsymptomatic group (serving as controls) are subtracted from the symptomatic group's overlap image. This method creates an image that shows regions that are damaged commonly in patients with the behavior of interest, regions that are damaged in the control patients, and regions that are damaged or spared in equal proportions between the two groups. As a further refinement, in VLSM, voxelwise statistical testing using χ^2 analysis can be performed between two groups of subjects for each and every voxel of the brain, with Bonferroni correction, a stringent correction for multiple comparisons whereby the P value is divided by the total number of χ^2 tests performed to determine the P value considered statistically significant. The results are presented as a density plot (www.MRIcro.com) (see Figure 8.16). Using this technique, for instance, Karnath et al. (2004) found that the right superior temporal cortex, the insula, putamen and caudate nucleus are the neural structures damaged more often in patients with spatial neglect.

Of greater importance, VLSM does not need to group patients by dichotomous behavioral cut off, but instead can make use of continuous behavioral and lesion information (Bates et al., 2003). For each voxel during the voxel-by-voxel analysis, patients must fall into a group either with or without damage in that voxel. Continuous behavior scores are then compared for these two groups, yielding a t-statistic for that voxel. Significant results, with Bonferroni correction in which the P value is divided by the total number of unique t-tests performed, implies that the region has significant relationship to the specific behavior of interest (see Figure 8.16). As an example, Bates et al. (2003) used VLSM and found that the anterior insula was critical for verbal fluency, and that the middle temporal gyrus was a significant factor in auditory comprehension in 101 left-hemisphere-damaged aphasic patients.

There are several reservations that bear on the interpretation of findings when using focal brain lesion approach to infer brain–behavior relationships. First, each brain region works in a plastic fashion as part of a dynamically changing network rather than having a fixed function (Farah et al., 1994; Raineteau & Schwab, 2001). Second, the same anatomical location may not have the same functional role in different individuals due to genetic–environmental interactions (Amunts et al.,

2004). Third, impaired function may be caused by injury to a distant brain region functionally connected to a region, a phenomenon called diaschisis, reflecting that the brain functions through interconnected networks (Silveri et al., 2001). Finally, a common area of lesion overlay could be simply that there are commonly damaged zones reflecting the same distribution of a blood supply; for example, strokes in the left middle cerebral artery territory often cause aphasia (Caviness et al., 2002). Regardless of how models of cognition are mapped onto brain regions, evidence from brain lesion studies must be taken into account. If focal lesions cause specific abnormalities, these lesions have disrupted a process, no matter whether it is through local or remote effect, or interruption of a network (Picton et al., 2006). Lesion data can determine what is necessary, if not sufficient, for particular cognitive functions (Fellows et al., 2005), and have played a major role in the development of cognitive neuroscience since the nineteenth-century clinicopathological studies, for example, when Broca correctly inferred a role for the left posterior inferior lateral frontal lobe in speech production (Dronkers et al., 2007) or Dejerine demonstrated the neural substrate of the disconnection syndrome, alexia without agraphia (Damasio & Damasio, 1989).

Hence an important step in planning any cognitive rehabilitation intervention is not only detailed behavioral analysis, but also a careful analysis of lesion parameters. Knowledge from the cumulative evidence base of multiple parallel single case and group studies can help guide expectations for recovery and choice of interventional approaches.

Summary

In summary, focal lesion analysis, especially utilizing modern computational techniques, can provide important information on structural brain damage–behavior relationships. New computational spatial normalization methods have improved the objectivity and accuracy of group comparisons. However,

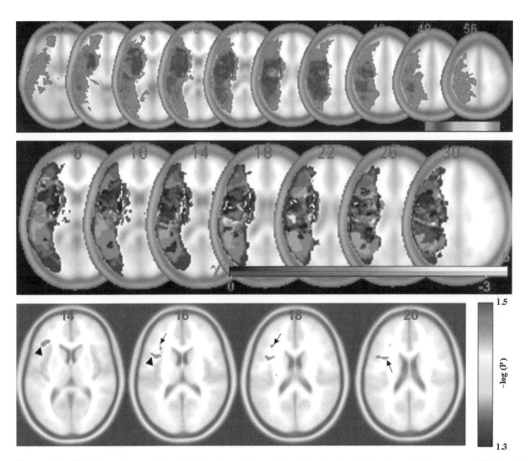

Figure 8.16. (This figure is reproduced in the color plate section at the front of this volume.) Upper panel: Simple lesion density plots from 25 patients with right hemisphere strokes, who were tested using the Sunnybrook Neglect Assessment Procedure (SNAP) (Leibovitch *et al.*, 1998) in a study of neglect. The number of overlapping lesions is illustrated by different colors coding increasing frequencies from violet (*n* = 1) to red (*n* = 25) in a standard template (Collins *et al.*, 1994).

Middle panel: Using the MRIcro lesion subtraction technique (Rorden & Brett, 2000), the overlapping lesions of the neglect patients (*n* = 15, SNAP score >4) after subtraction of the patients without neglect (*n* = 10, SNAP score 4) is illustrated by different color gradient corresponding with the χ^2 value (the upper color gradient of dark red to white for the neglect, and the lower color gradient from blue to green for the controls). The light yellow areas involving superior longitudinal fasciculus, frontooccipital fasciculus and superior temporal regions were more significantly damaged in the neglect patients than in controls at the level of $\chi^2 > 3.84$, $P < 0.05$, but they would not survive Bonferroni correction.

Lower panel: VLSM maps computed for continuous SNAP scores of the same 25 stroke patients on a voxel-by-voxel basis as recommended by Bates *et al.* (2003). Patients with lesion in a given voxel were compared with those without lesions in that voxel on measures of SNAP scores using t-statistic analysis, which can covary confounding factors. These VLSM maps of voxel-by-voxel ANCOVAs covarying out lesion size indicated SNAP scores were most affected by lesions in the anterior segment of the superior longitudinal fasciculus (SLF) (arrows) and the inferior frontal gyrus (BA44 and 45) (arrowheads). The maps are plotted with $-\log (P) \geq 1.3$ and $P < 0.05$, Bonferroni corrected, as shown by the color gradient.

the methods still require training and expertise; each step from scan acquisition, lesion mapping, and spatial normalization, to the final lesion-behavior analysis has to be separately and carefully processed. If such analyses are incorporated into both clinical care and research protocols, they can enhance the planning and execution of the custom-ised cognitive and physical rehabilitation needed by patients with focal brain injury.

As has been described in this chapter, computational methods can be used to extract quantitative information from scans obtained by standardized protocols to help in understanding underlying brain disease at the time of injury. Pure focal lesions can be traced and group comparisons are now conducted with objectivity and statistical rigor, greatly enhancing the ability to investigate the role of brain damage in cognitive outcome and potentially to understand the limitations and best avenues to follow for cognitive rehabilitation. Advanced imaging techniques are further enhancing our understanding of brain microstructural damage and in particular, tractography using diffusion tensor imaging is allowing us to directly appreciate network disruptions in cerebral white matter tracts. This will allow us to better understand the role of disconnections and direct cortical injury and in drawing inferences about which structures are necessary for particular cognitive functions. Recovery studies that utilize these lesion mapping techniques in conjunction with functional imaging methods inform us about pathways that are disrupted, and alternate pathways that may be intact and exploitable, potentially helping us to plan and monitor cognitive interventions.

Glossary of signal abnormalities in MRI

Virchow–Robin spaces (Figure 8.1)

The Virchow–Robin (VR) space, or perivascular space, is a CSF-filled extension of the subarachnoid space surrounding the arteries, arterioles, veins and venules entering the brain, usually seen in inferior slices in the basal ganglia region or on superior slices.

État criblé

État criblé refers to a dilatation or widening of the perivascular spaces as first observed by Durand-Fardel in 1842 (Barkhof, 2004; Braffman et al., 1988; Roman, 2002). Durand-Fardel believed this widening of the perivascular space was due to vascular congestion.

Lacunes (Figure 8.2)

The term lacune originates from the French, referring to a tiny hole, pit or cavity. Lacunes in the brain refer to a small cystic cavity of infarcted brain tissue caused by an occlusion of the small penetrating arteries (Fisher, 1982, 1991; Mohr, 1982; Roman, 2002). Lacunar infarcts generally appear hyperintense on both T2 and PD, and are classified as 1.5 cm or less in diameter.

Periventricular white matter hyperintensities (PVWMH) (Figure 8.3)

Periventricular white matter hyperintensities (PVWMH) are defined by their proximity to the ventricles. They are defined as hyperintensities found within an arbitrary distance from the edge of the ventricles or as any hyperintensity touching the ventricles. They can appear as smooth caps or as patches of irregularly shaped hyperintense patches.

Deep white subcortical hyperintensities (DWH) (Figure 8.4)

In contrast to PVWMH, deep white subcortical hyperintensities (DWH) are defined as discrete focal or small confluent hyperintensities which are not touching or in close proximity to the ventricles. Hyperintensities in the basal ganglia area and thalamus are also referred to by some as deep hyperintensities.

Amyloid angiopathy (Figure 8.5)

Cerebral amyloid angiopathy refers to the deposition of beta-amyloid in the media and adventitia of small and mid-sized arteries of the cortex and leptomeninges. These deposits are believed to contribute to blood vessel fragility and may lead to microbleeds and lobar intracerebral hemorrhage (ICH). Some subcortical hyperintensities in patients with Alzheimer's disease may relate to amyloid angiopathy (Kalaria, 2002; Pantoni & Garcia, 1997). Amyloidosis can be inferred from gradient echo MRI images, where hemosiderin deposits corresponding to old hemorrhages appear as hypointense dark spots which "bloom" and become more visible on this gradient echo MR sequence.

Multiple sclerosis (Figure 8.6)

In multiple sclerosis (MS), the punctate or confluent subcortical white matter hyperintensities seen on PD, T2-weighted and FLAIR images are believed to reflect a different pathogenesis, with multi-focal inflammation and demyelination as the main underlying causes for these lesions. Gliosis, demyelination, remyelination and axonal loss are also believed to contribute to the pathological changes underlying MS (Bermel & Bakshi, 2006).

Clasmatodendrosis (Figures 8.7 and 8.8)

A finding first described by Alzheimer in 1911 and termed clasmatodendrons (Greek for breaking up branches).

ACKNOWLEDGMENTS

We thank the following agencies/institutions for their support:

LC Campbell Cognitive Neurology Research Unit Figures 8.9–8.16 were courtesy of the Brain Imaging Laboratory of the Heart and Stroke Foundation Centre for Stroke Recovery

Sunnybrook Research Institute-Neuroscience
University of Toronto
Alzheimer Society of Canada
Alzheimer's Association US
Canadian Institutes of Health Research

REFERENCES

Admiraal-Behloul, F., van den Heuvel, D. M., Olofsen, H. *et al.* (2005). Fully automatic segmentation of white matter hyperintensities in MR images of the elderly. *NeuroImage*, **28**, 607–617.

Aggleton, J. P., & Brown, M. W. (1999). Episodic memory, amnesia, and the hippocampal-anterior thalamic axis. *Behavioral and Brain Sciences*, **22**, 425–444.

Amunts, K., Weiss, P. H., Mohlberg, H. *et al.* (2004). Analysis of neural mechanisms underlying verbal fluency in cytoarchitectonically defined stereotaxic space – the roles of Brodmann areas 44 and 45. *NeuroImage*, **22**, 42–56.

Anonymous (2000). The incidence of dementia in Canada. The Canadian Study of Health and Aging Working Group. *Neurology*, **55**, 66–73.

Ashburner, J., & Friston, K. J. (1999). Nonlinear spatial normalization using basis functions. *Human Brain Mapping*, **7**, 254–266.

Awad, I. A., Johnson, P. C., Spetzler, R. F., & Hodak, J. A. (1986). Incidental subcortical lesions identified on magnetic resonance imaging in the elderly. II. Postmortem pathological correlations. *Stroke*, **17**, 1090–1097.

Babikian, V., & Ropper, A. H. (1987). Binswanger's disease: a review. *Stroke*, **18**, 2–12.

Barkhof, F. (2004). Enlarged Virchow–Robin spaces: do they matter? *Journal of Neurology, Neurosurgery and Psychiatry*, **75**, 1516–1517.

Bates, E., Wilson, S. M., Saygin, A. P. *et al.* (2003). Voxel-based lesion-symptom mapping. *Nature Neuroscience*, **6**, 448–450.

Bermel, R. A., & Bakshi, R. (2006). The measurement and clinical relevance of brain atrophy in multiple sclerosis. *Lancet Neurology*, **5**, 158–170.

Blass, J. P., Hoyer, S., & Nitsch, R. (1991). A translation of Otto Binswanger's article, 'The delineation of the generalized progressive paralyses'. 1894. *Archives of Neurology*, **48**, 961–972.

Bocti, C., Swartz, R. H., Gao, F. Q. *et al.* (2005). A new visual rating scale to assess strategic white matter hyperintensities within cholinergic pathways in dementia. *Stroke*, **36**, 2126–2131.

Boone, K. B., Miller, B. L., Lesser, I. M. *et al.* (1992). Neuropsychological correlates of white-matter lesions in healthy elderly subjects. A threshold effect. *Archives of Neurology*, **49**, 549–554.

Braffman, B. H., Zimmerman, R. A., Trojanowski, J. Q. *et al.* (1988). Brain MR: Pathologic correlation with gross and histopathology. 1. Lacunar infarction and Virchow–Robin spaces. *American Journal of Roentgenology*, **151**, 551–558.

Brett, M., Leff, A. P., Rorden, C., & Ashburner, J. (2001). Spatial normalization of brain images with focal lesions using cost function masking. *NeuroImage*, **14**, 486–500.

Burton, E. J., Kenny, R. A., O'Brien, J. *et al.* (2004). White matter hyperintensities are associated with impairment of memory, attention, and global cognitive performance in older stroke patients. *Stroke*, **35**, 1270–1275.

Caviness, V. S., Makris, N., Montinaro, E. *et al.* (2002). Anatomy of stroke, Part I: an MRI-based topographic and volumetric system of analysis. *Stroke*, **33**, 2549–2556.

Chen, Y. W., Gurol, M. E., Rosand, J. *et al.* (2006). Progression of white matter lesions and hemorrhages in cerebral amyloid angiopathy. *Neurology*, **67**, 83–87.

Collins, D. L., Neelin, P., Peters, T. M., & Evans, A. C. (1994). Automatic 3D intersubject registration of MR volume data in standardized talairach space. *Journal of Computer Assisted Tomography*, **18**, 192–205.

Cordonnier, C., van der Flier, W. M., Sluimer, J. D. *et al.* (2006). Prevalence and severity of microbleeds in a memory clinic setting. *Neurology*, **66**, 1356–1360.

Dade, L. A., Gao, F. Q., Kovacevic, N. *et al.* (2004). Semiautomatic brain region extraction: a method of parcellating brain regions from structural magnetic resonance images. *NeuroImage*, **22**, 1492–1502.

Damasio, H., & Damasio, A. (1989). *Lesion Analysis in Neuropsychology*. New York, NY: Oxford University Press.

Davidson, P. S. R., Gao, F. Q., Mason, W. P., Winocur, G., & Anderson, N. D. (2008). Verbal fluency, trail making, and Wisconsin Card Sorting Test performance following right frontal lobe tumor resection. *Journal of Clinical and Experimental Neuropsychology*, **30**, 18–32.

de la Torre, J. C. (2002). Alzheimer disease as a vascular disorder: nosological evidence. *Stroke*, **33**, 1152–1162.

DeArmond, S. J., Fusco, M. M., & Dewey, M. M. (1989). *Structure of the Human Brain. A Photographic Atlas*. New York, NY: Oxford University Press.

DeCarli, C. (2003). The role of cerebrovascular disease in dementia. *Neurologist*, **9**, 123–136.

DeCarli, C., Murphy, D. G., Tranh, M. *et al.* (1995). The effect of white matter hyperintensity volume on brain structure, cognitive performance, and cerebral metabolism of glucose in 51 healthy adults. *Neurology*, **45**, 2077–2084.

DeCarli, C., Fletcher, E., Ramey, V., Harvey, D., & Jagust, W. J. (2005). Anatomical mapping of white matter hyperintensities (WMH): exploring the relationships between periventricular WMH, deep WMH, and total WMH burden. *Stroke*, **36**, 50–55.

Dronkers, N. F. (1996). A new brain region for coordinating speech articulation. *Nature Neuroscience*, **384**, 159–161.

Dronkers, N. F., Plaisant, O., Iba-Zizen, M. T., & Cabanis, E. A. (2007). Paul Broca's historic cases: high resolution MR imaging of the brains of Leborgne and Lelong. *Brain*, **130**, 1432–1441.

Eichenbaum, H., Otto, T., Cohen, N. J., & Aggleton, J. P. (1994). Two functional components of the hippocampal memory system. *Behavioral and Brain Sciences*, **17**, 449–518.

Farah, M. J., Bullinaria, J. A., Burton, A. M., & Bruce, V. (1994). Neuropsychological inference with an interactive brain: a critique of the locality assumption. *Behavioral and Brain Sciences*, **17**, 43–61.

Fein, G., Di Sclafani, V., Tanabe, J. *et al.* (2000). Hippocampal and cortical atrophy predict dementia in subcortical ischemic vascular disease. *Neurology*, **55**, 1626–1635.

Fellows, L. K., Heberlein, A. S., Morales, D. A., Shivde, G., Waller, S., & Wu, D. H. (2005). Method matters: an empirical study of impact in cognitive neuroscience. *Journal of Cognitive Neuroscience*, **17**, 850–858.

Fisher, C. M. (1982). Lacunar strokes and infarcts: a review. *Neurology*, **32**, 871–876.

Fisher, C. M. (1991). Lacunar infarcts – a review. *Cerebrovascular Diseases*, **1**, 311–320.

Forette, F., Seux, M. L., Staessen, J. A. *et al.* (1998). Prevention of dementia in randomized double-blind placebo-controlled systolic hypertension in Europe (Syst-Eur) trial. *Lancet*, **352**, 1347–1351.

Friston, K. J., Ashburner, J., Frith, C. D., Heather, J. D., & Frackowiak, R. S. J. (1995). Spatial registration and normalization of images. *Human Brain Mapping*, **3**, 165–189.

Gaffan, D. (1992a). Amnesia for complex naturalistic scenes and for objects following fornix transection in the rhesus monkey. *European Journal of Neuroscience*, **4**, 381–388.

Gaffan, D. (1992b). The role of the hippocampus-fornix-mammillary system in episodic memory. In L. R. Squire & N. Butters (Eds.), *Neuropsychology of Memory* (*2nd Edition*) (pp. 336–346). New York, NY: Guilford Press.

Gilboa, A., Winocur, G., Rosenbaum, R. S. *et al.* (2006). Hippocampal contributions to recollection in retrograde and anterograde amnesia. *Hippocampus*, **16**, 966–980.

Gosche, K. M., Velthuizen, R. P., Murtagh, F. R. *et al.* (1999). Automated quantification of brain magnetic resonance image hyperintensities using hybrid clustering and knowledge-based methods. *International Journal of Imaging Systems and Technology*, **10**, 287–293.

Gunning-Dixon, F. M., & Raz, N. (2000). The cognitive correlates of white matter abnormalities in normal aging: a quantitative review. *Neuropsychology*, **14**, 224–232.

Hachinski, V. C., Potter, P., & Merskey, H. (1987). Leukoaraiosis. *Archives of Neurology*, **44**, 21–23.

Hachinski, V., Iadecola, C., Petersen, R. C. *et al.* (2006). National Institute of Neurological Disorders and Stroke-Canadian Stroke Network vascular cognitive impairment harmonization standards. *Stroke*, **37**, 2220–2241.

Dejerine, J. (1892). Contribution à l'étude anatomo-pathologique et clinique des différentes variétés de cécité verbale. *Mémoires de la Société de Biologie*, **4**, 61–90.

Jack, C. R. J., O'Brien, P. C., Rettman, D. W. *et al.* (2001). FLAIR histogram segmentation for measurement of leukoaraiosis volume. *Journal of Magnetic Resonance Imaging*, **14**, 668–676.

Kabani, N. J., Sled, J. G., & Chertkow, H. (2002a). Magnetization transfer ratio in mild cognitive impairment and dementia of Alzheimer's type. *NeuroImage*, **15**, 604–610.

Kabani, N. J., Sled, J. G., Shuper, A., & Chertkow, H. (2002b). Regional magnetization transfer ratio changes in mild cognitive impairment. *Magnetic Resonance in Medicine*, **47**, 143–148.

Kalaria, R. N. (2002). Small vessel disease and Alzheimer's dementia: pathological considerations. *Cerebrovascular Diseases*, **13**, *Suppl. 2*, 48–52.

Kantarci, K., Smith, G. E., Ivnik, R. J. *et al.* (2002a). 1H magnetic resonance spectroscopy, cognitive function, and apolipoprotein E genotype in normal aging, mild cognitive impairment and Alzheimer's disease. *Journal of the International Neuropsychological Society*, **8**, 934–942.

Kantarci, K., Xu, Y., Shiung, M. M. *et al.* (2002b). Comparative diagnostic utility of different MR modalities in mild cognitive impairment and Alzheimer's disease. *Dementia and Geriatric Cognitive Disorders*, **14**, 198–207.

Karnath, H. O., Fruhmann, B. M., Kuker, W., & Rorden, C. (2004). The anatomy of spatial neglect based on voxel-wise statistical analysis: a study of 140 patients. *Cerebral Cortex*, **14**, 1164–1172.

Kaus, M. R., Warfield, S. K., Nabavi, A. *et al.* (2001). Automated segmentation of MR images of brain tumors. *Radiology*, **218**, 586–591.

Kovacevic, N., Lobaugh, N. J., Bronskill, M. J. *et al.* (2002). A robust method for extraction and automatic segmentation of brain images. *NeuroImage*, **17**, 1087–1100.

Launer, L. J., Ross, G. W., Petrovitch, H. *et al.* (2000). Midlife blood pressure and dementia: the Honolulu-Asia aging study. *Neurobiology of Aging*, **21**, 49–55.

Leibovitch, F. S., Black, S. E., Caldwell, C. B. *et al.* (1998). Brain-behavior correlations in hemispatial neglect CT and SPECT: the Sunnybrook Stroke Study. *Neurology*, **50**, 901–908.

Liao, D., Cooper, L., Cai, J. *et al.* (1996). Presence and severity of cerebral white matter lesions and hypertension, its treatment, and its control. The Atherosclerosis Risk in Communities Study. *Stroke*, **27**, 2262–2270.

Lim, A., Tsuang, D., Kukull, W. *et al.*, (1999). Clinico-neuropathological correlation of Alzheimer's disease in a community-based case series. *Journal of the American Geriatric Society*, **47**, 564–569.

Longstreth, W. T. J., Manolio, T. A., Arnold, A. *et al.* (1996). Clinical correlates of white matter findings on cranial magnetic resonance imaging of 3301 elderly people. The Cardiovascular Health Study. *Stroke*, **27**, 1274–1282.

Manolio, T. A., Kronmal, R. A., Burke, G. L. *et al.*, (1994). Magnetic resonance abnormalities and cardiovascular disease in older adults. The Cardiovascular Health Study. *Stroke*, **25**, 318–327.

Masdeu, J. C., Wolfson, L., Lantos, G. *et al.* (1989). Brain white-matter changes in the elderly prone to falling. *Archives of Neurology*, **46**, 1292–1296.

Mohr, J. P. (1982). Lacunes. *Stroke*, **13**, 3–11.

Mori, S., & Zhang, J. (2006). Principles of diffusion tensor imaging and its applications to basic neuroscience research. *Neuron*, **51**, 527–539.

MRC CFAS (2001). Pathological correlates of late-onset dementia in a multicentre, community-based population in England and Wales. Neuropathology Group of the Medical Research Council Cognitive Function and Ageing Study (MRC CFAS). *Lancet*, **357**, 169–175.

Mungas, D., Jagust, W. J., Reed, B. R. *et al.* (2001). MRI predictors of cognition in subcortical ischemic vascular disease and Alzheimer's disease. *Neurology*, **57**, 2229–2235.

Olszewski, J. (1962). Subcortical arteriosclerotic encephalopathy. Review of the literature on the so-called Binswanger's disease and presentation of two cases. *World Neurology*, **3**, 359–375.

Pantoni, L., & Garcia, J. H. (1995). The significance of cerebral white matter abnormalities 100 years after Binswanger's report. A review. *Stroke*, **26**, 1293–1301.

Pantoni, L., & Garcia, J. H. (1997). Pathogenesis of leukoaraiosis: a review. *Stroke*, **28**, 652–659.

Pantoni, L., & Lammie, G. A. (2002). Cerebral small vessel disease: pathological and pathophysiological aspects in relation to vascular cognitive impairment. In T. Erkinjuntti & S. Gaultier (Eds.), *Vascular Cognitive Impairment* (pp. 115–133). London, UK: Martin Dunitz.

Petrovitch, H., White, L. R., Izmirilian, G. *et al.* (2000). Midlife blood pressure and neuritic plaques, neurofibrillary tangles, and brain weight at death: the Honolulu-Asia Aging Study. *Neurobiology of Aging*, **21**, 57–62.

Picton, T. W., Stuss, D. T., Alexander, M. P. *et al.* (2007). Effects of focal frontal lesions on response inhibition. *Cerebral Cortex*, **17**, 826–838.

Picton, T. W., Stuss, D. T., Shallice, T., Alexander, M. P., & Gillingham, S. (2006). Keeping time: effects of focal frontal lesions. *Neuropsychologia*, **44**, 1195–1209.

Quddus, A., Lobaugh, N. J., Ramirez, J. *et al.* (2004). Robust protocol for the segmentation of subcortical hyperintensities on MRI scans. *Journal of Neurological Sciences*, **226**, 148–149.

Raineteau, O., & Schwab, M. E. (2001). Plasticity of motor systems after incomplete spinal cord injury. *Nature Reviews Neuroscience*, **2**, 263–273.

Ramirez, J., Levy, N., & Black, S. E. (2005). Lesion Explorer: an MRI segmentation processing technique for 3Dvolumetric analyses of lacunes, periventricular, and deep white matter hyperintensities. *VAS-COG*. Florence, Italy.

Robb, R. A., Hanson, D. P., Karwoski, R. A. *et al.* (1989). Analyze: a comprehensive, operator-interactive softward package for multidimensional medical image display and analysis. *Computerized Medical Imaging and Graphics*, **13**, 433–454.

Roman, G. C. (2002). On the history of lacunes, etat crible, and the white matter lesions of vascular dementia. *Cerebrovascular Diseases*, **13**, *Suppl. 2*, 1–6.

Rorden, C., & Brett, M. (2000). Stereotaxic display of brain lesions. *Behavioral Neurology*, **12**, 191–200.

Rosenbaum, R. S., Priselac, S., Kohler, S. *et al.* (2000). Remote spatial memory in an amnesic person with extensive bilateral hippocampal lesions. *Nature Neuroscience*, **3**, 1044–1048.

Rosenbaum, R. S., Kohler, S., Schacter, D. L. *et al.* (2005). The case of K.C.: Contributions of a memory-impaired person to memory theory. *Neuropsychologia*, **43**, 989–1021.

Roy, E. A., Black, S. E., Blair, N., & Dimeck, P. T. (1998). Analyses of deficits in gestural pantomime. *Journal of Clinical and Experimental Neuropsychology*, **20**, 628–643.

Sachdev, P. S., Wen, W., Christensen, H., & Jorm, A. F. (2005). White matter hyperintensities are related to physical disability and poor motor function. *Journal of Neurology, Neurosurgery and Psychiatry*, **76**, 362–367.

Sahlas, D. J., Bilbao, J. M., Swartz, R. H., & Black, S. E. (2002). Clasmatodendrosis correlating with periventricular hyperintensity in mixed dementia. *Annals of Neurology*, **52**, 378–381.

Scheltens, P., Barkhof, F., Leys, D. *et al.* (1993). A semi-quantitative rating scale for the assessment of signal hyperintensities on magnetic resonance imaging. *Journal of the Neurological Sciences*, **114**, 7–12.

Schmidt, R. (1992). Comparison of magnetic resonance imaging in Alzheimer's disease, vascular dementia and normal aging. *European Neurology*, **32**, 164–169.

Schmidt, R., Launer, L. J., Nilsson, L. G. *et al.* (2004). Magnetic resonance imaging of the brain in diabetes: the Cardiovascular Determinants of Dementia (CASCADE) Study. *Diabetes*, **53**, 687–692.

Schorer, C. E. (1992). Alzheimer and Kraepelin describe Binswanger's disease. *Journal of Neuropsychiatry and Clinical Neuroscience*, **4**, 55–58.

Silveri, M. C., Misciagna, S., & Terrezza, G. (2001). Right side neglect in right cerebellar lesion. *Journal of Neurology, Neurosurgery and Psychiatry*, **71**, 114–117.

Sled, J. G., Levesque, I., Santos, A. C. *et al.* (2004). Regional variations in normal brain shown by quantitative magnetization transfer imaging. *Magnetic Resonance in Medicine*, **51**, 299–303.

Snowdon, D. A. (2003). Healthy aging and dementia: findings from the Nun Study. *Annals of Internal Medicine*, **139**, 450–454.

Snowdon, D. A., Greiner, L. H., Mortimer, J. A. *et al.* (1997). Brain infarction and the clinical expression of Alzheimer disease. The Nun Study. *Journal of the American Medical Association*, **277**, 813–817.

Stanisz, G. J., Odrobina, E. E., Pun, J. *et al.* (2005). T1, T2 relaxation and magnetization transfer in tissue at 3T. *Magnetic Resonance in Medicine*, **54**, 507–512.

Starr, J. M., Leaper, S. A., Murray, A. D. *et al.* (2003). Brain white matter lesions detected by magnetic resonance imaging are associated with balance and gait speed. *Journal of Neurology, Neurosurgery and Psychiatry*, **74**, 94–98.

Steingart, A., Hachinski, V. C., Lau, C. *et al.* (1987). Cognitive and neurologic findings in subjects with diffuse white matter lucencies on computed tomographic scan (leuko-araiosis). *Archives of Neurology*, **44**, 32–35.

Stuss, D. T. (2006). Frontal lobes and attention: processes and networks, fractionation and integration. *Journal of the International Neuropsychological Society*, **12**, 261–271.

Stuss, D. T., Alexander, M. P., Shallice, T. *et al.* (2005). Multiple frontal systems controlling response speed. *Neuropsychologia*, **43**, 396–417.

Swartz, R. H., Black, S. E., Feinstein, A. *et al.* (2002). Utility of simultaneous brain, CSF and hyperintensity quantification in dementia. *Psychiatry Research*, **116**, 83–93.

Swartz, R. H., Stuss, D. T., Gao, F. Q., & Black, S. E. (2008). Independent cognitive effects of atrophy. Diffuse subcortical and thalamocortical cerebrovascular disease in dementia. *Stroke*, **39**, 822–830.

Talairach, J., & Tournoux, P. (1988). *Co-planar Stereotaxic Atlas of the Human Brain*. Stuttgart, Germany: Thieme Medical Publishers.

Thiebaut De Schotten, M., Kinkingnehun, S., Delmaire, C. *et al.* (2007). Visualization of Disconnection syndromes using diffusion tensor imaging tractography. *Neurology*, **68**, *Suppl. 1*, A215.

Tulving, E., Schacter, D. L., McLachlan, D. R., & Moscovitch, M. (1988). Priming of semantic autobiographical knowledge: a case study of retrograde amnesia. *Brain and Cognition*, **8**, 3–20.

van Dijk, E. J., Breteler, M. M., Schmidt, R. *et al.* (2004). The association between blood pressure, hypertension, and cerebral white matter lesions: cardiovascular determinants of dementia study. *Hypertension*, **44**, 625–630.

van Swieten, J. C., Geyskes, G. G., Derix, M. M. *et al.* (1991). Hypertension in the elderly is associated with white matter lesions and cognitive decline. *Annals of Neurology*, **30**, 825–830.

Wahlund, L. O., Agartz, I., Almqvist, O. *et al.* (1990). The brain in healthy aged individuals: MR imaging. *Radiology*, **174**, 675–679.

Webb, S., Munro, C. A., Midha, R., & Stanisz, G. J. (2003). Is multicomponent T2 a good measure of myelin content in peripheral nerve? *Magnetic Resonance in Medicine*, **49**, 638–645.

Wen, W., & Sachdev, P. (2004). The topography of white matter hyperintensities on brain MRI in healthy 60- to 64-year-old individuals. *NeuroImage*, **22**, 144–154.

Whitman, G. T., Tang, Y., Lin, A., & Baloh, R. W. (2001). A prospective study of cerebral white matter abnormalities in older people with gait dysfunction. *Neurology*, **57**, 990–994.

Woods, R. P., Cherry, S. R., & Mazziotta, J. C. (1992). Rapid automated algorithm for aligning and reslicing PET images. *Journal of Computer Assisted Tomography*, **16**, 620–633.

Ylikoski, R., Ylikoski, A., Erkinjuntti, T. *et al.* (1993). White matter changes in healthy elderly persons correlate with attention and speed of mental processing. *Archives of Neurology*, **50**, 818–824.

Zhang, Y., Schuff, N., Jahng, G. H. *et al.* (2007). Diffusion tensor imaging of cingulum fibers in mild cognitive impairment and Alzheimer disease. *Neurology*, **68**, 13–19.

9

Functional neuroimaging and cognitive rehabilitation: healthy aging as a model of plasticity

Cheryl L. Grady

Introduction

- After brain injury, there is short-term and long-term brain plasticity and reorganization.
- The brain also alters structurally and dynamically over the normal lifespan. Since more research has been completed in the area of aging, this knowledge serves as a model for understanding brain plasticity after cognitive rehabilitation.
- Changes in memory with aging have been extensively studied. Most functional neuroimaging research on brain plasticity with aging has been carried out in the memory domain.
- Both reduced and increased brain activity with aging has been reported. Each is reviewed.

The brain is not a static entity, but rather alters its structure and function dynamically over the lifespan (Grady *et al.*, 2006; Raz, 2000; Sowell *et al.*, 2001; Sullivan *et al.*, 1995). Changes also occur in the brain after damage, some of which are the result of the insult itself, and some of which are due to reorganization of neural pathways in response to the damage (Merzenich *et al.*, 1983; Ramachandran, 2005). Studies using functional neuroimaging techniques, such as positron emission tomography (PET) or functional magnetic resonance imaging (fMRI), to study brain plasticity have shown that there are changes in activity patterns due to learning new information or practicing a given task over some period of time (Karni *et al.*, 1995; Raichle *et al.*, 1994). These short-term changes are superimposed over the longer-term plasticity occurring naturally, and it is likely that the two types of plasticity interact with one another. Consideration

of all these factors when attempting to understand the effect of brain damage or injury on brain function and how this is influenced by rehabilitation thus becomes a complicated undertaking. Some of these issues have been addressed in functional neuroimaging studies of healthy older adults, so that aging can be used as a model of brain plasticity to help us understand the impact of cognitive rehabilitation on brain function.

It is well known in the field of cognitive aging that older adults, compared with young adults, often have poorer memory function. Older adults have particular difficulty with episodic memory (Craik & Jennings, 1992; Light, 1991; Park *et al.*, 2002; Zacks *et al.*, 2000), defined as the conscious recollection of events that have occurred in a person's experience (Tulving, 1983). In the laboratory, these age differences in episodic memory are seen in a reduced ability to learn and retrieve lists of stimuli, such as words or pictures of common objects (for a review see Craik & Bosman, 1992). Older adults have particular difficulty in retrieving accompanying information about stimuli learned during the course of an experiment, so-called "source" memory (Glisky *et al.*, 1995; Hashtroudi *et al.*, 1989; Schacter *et al.*, 1991; Spaniol *et al.*, 2006). For example, when learning a list of words presented verbally by either a male or female speaker, young adults are readily able to recall both the words and whether they were spoken by a man or woman, whereas older adults will have more difficulty remembering the speaker's gender than remembering the words. Older adults also recall fewer details about real-life, autobiographical memories (Levine *et al.*, 2002; Piolino *et al.*, 2002), and

Cognitive Neurorehabilitation, Second Edition: Evidence and Application, ed. Donald T. Stuss, Gordon Winocur and Ian H. Robertson. Published by Cambridge University Press. © Cambridge University Press 2008.

substantial age-related declines are seen on working memory tasks, i.e., tasks that require holding information on line for brief periods of time (Foos, 1995; Hasher & Zacks, 1988; Reuter-Lorenz *et al.*, 2000; Salthouse, 1990). In contrast, semantic memory, or the accumulation of knowledge about the world, is maintained or even increased in older adults, compared with younger adults (e.g., Craik & Jennings, 1992). Thus, not all aspects of memory function are affected adversely by older age.

In recent years, functional neuroimaging has been used to explore brain activity accompanying memory tasks in young and old adults, and to understand the neural mechanisms underlying behavioral differences. Not surprisingly, older adults often show less brain activity than do young adults when performing memory tasks, which can reasonably be assumed to reflect a reduced level of functioning, particularly when accompanied by poorer performance on the task. The major challenge in the field has been to interpret increased recruitment of task-related brain areas, or activation of unique brain regions in the elderly. Researchers have frequently concluded that more utilization of a given brain area in older adults represents compensatory activity, and it is this type of result that would be of most interest to those aiming to rehabilitate some cognitive function in a patient with brain damage. That is, one would like to know if it is possible to train a brain region or regions to take over a function that has been impaired due to damage in another region important for that function. The evidence, reviewed here, in healthy older adults would suggest that this may indeed be possible, but that a number of issues should be kept in mind.

Before reviewing the evidence of plasticity in the older brain, it is useful to describe the analytic approaches that have been used to study the brain mechanisms underlying cognitive aging. The most common approach has been a straightforward contrast of brain activity between young and old groups of participants and interpretation of the observed activity in the context of behavioral performance on the tasks. Much of this work has focused on the frontal lobes, which are thought to be particularly vulnerable to the effects of aging. Others have taken a multivariate approach to identify brain areas that show a common pattern of functional changes during the experimental tasks. Groups of regions thus identified can be thought of as the networks that underlie cognitive processing. Functional connectivity is another type of network-based approach and involves assessing how activity in a given region correlates with activity in other areas of the brain during a task. Connectivity approaches emphasize the functional interactions among brain areas and the ways in which these interactions mediate cognitive processing, rather than focusing on the activity in any individual brain region. This "whole-brain" type of approach has revealed that a number of brain areas, including the frontal lobes, appear to be critical sites of age-related change in function.

In this chapter I will review the evidence from functional neuroimaging studies for plasticity in the aging brain and how information gleaned from this work can inform the exploration of functional reorganization after brain damage. First, the evidence for reduced activity in older compared with younger adults will be discussed, followed by those studies finding increased activity in older adults. Finally, the application of network and multivariate approaches to cognitive aging will be reviewed. In each section, the relevance of this work done in aging to the use of imaging to study the effects of rehabilitation will be discussed.

Reduced brain activity in older adults

- Reduced activity in older, compared with younger adults, has been reported in left prefrontal cortex and medial temporal areas during encoding tasks.
- This finding may be due to a reduction in the frequency with which older adults use a deep or semantic encoding strategy spontaneously.
- Requiring older adults to use such strategies can lessen the age difference in brain activity during encoding.

Reduced brain activity in older adults typically has been noted during encoding, or learning new

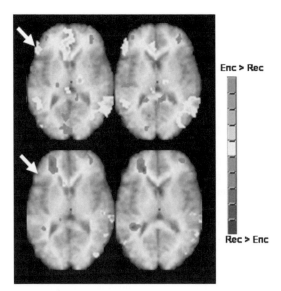

Enc > Rec

Rec > Enc

Figure 9.1. (This figure is reproduced in the color plate section at the front of this volume.) Areas with changes in activity during encoding (Enc) and recognition (Rec) of faces in young and old adults are shown on a standard structural MRI. Yellow/red areas are those with more activity during encoding, compared with recognition, and blue areas had more activity during recognition. Young adults (top) show increased activity during encoding in left inferior prefrontal cortex (white arrow), but older adults do not. Data are reprinted from Grady, C. L. *Encyclopedia of Neuroscience*, 2008, with permission from Elsevier.

material (see Figure 9.1). Younger adults have increased activity in left prefrontal cortex when learning new stimuli, and a common finding is that older adults show less activity in this area during encoding compared with younger adults (Cabeza *et al.*, 1997; Grady *et al.*, 1995; Logan *et al.*, 2002; Madden *et al.*, 1999). The reduced activity in left prefrontal cortex can be ameliorated to some extent by using encoding tasks that promote deep, or semantic processing of the to-be-remembered information (Grady *et al.*, 1999; Logan *et al.*, 2002). That is, both young and old adults show more left prefrontal activity during semantic encoding tasks, compared with those that do not require a focus on the semantic aspects of the stimulus, and this increase in older adults can be large enough to

remove most or all of the age difference (Logan *et al.*, 2002; Rosen *et al.*, 2002). This pattern of results is consistent with behavioral data suggesting that older adults may not spontaneously engage effective encoding strategies, e.g., those involving semantic processing by left inferior frontal cortex, but can use such strategies when required to do so (Craik & Bosman, 1992).

Frontal activity during memory retrieval is typically found in the right hemisphere (Cabeza & Nyberg, 2000; Lepage *et al.*, 2000; Rugg & Henson, 2002), and is often of the same magnitude regardless of age (e.g., Grady *et al.*, 1995). However, when the retrieval task places a heavy demand on memory search, without providing cues for retrieval, older adults show a reduction in right prefrontal activation (Anderson *et al.*, 2000; Cabeza *et al.*, 1997, 2002). Consistent with their reduced source memory, older adults also have less activation of prefrontal cortex during source retrieval compared with their younger counterparts (Cabeza *et al.*, 2000; Mitchell *et al.*, 2006).

Another area of memory that has been examined fairly extensively in the aging field is that of working memory. A number of working memory tasks have been used including delayed match-to-sample and n-back tasks. Some of these studies have reported less activity in some prefrontal regions in older adults (Grady *et al.*, 1998). When the different phases of the working memory task have been examined separately – memory set presentation, delay, and probe – age differences have been seen primarily during the presentation of the probe, i.e., when the memory decision is being made (Rypma & D'Esposito, 2000). This suggests that some aspects of working memory, such as rehearsal, might not be affected by age. Some recent work has shown that older adults are able to recruit prefrontal cortex at lower levels of working memory task load, but that this declines at higher task loads, whereas younger adults continue to increase prefrontal recruitment with increasing load (Mattay *et al.*, 2006). This finding is similar to that noted above for episodic retrieval, as both would suggest that tasks with high processing demands are likely to be associated with reduced brain activity in older adults, and potentially poorer performance as well. Another recent working memory study used pictures of faces and scenes and asked participants to remember one of the stimulus types while ignoring the other (Gazzaley *et al.*, 2005). Young adults either enhanced or suppressed activity in regions of occipital cortex that respond selectively to faces or scenes depending on whether the stimuli were attended or ignored. In contrast, older adults showed enhanced activity in these areas, but failed to reduce activity in face- and scene-selective regions when instructed to ignore them. Of particular interest, the ability of older adults to suppress activity to irrelevant information was correlated with their working memory performance. This result is consistent with the idea that reduced inhibitory function in older adults is related to age differences in working memory capacity (Hasher & Zacks, 1988).

In addition to prefrontal regions, less modulation of activity in older adults also has been found in other areas important for memory, including the hippocampus and the parahippocampal gyrus, and in visual areas of cortex (Grady *et al.*, 1995). Interestingly, when brain activity has been compared across different kinds of tasks, such as both working memory and episodic retrieval, similar age reductions in brain activity have been found in visual cortex and hippocampus (Cabeza *et al.*, 2004). Such a result is consistent with the idea that there is a "common cause" of cognitive aging, and indicate that reductions in both sensory processing and memory encoding could be involved in such a common cause. One thing to keep in mind, however, particularly when considering age differences in sensory cortex, is that less activity during a particular cognitive task in older adults may be due to more activity in these areas during the baseline condition. Thus, when activity during the baseline is subtracted from task activity, older adults will have a smaller task-related increase, but this does not mean that the region cannot be activated. Rather, the older adults are starting out from a higher level of activity. This in fact has been observed in visual cortex (Madden *et al.*, 2002).

Just as brain activity is reduced in older compared with younger adults under some experimental conditions, a patient with brain damage may show less activity in some areas compared with controls, even after rehabilitation. This might indicate that some aspect of function is still impaired, regardless of treatment. Of course, one would expect those areas with specific damage to have reduced or absent activation, but more distant regions might also be affected, particularly those that receive projections from the damaged area. It may also be the case, as mentioned above for aging, that the patients may simply have more activity in these regions during the baseline condition, and so not show any activation during the task of interest, unlike the controls. However, one would probably be more interested in those areas with *more* activity after rehabilitation, compared to a control group, as these would be the regions that presumably have taken over the function of the damaged regions. We now turn to the case of greater activity in older adults to explore this possibility.

Increased brain activity in older adults

- Increased brain activity in older adults, above that seen in young adults, has been reported most frequently in prefrontal cortex.
- This over-recruitment is often related to better performance in the older group, consistent with a compensatory mechanism.
- Similar over-recruitment is seen in patients with brain injury after some degree of recovery, suggesting that changes in brain activity reflect plasticity and/or the effects of rehabilitation.

Increased brain activity in older adults, compared with young adults, typically is found in the frontal lobes (see Figure 9.2), sometimes in areas of frontal cortex not active in young adults, or activation is seen bilaterally in the old, but unilaterally in the young (Cabeza, 2002). When brain activity has been measured during episodic memory retrieval, older adults frequently show activation in prefrontal regions bilaterally, even if frontal activation in

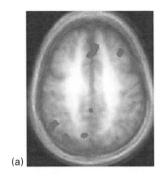
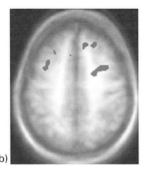

(a)   (b)

Figure 9.2. (This figure is reproduced in the color plate section at the front of this volume.) Areas of greater activity in older compared with younger adults during an auditory working memory task (a) and an auditory episodic memory task (b). Areas are shown on the average structural MRIs of the participants in the two experiments. Older adults showed more activity in right frontal and medial frontal cortex in both experiments. There were additional areas of greater activity in parietal regions during the working memory task. Data from the episodic memory task are reprinted from *Neuropsychologia* (2006), **44**, 2452–2464, with permission from Elsevier.

young adults is unilateral. Bilateral prefrontal activation during episodic retrieval has been found in older adults for a variety of stimuli, both verbal and nonverbal (Cabeza *et al.*, 2004; Grady *et al.*, 2002; Madden *et al.*, 1999). Another way of looking at the brain activity that supports retrieval is to see how activity during encoding of items that are later correctly remembered differs from that for encoding of items that are forgotten, known as the "subsequent memory effect." Using the subsequent memory effect, a number of investigators have found that activity in left inferior prefrontal cortex and the left medial temporal region in young adults is greater during encoding of subsequently remembered stimuli compared with activity for those items that are later forgotten (Brewer *et al.*, 1998; Otten & Rugg, 2001; Wagner *et al.*, 1998). A similar pattern has been found in old adults; however, older adults also have an association between more activity in right prefrontal cortex and subsequent recognition (Morcom *et al.*, 2003). Thus, older adults can show a more bilateral pattern of frontal activity during encoding, as they do during retrieval, when that encoding is sufficient to support later retrieval. A similar pattern has been found during some working memory tasks, where activation is unilateral in young adults, but in both hemispheres in older adults (Reuter-Lorenz *et al.*, 2000).

There is some evidence for greater activity during memory retrieval tasks in older adults in medial temporal areas outside of the hippocampus. In particular, studies of recognition memory have shown more activation of parahippocampal regions in older adults, compared with younger adults (Cabeza *et al.*, 2004; Grady *et al.*, 2005). Indeed, parahippocampal cortex in young adults often shows less activity when previously seen stimuli are presented during a recognition task, and this reduction in activity is thought to represent a signal of familiarity with the stimulus (Henson *et al.*, 2003). Increased activity in older adults in the parahippocampal gyrus may still indicate familiarity, but the nature of the signal may undergo a change with age. Interestingly, although hippocampal activity during memory retrieval is sometimes reduced with aging (Gutchess *et al.*, 2005; Mitchell *et al.*, 2000), bilateral activation of the hippocampus has been reported in older adults during an autobiographical memory retrieval task, whereas young adults had only left hippocampal activation (Maguire & Frith, 2003). This bilateral activation is similar to the bilateral prefrontal activity seen in older adults during other memory tasks, and may support those aspects of autobiographical retrieval which are maintained in the elderly.

There have been suggestions that additional recruitment of task-related brain areas, or engagement of unique areas not active in young adults, compensates for age-related changes in brain structure and function. Compensation has been invoked to explain greater brain activity in older adults when they are able to perform a particular task as well as younger adults (Grady *et al.*, 1994; McIntosh *et al.*, 1999), or when older adults who perform better on memory tasks recruit prefrontal cortex to a greater degree than those performing less well (Cabeza *et al.*, 2002). Older adults also may have more prefrontal activity than young adults when brain activity is examined just for those task trials where participants respond correctly (Morcom *et al.*, 2003). Such findings suggest that correct performance may be supported by this over-recruitment of frontal regions. Another approach has been to determine how brain activity is related to task performance by correlating these two measures in groups of young and old adults. Increased prefrontal activity is often correlated with better performance on memory tasks in older adults, but rarely in young adults (Grady *et al.*, 2005). In fact, in young adults prefrontal activity is usually correlated with poorer task performance (Grady *et al.*, 2005; Smith *et al.*, 2001), indicating that with age, the impact of brain activity on memory performance is altered.

On the other hand, some of this increased prefrontal activity in the elderly may reflect greater need or use of frontally mediated executive functions at lower levels of task demand than would be necessary for activation of this area in young adults. In this case the increased activity in prefrontal cortex might not be related to performance on the particular task, but would reflect a type of nonselective recruitment in older adults, perhaps related to task difficulty. Examples of this kind of scenario have been observed, and include increased activity in widely distributed areas of both lateral and medial portions of prefrontal cortex in older adults during tasks on which they perform worse than young adults (Fernandes *et al.*, 2006; Grady, 2002). These findings suggest that additional recruitment of prefrontal cortex in older adults may not always be associated with preserved cognitive performance in older adults.

These studies in healthy older adults provide strong evidence that over-recruitment of some brain areas, particularly in the frontal lobes, can be associated with preserved cognitive performance, and that those older adults who show this recruitment are those with the best memory. A similar result has been seen in people who are in the early stages of dementia (Grady *et al.*, 2003a; Stern *et al.*, 2000), suggesting that recruitment of alternative brain areas is a general response to brain dysfunction. Consistent with this idea, patients with strokes to various parts of the brain also have shown increased activity compared with controls, typically in areas contralateral to the stroke (Adair *et al.*, 2000; Chollet *et al.*, 1991; Johansson, 2000; Rijntjes, 2006; Weiller *et al.*, 1993, 1995). In most studies, this effect has not been tied to any particular rehabilitation effort (but see Hamzei *et al.*, 2006; Laatsch *et al.*, 2004; Musso *et al.*, 1999), so the specific effects of treatment largely are unknown. Nevertheless, this work suggests that changes in brain activity will be found after rehabilitation, and that these changes may involve recruitment of prefrontal regions that can be associated with improved performance. However, it would be important to assess whether there is a direct relation between over-recruitment of frontal areas and improvement in task performance, in order to rule out the possibility that increased activation is due to some other nonspecific factor rather than a result of the rehabilitation per se. In addition, there is evidence that greater activity in the areas nearby the damaged region may also be critical for recovery (Heiss *et al.*, 2003). Indeed, it may be that some functional interaction between these "recovered" regions and frontal cortex is important for improved performance, and the assessment of such interactions is discussed in the next section.

Different brain networks in older adults

- Recently, there has been increasing interest in using analytic approaches that address the functional inter-connectedness of brain areas.

- These network-based approaches have shown that younger and older adults engage different brain networks when carrying out cognitive tasks.
- It is likely that alterations in brain network function occur after injury and in response to rehabilitative efforts, but this has yet to be explored fully.

A relatively new approach to studying brain function is the focus on functional connectivity, or how activity in a given brain area is correlated with activity elsewhere in the brain, to identify networks of interacting regions. Studies using this approach have provided intriguing evidence that young and older adults recruit different brain networks, even when the measured behavior is the same. For example, when pictures of objects are used as stimuli in memory tasks, they are recognized well by both young and old adults. Encoding of these objects also is associated with increased activity in medial temporal regions in both young and old groups (Grady *et al.*, 1999). However, the areas that are functionally connected to the hippocampus during encoding vary with age (Gutchess *et al.*, 2003b, 2005). In young adults, during object encoding, hippocampal activity was correlated with activity in ventral prefrontal and occipitotemporal regions, whereas older adults showed correlations between hippocampal activity and more dorsal prefrontal, temporal and parietal regions (Grady *et al.*, 2003b). In addition, when putative networks were constructed based on these regions, age differences were seen. That is, younger adults showed the strongest interconnections between temporal and lateral frontal regions, whereas older adults showed stronger inputs from temporal regions into the hippocampus and from there to a region of medial frontal cortex (see Figure 9.3). Of particular interest is that these age-specific networks were associated with better memory performance. That is, those individuals in each age group who engaged the specific encoding network to a greater degree were the ones who later remembered the greatest number of objects.

Different functional connectivity of medial temporal regions in older adults, compared with young adults, also has been found during recognition

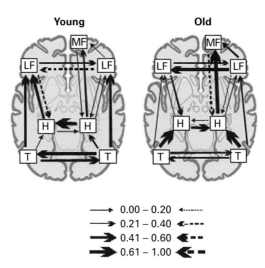

Figure 9.3. Network models for young and old adults during encoding of objects. Although the regions that went into the models were similar in the two groups, the effective connections between these regions differed across groups. For example, the influence of the right hippocampus (H) on the medial frontal region (MF) was stronger in the older group, whereas the inputs from the temporal regions (T) into the lateral frontal regions (LF) were larger in the young group. The strength of the connections is indicated by the size of the arrows (see key); solid arrows represent positive inputs and dashed arrows represent negative inputs. Reprinted with permission from *Hippocampus* (2003), **13**, 572–586, with permission from Wiley & Sons, Inc.

tasks. A recent study found that during recognition, the hippocampus showed stronger functional connections with cortical regions in young adults, whereas the entorhinal cortex showed stronger connections in older adults (Daselaar *et al.*, 2006). This finding was consistent with evidence that these two medial temporal areas mediate recollection and familiarity, respectively (Brown & Aggleton, 2001; Ranganath *et al.*, 2004), two aspects of memory that tap different qualitative experiences (Yonelinas, 2001), and with the many studies showing larger age differences in recollection than in familiarity (e.g., Davidson & Glisky, 2002; Prull *et al.*, 2006). Thus, age differences in recollective processes mediated by the hippocampus may be off-set by more reliance on familiarity mediated by networks involving medial temporal cortex adjacent to the hippocampus. Similar evidence for age differences in cognitive networks involving the hippocampus and its interactions with the cortex has been found in experiments tapping working memory as well (Della-Maggiore *et al.*, 2000). All of these studies that focus on network approaches to image analysis have provided evidence that aging results in the modification of large-scale network operations, in addition to affecting activity in specific brain regions, which in turn has an impact on memory ability.

As with aging, damage to the brain via stroke or other types of insult undoubtedly change the functional interactions among brain areas, thus altering the neural networks underlying cognitive function. This has been demonstrated in Alzheimer's disease (Grady *et al.*, 2003a; Greicius *et al.*, 2004; Stern *et al.*, 2000), Parkinson's disease (Nakamura *et al.*, 2001), and psychiatric disorders (Gilboa *et al.*, 2004; Goldapple *et al.*, 2004). This type of network approach has, with a few exceptions (Schoenfeld *et al.*, 2002), not been used to study reorganization of function after strokes, but would be ideal for exploring this phenomenon and how reorganization is influenced by rehabilitation training.

Conclusions

- A number of factors likely influence age differences in brain activity, including integrity of white matter fibers, education and personality.
- The same factors will affect the interpretation of differences in brain activity resulting from brain injury or rehabilitative training.
- Given the complexity of brain function, a full assessment of the impact of both age and rehabilitation on brain function will have to include examination of the dynamic interactions among brain regions, in conjunction with underlying structural changes.

It is clear that functional neuroimaging has opened a window into cognitive aging, shedding light on the roles of brain areas, such as prefrontal cortex and the hippocampus, in age-related differences in cognitive performance. However, a number of questions remain. For example, the extent to which alterations of brain activity or brain networks seen in older adults are due to changes in the function of the brain regions themselves or to changes in the white matter tracts that connect the regions is unknown. Both activity within brain areas and communication between cortical regions could be reduced or altered because the neurons in the regions themselves have altered function or because age affects the fibers that connect them (Nordahl *et al.*, 2006; Söderlund *et al.*, 2003). This is a particularly important issue to keep in mind when assessing brain function in the context of injury or degenerative disease, as these insults routinely impact white matter as well as gray matter. There are other factors that could influence brain activity in older and younger adults and these are just now beginning to receive attention. An example is education, which has been shown to have a protective effect against decline in cognitive function in older adults (Bennett *et al.*, 2003; Stern *et al.*, 1999). There is some evidence that education, or other indices of intellectual achievement, are related differently to brain activity in young vs. older adults (Stern *et al.*, 2005), such that education is positively correlated with frontal activity only in older adults (Springer *et al.*, 2005). In fact, in those frontal areas where activity is positively correlated with education in older adults, activity is negatively correlated with education in younger adults (see Figure 9.4). This finding is consistent with the evidence of greater frontal recruitment by older adults and suggests that frontal cortex is engaged particularly by those older adults who are highly educated. Thus, it may be that compensatory brain activity in older adults is most likely to be seen in those with higher education, but more work needs to be done in this area. The influence of other variables, such as personality traits or mood, on brain activity in older adults has yet to be examined, but as age differences have been found on these measures (Carstensen *et al.*, 2003; McCrae *et al.*, 1999), these factors also could be

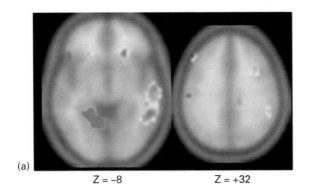

(a)

Z = −8   Z = +32

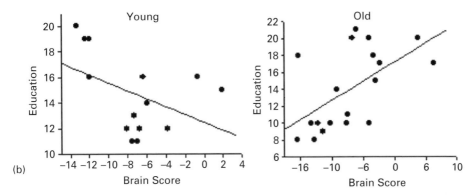

(b)

Figure 9.4. (This figure is reproduced in the color plate section at the front of this volume.) Brain areas where activity is correlated with years of education in young and old adults are shown on average MRIs in Panel (a). The brain scores plotted in (b) are scores that summarize activity seen in the images. As the brain scores increase, activity in the red/yellow areas increases, and as the brain score decreases, activity in the blue areas increases. More education in young adults is associated with more activity in left medial temporal areas (blue regions associated with negative brain scores) and less activity in frontal cortex. More years of education in older adults was associated with the opposite pattern, i.e., with more activity in frontal and right lateral temporal cortex (yellow/red regions associated with positive brain scores). Adapted with permission from *Neuropsychology* (2005), **19**, 181–192. Copyright © American Psychological Association.

influencing brain activity in older adults. There is some recent evidence that personality traits can modify brain activity during emotional or self-referential tasks in young adults (Canli *et al.*, 2001), so it will be of interest to pursue these effects in older adults as well.

Issues of how to interpret differences in brain activity between groups or even within a group between two points in time, are clearly relevant to interpreting differences in brain activity induced by cognitive training and rehabilitation programs. The age of the patients, their educational level, the demands of the task at hand, and the potential of the brain for plasticity are just some of the factors that could influence patterns of brain activity and cognitive networks. Finally, it is important to note that it is possible to identify a group difference in functional connectivity, or network interactions, involving a particular brain area even when no change in mean activation is seen in this area (e.g., Grady *et al.*, 2003a, 2003b). This indicates that a failure to find differences in brain activity between younger and older adults in a given region on a particular task does not mean that the functional communication of that region with other area is the same as well. Thus, one cannot always assume that the function of a brain area is unchanged with age merely by assessing its mean activity level. This would also be true when assessing brain activity after brain damage or cognitive training; one cannot assume that normal levels of activity in a brain region after some type of injury, or no change in activity after some type of training, means that the functional connections of that region are unchanged. A more detailed examination of the dynamic interactions among brain regions, in conjunction with underlying structural changes and assessment of the impact of network activity on behavioral performance, will likely be necessary to ultimately understand the impact of both age and rehabilitation on brain function.

REFERENCES

Adair, J. C., Nadeau, S. E., Conway, T. W. *et al.* (2000). Alterations in the functional anatomy of reading induced by rehabilitation of an alexic patient. *Neuropsychiatry, Neuropsychology and Behavioral Neurology*, **13**, 303–311.

Anderson, N. D., Iidaka, T., Cabeza, R. *et al.* (2000). The effects of divided attention on encoding- and retrieval-related brain activity: a PET study of younger and older adults. *Journal of Cognitive Neuroscience*, **12**, 775–792.

Bennett, D. A., Wilson, R. S., Schneider, J. A. *et al.* (2003). Education modifies the relation of AD pathology to level of cognitive function in older persons. *Neurology*, **60**, 1909–1915.

Brewer, J. B., Zhao, Z., Desmond, J. E., Glover, G. H., & Gabrieli, J. D. E. (1998). Making memories: brain activity that predicts how well visual experience will be remembered. *Science*, **281**, 1185–1187.

Brown, M. W., & Aggleton, J. P. (2001). Recognition memory: what are the roles of the perirhinal cortex and hippocampus? *Nature Reviews Neuroscience*, **2**, 51–61.

Cabeza, R. (2002). Hemispheric asymmetry reduction in older adults: the HAROLD model. *Psychology and Aging*, **17**, 85–100.

Cabeza, R., & Nyberg, L. (2000). Imaging cognition II: an empirical review of 275 PET and fMRI studies. *Journal of Cognitive Neuroscience*, **12**, 1–47.

Cabeza, R., Grady, C. L., Nyberg, L. *et al.* (1997). Age-related differences in neural activity during memory encoding and retrieval: a positron emission tomography study. *Journal of Neuroscience*, **17**, 391–400.

Cabeza, R., Anderson, N. D., Mangels, J. A., Nyberg, L., & Houle, S. (2000). Age-related differences in neural activity during item and temporal-order memory retrieval: a positron emission tomography study. *Journal of Cognitive Neuroscience*, **12**, 197–206.

Cabeza, R., Anderson, N. D., Locantore, J. K., & McIntosh, A. R. (2002). Aging gracefully: compensatory brain activity in high-performing older adults. *NeuroImage*, **17**, 1394–1402.

Cabeza, R., Daselaar, S. M., Dolcos, F. *et al.* (2004). Task-independent and task-specific age effects on brain activity during working memory, visual attention and episodic retrieval. *Cerebral Cortex*, **14**, 364–375.

Canli, T., Zhao, Z., Desmond, J. E. *et al.* (2001). An fMRI study of personality influences on brain reactivity to emotional stimuli. *Behavioral Neuroscience*, **115**, 33–42.

Carstensen, L. L., Fung, H. H., & Charles, S. T. (2003). Socioemotional selectivity theory and the regulation of emotion in the second half of life. *Motivation and Emotion*, **27**, 103–123.

Chollet, F., DiPiero, V., Wise, R. J. S. *et al.* (1991). The functional anatomy of motor recovery after stroke in humans: a study with positron emission tomography. *Annals of Neurology*, **29**, 63–71.

Craik, F. I. M., & Bosman, E. A. (1992). Age-related changes in memory and learning. In H. Bouma & J. Graafmans (Eds.), *Gerontechnology: Proceedings of the First International Conference on Technology and Aging* (pp. 79–92). Eindhoven, NL: IOS Press.

Craik, F. I. M., & Jennings, J. M. (1992). Human memory. In F. I. M. Craik & T. A. Salthouse (Eds.), *The Handbook of Aging and Cognition* (pp. 51–110). Hillsdale, NJ: Lawrence Erlbaum.

Daselaar, S. M., Fleck, M. S., Dobbins, I. G., Madden, D. J., & Cabeza, R. (2006). Effects of healthy aging on hippocampal and rhinal memory functions: an event-related fMRI study. *Cerebral Cortex*, **16**, 1771–1782.

Davidson, P. S. R., & Glisky, E. L. (2002). Neuropsychological correlates of recollection and familiarity in normal aging. *Cognitive, Affective, and Behavioral Neuroscience*, **2**, 174–186.

Della-Maggiore, V., Sekuler, A. B., Grady, C. L. *et al.* (2000). Corticolimbic interactions associated with performance on a short-term memory task are modified by age. *Journal of Neuroscience*, **20**, 8410–8416.

Fernandes, M. A., Pacurar, A., Moscovitch, M., & Grady, C. L. (2006). Neural correlates of auditory recognition under full and divided attention in younger and older adults. *Neuropsychologia*, **44**, 2452–2464.

Foos, P. W. (1995). Working memory resource allocation by young, middle-aged, and old adults. *Experimental Aging Research*, **21**, 239–250.

Gazzaley, A., Cooney, J. W., Rissman, J., & D'Esposito, M. (2005). Top-down suppression deficit underlies working memory impairment in normal aging. *Nature Neuroscience*, **8**, 1298–1300.

Gilboa, A., Shalev, A. Y., Laor, L. *et al.* (2004). Functional connectivity of the prefrontal cortex and the amygdala in posttraumatic stress disorder. *Biological Psychiatry*, **55**, 263–272.

Glisky, E. L., Polster, M. R., & Routhieaux, B. C. (1995). Double dissociation between item and source memory. *Neuropsychology*, **9**, 229–235.

Goldapple, K., Segal, Z., Garson, C. *et al.* (2004). Modulation of cortical-limbic pathways in major depression: treatment-specific effects of cognitive behavior therapy. *Archives of General Psychiatry*, **61**, 34–41.

Grady, C. L. (2002). Age-related differences in face processing: a meta-analysis of three functional neuroimaging experiments. *Canadian Journal of Experimental Psychology*, **56**, 208–220.

Grady, C. L. (2008). Functional neuroimaging studies of aging. In Squire, L. R. (Ed.-in-chief) *Encyclopedia of Neuroscience*. Oxford: Academic Press.

Grady, C. L., Maisog, J. M., Horwitz, B. *et al.* (1994). Age-related changes in cortical blood flow activation during visual processing of faces and location. *Journal of Neuroscience*, **14**, 1450–1462.

Grady, C. L., McIntosh, A. R., Horwitz, B. *et al.* (1995). Age-related reductions in human recognition memory due to impaired encoding. *Science*, **269**, 218–221.

Grady, C. L., McIntosh, A. R., Bookstein, F. *et al.* (1998). Age-related changes in regional cerebral blood flow during working memory for faces. *NeuroImage*, **8**, 409–425.

Grady, C. L., McIntosh, A. R., Rajah, M. N., Beig, S., & Craik, F. I. M. (1999). The effects of age on the neural correlates of episodic encoding. *Cerebral Cortex*, **9**, 805–814.

Grady, C. L., Bernstein, L. J., Beig, S., & Siegenthaler, A. L. (2002). The effects of encoding task on age-related differences in the functional neuroanatomy of face memory. *Psychology and Aging*, **17**, 7–23.

Grady, C. L., McIntosh, A. R., Beig, S. *et al.* (2003a). Evidence from functional neuroimaging of a compensatory prefrontal network in Alzheimer's disease. *Journal of Neuroscience*, **23**, 986–993.

Grady, C. L., McIntosh, A. R., & Craik, F. I. M. (2003b). Age-related differences in the functional connectivity of the hippocampus during memory encoding. *Hippocampus*, **13**, 572–586.

Grady, C. L., McIntosh, A. R., & Craik, F. I. M. (2005). Task-related activity in prefrontal cortex and its relation to recognition memory performance in young and old adults. *Neuropsychologia*, **43**, 1466–1481.

Grady, C. L., Springer, M. V., Hongwanishkul, D., McIntosh, A. R., & Winocur, G. (2006). Age-related changes in brain activity across the adult lifespan. *Journal of Cognitive Neuroscience*, **18**, 227–241.

Greicius, M. D., Srivastava, G., Reiss, A. L., & Menon, V. (2004). Default-mode network activity distinguishes Alzheimer's disease from healthy aging: evidence from functional MRI. *Proceedings of the National Academy of Sciences of the United States of America*, **101**, 4637–4642.

Gutchess, A. H., Welsh, R. C., Hedden, T. *et al.* (2005). Aging and the neural correlates of successful picture encoding: frontal activations compensate for decreased medial-temporal activity. *Journal of Cognitive Neuroscience*, **17**, 84–96.

Hamzei, F., Liepert, J., Dettmers, C. W., & Rijntjes, M. (2006). Two different reorganization patterns after rehabilitative therapy: an exploratory study with fMRI and TMS. *NeuroImage*, **31**, 710–720.

Hasher, L., & Zacks, R. T. (1988). Working memory, comprehension, and aging: a review and a new view. In G. H. Bower (Ed.), *The Psychology of Learning and Motivation, Vol. 22* (pp. 193–225). New York, NY: Academic Press.

Hashtroudi, S., Johnson, M. K., & Chrosniak, L. D. (1989). Aging and source monitoring. *Psychology and Aging*, **4**, 106–112.

Heiss, W.-D., Thiel, A., Winhuisen, L. *et al.* (2003). Functional imaging in the assessment of capability for recovery after stroke. *Journal of Rehabilitation Medicine*, **35**, 27–33.

Henson, R. N. A., Cansino, S., Herron, J. E., Robb, W. G. K., & Rugg, M. D. (2003). A familiarity signal in human anterior medial temporal cortex? *Hippocampus*, **13**, 301–304.

Johansson, B. B. (2000). Brain plasticity and stroke rehabilitation: the Willis Lecture. *Stroke*, **31**, 223–230.

Karni, A., Meyer, G., Jezzard, P. *et al.* (1995). Functional MRI evidence for adult motor cortex plasticity during motor skill learning. *Nature*, **377**, 155–158.

Laatsch, L. K., Thulborn, K. R., Krisky, C. M., Shobat, D. M., & Sweeney, J. A. (2004). Investigating the neurobiological basis of cognitive rehabilitation therapy with fMRI. *Brain Injury*, **18**, 957–974.

Lepage, M., Ghaffar, O., Nyberg, L., & Tulving, E. (2000). From the cover: prefrontal cortex and episodic memory retrieval mode. *Proceedings of the National Academy of Sciences of the United States of America*, **97**, 506–511.

Levine, B., Svoboda, E., Hay, J. F., Winocur, G., & Moscovitch, M. (2002). Aging and autobiographical memory: dissociating episodic from semantic retrieval. *Psychology and Aging*, **17**, 677–689.

Light, L. L. (1991). Memory and aging: four hypotheses in search of data. *Annual Review of Psychology*, **42**, 333–376.

Logan, J. M., Sanders, A. L., Snyder, A. Z., Morris, J. C., & Buckner, R. L. (2002). Under-recruitment and nonselective recruitment: dissociable neural mechanisms associated with aging. *Neuron*, **33**, 827–840.

Madden, D. J., Turkington, T. G., Provenzale, J. M. *et al.* (1999). Adult age differences in the functional neuroanatomy of verbal recognition memory. *Human Brain Mapping*, **7**, 115–135.

Madden, D. J., Turkington, T. G., Provenzale, J. M. *et al.* (2002). Aging and attentional guidance during visual search: functional neuroanatomy by positron emission tomography. *Psychology and Aging*, **17**, 24–43.

Maguire, E. A., & Frith, C. D. (2003). Aging affects the engagement of the hippocampus during autobiographical memory retrieval. *Brain*, **126**, 1511–1523.

Mattay, V. S., Fera, F., Tessitore, A. *et al.* (2006). Neurophysiological correlates of age-related changes in working memory capacity. *Neuroscience Letters*, **392**, 32–37.

McCrae, R. R., Costa, P. T. J., Pedrosa de Lima, M. *et al.* (1999). Age differences in personality across the adult life span: parallels in five cultures. *Developmental Psychology*, **35**, 466–477.

McIntosh, A. R., Sekuler, A. B., Penpeci, C. *et al.* (1999). Recruitment of unique neural systems to support visual memory in normal aging. *Current Biology*, **9**, 1275–1278.

Merzenich, M. M., Kaas, J. H., Wall, J. T. *et al.* (1983). Progression of change following median nerve section in the cortical representation of the hand in areas 3b and 1 in adult owl and squirrel monkeys. *Neuroscience*, **10**, 639–665.

Mitchell, K. J., Johnson, M. K., Raye, C. L., & D'Esposito, M. (2000). fMRI evidence of age-related hippocampal dysfunction in feature binding in working memory. *Cognitive Brain Research*, **10**, 197–206.

Mitchell, K. J., Raye, C. L., Johnson, M. K., & Greene, E. J. (2006). An fMRI investigation of short-term source memory in young and older adults. *NeuroImage*, **30**, 627–633.

Morcom, A. M., Good, C. D., Frackowiak, R. S. J., & Rugg, M. D. (2003). Age effects on the neural correlates of successful memory encoding. *Brain*, **126**, 213–229.

Musso, M., Weiller, C., Kiebel, S. *et al.* (1999). Training-induced brain plasticity in aphasia. *Brain*, **122**, 1781–1790.

Nakamura, T., Ghilardi, M. F., Mentis, M. *et al.* (2001). Functional networks in motor sequence learning: abnormal topographies in Parkinson's disease. *Human Brain Mapping*, **12**, 42–60.

Nordahl, C. W., Ranganath, C., Yonelinas, A. P. *et al.* (2006). White matter changes compromise prefrontal cortex function in healthy elderly individuals. *Journal of Cognitive Neuroscience*, **18**, 418–429.

Otten, L. J., & Rugg, M. D. (2001). Task-dependency of the neural correlates of episodic encoding as measured by fMRI. *Cerebral Cortex*, **11**, 1150–1160.

Park, D. C., Lautenschlager, G., Hedden, T. *et al.* (2002). Models of visuospatial and verbal memory across the adult life span. *Psychology and Aging*, **17**, 299–320.

Piolino, P., Desgranges, B., Benali, K., & Eustache, F. (2002). Episodic and semantic remote autobiographical memory in ageing. *Memory*, **10**, 239–257.

Prull, M. W., Dawes, L. L. C., Martin, A. M. I., Rosenberg, H. F., & Light, L. L. (2006). Recollection and familiarity in recognition memory: adult age differences and neuropsychological test correlates. *Psychology and Aging*, **21**, 107–118.

Raichle, M. E., Fiez, J. A., Videen, T. O. *et al.* (1994). Practice-related changes in human brain functional anatomy during nonmotor learning. *Cerebral Cortex*, **4**, 8–26.

Ramachandran, V. S. (2005). Plasticity and functional recovery in neurology. *Clinical Medicine*, **5**, 368–373.

Ranganath, C., Yonelinas, A. P., Cohen, M. X. *et al.* (2004). Dissociable correlates of recollection and familiarity within the medial temporal lobes. *Neuropsychologia*, **42**, 2–13.

Raz, N. (2000). Aging of the brain and its impact on cognitive performance: Integration of structural and functional findings. In F. I. M. Craik, & T. A. Salthouse (Eds.), *Handbook of Aging and Cognition – II* (pp. 1–90). Mahwah, NJ: Lawrence Erlbaum.

Reuter-Lorenz, P. A., Jonides, J., Smith, E. E. *et al.* (2000). Age differences in the frontal lateralization of verbal and spatial working memory revealed by PET. *Journal of Cognitive Neuroscience*, **12**, 174–187.

Rijntjes, M. (2006). Mechanisms of recovery in stroke patients with hemiparesis or aphasia: new insights, old questions and the meaning of therapies. *Current Opinion in Neurology*, **19**, 76–83.

Rosen, A. C., Prull, M. W., O'Hara, R. *et al.* (2002). Variable effects of aging on frontal lobe contributions to memory. *NeuroReport*, **13**, 2425–2428.

Rugg, M. D., & Henson, R. N. (2002). Episodic memory retrieval: An (event-related) functional neuroimaging perspective. In A. E. Parker, E. L. Wilding, & T. J. Bussey (Eds.), *The Cognitive Neuroscience of Memory Encoding and Retrieval* (pp. 3–37). London, UK: Psychology Press.

Rypma, B., & D'Esposito, M. (2000). Isolating the neural mechanisms of age-related changes in human working memory. *Nature Neuroscience*, **3**, 509–515.

Salthouse, T. A. (1990). Working memory as a processing resource in cognitive aging. *Developmental Review*, **10**, 101–124.

Schacter, D. L., Kaszniak, A. W., Kihlstrom, J. F., & Valdiserri, M. (1991). The relation between source memory and aging. *Psychology and Aging*, **6**, 559–568.

Schoenfeld, M. A., Noesselt, T., Poggel, D. *et al.* (2002). Analysis of pathways mediating preserved vision after striate cortex lesions. *Annals of Neurology*, **52**, 814–824.

Smith, E. E., Geva, A., Jonides, J. *et al.* (2001). The neural basis of task-switching in working memory: effects of performance and aging. *Proceedings of the National Academy of Sciences of the United States of America*, **98**, 2095–2100.

Söderlund, H., Nyberg, L., Adolfsson, R., Nilsson, L.-G., & Launer, L. J. (2003). High prevalence of white matter hyperintensities in normal aging: relation to blood pressure and cognition. *Cortex*, **39**, 1093–1105.

Sowell, E. R., Thompson, P. M., Tessner, K. D., & Toga, A. W. (2001). Mapping continued brain growth and gray matter density reduction in dorsal frontal cortex: inverse relationships during postadolescent brain maturation. *Journal of Neuroscience*, **21**, 8819–8829.

Spaniol, J., Madden, D. J., & Voss, A. (2006). A diffusion model analysis of adult age differences in episodic and semantic long-term memory retrieval. *Journal of Experimental Psychology: Learning, Memory, and Cognition*, **32**, 101–117.

Springer, M. V., McIntosh, A. R., Winocur, G., & Grady, C. L. (2005). The relation between brain activity during memory tasks and years of education in young and older adults. *Neuropsychology*, **19**, 181–192.

Stern, Y., Albert, S., Tang, M.-X., & Tsai, W.-Y. (1999). Rate of memory decline in AD is related to education and occupation. *Neurology*, **53**, 1942–1947.

Stern, Y., Moeller, J. R., Anderson, K. E. *et al.* (2000). Different brain networks mediate task performance in normal aging and AD: defining compensation. *Neurology*, **55**, 1291–1297.

Stern, Y., Habeck, C., Moeller, J. *et al.* (2005). Brain networks associated with cognitive reserve in healthy young and old adults. *Cerebral Cortex*, **15**, 394–402.

Sullivan, E. V., Marsh, L., Mathalon, D. H., Lim, K. O., & Pfefferbaum, A. (1995). Age-related decline in MRI volumes of temporal lobe gray matter but not hippocampus. *Neurobiology of Aging*, **16**, 591–606.

Tulving, E. (1983). *Elements of Episodic Memory*. New York, NY: Oxford University Press.

Wagner, A. D., Schacter, D. L., Rotte, M. *et al.* (1998). Building memories: remembering and forgetting of verbal experiences as predicted by brain activity. *Science*, **281**, 1188–1191.

Weiller, C., Ramsay, S. C., Wise, R. J. S., Friston, K. J., & Frackowiak, R. S. J. (1993). Individual patterns of functional reorganization in the human cerebral cortex after capsular infarction. *Annals of Neurology*, **33**, 181–189.

Weiller, C., Isensee, C., Rijntjes, M. *et al.* (1995). Recovery from Wernicke's aphasia: a positron emission tomographic study. *Annals of Neurology*, **37**, 723–732.

Yonelinas, A. P. (2001). Components of episodic memory: the contribution of recollection and familiarity. *Philosophical Transactions of the Royal Society of London, Series B: Biological Sciences*, **356**, 1363–1374.

Zacks, R. T., Hasher, L., & Li, K. Z. H. (2000). Human memory. In F. I. M. Craik & T. A. Salthouse (Eds.), *The Handbook of Aging and Cognition* (pp. 293–357). Mahwah, NJ: Lawrence Erlbaum.

10

Functional brain imaging and neurological recovery

Maurizio Corbetta

The problem of neurological recovery after injury

It is unwise to prophesy either death or recovery in acute diseases. (Hippocrates: Aphorisms II-19 *c*. 500 BC)

- Neurological recovery occurs commonly, and is mediated by many mechanisms from cells to systems.
- Research is currently trying to clarify which neural mechanisms of recovery are behaviorally significant.

It is a common observation on neurology wards that most patients improve after a stroke or a traumatic brain injury. About 80–90% of all stroke patients have motor deficits (or hemiparesis) at onset, while only 40–60% of them have a persistent deficit at 6 months to 1 year (Dobkin, 2005). Similar degrees of recovery occur for language and visuospatial perception (Sarno & Levita, 1971; Stone *et al.*, 1993). Whereas early (1–3 days) recovery may be explained by vascular changes, such as early canalization of an obstructed vessel or reduction in the amount of edema surrounding an ischemic area, recovery that occurs in the weeks and months following the stroke must be explained by different mechanisms.

The central nervous system reacts to injuries (stroke, trauma) through changes that occur at the level of brain networks, areas, neurons, connections, molecules and even genes (Carmichael, 2003a; Nudo, 1999; Weiller, 1998). Many of these changes represent "house-keeping" operations unrelated to behavioral recovery. For instance, in the area

of ischemic damage an inflammatory reaction is mounted within 24–48 hours that leads to the elimination of vascular and cellular debris. At the level of brain networks, damage to one area may lead to a decrement of synaptic activity downstream in a connected area, which will in turn downregulate its metabolic demands (diaschisis) (Baron *et al.*, 1980).

Hence, a fundamental goal of current neurobiological research on recovery of function is "to separate the wheat from the chaff," that is, determine which changes are triggered by brain injury and which of those changes are actually related to behavioral recovery. Once and if that goal is achieved, it will be possible to use information about mechanisms of recovery to categorize patients, predict outcome, and develop novel interventions. This research program is hampered by incredible theoretical and pragmatic challenges. The problem is multidimensional, as illustrated in Figure 10.1. One dimension is the brain with its different levels of organization (molecules to networks), where changes putatively related to recovery occur at different levels, but must be related across levels to be helpful. For instance, going from brain to molecules, we would like to understand how changes recorded at the level of brain networks relate to changes recorded from single neurons near the lesion or in distant but connected neuronal populations, and how in turn these neuronal changes are related to upregulation or downregulation of receptors involved in neural transmission (e.g., N-methyl-D-aspartate (NMDA) or gamma-aminobutyric acid (GABA) receptors).

Cognitive Neurorehabilitation, Second Edition: Evidence and Application, ed. Donald T. Stuss, Gordon Winocur and Ian H. Robertson. Published by Cambridge University Press. © Cambridge University Press 2008.

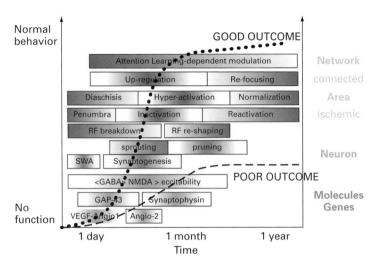

Figure 10.1. Three-dimensional-problem space for studying recovery of function: RF = receptive field; SWA = slow wave activation; GAP = growth-associated protein; VEGF = vascular endothelial growth factor; Angio-2 = angiopoietin 2.

A second dimension is the timing of these changes in relation to the time course of recovery. Ideally, one would like to concentrate on mechanisms that have a temporal profile matching or paralleling the time course of recovery. A final important and critical dimension is the behavioral relevance of these mechanisms. How do these mechanisms relate to good or poor level of function? How do they relate to the degree of recovery, that is, the amount of change from acute to chronic?

The role of functional brain imaging

- Functional brain imaging allows the visualization of neural mechanisms of recovery at the systems level.
- Different experimental strategies are used to study after injury the relationship between neural activity and behavior.
- The interpretation of brain-imaging findings in nonhealthy subjects must be cautious in light of many possible experimental and biological artifacts due to the injury or other associated factors.

Functional brain imaging techniques allow the visualization of the living human brain at the level of areas

and networks (Figure 10.1). Some of these techniques (positron emission tomography (PET) or magnetic resonance imaging (MRI)) are based on measuring regional metabolic signals (blood flow: PET; oxygen metabolism, glucose metabolism: PET; oxygen concentration: PET/fMRI) that are indirectly related to the level of neuronal activity (see Prichard & Rosen, 1994 and Raichle, 1987 for reviews). While the exact cellular mechanisms linking neuronal activity to metabolic changes are not fully understood, the current theory is that task-related increases or decreases in blood flow, glucose metabolism, and oxygen concentration are related to the sum of the excitatory and inhibitory inputs to and within an area (Lauritzen & Gold, 2003; Logothetis *et al.*, 2001). In other words it is assumed that the majority of the metabolic demands within a cortical area reflect the input and the local integration of information. Functional brain imaging methods are hence ideally suited to identify changes at the level of areas or brain networks related to functional recovery (Figure 10.1).

Experimental strategies

Three main strategies have been applied to the study of neurological recovery. The first strategy involves the correlation of behavioral scores on neuropsychological tests with regional measurements of blood flow or glucose metabolism in the resting state (Hillis *et al.*, 2002; Metter, 1991). Resting measurements are relatively simple to obtain, and permit testing of large numbers of patients with a wide range of behavioral deficits. However, they require a priori definition of regions of interest, which may or may not be known for a certain function. Moreover, they do not allow a direct correlation of task-evoked activity with behavioral performance measured simultaneously in the scanner. Recent studies have relied on changes of resting blood flow in a given area induced either by spontaneous recovery or pharmacological manipulation of systemic blood pressure to link more directly dysfunction in one area with specific cognitive deficits (Hillis *et al.*, 2003, 2005).

A second strategy involves measurements of whole brain activity during the performance of a task (Chollet *et al.*, 1991; Weiller *et al.*, 1995). This is the strategy most often utilized in studies of neurological recovery. The main disadvantage is that only patients with mild or moderate impairment who are able to perform at some level of proficiency can participate. This requirement severely limits the number of potential participants, and makes it almost impossible to study large samples (typically not more than 10–20 patients are scanned per study). An additional problem is that it is difficult to interpret differences in patterns of brain activation with healthy subjects unless patients and controls perform similarly (see Price *et al.*, 2006 for a recent review on fMRI scanning of neurologically impaired subjects). The ability to image the whole brain is invaluable because most studies are still exploratory, and the function of most brain areas is unknown even in healthy subjects.

A third approach considers the functional interaction between brain regions and their influence on behavior. This approach is based on the analysis of how the temporal correlation of signals between different regions changes during a task. These methods require strong assumptions regarding either the task or the existence of anatomical connections between regions (structural equation modeling, dynamic causal modeling) (Price *et al.*, 2006). A much simpler approach is to consider inter-regional temporal correlations in the resting state, i.e., in the absence of any active behavior. A number of recent studies show that this approach is very powerful in identifying healthy brain networks (Fox *et al.*, 2005), and may be also quite sensitive in defining pathological conditions (Greicius *et al.*, 2004).

Pitfalls

The use of functional brain imaging to study neurological recovery is predicated on the fact that the physiological relationship between neuronal activity and hemodynamic (blood flow, oxygenation) signals, so called "neurovascular coupling," is normal. However, since this is hardly the case in elderly patients with significant cerebrovascular or degenerative diseases, one has to be aware of the many factors that can influence the interpretation of brain-imaging signals in neurologically impaired subjects.

One factor is the effect of aging on blood vessels. Aging may influence the structure of blood vessels, interfere with signaling underlying neurovascular coupling, or directly impair neuronal function. Moreover, widespread cerebral activations, similar to those reported in recovering stroke patients, have been reported in aging subjects and correlated with cognitive compensation (Buckner, 2004; Reuter-Lorenz, 2002). Atherosclerosis may also change the structure of the brain blood vessels and impair neurovascular coupling. The blood flow response to a stimulus may be suppressed even when behavior is normal, and neuronal activity is present (Pineiro *et al.*, 2002; Powers *et al.*, 1988; Rossini *et al.*, 2004; Röther *et al.*, 2002) or the temporal dynamics of the blood-oxygen level dependent (BOLD) response recorded with fMRI may be abnormal (D'Esposito *et al.*, 2003). A third factor is the potential effect of angiogenesis (Carmichael, 2003a). Angiogenesis defines a sequence of events including vascular permeability, extravasation of plasma proteins, destabilization of mature vessels, endothelial cell division

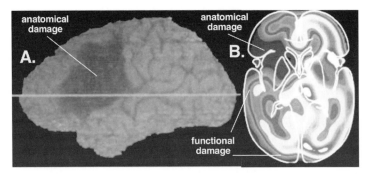

Figure 10.2. (This figure is reproduced in the color plate section at the front of this volume.) (A) Three-dimensional anatomical MRI reconstruction of stroke; (B) corresponding PET blood flow slice. Note decreased blood flow from the damaged area (blue) and structurally normal temporal and occipital lobes of the damaged hemisphere.

and budding, the formation of new vascular trees, and then finally new patterns of local blood flow. These changes occur in the perilesional area in the first 1–2 weeks after a stroke, and co-localize with sites of synaptic sprouting and post-stroke stem cell response. It is commonly reported that task induced blood flow or BOLD signals may be weak or not present at the subacute stage (3–4 weeks), and become more detectable at the chronic stage (3–6 months) (Heiss *et al.*, 1999). Although these results are considered evidence of local neural reorganization, it is possible that at the acute stage neuronal activity in the perilesional area may be present but not detectable with neuroimaging methods because of lack of a mature vascular system capable of sustaining a normal neurovascular coupling.

A final factor is the effect of diaschisis on task-evoked BOLD or blood-flow signals. Diaschisis is defined as a decrement in neuronal activity and metabolism within an area produced by lack of excitatory input from a connected area that is injured (Baron *et al.*, 1980; Feeney & Baron, 1986; von Monakow, 1911). Diaschisis can occur in cortex after thalamic or basal ganglia lesions; in homologous areas of the contralesional hemisphere via callosal connections; and, in distant areas within the same hemisphere through long-range cortico-cortical connections. Figure 10.2 shows diaschisis in the occipito temporal lobe at 6 months post-onset after a stroke in the frontal lobe. It is currently

unknown whether changes of the neuronal and metabolic baseline of an area affect stimulus- or task-evoked activity.

Although there are numerous artifacts affecting the interpretation of brain-imaging signals in pathological conditions, and there is little defense against false negatives, as for example in the case of preserved neural activity in the absence of metabolic changes (Rossini *et al.*, 2004), the best protection against false positive remains a careful analysis of behavioral conditions and of their correlation with brain-imaging data. In other words, if a pattern of brain activation robustly correlates with behavior then one can worry less about artifacts. Nonetheless, progress in this field is slow. A recent review on aphasia recovery noted that in a 1-year period only 35 patients had been reported across eight studies (Price & Crinion, 2005).

Summary

Brain imaging is a powerful approach to visualize the neural changes triggered by an injury at the level of individual areas or brain networks. A critical goal is to concentrate on changes that are behaviorally relevant, associated with either the level of a function or a change in function. Studies in nonhealthy brains are complicated by many confounding factors such as changes in the structure of the vessels associated with aging or other associated clinical conditions. These vascular changes may affect the fidelity with which the local neural activity is transformed in a measurable hemodynamic response. There are also anatomical and physiological changes associated with the injury, be it ischemic, neoplastic, degenerative or traumatic. Although we have concentrated on ischemic lesions, each condition has its own caveats that need to be understood in detail before embarking in a neuroimaging study. It is the author's opinion that behavioral controls and the constant search of associations between brain changes and behavior is the best protection against artifactual results.

Neural correlates of motor recovery

- Improvements in motor function commonly occur in the first 3 months post-injury; however, it is more correct to speak of motor reorganization rather than of motor recovery, given the pattern of movements is never the same after a lesion.
- Motor reorganization involves different mechanisms: the bilateral recruitment and over-activation of nonprimary motor and attention areas early on after injury.
- The normalization and focusing of activity within primary motor circuits that correlates with behavioral recovery.
- Shifts in the topography of motor areas that may reflect permanent changes in neural organization and that are of uncertain behavioral significance.

The large majority of patients with a stroke invariably show some degree of recovery ranging from minimal to complete (Twitchell, 1951). The degree of recovery depends on initial severity, being more complete in patients with milder deficits at onset, and occurs largely in the first 3 months post-stroke tapering off by about 6 months. Importantly, the recovered movements are not identical to the original movements in terms of dynamics (speed, accuracy, trajectories) and thus pattern of muscle recruitment, even when the lesions are circumscribed to parts of sensory-motor cortex (Friel &

Nudo, 1998). It is therefore more correct to speak of "motor reorganization."

Three main physiological changes have been identified in the motor system: (i) over-activation and bilateral recruitment of motor, pre-motor and attention-related areas; (ii) a focusing of activity over time; (iii) topographic shifts in sensory-motor representations.

Over-activation and bilateral recruitment of motor, pre-motor and attention-related areas

The normal pattern of activation during simple actions (e.g., repetitive finger opposition) involves a relatively small number of areas including the contra-lateral sensory-motor, pre-motor, and supplementary motor cortices, thalamus, and ipsilateral cerebellum. When movements are more attention-demanding, as during a sequence of finger movements, or when movements are unskilled, the basic contra-lateral organization becomes more bilateral with recruitment of prefrontal, parietal and cingulate areas that control, monitor and correct performance (Kim et al., 1993; Passingham, 1996).

A lesion that damages motor cortex or the descending cortico-spinal fibers causes an acute inactivation of the motor cortex accompanied by a decrement of cortical excitability both near lesion and at distance (Neumann-Haefelin & Witte, 2000). The level of residual motor excitability, i.e., the ability to drive movement-evoked potentials peripherally, is predictive of outcome (Delvaux et al., 2003; Pennisi et al., 1999; Rapisarda et al., 1996). In patients that attempt to move their paretic limb early on after a stroke several studies have shown a relative over-activation and bilateral recruitment of motor, pre-motor and attention-controlling areas in the damaged and normal hemisphere (Figure 10.3). This early increase is followed by a decrease in task-related activity several months later (Calautti et al., 2001; Marshall et al., 2000). However, even in patients with excellent recovery of motor function a number of studies show at the chronic stage a persistence of over-activation, as compared with healthy controls, during movements of the affected

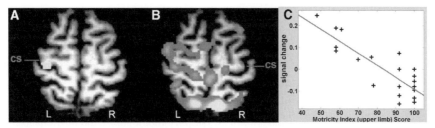

Figure 10.3. (This figure is reproduced in the color plate section at the front of this volume.) (A) Activation of left motor cortex in a healthy subject for right-hand movements; (B) bilateral activation of motor cortex and accessory motor areas for same movement in patient with subcortical stroke in left hemisphere; (C) inverse relationship between motor outcome and level of activation in supplementary motor area. Picture kindly provided by Nick Ward.

upper extremity (Chollet *et al.*, 1991; Cramer *et al.*, 1997; Seitz *et al.*, 1998; Weiller *et al.*, 1992). When these observations were originally made, it was suggested that this over-activation reflected the compensatory recruitment of accessory motor systems in pre-motor, supplementary and ipsi-lesional motor cortices that are known to project in parallel to the spinal cord (Dum & Strick, 2002) and that may be used to circumvent the blockage of transmission from the damaged motor cortex.

However, subsequent studies showed that a bilateral (and over-active) pattern of motor activation correlates with a less complete recovery of motor function. In fact patients with no residual impairment tend to have relatively normal maps of motor activation with weak or no bilateral recruitment, whereas patients with lesser recovery tend to activate more strongly and more bilaterally the motor system (Calautti *et al.*, 2001, 2003; Johansen-Berg *et al.*, 2002a; Ward *et al.*, 2003a). Moreover, at a time (>3 months post-stroke) in which recovery is deemed to be near complete, the degree of activation in the motor system negatively correlates with outcome (Figure 10.3).

Why does the motor system become over- and bilaterally active after a stroke? A number of control experiments suggest that over-activity does not depend on perceived effort or increased attention to the task, which are known to boost neural activity (Johansen-Berg & Matthews, 2002; Passingham, 1996), but that it reflects an upregulation of the motor system trying to overcome a defective motor

output (Ward *et al.*, 2003a, 2003b). The bilateral recruitment of motor networks may be especially important as a compensatory mechanism for patients whose recovery is not complete. In fact the recruitment is greater in patients with greater cortico-spinal dysfunction as assessed by transcranial magnetic stimulation (TMS) (Ward, 2006). Moreover, inhibitory TMS of the pre-motor cortex, both on the same (Fridman *et al.*, 2004) and opposite side of a lesion (Johansen-Berg *et al.*, 2002b) disrupts motor performance of the paretic hand especially in patients with non optimal recovery, whereas stimulation in healthy controls does not have any measurable effect.

A possible exception is represented by activity in the motor cortex opposite the lesion. A number of recent studies suggest that activity from the intact motor cortex may be inhibitory onto the damaged motor cortex; that this inhibition may be mediated through callosal connections (Meyer *et al.*, 1995; Shimizu *et al.*, 2002) and that removal of this inhibition by either electrical or magnetic stimulation may partially improve hand function (Murase *et al.*, 2004).

These findings illustrate an important principle currently not well appreciated by clinicians. The observed motor deficits do not only reflect the structural damage due to stroke, but also the induced physiological dysfunction on anatomically intact tissue. At the neuronal level these physiological changes may be due to the disorganization of motor receptive fields that have been described in the tissue surrounding an ischemic area in motor cortex (Carmichael, 2003b; Nudo, 1999) and in distant areas like the ventral premotor cortex (Dancause *et al.*, 2005; Frost *et al.*, 2003).

Focusing and normalization of activity over time

In the weeks and months following a stroke, motor performance improves with practice. Sometimes in patients with excellent recovery the reorganized motor patterns achieve near normal performance, although it is more correct to describe this process as "reorganization" given that the recovered behavioral pattern is never identical to the original one. In other patients the reorganized motor patterns are quite abnormal and inefficient.

These behavioral differences in the level of final outcome are captured by changes over time in the magnitude and topography of activation in the motor systems. Patients who recover motor function to a greater extent show stronger task-related decreases in motor networks than patients who recover less completely. Importantly, this relationship is independent of the rate of recovery or initial severity of the deficit (Ward *et al.*, 2003a). Furthermore, patients with better recovery tend to activate their motor system with a stronger contra-lateral than ipsilateral pattern, whereas patients with poorer recovery tend to maintain a more bilateral distribution of activity (Feydy *et al.*, 2002; Small *et al.*, 2002; Ward *et al.*, 2003a). Therefore recovery appears to be associated with a "focusing" of activity within motor networks of the damaged hemisphere, and a restriction of activity in the undamaged hemisphere and outside of the motor system. This process is similar to what is described during motor learning in healthy subjects (Poggio & Bizzi, 2004). Naïve performance is associated with a strong bilateral recruitment of higher-order areas, including the prefrontal cortices, which tends to decrease as learning progresses. Even highly complicated movements like piano playing may be carried out with relatively simple motor circuits when they are highly trained and over-learned (Karni *et al.*, 1998; Merzenich *et al.*, 1996).

Shifts in the topography of sensory-motor representations

Functional reorganization may also occur within the sensory-motor cortex and takes the form of a relative shift in the topography of activation (Calautti *et al.*, 2001, 2003; Pineiro *et al.*, 2001; Weiller *et al.*, 1992). During the execution of finger movements, activity is normally centered in the hand representation of sensory-motor cortex, although considerable variability has been reported (Cramer *et al.*, 2003). In patients with subcortical strokes and recovered upper extremity function, some studies have reported a ventral shift toward the face representation, while other studies have reported a posterior shift toward the post-central gyrus (primary somatosensory cortex). These topographical shifts (or "remapping") are not unique to stroke patients, but have been observed in patients with peripheral deafferentation such as limb amputees or patients with spinal cord injury (SCI) (Corbetta *et al.*, 2002; Flor *et al.*, 1995; Ramachandran, 1993).

What are the neuronal bases of these topographic shifts in functional activation? In patients with limb amputation or sensory deafferentation, cortical remapping is related to anatomical changes at the subcortical and thalamic levels with re-routing of inputs from the deafferented limb to relay nuclei that code inputs from the face (Jones & Pons, 1998; Pons *et al.*, 1991). In the case of cortical lesions, remapping may be related to local sprouting and a change in the organization of intra-area connections (Carmichael, 2003b). At the physiological level, Nudo *et al.* have discovered that after small lesions in the somatosensory or motor cortex, monkeys recover the use of the injured fingertips (Nudo, 1999; Nudo *et al.*, 1996a, 1996b). In parallel, there is a re-emergence of the injured fingertip representation in the territory adjacent to the lesion. It remains unknown what determines the variability of shift direction (dorso-ventral, antero-posterior), and whether these shifts have any behavioral consequence in terms of recovery or final outcome.

Summary

Studies of motor reorganization offer a roadmap for what neuroimaging may offer to neurorehabilitation. Both cross-sectional and longitudinal studies have established a set of mechanisms – initial over-activation and recruitment of both motor and non-motor areas followed by refocusing of activity within the motor networks – that are behaviorally relevant (Ward *et al.*, 2003a, 2003b). Importantly, these mechanisms capture the final level of motor competence of a subject, such that the more abnormal the strength and topography of brain activation at the chronic stage, the lesser the level of motor recovery, as well as the potential for improvement over time, such that the more normal the pattern of activity becomes from acute to chronic stage, the more improvement can be expected in that particular patient. While the predictive power of these physiological indicators remains to be tested, these results suggest that in principle brain scans can predict final outcome and changes of motor function over time. This is important not only for diagnosis or prognosis, but also for monitoring the effects of novel rehabilitative interventions. Does a specific treatment improve the level of over-activation in the brain, and correspondingly does it improve behavior? The importance of having identified a physiological, and behaviorally significant, mechanism is critical because it should allow the design of interventions that do not try to improve behavior specifically, but rather that target a specific neural mechanism. The hope is that this strategy may be more effective.

Neural correlates of aphasia recovery

- Language can improve for a longer time than motor function, up to 2 years post-injury.
- The reorganization of language depends on the recruitment of regions in the right hemisphere homologous to the language areas damaged in the left hemisphere.

- Another mechanism is the reactivation of left hemisphere regions initially rendered dysfunctional by the lesion.
- As in the case of motor function, the best outcome can be expected when the reorganized pattern of activation closely resembles the normal pattern.

The majority of aphasic patients also show recovery ranging from minimal to complete (Kertesz & McCabe, 1977). The time course for language recovery, however, is more protracted than for motor recovery. Language recovery is largely complete by 1 year post-onset with diminished rate of recovery by the 2-year mark (Basso *et al.*, 1982l; Kertesz & McCabe, 1977; Sarno & Levita, 1979). As in the motor system, it is more correct to speak of reorganization than of true recovery of function. Clearly, in individuals with poor recovery, language production is not identical to the original output; articulation is of poorer quality, grammatical structures are not well preserved and word choice is affected.

Recruitment of right hemisphere and shift toward the left hemisphere

Two theories have been traditionally proposed to explain the recovery of aphasia. In light of current evidence, it is clear that these two theories are not mutually exclusive, but rather represent a continuum.

The first theory, originally proposed by Carl Wernicke (Wernicke, 1908) posits that activity in the right hemisphere plays a major role in allowing the return of language. There is considerable support for this view. Some recovery occurs in patients with very large lesions of the left hemisphere (Cummings *et al.*, 1979). Electrophysiological and early blood flow studies with Xenon methods reported "abnormal" right hemisphere activity in recovered aphasics during language tasks (Papanicolaou *et al.*, 1988). Several functional activation studies with PET and fMRI have also reported recruitment of right hemisphere regions homologous to those active during language processing in

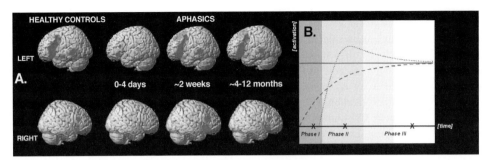

Figure 10.4. (This figure is reproduced in the color plate section at the front of this volume.) (A) Longitudinal changes in brain activation in aphasic patients and healthy controls on a semantic judgment task in left (top) and right (bottom) hemispheres; (B) time course of activity in left and right hemispheres from acute to chronic stage. Picture kindly provided by Cornelius Weiller.

the left hemisphere in healthy adults (Belin *et al.*, 1996; Blasi *et al.*, 2002; Buckner *et al.*, 1996; Cao *et al.*, 1999; Gold & Kertesz, 2000; Rosen *et al.*, 2000; Thulborn *et al.*, 1999; Warburton *et al.*, 1999; Weiller *et al.*, 1995), though right hemisphere recruitment may depend on the extent of lesion in critical language structures in the left hemisphere (Blank *et al.*, 2003).

The second theory proposes that aphasia recovery depends on regions in the left hemisphere. Support comes from studies that have combined neuropsychological testing and resting/activation measurements of regional metabolic glucose metabolism (rCMRGl) (Heiss *et al.*, 1993; Metter *et al.*, 1989; 1990; Mimura *et al.*, 1998; Vallar *et al.*, 1988). These studies have demonstrated that hypo-metabolism of regions in the left hemisphere measured within 2 to 3 weeks from the onset of the stroke correlates with the rate of improvement on selected language scales. For example, low acute rCMRGl in the left superior temporal gyrus predicted poor performance on a follow-up test of auditory comprehension (Heiss *et al.*, 1993). Figure 10.2 shows an example of left hemisphere hypo-metabolism (in this case low blood flow) at rest after a stroke in the frontal lobe. Heiss and colleagues (Heiss *et al.*, 1999) showed that favorable recovery of auditory comprehension in frontal-subcortical patients was correlated with activation of the right superior temporal gyrus and right inferior frontal gyrus at baseline, followed by

activation of left superior temporal gyrus at follow-up during auditory word repetition. Unfavorable outcome was associated with persistent activity in the right frontal gyrus.

A recent longitudinal fMRI study provides a possible reconciliation between these two theories, and a link with studies in the motor system (Saur *et al.*, 2006). Patients with aphasia and left hemisphere strokes in perisylvian cortex were studied at 0–4 days, ~2 weeks, and ~4–12 months post-stroke (Figure 10.4). No or weak activity in language-related regions of either hemisphere was found at 0–4 days; at ~2 weeks there was a sharp rise of activity in homologous right hemisphere regions; at the chronic stage there was a relative decrement of right hemisphere activity in parallel with a monotonic rise of activity in left hemisphere regions, which approximated the normal pattern of lateralisation observed in healthy brains. This temporal profile parallels that observed in the motor system with an early bilateral recruitment of accessory motor and attention regions followed at the chronic stage by a focusing of activity toward the motor system in the damaged hemisphere.

Both right- and left-hemisphere reorganized activity may be functionally significant post-stroke. Some patients with a left hemisphere lesion and recovery of language can return aphasic after the right hemisphere is subsequently inactivated (Kinsbourne, 1971) or damaged (Basso *et al.*, 1989).

Selected patients with left frontal cortex stroke and excellent recovery show abnormally strong activation of the homologous regions in the right inferior frontal gyrus (Buckner *et al.*, 1996), a result consistent with compensation. Several experiments find a correlation between language comprehension and right hemisphere activation (Crinion & Price, 2005; Musso *et al.*, 1999; Sharp *et al.*, 2004; Weiller *et al.*, 1995). However, a number of studies on speech production either failed to find any consistent relationship with right hemisphere activations (e.g., Rosen *et al.*, 2000), or found a negative correlation with language recovery (Belin *et al.*, 1996; Cao *et al.*, 1999; Heiss *et al.*, 1999; Warburton *et al.*, 1999). It is generally believed that the presence of left hemisphere activation in language areas tends to correlate with a more complete recovery (Rosen *et al.*, 2000). Left temporal cortex re-activation has been associated in several studies with good language outcome (Fernandez *et al.*, 2004; Heiss *et al.*, 1993, 1999). The degree of left (but also right) IFG activation at the acute stage (~2 days) has been associated with the level of language function (Saur *et al.*, 2006).

In individual patients the functional contribution of left vs. right hemisphere language areas will vary as a function of many variables such as size and etiology of the lesion, involvement of the white matter connecting posterior-to-anterior areas, time of measurement, original degree of language lateralization, and language function considered. As an example, let us consider the effect of measuring brain–behavior relationships at different time points in the course of recovery. In Saur *et al.* (2006), language function correlated at 0–4 days with the degree of activation in both left and right Broca's area and supplementary motor area (SMA). Some of these regions were presumably within the area of penumbra, i.e., the area of decreased blood flow in structurally intact tissue neighboring the stroke. Hillis and colleagues also reported that in the acute stage the degree of hypo-perfusion near the infarct correlates with specific language impairment, i.e., decreased blood flow in posterior superior temporal gyrus correlates with poor word comprehension (Hillis *et al.*, 2001, 2006). Hence, early on the functional status of the penumbra is critical for performance.

Conversely, longitudinal gains in language from 0–4 days to 2 weeks strongly correlated with increases of activity in right Broca homologue and SMA (Saur *et al.*, 2006). Therefore at this sub-acute stage the level of activation in the homologous right hemisphere cortices appears highly significant. This conclusion is consistent with the observation that at 2 weeks disruption of activity by TMS in the right Broca homologue impairs language in five out of eight patients that have a bilateral pattern of language-related activation, whereas it is not effective in the few patients that maintain a left hemisphere pattern (Winhuisen *et al.*, 2005). As in the motor system the persistence of an over-active right hemisphere language system may not represent an optimal mechanism for language recovery. Patients whose language is affected by right frontal TMS do not recover as well as patients who are able to reactivate their left hemisphere (Winhuisen *et al.*, 2005). Along the same lines it has been hypothesized that late right hemisphere over-activity actually plays a maladaptive role. Recent experiments show that inhibitory rTMS applied at the chronic stage to right hemisphere frontal regions produces some limited but persistent gains of naming in patients with severe aphasia (Naeser *et al.*, 2005a, 2005b).

Summary

The current consensus is that right hemisphere activity alone is the least effective mechanism for the recovery of speech production, followed by a bilateral activation of language networks, and in turn the best mechanism remains a left lateralized pattern of activation. For speech comprehension, right hemisphere activity alone may also lead to good outcome possibly due to a more bilateral representation of comprehension mechanisms. It is the author's opinion that research on language recovery is currently hampered by the lack of a good neural model of language function that takes in to account neurological, neuropsychological, linguistic and functional information. To study recovery we are still anchored to paradigms and theories developed in the 1800s, while at the same time it has not been easy to find straightforward relationships between patterns of language activation and mechanisms based in linguistics and neuropsychology (but see Price, 2000).

Neural correlates of spatial neglect recovery

- Spatial neglect tends to spontaneously improve but has long-term effects on disability.
- At the sub-acute stage (~3 weeks) brain activity is bilaterally depressed throughout the cortex, although specific regions in posterior parietal and occipital visual cortex show an inter-hemispheric functional imbalance.
- At the chronic stage (~9 months) the cortex is overall more responsive, and the occipito-parietal functional imbalance has normalized. The acute imbalance and chronic normalization correlate, respectively, with initial severity and subsequent recovery of attention in the left visual field.
- Disturbance of resting functional connectivity, i.e., temporal interaction between regions independently of task performance, have been recently demonstrated in stroke patients with spatial neglect. This opens up the possibility to study more severe patients that cannot perform a behavioral task in the scanner.

Unilateral spatial neglect (or neglect) occurs in about 25–30% of all patients (Appelros et al., 2002; Buxbaum et al., 2004; Pedersen et al., 1997). It occurs for lesions to either the left or the right hemisphere, but it is more severe and enduring after right hemisphere damage (Stone et al., 1993). Although neglect tends to partially improve spontaneously, it is associated with poor motor recovery, higher disability and poor response to rehabilitation (Buxbaum et al., 2004; Cherney et al., 2001; Katz et al., 1999; Paolucci et al., 2001). Although several behavioral dissociations have been reported in neglect, a clinically helpful distinction is between

spatially lateralized (left side neglect) and non-lateralized deficits (arousal, spatial and temporal capacity) (Barrett et al., 2006; Husain & Rorden, 2003; Robertson, 2001). It is currently under investigation whether lateralized or nonlateralized deficits are more significant in terms of recovery and final outcome (Barrett et al., 2006; Buxbaum et al., 2004; Farné et al., 2004).

Early work showed that the recovery of neglect was associated with the restoration of normal activity in ipsilateral subcortical nuclei after frontal damage in monkeys (Deuel & Collins, 1984), or right hemisphere regions after cortical-subcortical damage in humans (Hillis et al., 2005; Karnath et al., 2005; Pizzamiglio et al., 1998; Vallar et al., 1988). These findings had been interpreted according to the theory that neglect reflected damage of key brain areas involved in spatial processing, i.e., inferior parietal lobule (IPL) (Mort et al., 2003; Vallar & Perani, 1987), superior temporal gyrus (STG) (Karnath et al., 2001, 2004), subcortical nuclei (Karnath et al., 2002; Vallar & Perani, 1987), and the inferior frontal cortex (Husain & Kennard, 1996; Vallar & Perani, 1987). Only recently has it been possible to measure task-evoked brain activity in the course of recovery, and these studies have instead emphasized the importance of distributed dysfunction in frontoparietal cortical networks (Corbetta et al., 2005; Thiebaut de Schotten et al., 2005).

Bi-hemispheric acute suppression and chronic reactivation

A recent study (Corbetta et al., 2005) showed that patients suffer from a widespread suppression of task-evoked activity in both hemispheres about 3 weeks after a right hemisphere stroke causing clinical neglect (Figure 10.5). Interestingly, all of these regions were structurally intact and tens of centimeters away from the site of damage. At a follow-up measurement 39 weeks post-stroke, most regions had recovered a normal level of activation (Figure 10.5b), which qualitatively paralleled the recovery of neglect.

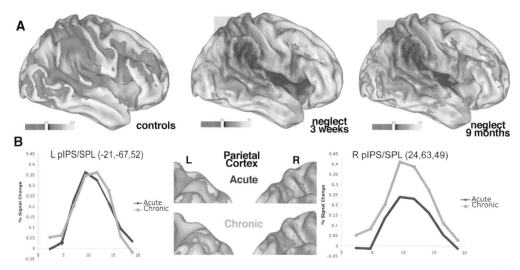

Figure 10.5. (This figure is reproduced in the color plate section at the front of this volume.) (A) Activity in right hemisphere of controls and patients with spatial neglect at 3 weeks and ~9 months during a spatial orienting task; (B) time course of activity in left and right parietal cortex at acute and chronic stage.

This widespread suppression is in contrast with the widespread over-activation reported in studies of motor and aphasia recovery. There are several possible explanations for this difference. One possibility is that neglect patients, who suffer from a general decrement in the level of vigilance (Heilman *et al.*, 1985), may have a reduced level of activation throughout the brain. Another intriguing possibility is that activity spreads in sensory and motor systems differently. Sensory signals may be broadcasted widely, and a lesion may block this "spreading" activation to widely distributed networks of areas. Conversely, motor signals may require a greater extent of focusing onto the appropriate response mechanism, which may involve the inhibition of other response areas. A lesion may thus lead to a decrement of this inhibition and a secondary over-activation of accessory motor areas. A final possibility is that lesions causing neglect impair more diffusely posterior sensory and anterior motor systems that are strongly integrated during spatial processing, the core problem in this syndrome.

Inter-hemispheric imbalance

A different mechanism is a functional imbalance of task-evoked activity. The imbalance involves a relatively stronger activation of the left (intact) hemisphere over the right (damaged) hemisphere at the acute stage, which normalizes at the chronic stage. This *"push-pull"* imbalance occurs in parietal and occipital cortices that are structurally intact, and correlates with the degree of spatial neglect (Corbetta *et al.*, 2005).

These results are interesting in many respects. Many years ago, based on observations in neurologically damaged patients, Marcel Kinsbourne proposed that neglect underlies an imbalance of opposing and reciprocally competing orienting mechanisms in each hemisphere (Kinsbourne, 1977). The idea is that each hemisphere is responsible for directing attention and sensory-motor actions toward the contra-lateral side of space, and that each hemisphere competes for the allocation of attention. For example, right hemisphere damage will impair leftward orienting, which will be made worse by the rightward orienting generated by an unopposed left hemisphere. The notion of inter-hemispheric competition is a powerful physiological concept that may also apply to the motor system for explaining the inhibitory effects of the intact motor cortex, and to the language system to explain the apparently beneficial effect of right frontal TMS. It may then represent a unifying hypothesis to explain different neurological deficits and their recovery.

Breakdown of functional connectivity

A third mechanism, which we think will fundamentally change the way we think about neurological systems and their recovery in focal (e.g., stroke) and diffuse (e.g., TBI) brain injuries, is a breakdown of functional connectivity. As discussed in the introduction, functional connectivity refers to inter-regional temporal correlations of the blood-oxygen level dependent (BOLD) signal in the resting state (i.e., in the absence of an explicit task) (Biswal *et al.*, 1995). Coherent low-frequency (< 0.01 Hz) (Cordes *et al.*, 2001) BOLD fluctuations occur within widely distributed but anatomically discrete networks that recapitulate the spatial topography of task-evoked BOLD responses commonly observed with a variety of behavioral paradigms, e.g., somatosensory (Biswal *et al.*, 1995), language (Hampson *et al.*, 2002, 2006) default (Fox *et al.*, 2005, Greicius *et al.*, 2004; Laufs *et al.*, 2003) and attention (Fox *et al.*, 2005, 2006). To date the neurophysiological correlates of these metabolic fluctuations are unknown, but they may reflect low frequency fluctuations of the band-limited power of oscillating neuronal signals (Leopold & Logothetis, 2003; Leopold *et al.*, 2003).

We have recently reported a breakdown of inter-hemispheric functional connectivity in patients with spatial neglect. The breakdown of functional connectivity was behaviorally significant, and occurred in the same posterior parietal regions in which an imbalance of task-evoked activity had been reported (He *et al.*, in press). The posterior parietal cortex is part of a distributed dorsal frontoparietal network for the selection of stimuli and responses (Corbetta & Shulman, 2002). Interestingly, this region is almost never directly

damaged by lesions causing neglect, which are typically located more ventrally either in temporo-parietal junction or inferior frontal cortex, but its response characteristics are dramatically changed, and account for a great deal of the clinical symptoms. This is yet another example of a neurological deficit and its recovery controlled not by structural but physiological dysfunction.

Summary

Research on spatial neglect has recently taken advantage of the development of functional-anatomical models of attentional controls developed in healthy subjects (Corbetta *et al.*, 2005; Corbetta & Shulman, 2002; Hillis, 2006). Based on this model neglect is mediated by the distributed dysfunction of at least two cortico-cortical systems, a dorsal frontoparietal network centered in intraparietal and dorsal frontal cortex controlling the distribution of attention in extra-personal space, and a ventral frontoparietal network, lateralized to the right hemisphere, that is activated by the sudden appearance of novel and unexpected targets anywhere in the visual field. We have proposed that the former system mediates lateralized deficits of neglect, while the latter system controls non-lateralized deficits such as deficits of arousal and capacity that are influenced by nonlateralized sensory information. The research reviewed above points to the activity imbalance in dorsal parietal cortex as a possible neural mediator of the left-right behavioral imbalance that is the hallmark of neglect. Hence, modulation of this neural imbalance either by behavioral interventions such as prisms (Rossetti *et al.*, 1998), drugs (Malhotra *et al.*, 2006), or physical manipulation as in the case of trans-cranial magnetic stimulation (Brighina *et al.*, 2003) should be tested as a possible strategy to improve neglect.

Conclusions

There are several important take-home messages from brain-imaging research on the recovery of neurological function. The most important lesson is that neurological deficits observed after focal brain injury do not reflect only local neuronal injury, but also physiological dysfunction in a connected network of brain areas, both near and far away from the lesion.

This insight has both theoretical and clinical consequences. Theoretically, one of the most powerful logical instruments to understand the architecture of the mind is the double dissociation of symptoms (Caramazza, 1992). If patient A has deficit 1, but not deficit 2, while patient B has deficit 2, but not 1, then one can conclude that the processes underlying deficits 1 and 2 are independent, i.e., constitute different mind modules. A common anatomical extension of this syllogism is that if patients A and B have different lesions in the brain, processes 1 and 2 are also localized to different neurological modules. However, given any lesion has distributed effect on a widespread network of areas, this modular view cannot any longer be sustained. At the anatomical level both deficits 1 and 2 may arise because of dysfunction of a third party area that is affected by both lesions. Furthermore, any behavioral deficit will reflect the dysfunction of multiple modules at once. A more modern view suggests that two different behavioral deficits arise because of different functional states of brain networks that may even be shared.

From a clinical standpoint, for over 150 years, we have trained our students to localize behavioral deficits, and the principle of functional localization is one of the cornerstones of neurology and neuropsychology. These results indicate that the whole field of functional localization should be re-visited considering the functional effects of lesions on brain networks. The dynamic adjustments of task- or resting activity in areas connected to the site of injury are the most likely mechanism underlying recovery of function, and the persistence of abnormal functional states the most likely cause of poor outcome. While neural plasticity in the form of sprouting and formation of new connections may certainly occur at the local level and perhaps even between distant

regions (Dancause et al., 2005), it is likely that in the adult brain they do not represent a majority mechanism. Conversely, physiological changes in widely distributed networks have been easily and robustly found in every patient studied. This should move the emphasis of treatment and restorative trials toward modulating the level of activity in pre-existing networks.

Finally, as earlier suggested, progress in this field of research is relatively slow and incremental. Experiments are hard for both researchers and willing patients, and significant breakthroughs are difficult to attain when considering only one level of analysis. Quicker progress shall occur when we will be able to integrate observations about brain networks and areas with information about neurons, synapses and molecules. In no small part, difficulties in advancing this field have been related to the lack of animal models of human cognitive functions, and the different spatio-temporal scales at which brain activity has been investigated in humans and experimental animals. A potential breakthrough is offered by the introduction of fMRI in small animals to study post-stroke recovery. Surprisingly, the fMRI patterns in these animals are very similar to those observed in human subjects (Dijkhuizen et al., 2001, 2003). This is very significant as the pattern of functional activation may be independent of function (sensory-motor vs. language) or species (rat vs. humans), and mainly related to the pattern of connectivity that is likely to be largely preserved in its essential organization across species. If that is true then it will be possible to use animal models to generate predictions about human data and vice versa, both in terms of mechanisms and interventions. Linking information across level is critical to generate a brain theory of recovery of function that will hopefully improve human health.

ACKNOWLEDGMENTS

This work is supported by NINDS, NIMH and JS McDonnell Foundation.

REFERENCES

Appelros, P., Karlsson, G. M., Seiger, Å., & Nydevik, I. (2002). Neglect and anosognosia after first-ever stroke: incidence and relationship to disability. *Journal of Rehabilitation Medicine*, **34**, 215–220.

Baron, J. C., Bousser, M.-G., Comar, D., & Castaigne, P. (1980). Crossed cerebellar diaschisis in human supratentorial brain infarction. *Transactions of the American Neurological Association*, **105**, 459–461.

Barrett, A. M., Buxbaum, L. J., Coslett, H. B. *et al.* (2006). Cognitive rehabilitation interventions for neglect and related disorders: moving from bench to bedside in stroke patients. *Journal of Cognitive Neuroscience*, **18**, 1223–1236.

Basso, A., Capitani, E., & Zanobio, M. E. (1982). Pattern of recovery of oral and written expression and comprehension in aphasic patients. *Behavioural Brain Research*, **6**, 115–128.

Basso, A., Gardelli, M., Grassi, M. P., & Mariotti, M. (1989). The role of the right hemisphere in recovery from aphasia. Two case studies. *Cortex*, **25**, 555–566.

Belin, P., Van Eeckhout, P., Zilbovicius, M. *et al.* (1996). Recovery from nonfluent aphasia after melodic intonation therapy: a PET study. *Neurology*, **47**, 1504–1511.

Biswal, B., Yotkin, F. Z., Haughton, V. M., & Hyde, J. S. (1995). Functional connectivity in the motor cortex of resting human brain using echo-planar MRI. *Magnetic Resonance in Medicine*, **34**, 537–541.

Blank, S. C., Bird, H., Turkheimer, F., & Wise, R. J. S. (2003). Speech production after stroke: the role of the right pars opercularis. *Annals of Neurology*, **54**, 310–320.

Blasi, V., Young, A. C., Tansy, A. P. *et al.* (2002). Word retrieval learning modulates right frontal cortex in patients with left frontal damage. *Neuron*, **36**, 159–170.

Brighina, F., Bisiach, E., Oliveri, M. *et al.* (2003). 1 Hz repetitive transcranial magnetic stimulation of the unaffected hemisphere ameliorates contralesional visuospatial neglect in humans. *Neuroscience Letters*, **336**, 131–133.

Buckner, R. L. (2004). Memory and executive function in aging and AD: multiple factors that cause decline and reserve factors that compensate. *Neuron*, **44**, 195–208.

Buckner, R. L., Corbetta, M., Schatz, J., Raichle, M. E., & Petersen, S. E. (1996). Preserved speech abilities and compensation following prefrontal damage. *Proceedings of the National Academy of Sciences of the United States of America*, **93**, 1249–1253.

Buxbaum, L. J., Ferraro, M. K., Veramonti, T. *et al.* (2004). Hemispatial neglect: subtypes, neuroanatomy, and disability. *Neurology*, **62**, 749–756.

Calautti, C., Leroy, F., Guincestre, J.-Y., Marie, R.-M., & Baron, J. C. (2001). Sequential activation brain mapping after subcortical stroke: changes in hemispheric balance and recovery. *NeuroReport*, **12**, 3883–3886.

Calautti, C., Leroy, F., Guincestre, J.-Y., & Baron, J. C. (2003). Displacement of primary sensorimotor cortex activation after subcortical stroke: a longitudinal PET study with clinical correlation. *NeuroImage*, **19**, 1650–1654.

Cao, Y., Vikingstad, E. M., George, K. P., Johnson, A. F., & Welch, K. M. A. (1999). Cortical language activation in stroke patients recovering from aphasia with functional MRI. *Stroke*, **30**, 2331–2340.

Caramazza, A. (1992). Is cognitive neuropsychology possible? *Journal of Cognitive Neuroscience*, **4**, 80–95.

Carmichael, S. T. (2003a). Gene expression changes after focal stroke, traumatic brain and spinal cord injuries. *Current Opinion in Neurology*, **16**, 699–704.

Carmichael, S. T. (2003b). Plasticity of cortical projections after stroke. *Neuroscientist*, **9**, 64–75.

Cherney, L. R., Halper, A. S., Kwasnica, C. M., Harvery, R. L., & Zhang, M. (2001). Recovery of functional status after right hemisphere stroke: relationship with unilateral neglect. *Archives of Physical Medicine and Rehabilitation*, **82**, 322–328.

Chollet, F., DiPiero, V., Wise, R. J. S. *et al.* (1991). The functional anatomy of motor recovery after stroke in humans: a study with positron emission tomography. *Annals of Neurology*, **29**, 63–71.

Corbetta, M., & Shulman, G. L. (2002). Control of goal-directed and stimulus-driven attention in the brain. *Nature Reviews Neuroscience*, **3**, 201–215.

Corbetta, M., Burton, H., Sinclair, R. J. *et al.* (2002). Functional reorganization and stability of somatosensory-motor cortical topography in a tetraplegic subject with late recovery. *Proceedings of the National Academy of Sciences of the United States of America*, **99**, 17066–17071.

Corbetta, M., Kincade, M. J., Lewis, C., Snyder, A. Z., & Sapir, A. (2005). Neural basis and recovery of spatial attention deficits in spatial neglect. *Nature Neuroscience*, **8**, 1603–1610.

Cordes, D., Haughton, V. M., Arfanakis, K. *et al.* (2001). Frequencies contributing to functional connectivity in the cerebral cortex in "resting state" data. *American Journal of Neuroradiology*, **22**, 1326–1333.

Cramer, S. C., Nelles, G., Benson, R. R. *et al.* (1997). A functional MRI study of subjects recovered from hemiparetic stroke. *Stroke*, **28**, 2518–2527.

Cramer, S. C., Benson, R. R., Burra, V. C. *et al.* (2003). Mapping individual brains to guide restorative therapy after stroke: rationale and pilot studies. *Neurological Research*, **8**, 811–814.

Crinion, J., & Price, C. J. (2005). Right anterior superior temporal activation predicts auditory sentence comprehension following aphasic stroke. *Brain*, **128**, 2858–2871.

Cummings, J. L., Benson, D. F., Walsh, M. J., & Levine, H. L. (1979). Left-to-right transfer of language dominance: case-study. *Neurology*, **29**, 1547–1550.

Dancause, N., Barbay, S., Frost, S. B. *et al.* (2005). Extensive cortical rewiring after brain injury. *Journal of Neuroscience*, **25**, 10167–10179.

Delvaux, V., Alagona, G., Gérard, P. *et al.* (2003). Post-stroke reorganization of hand motor area: a 1-year prospective follow-up with focal transcranial magnetic stimulation. *Clinical Neurophysiology*, **114**, 1217–1225.

D'Esposito, M., Deouell, L. Y., & Gazzaley, A. (2003). Alterations in the BOLD fMRI signal with ageing and disease: a challenge for neuroimaging. *Nature Reviews Neuroscience*, **4**, 863–872.

Deuel, R. K., & Collins, R. C. (1984). The functional anatomy of frontal lobe neglect in the monkey: Behavioral and quantitative 2-deoxyglucose studies. *Annals of Neurology*, **15**, 521–529.

Dijkhuizen, R. M., Ren, J., Mandeville, J. B. *et al.* (2001). Functional magnetic resonance imaging of reorganization in rat brain after stroke. *Proceedings of the National Academy of Sciences of the United States of America*, **98**, 12766–12771.

Dijkhuizen, R. M., Singhal, A. B., Mandeville, J. B. *et al.* (2003). Correlation between brain reorganization, ischemic damage, and neurologic status after transient focal cerebral ischemia in rats: a functional magnetic resonance imaging study. *Journal of Neuroscience*, **23**, 510–517.

Dobkin, B. H. (2005). Rehabilitation after stroke. *New England Journal of Medicine*, **352**, 1677–1684.

Dum, R. P., & Strick, P. L. (2002). Motor areas in the frontal lobe of the primate. *Physiology and Behavior*, **77**, 677–682.

Farné, A., Buxbaum, L. J., Ferraro, M. *et al.* (2004). Patterns of spontaneous recovery of neglect and associated disorders in acute right brain-damaged patients. *Journal of Neurology, Neurosurgery and Psychiatry*, **75**, 1401–1410.

Feeney, D. M., & Baron, J. C. (1986). Diaschisis. *Stroke*, **17**, 817–830.

Fernandez, B., Cardebat, D., Demonet, J.-F. *et al.* (2004). Functional MRI follow-up study of language processes in healthy subjects and during recovery in a case of aphasia. *Stroke*, **35**, 2171–2176.

Feydy, A., Carlier, R., Roby-Brami, A. *et al.* (2002). Longitudinal study of motor recovery after stroke: recruitment and focusing of brain activation. *Stroke*, **33**, 1610–1617.

Flor, H., Elbert, T., Knecht, S. *et al.* (1995). Phantom-limb pain as a perceptual correlate of cortical reorganization following arm amputation. *Nature*, **375**, 482–484.

Fox, M. D., Snyder, A. Z., Vincent, J. L. *et al.* (2005). The human brain is intrinsically organized into dynamic, anticorrelated functional networks. *Proceedings of the National Academy of Sciences of the United States of America*, **102**, 9673–9678.

Fox, M. D., Corbetta, M., Snyder, A. Z., Vincent, J. L., & Raichle, M. E. (2006). Spontaneous neuronal activity distinguishes human dorsal and ventral attention systems. *Proceedings of the National Academy of Sciences of the United States of America*, **103**, 10046–10051.

Fridman, E. A., Hanakawa, T., Chung, M. *et al.* (2004). Reorganization of the human ipsilesional premotor cortex after stroke. *Brain*, **127**, 747–758.

Friel, K. M., & Nudo, R. J. (1998). Recovery of motor function after focal cortical injury in primates: compensatory movement patterns used during rehabilitative training. *Somatosensory and Motor Research*, **15**, 173–189.

Frost, S. B., Barbay, S., Friel, K. M., Plautz, E. J., & Nudo, R. J. (2003). Reorganization of remote cortical regions after ischemic brain injury: a potential substrate for stroke recovery. *Journal of Neurophysiology*, **89**, 3205–3214.

Gold, B. T., & Kertesz, A. (2000). Right hemisphere semantic processing of visual words in an aphasic patient: an fMRI study. *Brain and Language*, **73**, 456–465.

Greicius, M. D., Srivastava, G., Reiss, A. L., & Menon, V. (2004). Default-mode network activity distinguishes Alzheimer's disease from healthy aging: evidence from functional MRI. *Proceedings of the National Academy of Sciences of the United States of America*, **101**, 4637–4642.

Hampson, M., Peterson, B. S., Skudlarski, P., Gatenby, J. C., & Gore, J. C. (2002). Detection of functional connectivity using temporal correlations in MR images. *Human Brain Mapping*, **15**, 247–262.

Hampson, M., Tokoglu, F., Sun, Z. *et al.* (2006). Connectivity-behavior analysis reveals that functional connectivity between left BA39 and Broca's area varies with reading ability. *NeuroImage*, **31**, 513–519.

He, B. J., Snyder, A. Z., & Vincent, J. L. (in press). Breakdown on intrinsic brain synchrony in spatial neglect: a novel mechanism to explain brain-behavior relationships after stroke. *Neuron*.

Heilman, K. M., Watson, R. T., & Valenstein, E. (1985). Neglect and related disorders. In K. M. Heilman & E. Valenstein (Eds.), *Clinical Neuropsychology* (pp. 243–293). New York, NY: Oxford University Press.

Heiss, W.-D., Kessler, J., Karbe, H., Fink, G. R., & Pawlik, G. (1993). Cerebral glucose metabolism as a predictor of recovery from aphasia in ischemic stroke. *Archives of Neurology*, **50**, 958–964.

Heiss, W.-D., Kessler, J., Thiel, A., Ghaemi, M., & Karbe, H. (1999). Differential capacity of left and right hemispheric areas for compensation of poststroke aphasia. *Annals of Neurology*, **45**, 430–438.

Hillis, A. E. (2006). Neurobiology of unilateral spatial neglect. *Neuroscientist*, **12**, 153–163.

Hillis, A. E., Wityk, R. J., Tuffiash, E. *et al.* (2001). Hypoperfusion of Wernicke's area predicts severity of semantic deficit in acute stroke. *Annals of Neurology*, **50**, 561–566.

Hillis, A. E., Wityk, R. J., Barker, P. B. *et al.* (2002). Subcortical aphasia and neglect in acute stroke: the role of cortical hypoperfusion. *Brain*, **125**, 1094–1104.

Hillis, A. E., Ulatowski, J. A., Barker, P. B. *et al.* (2003). A pilot randomized trial of induced blood pressure elevation: effects on function and focal perfusion in acute and subacute stroke. *Cerebrovascular Diseases*, **16**, 236–246.

Hillis, A. E., Newhart, M., Heidler, J. *et al.* (2005). Anatomy of spatial attention: insights from perfusion imaging and hemispatial neglect in acute stroke. *Journal of Neuroscience*, **25**, 3161–3167.

Hillis, A. E., Kleinman, J. T., Newhart, M. *et al.* (2006). Restoring cerebral blood flow reveals neural regions critical for naming. *Journal of Neuroscience*, **26**, 8069–8073.

Husain, M., & Kennard, C. (1996). Visual neglect associated with frontal lobe infarction. *Journal of Neurology*, **243**, 652–657.

Husain, M., & Rorden, C. (2003). Non-spatially lateralized mechanisms in hemispatial neglect. *Nature Reviews Neuroscience*, **4**, 26–36.

Johansen-Berg, H., & Matthews, P. M. (2002). Attention to movement modulates activity in sensori-motor areas, including primary motor cortex. *Experimental Brain Research*, **142**, 13–24.

Johansen-Berg, H., Dawes, H., Guy, C. *et al.* (2002a). Correlation between motor improvements and altered fMRI activity after rehabilitative therapy. *Brain*, **125**, 2731–2742.

Johansen-Berg, H., Rushworth, M. F. S., Bogdanovic, M. D. *et al.* (2002b). The role of ipsilateral premotor cortex in hand movement after stroke. *Proceedings of the National Academy of Sciences of the United States of America*, **99**, 14518–14523.

Jones, E. G., & Pons, T. P. (1998). Thalamic and brainstem contributions to large-scale plasticity of primate somatosensory cortex. *Science*, **282**, 1121–1125.

Karnath, H.-O., Ferber, S., & Himmelbach, M. (2001). Spatial awareness is a function of the temporal not the posterior parietal lobe. *Nature*, **411**, 950–953.

Karnath, H.-O., Himmelbach, M., & Rorden, C. (2002). The subcortical anatomy of human spatial neglect: putamen, caudate nucleus and pulvinar. *Brain*, **125**, 350–360.

Karnath, H.-O., Fruhmann Berger, M., Küker, W., & Rorden, C. (2004). The anatomy of spatial neglect based on voxelwise statistical analysis: a study of 140 patients. *Cerebral Cortex*, **14**, 1164–1172.

Karnath, H.-O., Zopf, R., Johannsen, L. *et al.* (2005). Normalized perfusion MRI to identify common areas of dysfunction: patients with basal ganglia neglect. *Brain*, **128**, 2462–2469.

Karni, A., Meyer, G., Rey-Hipolito, C. *et al.* (1998). The acquisition of skilled motor performance: fast and slow experience-driven changes in primary motor cortex. *Proceedings of the National Academy of Sciences of the United States of America*, **95**, 861–868.

Katz, N., Hartman-Maeir, A., Ring, H., & Soroker, N. (1999). Functional disability and rehabilitation outcome in right hemisphere damaged patients with and without unilateral spatial neglect. *Archives of Physical Medicine and Rehabilitation*, **80**, 379–384.

Kertesz, A., & McCabe, P. (1977). Recovery patterns and prognosis in aphasia. *Brain*, **100**, 1–18.

Kim, S.-G., Ashe, J., Georgopoulos, A. P. *et al.* (1993). Functional imaging of human motor cortex at high magnetic field. *Journal of Neurophysiology*, **69**, 297–302.

Kinsbourne, M. (1971). Minor cerebral hemisphere as a source of aphasic speech. *Archives of Neurology*, **25**, 302–306.

Kinsbourne, M. (1977). Hemi-neglect and hemisphere rivalry. In E. A. Weinstein & R. L. Friedland (Eds.), *Hemi-inattention and Hemispheric Specialization, Vol. 18* (pp. 41–52). New York, NY: Raven Press.

Laufs, H., Krakow, K., Sterzer, P. *et al.* (2003). Electroencephalographic signatures of attentional and cognitive default modes in spontaneous brain activity fluctuations at rest. *Proceedings of the National Academy of Sciences of the United States of America*, **100**, 11053–11058.

Lauritzen, M., & Gold, L. (2003). Brain function and neurophysiological correlates of signals used in functional neuroimaging. *Journal of Neuroscience*, **23**, 3972–3980.

Leopold, D. A., & Logothetis, N. K. (2003). Spatial patterns of spontaneous local field activity in the monkey visual cortex. *Reviews in the Neurosciences*, **14**, 195–205.

Leopold, D. A., Murayama, Y., & Logothetis, N. K. (2003). Very slow activity fluctuations in monkey visual cortex: implications for functional brain imaging. *Cerebral Cortex*, **13**, 422–433.

Logothetis, N. K., Pauls, J., Augath, M., Trinath, T., & Oeltermann, A. (2001). Neurophysiological investigation of the basis of the fMRI signal. *Nature*, **412**, 150–157.

Malhotra, P. A., Parton, A. D., Greenwood, R., & Husain, M. (2006). Noradrenergic modulation of space exploration in visual neglect. *Annals of Neurology*, **59**, 186–190.

Marshall, R. S., Perera, G. M., Lazar, R. M. *et al.* (2000). Evolution of cortical activation during recovery from corticospinal tract infarction. *Stroke*, **31**, 656–661.

Merzenich, M., Wright, B., Jenkins, W. *et al.* (1996). Cortical plasticity underlying perceptual, motor, and cognitive skill development: implications for neurorehabilitation. *Cold Spring Harbor Symposium on Quantitative Biology*, **61**, 1–8.

Metter, E. J. (1991). Brain-behavior relationships in aphasia studied by positron emission tomography. *Annals of the New York Academy of Sciences*, **620**, 153–164.

Metter, E. J., Kempler, D., Jackson, C. *et al.* (1989). Cerebral glucose metabolism in Wernicke's, Broca's, and conduction aphasia. *Archives of Neurology*, **46**, 27–34.

Metter, E. J., Hanson, W. R., Jackson, C. A. *et al.* (1990). Temporoparietal cortex in aphasia: evidence from positron emission tomography. *Archives of Neurology*, **47**, 1235–1238.

Meyer, B.-U., Röricht, S., Gräfin von Einsiedel, H., Kruggel, F., & Weindl, A. (1995). Inhibitory and excitatory interhemispheric transfers between motor cortical areas in normal humans and patients with abnormalities of the corpus callosum. *Brain*, **118**, 429–440.

Mimura, M., Kato, M., Kato, M. *et al.* (1998). Prospective and retrospective studies of recovery in aphasia: changes in cerebral blood flow and language functions. *Brain*, **121**, 2083–2094.

Mort, D. J., Malhotra, P., Mannan, S. K. *et al.* (2003). The anatomy of visual neglect. *Brain*, **126**, 1986–1997.

Murase, N., Duque, J., Mazzocchio, R., & Cohen, L. G. (2004). Influence of interhemispheric interactions on motor function in chronic stroke. *Annals of Neurology*, **55**, 400–409.

Musso, M., Weiller, C., Kiebel, S. *et al.* (1999). Training-induced brain plasticity in aphasia. *Brain*, **122**, 1781–1790.

Naeser, M., Martin, P., Nicholas, M. *et al.* (2005a). Improved naming after TMS treatments in a chronic, global aphasia patient: case report. *Neurocase*, **11**, 182–193.

Naeser, M., Martin, P. I., Nicholas, M. *et al.* (2005b). Improved picture naming in chronic aphasia after TMS to part of right Broca's area: an open-protocol study. *Brain and Language*, **93**, 95–105.

Neumann-Haefelin, T., & Witte, O. W. (2000). Periinfarct and remote excitability changes after transient middle cerebral artery occlusion. *Journal of Cerebral Blood Flow and Metabolism*, **20**, 45–52.

Nudo, R. J. (1999). Recovery after damage to motor cortical areas. *Current Opinion in Neurobiology*, **9**, 740–747.

Nudo, R. J., Milliken, G. W., Jenkins, W. M., & Merzenich, M. M. (1996a). Use-dependent alterations of movement representations in primary motor cortex of adult squirrel monkeys. *Journal of Neuroscience*, **16**, 785–807.

Nudo, R. J., Wise, B. M., SiFuentes, F., & Milliken, G. W. (1996b). Neural substrates for the effects of rehabilitative training on motor recovery after ischemic infarct. *Science*, **272**, 1791–1794.

Paolucci, S., Grasso, M. G., Antonucci, G. *et al.* (2001). Mobility status after inpatient stroke rehabilitation: 1-year follow-up and prognostic factors. *Archives of Physical Medicine and Rehabilitation*, **82**, 2–8.

Papanicolaou, A. C., Moore, B. D., Deutsch, G., Levin, H. S., & Eisenberg, H. M. (1988). Evidence for right-hemisphere involvement in recovery from aphasia. *Archives of Neurology*, **45**, 1025–1029.

Passingham, R. E. (1996). Attention to action. *Philosophical Transactions of the Royal Society of London, Series B: Biological Sciences*, **351**, 1473–1479.

Pedersen, P. M., Jorgensen, H. S., Nakayama, H., Raaschou, H. O., & Olsen, T. S. (1997). Hemineglect in acute stroke-incidence and prognostic implications. The Copenhagen Stroke Study 1. *American Journal of Physical Medicine and Rehabilitation*, **76**, 122–127.

Pennisi, G., Rapisarda, G., Bella, R. *et al.* (1999). Absence of response to early transcranial magnetic stimulation in ischemic stroke patients: prognostic value for hand motor recovery. *Stroke*, **30**, 2666–2670.

Pineiro, R., Pendlebury, S., Johansen-Berg, H., & Matthews, P. M. (2001). Functional MRI detects posterior shifts in primary sensorimotor cortex activation after stroke: evidence of local adaptive reorganization? *Stroke*, **32**, 1134–1139.

Pineiro, R., Pendlebury, S., Johansen-Berg, H., & Matthews, P. M. (2002). Altered hemodynamic responses in patients after subcortical stroke measured by functional MRI. *Stroke*, **33**, 103–109.

Pizzamiglio, L., Perani, D., Cappa, S. F. *et al.* (1998). Recovery of neglect after right hemispheric damage: H215 O positron emission tomographic activation study. *Archives of Neurology*, **55**, 561–568.

Poggio, T., & Bizzi, E. (2004). Generalization in vision and motor control. *Nature*, **431**, 768–774.

Pons, T. P., Garraghty, P. E., Ommaya, A. K. *et al.* (1991). Massive cortical reorganization after sensory deafferentation in adult macaques. *Science*, **252**, 1857–1860.

Powers, W. J., Fox, P. T., & Raichle, M. E. (1988). The effect of carotid artery disease on the cerebrovascular response to physiologic stimulation. *Neurology*, **38**, 1475–1478.

Price, C. J. (2000). The anatomy of language: contributions from functional neuroimaging. *Journal of Anatomy*, **197**, 335–359.

Price, C. J., & Crinion, J. (2005). The latest on functional imaging studies of aphasic stroke. *Current Opinion in Neurology*, **18**, 429–434.

Price, C. J., Crinion, J., & Friston, K. J. (2006). Design and analysis of fMRI studies with neurologically impaired patients. *Journal of Magnetic Resonance Imaging*, **23**, 816–826.

Prichard, J. W., & Rosen, B. R. (1994). Functional study of the brain by NMR. *Journal of Cerebral Blood Flow and Metabolism*, **14**, 365–372.

Raichle, M. E. (1987). Circulatory and metabolic correlates of brain function in normal humans. In V. B. Mountcastle & F. Plum (Eds.), *Handbook of Physiology, The Nervous System V. Higher Functions of the Brain, Part 2.* (pp. 643–674). Bethesda, MD: American Physiological Society.

Ramachandran, V. S. (1993). Behavioral and magnetoencephalographic correlates of plasticity in the adult human brain. *Proceedings of the National Academy of Sciences of the United States of America*, **90**, 10413–10420.

Rapisarda, G., Bastings, E., Maertens de Noordhout, A., Pennisi, G., & Delwaide, P. J. (1996). Can motor recovery in stroke patients be predicted by early transcranial magnetic stimulation? *Stroke*, **27**, 2191–2196.

Reuter-Lorenz, P. A. (2002). New visions of the aging mind and brain. *Trends in Cognitive Sciences*, **6**, 394–400.

Robertson, I. H. (2001). Do we need the "lateral" in unilateral neglect? Spatially nonselective attention deficits in unilateral neglect and their implications for rehabilitation. *NeuroImage*, **14**, S85–S90.

Rosen, H. J., Petersen, S. E., Linenweber, M. R. *et al.* (2000). Neural correlates of recovery from aphasia after damage to left inferior frontal cortex. *Neurology*, **55**, 1883–1894.

Rossetti, Y., Rode, G., Pisella, L. *et al.* (1998). Prism adaptation to a rightward optical deviation rehabilitates left hemispatial neglect. *Nature*, **395**, 166–169.

Rossini, P. M., Altamura, C., Ferretti, A. *et al.* (2004). Does cerebrovascular disease affect the coupling between neuronal activity and local haemodynamics? *Brain*, **127**, 99–110.

Röther, J., Knab, R., Hamzei, F. *et al.* (2002). Negative dip in BOLD fMRI is caused by blood flow – oxygen consumption uncoupling in humans. *NeuroImage*, **15**, 98–102.

Sarno, M. T., & Levita, E. (1971). Natural course of recovery in severe aphasia. *Archives of Physical Medicine and Rehabilitation*, **52**, 175–178.

Sarno, M. T., & Levita, E. (1979). Recovery in treated aphasia in the first year post-stroke. *Stroke*, **10**, 663–670.

Saur, D., Lange, R., Baumgaertner, A. *et al.* (2006). Dynamics of language reorganization after stroke. *Brain*, **129**, 1371–1384.

Seitz, R. J., Hoflich, P., Binkofski, F. *et al.* (1998). Role of the premotor cortex in recovery from middle cerebral artery infarction. *Archives of Neurology*, **55**, 1081–1088.

Sharp, D. J., Scott, S. K., & Wise, R. J. S. (2004). Retrieving meaning after temporal lobe infarction: the role of the basal language area. *Annals of Neurology*, **56**, 836–846.

Shimizu, T., Hosaki, A., Hino, T. *et al.* (2002). Motor cortical disinhibition in the unaffected hemisphere after unilateral cortical stroke. *Brain*, **125**, 1896–1907.

Small, S. L., Hlustik, P., Noll, D. C., Genovese, C., & Solodkin, A. (2002). Cerebellar hemispheric activation ipsilateral to the paretic hand correlates with functional recovery after stroke. *Brain*, **125**, 1544–1557.

Stone, S. P., Halligan, P. W., & Greenwood, R. J. (1993). The incidence of neglect phenomena and related disorders in patients with an acute right or left hemisphere stroke. *Age and Ageing*, **22**, 46–52.

Thiebaut de Schotten, M., Urbanski, M., Duffau, H. *et al.* (2005). Direct evidence for a parietal-frontal pathway subserving spatial awareness in humans. *Science*, **309**, 2226–2228.

Thulborn, K. R., Carpenter, P. A., & Just, M. A. (1999). Plasticity of language-related brain function during recovery from stroke. *Stroke*, **30**, 749–754.

Twitchell, T. E. (1951). The restoration of motor function following hemiplegia in man. *Brain*, **74**, 443–480.

Vallar, G., & Perani, D. (1987). The anatomy of spatial neglect in humans. In M. Jeannerod (Ed.), *Neurophysiological and Neuropsychological Aspects of Spatial Neglect* (pp. 235–258). Amsterdam, the Netherlands: Elsevier Science Publishers (North-Holland).

Vallar, G., Perani, D., Cappa, S. F. *et al.* (1988). Recovery from aphasia and neglect after subcortical stroke: neuropsychological and cerebral perfusion study. *Journal of Neurology, Neurosurgery and Psychiatry*, **51**, 1269–1276.

von Monakow, C. (1911). Lokalisation der Hirnfunktionen [Localization of brain functions]. *Journal fur Psychologie and Neurologie*, **17**, 185–200.

Warburton, E., Price, C. J., Swinburn, K., & Wise, R. J. S. (1999). Mechanisms of recovery from aphasia: evidence from positron emission tomography studies. *Journal of Neurology, Neurosurgery and Psychiatry*, **66**, 155–161.

Ward, N. S. (2006). The neural substrates of motor recovery after focal damage to the central nervous system. *Archives of Physical Medicine and Rehabilitation*, **87**, Suppl. 2, 30–35.

Ward, N. S., Brown, M. M., Thompson, A. J., & Frackowiak, R. S. J. (2003a). Neural correlates of outcome after stroke: a cross-sectional fMRI study. *Brain*, **126**, 1430–1448.

Ward, N. S., Brown, M. M., Thompson, A. J., & Frackowiak, R. S. J. (2003b). Neural correlates of motor recovery after stroke: a longitudinal fMRI study. *Brain*, **126**, 2476–2496.

Weiller, C. (1998). Imaging recovery from stroke. *Experimental Brain Research*, **123**, 13–17.

Weiller, C., Chollet, F., Friston, K. J., Wise, R. J. S., & Frackowiak, R. S. J. (1992). Functional reorganization of the brain in recovery from striatocapsular infarction in man. *Annals of Neurology*, **31**, 463–472.

Weiller, C., Isensee, C., Rijntjes, M. *et al.* (1995). Recovery from Wernicke's aphasia: a positron emission tomographic study. *Annals of Neurology*, **37**, 723–732.

Wernicke, C. (1908). The symptom complex of aphasia. In E. D. Church (Ed.), *Modern Clinical Medicine: Diseases of the Nervous System* (pp. 265–325). New York, NY: Appleton-Century-Crofts.

Winhuisen, L., Thiel, A., Schumacher, B. *et al.* (2005). Role of the contralateral inferior frontal gyrus in recovery of language function in poststroke aphasia: a combined repetitive transcranial magnetic stimulation and positron emission tomography study. *Stroke*, **36**, 1759–1763.

11

The role of neuroelectric and neuromagnetic recordings in assessing learning and rehabilitation effects

Claude Alain and Bernhard Ross

Introduction

- The functional organization of the adult sensory system is dynamic and modifiable by training.
- Scalp recording of EEG and extra-cranial MEG recording are noninvasive techniques for investigating neuroplastic changes in humans.

Learning and rehabilitation can result in improvement in motor controls, general cognitive functioning including attention and memory, and improvement in observers' ability to discriminate differences in the attributes of sensory stimuli. In this chapter, we focus our review of the literature on studies that examine neuroplastic changes associated with behavioral improvement in perceptual skills. This is a research area with great cross-pollination between basic neurophysiological studies revealing fundamental properties of neurons and cortical reorganization following extended training, and neuroimaging studies in humans showing neuroplastic changes in larger intertwining systems or networks rather than a specific sub-population of neurons.

It is now well accepted that the adult brain is malleable and shows an amazing ability to adapt to a novel environment or the drastic changes caused by injury. Indeed, during the last decade converging evidence from animal neurophysiology and human neuropsychological and neuroimaging research has revealed a remarkable degree of brain plasticity in the sensory and motor systems during adulthood. In hindsight, such plasticity is no surprise given that the adult brain needs to meet the processing demands of an ever-changing environment: learning-induced changes in mature sensory cortices may occur in a task-dependent manner, and can include rapid and highly specific changes in the response properties of cells (Edeline et al., 1993; Fritz et al., 2003). For instance, changes in the receptive fields of ferret auditory cortex can occur within the first minutes of a tone discrimination task that was previously learned (Fritz et al., 2003, 2005a, 2005b). However, these neuroplastic changes were smaller or absent when the animal listened passively to the same sounds. Such rapid changes in the receptive fields of sensory neurons have been observed in a wide variety of situations including classical conditioning (Bakin & Weinberger, 1990; Edeline et al., 1993), instrumental avoidance conditioning (Bakin et al., 1996) and auditory discrimination learning (Fritz et al., 2003). These findings suggest that learning and memory are not static but rather allow for dynamic adjustments that likely depend on various factors like goal-directed behavior, experience or injury. These changes can occur quickly with only a few trials. However, as the training regimen or rehabilitation continues, more permanent changes are likely to take place.

Evidence from single cell recordings suggests that extended training involving daily practice sessions over a long period is associated with changes in the topographical organization representing the trained sensory attributes (Recanzone et al., 1992, 1993).

Cognitive Neurorehabilitation, Second Edition: Evidence and Application, ed. Donald T. Stuss, Gordon Winocur and Ian H. Robertson. Published by Cambridge University Press. © Cambridge University Press 2008.

These more permanent changes in sensory and/or motor representations following extended training may involve the expression of new synaptic connections, thereby resulting in an enlarged cortical representation of a specific stimulus after training (Recanzone *et al.*, 1993; Rutkowski & Weinberger, 2005). For example, extensive frequency discrimination training of tactile vibration stimuli applied to a digit in nonhuman primates was found to enhance stimulus representation that was restricted to the trained skin location compared with control digits (Recanzone *et al.*, 1992). In a subsequent study, Recanzone *et al.* (1993) trained nonhuman primates to make fine pitch discriminations over several daily training sessions and found enlarged cortical maps and sharper tuning of receptive fields at the trained frequency, which correlated with increased perceptual acuity. Although such topographical changes in auditory cortices have been reported for various animals including rats (Polley *et al.*, 2006) and barn owls (Bergan *et al.*, 2005), other studies have failed to find topographical changes in the auditory cortex following extended training (e.g., Brown *et al.*, 2004; Witte & Kipke, 2005). The lack of enlarged representation could be related to several factors such as the species (e.g., cats, Brown *et al.*, 2004; Witte & Kipke, 2005), the duration of training (Witte & Kipke, 2005) and/or different stimulus configurations and training paradigms. The way the enlarged areas are calculated may have been a factor given that the total size of a sensory map may not always have been enlarged but rather a region responding to a particular frequency may expand at the expense of another. Notwithstanding sporadic discrepancies in the literature, evidence from animal research strongly supports the notion that functional reorganization after training can take place in the adult's brain.

In spite of the tremendous progress made in understanding the neural underpinnings associated with animal learning, there remain major gaps between basic animal learning and memory research and more applied research on behavioral and cognitive rehabilitation in individuals suffering from psychiatric or neurological diseases.

Researchers and clinicians are challenged by the constant need to monitor and enhance the effect of rehabilitation. Electroencephalography (EEG) and magnetoencephalography (MEG) recordings of neuroelectric and neuromagnetic activity respectively are increasingly used in investigating the neuroplastic changes associated with extended training and may prove to be valuable tools in assessing the impact of rehabilitation techniques on structural and functional brain activity in humans. Both recording methods are completely noninvasive and provide a means to evaluate the activity of the human brain, as we perceive stimuli, make decisions and generate motor commands. Electroencephalography and MEG can be used in multiple repeated sessions, and they are less expensive than other imaging techniques such as functional magnetic resonance imaging (fMRI).

Moreover, EEG and MEG provide very accurate temporal information about the sequence of neural events underlying perception and cognition as well as response selection, preparation and execution. Such temporal resolution is particularly helpful when investigating the level at which training regimens modulate brain activity. Because brain responses can be recorded for stimuli presented either within or outside the focus of attention, these techniques may contribute important information in assessing the impact of top-down controlled processes in brain plasticity and rehabilitation. Lastly, recent advances in brain electrical and magnetic source analysis have improved our understanding of the neural generators of sensory (exogenous) and cognitive (endogenous) evoked responses, making these techniques ideal for assessing the impact of learning and rehabilitation programs on functional brain reorganization.

In the following sections, we review the evidence from various paradigms and approaches suggesting that the recording of neuroelectric and neuromagnetic activity can provide objective markers of recovery of cortical mechanisms, with an emphasis on perceptual learning. Perceptual learning occurs when two stimuli that at first appear identical, become differentiated with practice. This is a true change in perception – not just a change in strategy or a change in response criterion. Importantly, the presence and characteristics of ERPs (event-related potentials, obtained by averaging EEG segments time-locked to the stimulus onset) and ERFs (event-related fields, the complement to ERP obtained with MEG) in terms of latency and amplitude can be quantified during the course of training and recovery following a stroke or closed head injury. In conjunction with behavioral measures, recording of neuroelectric and neuromagnetic activity can highlight neuroplastic changes associated with the recovery of motor, perceptual and cognitive functions. We propose that the recording of ERPs and ERFs can be particularly useful in the framework of cortical remodeling following training procedures and as a monitor of cortical repair that parallels clinical improvements. The goal of this chapter is to assess the role of neuroelectric and neuromagnetic measurements as potential tools in assessing the brain plasticity associated with training and/or following brain damage. This review may assist in the development of more effective ways to assess and monitor the impact of training regimens during rehabilitation by evaluating the role of EEG and MEG in identifying neuroplastic changes in human observers. We now consider some of the methodological considerations with respect to the application of these techniques in basic and applied research, before going on to discuss studies that used these techniques in investigating neuroplastic changes following extended training in various perceptual and cognitive tasks.

Methodological and technical considerations

- The EEG/MEG signal is directly related to the number of synchronously activated cortical neurons.
- Relevant measures for training induced plasticity include changes in amplitude and latency of sensory evoked responses, oscillatory activity, intracortical coherence and source localization.

- Dipole source analysis aims at explaining the scalp-recorded data with a small number of generators.

Introduction to neuroelectric and neuromagnetic signals

Common primary sources of neuroelectric and neuromagnetic signals are current flows within apical dendrites of pyramidal neurons in the cerebral cortex. The intracellular currents are associated with magnetic fields that propagate through the brain tissue and the skull and are detected extra-cranially using MEG. Corresponding extra-cellular electric currents spread through the conductive brain tissue, the cerebrospinal fluid, the skull and the skin and result in voltage differences at the scalp surface, which are recorded with electrodes attached to the head using EEG. Since the dendrites of adjacent cortical neurons are aligned in parallel, the magnetic fields of single neurons are superimposed and result in a larger measurable magnetic field. The corresponding volume currents superimpose in a similar way and contribute to the expression of the voltage distribution on the scalp surface. Consequently, the EEG and MEG signals can be viewed as direct and complementary measures of the number of synchronously activated cortical neurons at the time of recording. Some 1000 to 100 000 neurons must be synchronously active in order to be registered with EEG or MEG (Williamson et al., 1991).

Modern MEG systems measure brain activity simultaneously at 150 to 300 positions above the head. The detection coils of 10 to 20 mm diameter are equidistantly spaced on a helmet-shaped array. Participants are required to keep their head in a fixed position inside the helmet and to minimize as much as possible any head movement during the measurement. Most MEG systems measure the difference of magnetic flow through two coils, which are either arranged in an axial direction or side by side in the plane. Such axial or planar gradiometers measure the magnetic field gradient perpendicular to the head or in tangential direction, respectively. The exceptionally high sensitivity for detecting small magnetic field changes is achieved by using superconducting quantum interference devices (SQUID), which convert magnetic field changes into recordable voltage changes. The SQUID devices operate near absolute zero temperature and need continuous cooling with liquid helium. Typical whole-head MEG systems are mounted in a large dewar positioned above the head of the participant. The size of detectable magnetic fields of brain activity is one to several hundred fT (femto Tesla, 10^{-15} T), which is 8–10 orders of magnitude smaller than the earth's magnetic field. To reduce the effects of environmental magnetic fields, MEG systems need special magnetically shielded rooms and noise cancellation techniques. Because the strength of the magnetic field decreases with increasing distance from the sensors, MEG is more sensitive to cortical sources than "deeper" subcortical sources. Furthermore, MEG is more sensitive to magnetic fields perpendicular to the coils (tangential sources). For example, a source at the center of the sphere (i.e., the head) produces magnetic fields almost in parallel with all sensor coils (radial sources) and is almost not visible in MEG. This is in contrast with EEG, which is sensitive to both radial and tangential sources, highlighting the importance of combining EEG with MEG recordings, especially in cases where complex source configurations are suspected.

Modern EEG systems contain 32–256 electrodes, which are usually mounted on a cap. High-density integration of the EEG amplifier makes the system portable. This is important given that clinical studies may require measurements at the bed site. Also, some of the new developments in using biofeedback techniques and EEG for assistance of individuals suffering from language and motor impairment depends on the portability of the EEG system.

The most common data analysis technique for separating relevant neuroelectric and neuromagnetic activity from the background neuronal activity consist of averaging epochs of brain waves that are time-locked to either external sensory events such as auditory, visual or somatosensory stimuli or internal events such as perception and decision-making processes. Some of these brain waves are exogenous (i.e., obligatory) in the sense that they occur regardless of the observer's intention and motivation, reflecting the physical properties of the external events, whereas others are endogenous because they are determined by psychological factors such as attention and expectation. The amplitudes of the event-related brain waves index the strength of the response, whereas the latency refers to the amount of time, in milliseconds (ms), that is taken to generate the bioelectrical response following the onset of the event. The latency of sensory responses is therefore related to neural conduction time and site of excitation; the time it takes for the sensory input to travel through the peripheral sensory system to the place of excitation in the sensory cortex.

Source analysis

Determining the intra-cerebral sources for neuroelectric and neuromagnetic activities measured outside the head is referred to as the bioelectromagnetic inverse problem. For this analysis, the head is modeled in first approximation as a spherical volume (Sarvas, 1987). Often the cerebral sources can be modeled with only a small number of dipoles, for example single sources in the left and right auditory cortices. For estimation of the dipole location, orientation and strength, the difference between the measured magnetic or electric field and the calculated field is minimized by varying the dipole parameters (Hämäläinen et al., 1993). Since the magnetic and electric fields sum linearly, more complicated source configurations may be composed by adding the contributions of several dipoles. More general approaches modeling brain activity with spatially distributed sources can be accessed with methods like minimum-norm solutions (Lin et al., 2006) or beamformer techniques (Hillebrand & Barnes, 2005). For minimum-norm source estimation, the field of a large number of dipoles at fixed positions, for example equally spaced on the cortical surface, is approximated to the measured field with the constraint of minimal current densities (Wang, 1993). Beamformer methods are spatial filters that identify for each volume element in the brain the unique contribution of a source, which is not coherent with other sources (Sekihara *et al.*, 2001; Vrba & Robinson, 2001).

After localizing the sources, time-series of brain activity at the source location can be calculated to illustrate the time course of neural activity (Figure 11.1). This source space projection method transforms the hundreds of electric and magnetic field waveforms into a small number of source waveforms. This improves the signal-to-noise ratio by reducing the overlap from other possible sources and filtering out the effect of sensor noise (Ross *et al.*, 2000; Tesche *et al.*, 1995). Although the source space projection method is more commonly used for analysing MEG data, a similar approach has also been applied to EEG data (Heinrich *et al.*, 2004; McDonald & Alain, 2005).

Summary

Electroencephalography and magnetoencephalography are powerful techniques for investigating neuroplastic changes associated with learning and rehabilitation because they permit the opportunity to study brain activity with precise temporal resolution. Moreover, scalp recordings of ERPs or ERFs can be used to examine both exogenous (sensory representation) and endogenous (attention and learning) aspects of information processing. The development of new dipole source modeling algorithms can help localise the neural generators allowing researchers to identify which brain areas support behavioral improvement following training and rehabilitation programs. We now turn to the effects of training and expertise on sensory evoked responses as measured by EEG and MEG.

Perceptual learning and neuroplastic changes in sensory evoked responses

- Perceptual learning modulates amplitude and latency of sensory evoked responses.

- Practice-related changes in sensory evoked responses could be expressed as:
  (1) increase in the size of cortical areas representing the trained attribute;
  (2) higher degrees of synchronization within a particular neural ensemble;
  (3) sharpening the tuning of cells for the task-relevant (trained) attributes; and
  (4) changes in cortical maps (locus) representing the trained attribute.

In the past 10 years, there has been a growing interest in using EEG and MEG techniques to investigate brain plasticity in human adults. In this section, we review several studies that have used EEG and/or MEG to reveal neuroplastic changes in auditory, visual and motor systems in normal healthy adults. Then, we examine studies that have used these techniques to assess and monitor recovery following a stroke or closed head injury.

Measuring neural activity during auditory learning

The effects of practice on auditory processing have been extensively studied by comparing amplitude and latency of auditory evoked potentials (AEPs) and auditory evoked fields (AEFs). Auditory evoked potentials and AEFs are comprised of sequences of several positive and negative deflections (i.e., waves). Each deflection reflects synchronous activity from large neuronal ensembles that are time-locked to sound onset. The sequence of AEPs tracks neuronal processing as the information ascends the auditory system from the cochlea, through early brainstem response (1–10 ms after sound onset) to the primary auditory cortex (middle-latency evoked responses, 10–50 ms) and onto higher auditory cortical areas. Long-latency evoked potentials take place after 50 ms and include the P1, N1 and P2 waves. The P1-N1-P2 complex is related to signal detection and is present only when a transient auditory stimulus is audible (Hillyard *et al.*, 1971; Martin *et al.*, 1997). However, the conscious discrimination of an auditory event is often associated with an

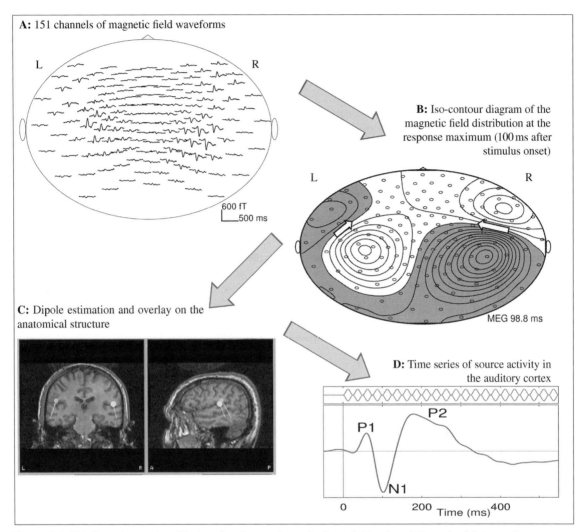

Figure 11.1. (This figure is reproduced in the color plate section at the front of this volume.) Example of data transform during magnetoencephalography (MEG) analysis. (A) This panel shows an average auditory event-related field recorded in a representative participant. The evoked response comprises a negative wave that is maximal over the left (L) and right (R) hemispheres. (B) Iso-contour maps illustrating the amplitude distribution of this negative wave peaking at about 100 ms (i.e., N1m). The shaded areas indicate the outgoing field. (C) The amplitude distribution can be accounted for by a pair of dipoles located in the temporal lobe near Heschl's gyrus. The dipoles are superimposed on the magnetic resonance image (MRI) obtained from the participants. (D) This panel shows the source waveform activity from the right auditory cortex. The source waveform comprises an early positive peak at about 50 ms (P1), followed by the N1 and P2 wave peaking at about 100 and 180 ms post-stimulus, respectively. The red drawing at the top of the panel illustrates the amplitude-modulated tone used to elicit the response.

additional late positive wave peaking between 250 and 600 ms post-stimulus, referred to as the P300 or P3b (Hillyard et al., 1971; Martin et al., 1997; Parasuraman & Beatty, 1980).

One way to assess the impact of extended training on brain plasticity is to compare individuals that differ in terms of their expertise with the material presented, such as in the case where musicians and non-musicians are presented with auditory stimuli. Shahin et al. (2003) examined the effects of long-term musical training on ERPs and found larger N1c amplitudes (~140 ms) to pure tone, piano tones or violin tones in musicians relative to non-musicians. The N1c is an ERP component thought to reflect the activation of the lateral portion of the superior temporal gyrus. This effect of musical training on the N1c was accompanied by enhancement of the P2 (~185 ms) wave, an ERP component that is maximal at central sites (Shahin et al., 2003). The enhanced P2 amplitude in musicians compared with non-musicians was recently replicated using MEG (Kuriki et al., 2006). Musicians also showed enhanced early cortical activity (19–30 ms), which was paralleled by an increase in gray matter volume (Schneider et al., 2002). Larger N1m (the magnetic counterpart of the electric N1) has also been found for piano tone compared with pure tone in musicians, whereas no such difference in brain response was found in non-musicians (Pantev et al., 1998). Neuromagnetic recordings have also revealed enhanced N1m that was specific to the principal instrument played by the musician (Pantev et al., 2001b). Although such findings are in accordance with the notion that timbre-specific enhancements in cortical representation are attributable to musical practice rather than a predisposition to music (Pantev et al., 2001a), subsequent studies could not consistently demonstrate differences in N1m amplitude elicited by piano tones and pure tones between musicians and non-musicians (Hirata et al., 1999; Lütkenhöner et al., 2006; Schneider et al., 2002). This discrepancy in the literature may reflect procedural differences. Studies that revealed enhanced N1 amplitude in musicians usually adjusted sound intensity on an individual basis based on hearing

thresholds for each stimulus type (Pantev et al., 1998) whereas those failing to show differences between musicians and non-musicians presented stimuli at the same intensity level for all participants (Hirata et al., 1999).

Another way to assess the neuroplastic changes associated with learning and rehabilitation involves comparing performance and brain activity prior to and after training in discriminating stimuli that originally appear very similar. Training-related changes in auditory evoked responses have been reported for a wide range of tasks requiring a discrimination between tones of different frequencies (Bosnyak et al., 2004; Brattico et al., 2003; Menning et al., 2000), consonant vowel stimuli varying in voice onset time (Tremblay et al., 1997, 2001), as well as in tasks requiring segregation and identification of concurrent vowels (Reinke et al., 2003). Prior studies focusing on auditory perceptual learning have shown a decrease in N1 latency (Bosnyak et al., 2004; Reinke et al., 2003) as well as an augmentation of N1m amplitude (Menning et al., 2000) following extended training. The training-related enhancement in N1m may either indicate that more neurons are activated or that neurons representing the stimulus were firing more synchronously. In addition, the N1c component showed an increase in amplitude with extended practice (Bosnyak et al., 2004). Interestingly, the N1c amplitude continued to increase over 15 training sessions (Bosnyak et al., 2004). In addition, extended training has been found to enhance the amplitude of the P2 wave (Atienza et al., 2002; Bosnyak et al., 2004; Reinke et al., 2003; Tremblay et al., 2001) which can appear after two (Atienza et al., 2002) or three (Bosnyak et al., 2004) daily test sessions. Figure 11.2 shows the effects of four daily training sessions on N1 and P2 waves elicited by two vowels presented simultaneously. In that study, the enhanced P2 amplitude paralleled behavioral improvement in identifying both vowels presented concurrently (Reinke et al., 2003). The enhancement in P2 amplitude was preceded by rapid neuroplastic changes over the right auditory cortex during the first hour of testing, which occurred only when listeners were

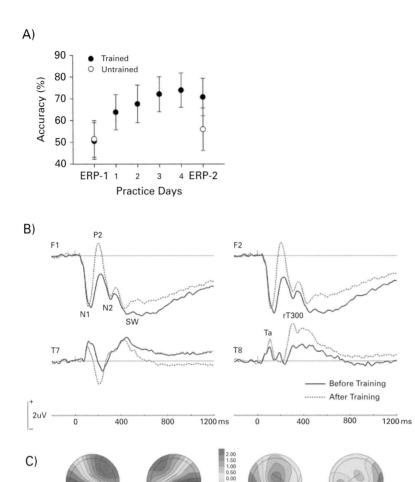

A)

B)

C)

Figure 11.2. (This figure is reproduced in the color plate section at the front of this volume.) Effects of training on auditory ERPs. (A) Group mean accuracy in identifying two vowels presented simultaneously during the first (ERP-1) and second ERP (ERP-2) recording sessions in trained and untrained individuals as well as during the four daily training sessions in the trained group. Error bars reflect standard error of the mean. (B) Group mean ERPs recorded before and after 4 days training period in the trained group. Note the large increase in P2 amplitude over the frontal electrodes (i.e., F1 and F2). Behavioral improvement was also paralleled by an increase in amplitude recorded over the right temporal cortex (i.e., T8). F1 = Left Frontal; F2 = Right Frontal; T7 = Left Temporal; T8 = Right Temporal. (C) Isocontour maps of the difference in ERP amplitude between the first and second ERP testing sessions. Adapted with permission from Reinke *et al.* (2003).

attending to the stimuli (Alain *et al.*, 2007). There was no significant increase in P2 amplitude within the first hour of testing (Alain *et al.*, 2007), suggesting that the P2 effects index a relatively slow learning process that may depend on consolidation over several days. However, it has been reported that exposure to the stimulus material without discrimination training can also result in P2 amplitude changes (Sheehan *et al.*, 2005). In summary, the majority of EEG and MEG studies show that learning-related changes in sensory evoked responses (i.e., N1, N1c and P2) can be observed in a wide range of carefully designed auditory tasks.

Another auditory ERP component that has been used to investigate the impact of training on sensory representation is the mismatch negativity (MMN). The MMN is elicited by infrequent deviant stimuli embedded in a sequence of otherwise homogenous stimuli (Picton *et al.*, 2000). Sounds that deviate in terms of their pitch, spatial location, duration, and intensity from repeating standard stimuli elicit an MMN wave. Also, infrequent disruptions in the temporal organization of sounds such as in a sequence of sounds that alternate in pitch (Alain *et al.*, 1994, 1999) or during the violation of musical contours or intervals (Fujioka *et al.*, 2004; Trainor *et al.*, 2002) generate MMN waves. The MMN is thought to index automatic detection of stimulus invariance, with its amplitude and latency increasing and decreasing respectively, as the deviant stimulus becomes more discriminable (Alain *et al.*, 1994, 2004; Javitt *et al.*, 1998; Sams *et al.*, 1985).

Previous research has shown that musical expertise is associated with enhanced MMN amplitude (Fujioka *et al.*, 2004, 2005; Lopez *et al.*, 2003; Nager *et al.*, 2003; Tervaniemi *et al.*, 1997). Moreover, studies of language processing in healthy adults have found enhanced MMN amplitude in response to phoneme changes that are relevant to listeners' native language (Näätänen *et al.*, 1997; Ylinen *et al.*, 2006), providing further support that MMN amplitude is sensitive to observers' expertise. The MMN latency decreases and its amplitude increases following pitch (Menning *et al.*, 2000) and speech (Kraus *et al.*, 1995) discrimination training. Enhanced MMN amplitude has also been reported within a single daily training session (Atienza *et al.*, 2002; Gottselig *et al.*, 2004; Tremblay *et al.*, 1997). In these studies, the MMN was recorded during passive listening prior to and after a brief training session that involved an active listening task. Although the MMN is thought to index a pre-attentive change detection process (Näätänen, 1992), evidence from many studies has suggested that attention to auditory stimuli enhances the MMN amplitude (Alain &

Izenberg, 2003; Alain & Woods, 1997; Arnott & Alain, 2002; Woldorff *et al.*, 1991, 1998). Therefore, it is still debated whether an enhanced MMN amplitude following training is related to learning per se or whether it indexes participants' increased attention to recently learned auditory material. However, the fact that training-related changes in MMN amplitude are seen in response to speech stimuli that share the trained acoustic cue but were *not* used in the training session suggests that attention alone might not be responsible for training-related changes in MMN (Tremblay *et al.*, 1997). The effects of training on MMN occur quickly, being present after 105 minutes of practice (Tremblay *et al.*, 1998). This rapid training-related change in MMN amplitude was followed by behavioral improvement in speech discrimination. Together, these findings suggest that the MMN wave could be used to assess the efficacy of training in the absence of a behavioral response. This is particularly important in cases where the effectiveness of auditory training can be difficult to assess using behavioral methods such as in infants, young children and individuals with aphasia.

Although studies employing the MMN as the dependent measure may provide important insights into the physiological processes underlying stimulus representation, auditory discrimination and learning, this ERP/ERF component is not necessarily suitable to assess the impact of recovery and rehabilitation on a single patient basis. The MMN is relatively small in amplitude and elicited by infrequent events thereby requiring relatively long recording sessions in order to obtain a reliable signal/noise ratio. Also, there is no one-to-one relationship between behavioral improvement and neuroplastic change in stimulus representation because the MMN is recorded during passive listening and changes in amplitude may reflect stimulus exposure or top-down modulations as mentioned earlier.

In summary, ERPs or ERFs can be used to assess the impact of auditory training regimens. Notwithstanding some inconsistencies in the literature, the bulk of the research comparing musicians and non-musicians, as well as those directly assessing neuroplastic changes during the auditory perceptual learning, reveals reliable changes in sensory evoked responses that parallel behavioral improvement. Moreover, our review of the literature shows that rapid and slow perceptual learning is associated with a distinct pattern of neural activity, with the training-related P2 enhancement requiring several daily practice sessions. The extent to which these neuroplastic changes are modality-specific is examined by reviewing the effects of practice and expertise on visual evoked responses.

Visual evoked responses

Visual evoked potentials are comprised of positive, negative, positive deflections peaking at about 100 (P1), 170 (N1) and 240 (P2) ms respectively after stimulus onset over the occipital and inferior parietal regions. The amplitude of the P1 wave is sensitive to spatial attention (Woldorff et al., 2002), whereas the N1 amplitude is modulated by the nature of the visual input such as a face or an object (Itier & Taylor, 2004).

The fact that the N170 is larger for some classes of stimuli over others may reflect the viewer's expertise with the material. Indeed, larger N170 has been observed in bird watchers for bird stimuli (Tanaka & Curran, 2001), and for car experts viewing cars (Gauthier et al., 2003). Similarly, when English readers were presented with Roman and Chinese characters, Chinese characters elicited smaller N170 than Roman characters (Wong et al., 2005). This language-specific effect was not present in Chinese–English bilinguals. These findings suggest that the visual N170 reflects long-term experience with visual material and, perhaps, could be used to assess the integrity of long-term representations following brain injury.

In comparison with hearing research, fewer studies have examined the impact of an explicit training regimen on visual evoked responses and those that examine training-induced plasticity have yielded mixed results. For instance, some studies reported an enhancement of visual N170 amplitude elicited by nonface objects (e.g., greebles, vernier stimuli) following extended training (Rossion et al., 2004; Shoji & Skrandies, 2006). However, other studies found reduced N1 amplitude over the parietal region (Song et al., 2002, 2005) that was generalised over differently oriented stimuli (Ding et al., 2003). Learning to detect degraded images, which were not recognized unless previously associated with its nondegraded version, also resulted in enhanced amplitude of induced gamma oscillation at about 250 ms after stimulus onset (Goffaux et al., 2004).

In addition, training on a simple visual discrimination task has been associated with enhanced P2 amplitude, which was paralleled by a decrease in response time (Ding et al., 2003; Song et al., 2005). Both the P2 enhancement and RT training-related improvement were specific to the trained stimuli (Ding et al., 2003). The P2 enhancement was not present when participants were trained with slightly more complex stimuli (e.g., arrow as opposed to line segments) (Song et al., 2005). For the arrow stimuli, training resulted in an increased P3 (350–550 ms) amplitude over the central/parietal areas (Song et al., 2005). These findings suggest that perceptual learning modifies the response at different levels of visual cortical processing related to the complexity of the stimulus. The neuronal mechanisms involved in perceptual learning may depend on the nature (e.g., the complexity) of the stimuli used in the discrimination task.

As in the auditory modality, learning to discriminate between various classes of visual stimuli results in enhanced visual evoked responses. Interestingly, the P2 enhancement was also observed after daily practice sessions. While the early neuroplastic changes in N1 amplitude may reflect modality-specific effects, the later modulation occurring during the P2 interval may be reflecting more general aspects of learning common across different modalities. The pattern of changes in both auditory and visual modalities is consistent with the proposal that the P2 indexes consolidation during learning.

Somatosensory evoked responses

Tactile stimulations generate somatosensory evoked responses over the central scalp region that include early (e.g., N20, P27 and P45 wave) and late responses (N70, N140 and P220) whose latency and amplitude vary as a function of the site of stimulation (e.g., finger vs. foot). In comparison with auditory and visual evoked responses, which mainly showed changes in the response size, the effects of laboratory training on somatosensory evoked responses seems more likely to be expressed in changes in source locations than in response amplitudes. For instance, Schwenkreis *et al.* (2001) showed short-term changes in dipole location of the N20 after one hour of training, but no difference in amplitude between pre- and post-training recordings. Another MEG study examining the effect of a 30-day training regimen in discriminating the frequency of vibro-tactile finger stimulation resulted in significant improvement of behavioral performance that can even be generalized to the untrained hand, but failed to produce reliable changes in somatosensory evoked responses (Imai *et al.*, 2003). In comparison, Braun *et al.* (2002) used the more reliable within-subject, within-session measure of distance in the representation of digit 2 and 5 and found an increase in distance after vibro-tactile discrimination training without a measurable change in the amplitude of the somatosensory evoked field. Another study has shown improved discrimination performance with training that was paralleled by changes in MEG signal spectral power around 10 and 20 Hz, but found no reliable change in the amplitude of somatosensory evoked responses and their localization (Liu & Ioannides, 2004). Pleger *et al.* (2001) showed improvement in spatial discrimination thresholds, which were paralleled by a shift in the localization of the N20-dipole of the index finger that was stimulated. The distance between the dipole pre- and post-training was significantly larger on the trained side than on the control side, revealing a highly selective effect with no transfer to the index finger of the opposite, non-trained hand. The improvement in discrimination abilities was predicted by the changes in dipole localization.

Summary

Improvement in tactile discrimination is associated with neuroplastic changes in the primary somatosensory area generating early sensory responses. These changes occur after extended training and appear to be highly specific to the trained area. The studies reviewed above demonstrate that behavioral improvement during tactile discrimination training is paralleled by changes in cortical networks. However, further work is needed to identify robust measures in the recorded EEG or MEG, which reflect reliably the training induced changes. The most promising candidates seem to be within-subject localization measures like the extension of the hand area and changes in the EEG/MEG signal spectrum.

ERP/ERF measurements during rehabilitation and treatment

- Stroke recovery and rehabilitation are associated with neuroplastic changes in sensory evoked responses and cognitive evoked potentials.

Scalp recording of ERPs and ERFs have been used extensively in clinical research. More recently, there has been a growing interest in examining whether ERPs and ERFs could be useful prognostic tools in predicting recovery following moderate and severe brain injury (for a review see Giaquinto, 2004; Lew *et al.*, 2006). As we mentioned earlier, we believe that ERPs and ERFs could be very useful for longitudinal monitoring and assessing cortical remodeling following rehabilitation. In the previous section, we reviewed evidence supporting neuroplastic changes in the auditory, visual and somatosensory systems, revealing a high level of brain plasticity in sensory systems of healthy adults. In most studies, improvements in performance were associated with an enhancement in the amplitude of neuroelectric or neuromagnetic activity. The latter is consistent with recruitment of additional neurons representing the trained attribute and/or higher degree of synchronization within a particular neural ensemble. Topographical changes were also observed in some studies indicating that training can also generate changes in cortical maps (loci) representing the trained attribute. More importantly, findings from these studies reveal neuroplastic changes in the adults' brain following various training regimens, which can be documented using EEG and MEG.

In spite of evidence showing training-related induced brain plasticity in healthy adults, the literature contains relatively few articles dealing with the use of ERPs and/or ERFs in assessing rehabilitation and plasticity in disordered systems. Keren et al. (1998) recorded ERPs from patients with closed head injury 2, 3 and 3.5 or more months after injury. Patients with severe closed head injury (significant degree of impaired consciousness greater than 24 hours) were divided into two groups according to severity using the Glasgow Coma Scale, which quantifies the level of consciousness following traumatic brain injury. Event-related potentials were elicited using the standard auditory P3 "oddball" paradigm, including targets defined by their higher pitch. At the initial test, the more severely injured group showed significantly longer P3 latencies than the less severely injured patients. In subsequent recordings, P3 latency was found to be significantly shorter compared with the initial P3 latency, and the difference in P3 latency between the two patient groups was no longer statistically significant by the time of the third recording. For the group as a whole, P3 latency decreased significantly on each repeated recording, and may reflect a decrease in stimulus evaluation time. In addition, the N2 latency was found to be significantly shorter between the first and third recordings. These changes in P3 latency correlated with improvement in neuropsychological tests such as short- and long-term story recall, word recall and Raven's progressive matrices. Although this study suggests that the P3 wave may be used as a physiologic index of brain activity that correlates with recovery from closed

head injury, this finding should be interpreted with caution since a recent study failed to find reliable changes in P3 amplitude or latency in post-stroke global aphasics as a function of recovery (Nolfe et al., 2006). However, the lack of a clear relationship between ERP measurement and recovery may be attributed to the nature of the paradigm used by Nolfe et al. (2006), which did not emphasize focus of attention and learning.

Evidence suggests that ERPs can be very helpful in assessing the reorganization of language following brain lesions even in patients with chronic aphasia. For instance, Pulvermüller et al. (2005) examined the impact of intense language therapy for 2 weeks on performance and brain activity elicited by visually presented words and pseudo-words. They found significant improvement in speech comprehension, which was paralleled by enhanced P2 amplitude elicited by words following treatment. Brain responses elicited by meaningless pseudo-words were not modulated by the language therapy, suggesting that the neurophysiological changes were specific to words. In an effort to determine the recovery of cortical auditory discrimination in eight aphasic left-hemisphere-stroke patients, Ilvonen et al. (2003) measured the MMN wave to duration and frequency changes in a repetitive, harmonically rich tone, 4 and 10 days and again 3 and 6 months after their first unilateral stroke. Relative to the initial testing session, they found increasing MMN amplitudes during the 3–6 months follow-up, which were accompanied by progressive improvement in speech-comprehension tests. This suggests that the MMN reflects spontaneous recovery and/or recruitment of auditory cortex spared by the lesion.

Perceptual training with nonlinguistic audiovisual stimuli in dyslexic children has also been found to improve sound discrimination as indexed by the MMN, which was accompanied by improvements in reading skills (Kujala et al., 2001). Similar neuroplastic changes in auditory cortex were recently observed for a phonological intervention applied to preschool children diagnosed with a specific language impairment (Pihko et al., 2007). These results are very encouraging and suggest that behavioral improvements in language function during rehabilitation are paralleled by changes in the amplitude of ERP components.

Event-related potentials have also been used to assess clinical improvement associated with processing somatosensory and visual stimuli. For instance, Giaquinto & Fraioli (2003) measured the N140 and P3 waves elicited by standard and target cutaneous electrical stimuli in patients suffering from a stroke in the middle cerebral artery area. The target stimuli were presented on the elbow of the paralyzed side whereas the standard stimuli were applied on the ipsilateral shoulder. Participants indicated, by pressing a button, whenever they noticed the target stimulus. Patients in the trained group performed this discrimination task five times a week for 3 consecutive weeks whereas those in the control group were tested twice; once at the beginning and again at the end of 3 weeks. The main finding of that study was that daily practice significantly improved the recovery of N140 for stimuli presented contralateral to the paralyzed side. While 15% of the patients showed an N140 during the first testing session, the proportion increased to 80% at the end of the training regimen. In the control group, there was no difference in the proportion of patients showing the N140 response. Similarly, behavioral improvement associated with rehabilitation of chronic post-stroke visual field defects has been associated with a recovery of the P1 wave from the visual evoked responses (Julkunen *et al.*, 2003). Henriksson *et al.* (2007) examined the effects of extended training on cortical reorganization and found that weekly stimulation of the blind hemifield can induce cortical reorganization of visual areas in the intact hemisphere. These studies demonstrate that training-related improvements in the detection of sensory stimuli are accompanied by neuroplastic changes in sensory evoked responses, highlighting the fact that neuroelectric brain activity can be used to monitor and assess the impact of rehabilitation at the cortical level.

Magnetoencephalography has recently been applied to assess the impact of a rehabilitation technique for musicians suffering from focal hand dystonia, a disorder involving cramps and uncoordinated movements of the hand and fingers. Improvement in symptoms following treatment was paralleled by alteration in the functional organization of the somatosensory cortex (Candia *et al.*, 2003). Other MEG studies demonstrated that the cortical reorganization related to the writer's cramp is task specific (Braun *et al.*, 2003) and that specific changes in cortical networks can be identified using measures of coherence between brain regions (Butz *et al.*, 2006). Magnetoencephalography is sensitive to hemispheric differences and this property is useful for observing cortical plasticity during recovery from unilateral stroke. Comparing somatosensory responses from the affected and un-affected hemisphere is a sensitive within-subject measure and gives insight into stroke-related plastic changes despite possible large inter-subject variability in the responses (Rossini *et al.*, 2001).

Summary

Recent longitudinal studies combining behavioral methods with recording of neuroelectric and/or neuromagnetic brain activity provide new insight regarding the nature and the level at which rehabilitation can impact brain function. The technique can be used to assess a wide range of treatment and shows promise in assessing the impact of rehabilitation on perceptual, cognitive and motor functions.

Overall summary and future directions

Neurophysiological studies in nonhuman primates as well as neuroimaging research in humans have revealed a remarkable degree of brain plasticity. This discovery of a highly dynamic and malleable brain in adulthood opens new areas and provides hope in treating individuals with brain dysfunctions. However, there are major challenges for research in rehabilitation. The ability to objectively assess and monitor the efficacy of rehabilitation techniques is central for developing more effective rehabilitation programs. The evidence reviewed in this chapter suggests that EEG and MEG techniques may prove to be useful tools in assessing and monitoring brain plasticity in some situations. Recording of neuroelectric and neuromagnetic activity is versatile and easy to use in conjunction with behavioral methods. The portability of the EEG system may promote research at the bedside or in more natural settings, such as someone's house. Both techniques can be used to examine whether newly acquired skills can be generalized to other situations.

Further research is needed to explore the characteristics of this remarkably adaptable cortical activity and to uncover its boundary conditions. For instance, what are the links between early and rapid neuroplastic changes that occur within the first hours of training and those that take place following several daily practice sessions? Is the brain of middle-aged adults and/or older adults as plastic as those of young adults? If so, can such extended training be used to alleviate perceptual and cognitive "problems" that occur with normal aging? Answers to these and related questions will advance our knowledge of learning and cortical plasticity and have important implications for rehabilitation.

ACKNOWLEDGMENTS

The preparation of this book chapter was supported by grants from the Canadian Institutes of Health Research, the Natural Sciences and Engineering Research Council of Canada, and the Hearing Foundation of Canada. We are grateful to the volunteers who participated in the experiments reviewed here from our laboratory and the support from the Canadian Foundation for Innovation and the Ontario Innovation Trust for the purchase of equipment needed to carry out these experiments. Special thanks to Lori Bernstein, Tony Shahin, Kelly McDonald, Karen Reinke and Kelly Tremblay for helpful comments on earlier versions of this chapter.

REFERENCES

Alain, C., & Izenberg, A. (2003). Effects of attentional load on auditory scene analysis. *Journal of Cognitive Neuroscience*, **15**, 1063–1073.

Alain, C., & Woods, D. L. (1997). Attention modulates auditory pattern memory as indexed by event-related brain potentials. *Psychophysiology*, **34**, 534–546.

Alain, C., Woods, D., & Ogawa, K. (1994). Brain indices of automatic pattern processing. *NeuroReport*, **6**, 140–144.

Alain, C., Cortese, F., & Picton, T. W. (1999). Event-related brain activity associated with auditory pattern processing. *NeuroReport*, **10**, 2429–2434.

Alain, C., McDonald, K. L., Ostroff, J. M., & Schneider, B. (2004). Aging: a switch from automatic to controlled processing of sounds? *Psychology and Aging*, **19**, 125–133.

Alain, C., Snyder, J. S., He, Y., & Reinke, K. S. (2007). Changes in auditory cortex parallel rapid perceptual learning. *Cerebral Cortex*, **17**, 1074–1084.

Arnott, S. R., & Alain, C. (2002). Stepping out of the spotlight: MMN attenuation as a function of distance from the attended location. *NeuroReport*, **13**, 2209–2212.

Atienza, M., Cantero, J. L., & Dominguez-Marin, E. (2002). The time course of neural changes underlying auditory perceptual learning. *Learning and Memory*, **9**, 138–150.

Bakin, J. S., & Weinberger, N. M. (1990). Classical conditioning induces CS-specific receptive field plasticity in the auditory cortex of the guinea pig. *Brain Research*, **536**, 271–286.

Bakin, J. S., South, D. A., & Weinberger, N. M. (1996). Induction of receptive field plasticity in the auditory cortex of the guinea pig during instrumental avoidance conditioning. *Behavioral Neuroscience*, **110**, 905–913.

Bergan, J. F., Ro, P., Ro, D., & Knudsen, E. I. (2005). Hunting increases adaptive auditory map plasticity in adult barn owls. *Journal of Neuroscience*, **25**, 9816–9820.

Bosnyak, D. J., Eaton, R. A., & Roberts, L. E. (2004). Distributed auditory cortical representations are modified when non-musicians are trained at pitch discrimination with 40 Hz amplitude modulated tones. *Cerebral Cortex*, **14**, 1088–1099.

Brattico, E., Tervaniemi, M., & Picton, T. W. (2003). Effects of brief discrimination-training on the auditory N1 wave. *NeuroReport*, **14**, 2489–2492.

Braun, C., Haug, M., Wiech, K. *et al.* (2002). Functional organization of primary somatosensory cortex depends on the focus of attention. *NeuroImage*, **17**, 1451–1458.

Braun, C., Schweizer, R., Heinz, U., Wiech, K., Birbaumer, N., & Topka, H. (2003). Task-specific plasticity of somatosensory cortex in patients with writer's cramp. *NeuroImage*, **20**, 1329–1338.

Brown, M., Irvine, D. R. F., & Park, V. N. (2004). Perceptual learning on an auditory frequency discrimination task by cats: association with changes in primary auditory cortex. *Cerebral Cortex*, **14**, 952–965.

Butz, M., Timmermann, L., Gross, J. *et al.* (2006). Oscillatory coupling in writing and writer's cramp. *Journal of Physiology-Paris*, **99**, 14–20.

Candia, V., Wienbruch, C., Elbert, T., Rockstroh, B., & Ray, W. (2003). Effective behavioral treatment of focal hand dystonia in musicians alters somatosensory cortical organization. *Proceedings of the National Academy of Sciences of the United States of America*, **100**, 7942–7946.

Ding, Y., Song, Y., Fan, S., Qu, Z., & Chen, L. (2003). Specificity and generalization of visual perceptual learning in humans: an event-related potential study. *NeuroReport*, **14**, 587–590.

Edeline, J. M., Pham, P., & Weinberger, N. M. (1993). Rapid development of learning-induced receptive field plasticity in the auditory cortex. *Behavioral Neuroscience*, **107**, 539–551.

Fritz, J., Shamma, S., Elhilali, M., & Klein, D. (2003). Rapid task-related plasticity of spectrotemporal receptive fields in primary auditory cortex. *Nature Neuroscience*, **6**, 1216–1223.

Fritz, J., Elhilali, M., & Shamma, S. (2005a). Active listening: task-dependent plasticity of spectrotemporal receptive fields in primary auditory cortex. *Hearing Research*, **206**, 159–176.

Fritz, J. B., Elhilali, M., & Shamma, S. A. (2005b). Differential dynamic plasticity of A1 receptive fields during multiple spectral tasks. *Journal of Neuroscience*, **25**, 7623–7635.

Fujioka, T., Trainor, L. J., Ross, B., Kakigi, R., & Pantev, C. (2004). Musical training enhances automatic encoding of melodic contour and interval structure. *Journal of Cognitive Neuroscience*, **16**, 1010–1021.

Fujioka, T., Trainor, L. J., Ross, B., Kakigi, R., & Pantev, C. (2005). Automatic encoding of polyphonic melodies in musicians and nonmusicians. *Journal of Cognitive Neuroscience*, **17**, 1578–1592.

Gauthier, I., Curran, T., Curby, K. M., & Collins, D. (2003). Perceptual interference supports a non-modular account of face processing. *Nature Neuroscience*, **6**, 428–432.

Giaquinto, S. (2004). Evoked potentials in rehabilitation. A review. *Functional Neurology*, **19**, 219–225.

Giaquinto, S., & Fraioli, L. (2003). Enhancement of the somatosensory N140 component during attentional training after stroke. *Clinical Neurophysiology*, **114**, 329–335.

Goffaux, V., Mouraux, A., Desmet, S., & Rossion, B. (2004). Human non-phase-locked gamma oscillations in experience-based perception of visual scenes. *Neuroscience Letters*, **354**, 14–17.

Gottselig, J. M., Brandeis, D., Hofer-Tinguely, G., Borbely, A. A., & Achermann, P. (2004). Human central auditory plasticity associated with tone sequence learning. *Learning and Memory*, **11**, 162–171.

Hämäläinen, M., Hari, R., Ilmoniemi, R. J., Knuutila, J., & Ov, L. (1993). Magnetoencephalography – theory, instrumentation, and applications to noninvasive studies of the working human brain. *Reviews of Modern Physics*, **65**, 413–505.

Heinrich, A., Alain, C., & Schneider, B. A. (2004). Within- and between-channel gap detection in the human auditory cortex. *NeuroReport*, **15**, 2051–2056.

Henriksson, L., Raninen, A., Näsänen, R., Hyvärinen, L., & Vanni, S. (2007). Training-induced cortical representation of a hemianopic hemifield. *Journal of Neurology, Neurosurgery and Psychiatry*, **78**, 74–81.

Hillebrand, A., & Barnes, G. R. (2005). Beamformer analysis of MEG data. *International Review of Neurobiology*, **68**, 149–171.

Hillyard, S. A., Squires, K. C., Bauer, J. W., & Lindsay, P. H. (1971). Evoked potential correlates of auditory signal detection. *Science*, **172**, 1357–1360.

Hirata, Y., Kuriki, S., & Pantev, C. (1999). Musicians with absolute pitch show distinct neural activities in the auditory cortex. *NeuroReport*, **10**, 999–1002.

Ilvonen, T.-M., Kujala, T., Kiesiläinen, A. *et al.* (2003). Auditory discrimination after left-hemisphere stroke: a mismatch negativity follow-up study. *Stroke*, **34**, 1746–1751.

Imai, T., Kamping, S., Breitenstein, C., *et al.* (2003). Learning of tactile frequency discrimination in humans. *Human Brain Mapping*, **18**, 260–271.

Itier, R. J., & Taylor, M. J. (2004). N170 or N1? Spatiotemporal differences between object and face processing using ERPs. *Cerebral Cortex*, **14**, 132–142.

Javitt, D. C., Grochowski, S., Shelley, A. M., & Ritter, W. (1998). Impaired mismatch negativity (MMN) generation in schizophrenia as a function of stimulus deviance, probability, and interstimulus/interdeviant interval. *Electroencephalography and Clinical Neurophysiology*, **108**, 143–153.

Julkunen, L., Tenovuo, O., Jääskeläinen, S., & Hämäläinen, H. (2003). Rehabilitation of chronic post-stroke visual field defect with computer-assisted training. *Restorative Neurology and Neuroscience*, **21**, 19–28.

Keren, O., Ben-Dror, S., Stern, M. J., Goldberg, G., & Groswasser, Z. (1998). Event-related potentials as an index of cognitive function during recovery from severe closed head injury. *Journal of Head Trauma Rehabilitation*, **13**, 15–30.

Kraus, N., McGee, T., Carrell, T. D. *et al.* (1995). Central auditory system plasticity associated with speech discrimination training. *Journal of Cognitive Neuroscience*, **7**, 25–32.

Kujala, T., Karma, K., Ceponiene, R. *et al.* (2001). Plastic neural changes and reading improvement caused by audiovisual training in reading-impaired children. *Proceedings of the National Academy of Sciences of the United States of America*, **98**, 10509–10514.

Kuriki, S., Kanda, S., & Hirata, Y. (2006). Effects of musical experience on different components of MEG responses elicited by sequential piano-tones and chords. *Journal of Neuroscience*, **26**, 4046–4053.

Lew, H. L., Poole, J. H., Castandeda, A., Salerno, R. M., & Gray, M. (2006). Prognostic value of evoked and event-related potentials in moderate to severe brain injury. *Journal of Head Trauma Rehabilitation*, **21**, 350–360.

Lin, F. H., Witzel, T., Ahlfors, S. P. *et al.* (2006). Assessing and improving the spatial accuracy in MEG source localization by depth-weighted minimum-norm estimates. *NeuroImage*, **31**, 160–171.

Liu, L., & Ioannides, A. A. (2004). MEG study of short-term plasticity following multiple digit frequency discrimination training in humans. *Brain Topography*, **16**, 239–243.

Lopez, L., Jürgens, R., Diekmann, V. *et al.* (2003). Musicians versus nonmusicians: a neurophysiological approach. *Annals of the New York Academy of Sciences*, **999**, 124–130.

Lütkenhöner, B., Seither-Preisler, A., & Seither, S. (2006). Piano tones evoke stronger magnetic fields than pure tones or noise, both in musicians and non-musicians. *NeuroImage*, **30**, 927–937.

Martin, B. A., Sigal, A., Kurtzberg, D., & Stapells, D. R. (1997). The effects of decreased audibility produced by high-pass noise masking on cortical event-related potentials to speech sounds /ba/ and /da/. *Journal of the Acoustical Society of America*, **101**, 1585–1599.

McDonald, K. L., & Alain, C. (2005). Contribution of harmonicity and location to auditory object formation in free field: evidence from event-related brain potentials. *Journal of the Acoustical Society of America*, **118**, 1593–1604.

Menning, H., Roberts, L. E., & Pantev, C. (2000). Plastic changes in the auditory cortex induced by intensive frequency discrimination training. *NeuroReport*, **11**, 817–822.

Näätänen, R. (1992). *Attention and Brain Function*. Hillsdale, NJ: Lawrence Erlbaum.

Näätänen, R., Lehtokoski, A., Lennes, M. *et al.* (1997). Language-specific phoneme representations revealed by electric and magnetic brain responses. *Nature*, **385**, 432–434.

Nager, W., Kohlmetz, C., Altenmüller, E., Rodriguez-Fornells, A., & Münte, T. F. (2003). The fate of sounds in conductors' brains: an ERP study. *Cognitive Brain Research*, **17**, 83–93.

Nolfe, G., Cobianchi, A., Mossuto-Agatiello, L., & Giaquinto, S. (2006). The role of P300 in the recovery of post-stroke global aphasia. *European Journal of Neurology*, **13**, 377–384.

Pantev, C., Oostenveld, R., Engelien, A., Ross, B., Roberts, L. E., & Hoke, M. (1998). Increased auditory cortical representation in musicians. *Nature Neuroscience*, **392**, 811–814.

Pantev, C., Engelien, A., Candia, V., & Elbert, T. (2001a). Representational cortex in musicians. Plastic alterations in response to musical practice. *Annals of the New York Academy of Sciences*, **930**, 300–314.

Pantev, C., Roberts, L. E., Schulz, M., Engelien, A., & Ross, B. (2001b). Timbre-specific enhancement of auditory cortical representations in musicians. *NeuroReport*, **12**, 169–174.

Parasuraman, R., & Beatty, J. (1980). Brain events underlying detection and recognition of weak sensory signals. *Science*, **210**, 80–83.

Picton, T. W., Alain, C., Otten, L., Ritter, W., & Achim, A. (2000). Mismatch negativity: different water in the same river. *Audiology and Neurootology*, **5**, 111–139.

Pihko, E., Mickos, A., Kujala, T. *et al.* (2007). Group intervention changes brain activity in bilingual language-impaired children. *Cerebral Cortex*, **17**, 849–858.

Pleger, B., Dinse, H. R., Ragert, P., Schwenkreis, P., Malin, J.-P., & Tegenthoff, M. (2001). Shifts in cortical representations predict human discrimination improvement. *Proceedings of the National Academy of Sciences of the United States of America*, **98**, 12255–12260.

Polley, D. B., Steinberg, E. E., & Merzenich, M. M. (2006). Perceptual learning directs auditory cortical map reorganization through top-down influences. *Journal of Neuroscience*, **26**, 4970–4982.

Pulvermüller, F., Hauk, O., Zohsel, K., Neininger, B., & Mohr, B. (2005). Therapy-related reorganization of language in both hemispheres of patients with chronic aphasia. *NeuroImage*, **28**, 481–489.

Recanzone, G. H., Jenkins, W. M., Hradek, G. T., & Merzenich, M. M. (1992). Progressive improvement in discriminative abilities in adult owl monkeys performing a tactile frequency discrimination task. *Journal of Neurophysiology*, **67**, 1015–1030.

Recanzone, G. H., Schreiner, C. E., & Merzenich, M. M. (1993). Plasticity in the frequency representation of primary auditory cortex following discrimination training in adult owl monkeys. *Journal of Neuroscience*, **13**, 87–103.

Reinke, K. S., He, Y., Wang, C., & Alain, C. (2003). Perceptual learning modulates sensory evoked response during vowel segregation. *Cognitive Brain Research*, **17**, 781–791.

Ross, B., Borgmann, C., Draganova, R., Roberts, L. E., & Pantev, C. (2000). A high-precision magnetoencephalographic study of human auditory steady-state responses to amplitude-modulated tones. *Journal of the Acoustic Society of America*, **108**, 679–691.

Rossini, P. M., Tecchio, F., Pizzella, V. *et al.* (2001). Interhemispheric differences of sensory hand areas after monohemispheric stroke: MEG/MRI integrative study. *NeuroImage*, **14**, 474–485.

Rossion, B., Kung, C. C., & Tarr, M. J. (2004). Visual expertise with nonface objects leads to competition with the early perceptual processing of faces in the human occipitotemporal cortex. *Proceedings of the National Academy of Sciences of the United States of America*, **101**, 14521–14526.

Rutkowski, R. G., & Weinberger, N. M. (2005). Encoding of learned importance of sound by magnitude of representational area in primary auditory cortex. *Proceedings of the National Academy of Sciences of the United States of America*, **102**, 13664–13669.

Sams, M., Paavilainen, P., Alho, K., & Näätänen, R. (1985). Auditory frequency discrimination and event-related potentials. *Electroencephalography and Clinical Neurophysiology*, **62**, 437–448.

Sarvas, J. (1987). Basic mathematical and electromagnetic concepts of the biomagnetic inverse problem. *Physics in Medicine and Biology*, **32**, 11–22.

Schneider, P., Scherg, M., Dosch, H. G. *et al.* (2002). Morphology of Heschl's gyrus reflects enhanced activation in the auditory cortex of musicians. *Nature Neuroscience*, **5**, 688–694.

Schwenkreis, P., Pleger, B., Höffken, O., Malin, J.-P., & Tegenthoff, M. (2001). Repetitive training of a synchronised movement induces short-term plastic changes in the human primary somatosensory cortex. *Neuroscience Letters*, **312**, 99–102.

Sekihara, K., Nagarajan, S. S., Poeppel, D., Marantz, A., & Miyashita, Y. (2001). Reconstructing spatio-temporal activities of neural sources using an MEG vector beamformer technique. *IEEE Transactions on Biomedical Engineering*, **48**, 760–771.

Shahin, A., Bosnyak, D. J., Trainor, L. J., & Roberts, L. E. (2003). Enhancement of neuroplastic P2 and N1c auditory evoked potentials in musicians. *Journal of Neuroscience*, **23**, 5545–5552.

Sheehan, K. A., McArthur, G. M., & Bishop, D. V. M. (2005). Is discrimination training necessary to cause changes in the P2 auditory event-related brain potential to speech sounds? *Cognitive Brain Research*, **25**, 547–553.

Shoji, H., & Skrandies, W. (2006). ERP topography and human perceptual learning in the peripheral visual field. *International Journal of Psychophysiology*, **61**, 179–187.

Song, Y., Ding, Y., Fan, S., & Chen, L. (2002). An event-related potential study on visual perceptual learning under short-term and long-term training conditions. *NeuroReport*, **13**, 2053–2057.

Song, Y., Ding, Y., Fan, S. *et al.* (2005). Neural substrates of visual perceptual learning of simple and complex stimuli. *Clinical Neurophysiology*, **116**, 632–639.

Tanaka, J. W., & Curran, T. (2001). A neural basis for expert object recognition. *Psychological Science*, **12**, 43–47.

Tervaniemi, M., Ilvonen, T., Karma, K., Alho, K., & Näätänen, R. (1997). The musical brain: brain waves reveal the neurophysiological basis of musicality in human subjects. *Neuroscience Letters*, **226**, 1–4.

Tesche, C. D., Uusitalo, M. A., Ilmoniemi, R. J. *et al.* (1995). Signal-space projections of MEG data characterize both distributed and well-localized neuronal sources. *Electroencephalography and Clinical Neurophysiology*, **95**, 189–200.

Trainor, L. J., McDonald, K. L., & Alain, C. (2002). Automatic and controlled processing of melodic contour and interval information measured by electrical brain activity. *Journal of Cognitive Neuroscience*, **14**, 430–442.

Tremblay, K., Kraus, N., Carrell, T. D., & McGee, T. (1997). Central auditory system plasticity: generalization to novel stimuli following listening training. *Journal of the Acoustical Society of America*, **102**, 3762–3773.

Tremblay, K., Kraus, N., & McGee, T. (1998). The time course of auditory perceptual learning: neurophysiological changes during speech-sound training. *NeuroReport*, **9**, 3556–3560.

Tremblay, K., Kraus, N., McGee, T., Ponton, C., & Otis, B. (2001). Central auditory plasticity: changes in the N1-P2 complex after speech-sound training. *Ear and Hearing*, **22**, 79–90.

Vrba, J., & Robinson, S. E. (2001). Signal processing in magnetoencephalography. *Methods*, **25**, 249–271.

Wang, J. Z. (1993). Minimum-norm least-squares estimation: magnetic source images for a spherical model head. *IEEE Transactions on Biomedical Engineering*, **40**, 387–396.

Williamson, S. J., Lu, Z. L., Karron, D., & Kaufman, L. (1991). Advantages and limitations of magnetic source imaging. *Brain Topography*, **4**, 169–180.

Witte, R. S., & Kipke, D. R. (2005). Enhanced contrast sensitivity in auditory cortex as cats learn to discriminate sound frequencies. *Cognitive Brain Research*, **23**, 171–184.

Woldorff, M. G., Hackley, S. A., & Hillyard, S. A. (1991). The effects of channel-selective attention on the mismatch negativity wave elicited by deviant tones. *Psychophysiology*, **28**, 30–42.

Woldorff, M. G., Hillyard, S. A., Gallen, C. C., Hampson, S. R., & Bloom, F. E. (1998). Magnetoencephalographic recordings demonstrate attentional modulation of mismatch-related neural activity in human auditory cortex. *Psychophysiology*, **35**, 283–292.

Woldorff, M. G., Liotti, M., Seabolt, M. *et al.* (2002). The temporal dynamics of the effects in occipital cortex of visual-spatial selective attention. *Cognitive Brain Research*, **15**, 1–15.

Wong, A. C. N., Gauthier, I., Woroch, B., DeBuse, C., & Curran, T. (2005). An early electrophysiological response associated with expertise in letter perception. *Cognitive, Affective and Behavioral Neuroscience*, **5**, 306–318.

Ylinen, S., Shestakova, A., Huotilainen, M., Alku, P., & Näätänen, R. (2006). Mismatch negativity (MMN) elicited by changes in phoneme length: a cross-linguistic study. *Brain Research*, **1072**, 175–185.

Factors affecting successful outcome

Introduction to Section 3

Ian H. Robertson

The term "holistic" can sometimes be used in a rather unscientific manner, but its use in this part of the book is appropriate, as here we consider a number of factors which can sometimes be neglected in discussions of cognitive rehabilitation. This is particularly true when rehabilitation researchers are trying to integrate practical rehabilitation efforts into theoretical models of brain function, an extremely complex and difficult task; but it is also true even in clinical rehabilitation contexts that factors such as diet, exercise, psychosocial environment, motivation, awareness and mood are not systematically considered.

We are fortunate to have five excellent chapters in this part of the book, which covered a range of areas that have not been considered together in previous textbooks of cognitive rehabilitation. Ghaffar and Feinstein give comprehensive and first-class account of brain–behavior relationships in the area of mood and motivation. These domains are extremely "hot topics" in basic cognitive neuroscience and have been applied to clinical conditions such as depression and drug addiction, but hitherto have not been actively considered in great detail in the field of cognitive rehabilitation.

Why should this be? In part, it may be because of the disciplinary background of those carrying out cognitive rehabilitation, which often focuses on the neurological and neuropsychological aspects of brain function. While mood and motivation would be central concepts in problems such as drug addiction and emotional disorder, they have been much less central issues in cognitive rehabilitation.

Another factor may be the sheer complexity of trying to understand complex relationships within cognitive systems which mitigate against compounding the complexity by introducing emotional and motivational factors to the explanatory system.

Yet the more that cognitive neuroscience demonstrates the role a key brain region (identified by Ghaffar and Feinstein as central to motivation) as the anterior cingulate in mediating between cognitive and emotional functioning in domains such as error processing (Magno *et al.*, 2006), the more it is clear that cognitive rehabilitation has no choice but to try to integrate these key concepts into the development of models of rehabilitation.

Prigatano has been a pioneer in considering issues of awareness and motivation in rehabilitation, and indeed has placed them at the very center of the influential models of rehabilitation that he has developed. In many ways his research predated modern brain imaging approaches to studying self-awareness and motivation, and the field of cognitive rehabilitation has been fortunate to benefit from his prescient theorizing.

There are grounds for believing that the starting point of cognitive rehabilitation should perhaps lie in systematic evaluation of motivation and self-awareness, as the evidence is strong that recovery of function depends on the recognition that a deficit exists (Gialanella *et al.*, 2005). Furthermore, intellectual recognition does not necessarily entail an appropriate emotional response to the deficit or to the errors that arise from it; recent research on error processing, for instance, has shown that it is

Cognitive Neurorehabilitation, Second Edition: Evidence and Application, ed. Donald T. Stuss, Gordon Winocur and Ian H. Robertson. Published by Cambridge University Press. © Cambridge University Press 2008.

possible to differentiate between an unconscious processing of errors and a conscious processing, which are subserved by different brain regions and can thus be differentially affected by brain damage (O'Connell *et al.*, 2007).

Motivation must in part rise from the emotional and intellectual response to the recognition of errors, as well as from more basic components of "drive" as outlined by Ghaffar and Feinstein; they have shown how it is possible to differentiate between different possible brain circuits, underpinning different aspects of these complex states and processes, namely: a dorsolateral prefrontal (DLPF) circuit subserving executive cognitive tasks; an orbitofrontal circuit linked to mood, behavior and personality change; and an anterior cingulate pathway associated with motivation.

Dawson and Winocur review seminal work on the role of psychosocial factors on cognitive function, and on the recovery of cognitive deficit following brain damage. Their original findings that environmental changes that are common among elderly people, such as moving into supported accommodation, can produce significant changes in cognitive function, are extremely important, as are the findings that the perception of loss of control is a major psychological variable mediating between these changes and the cognitive consequences.

The relationship between psychological variables such as loss of control and self-esteem on the one hand, and neuropsychological variables such as memory and attention on the other, is largely unexplored in cognitive rehabilitation research. Dawson and Winocur's contribution to this area is seminal and represents a very important and novel approach to cognitive rehabilitation.

Scherder and Eggermont give a thoughtful and important review of the role of exercise in the progress and rehabilitation of neurodegenerative disorders. This chapter complements nicely the review in Chapter 24 by Kramer, Erickson and McAuley of the effects of exercise on cognition. Interestingly, Scherder and Eggermont suggest that factors such as executive deficits and gait dysfunction may result in losses of physical activity, which deprive the brain of enhancing stimulation.

Parrott and Greenwood bring another dimension to this "holistic" approach to cognitive rehabilitation, namely the question of diet. While considerable discussion has taken place about the role of pharmaceutical agents in potentiating rehabilitative methods (see Chapters 17, 18 and 19), there has been virtually no discussion about how the major source of brain chemistry – food – may impact on cognitive recovery and rehabilitation. Parrott and Greenwood comprehensively review both the acute and chronic effects of diet on cognitive function, and give compelling evidence that this is a long neglected aspect of rehabilitation that must now be actively considered.

Mood, motivation, awareness, exercise, diet and the psychosocial environment may have been peripheral or absent from previous textbooks of cognitive rehabilitation, but these five chapters in this section surely demonstrate that these should be center stage in the future development of cognitive rehabilitation.

REFERENCES

Gialanella, B., Monguzzi, V., Santoro, R., & Rocchi, S. (2005). Functional recovery after hemiplegia in patients with neglect: the rehabilitative role of anosognosia. *Stroke*, **36**, 2687–2690.

Magno, E., Foxe, J., Molholm, S., Robertson, I. H., & Garavan, H. (2006). The anterior cingulate and error avoidance. *Journal of Neuroscience*, **26**, 4769–4773.

O'Connell, R. G., Dockree, P. M., Bellgrove, M. A. *et al.* (2007). The role of cingulate cortex in the detection of errors with and without awareness: a high-density electrical mapping study. *European Journal of Neuroscience*, **25**, 2571–2579.

12

Mood, affect and motivation in rehabilitation

Omar Ghaffar and Anthony Feinstein

Introduction

Patients with an acquired brain injury may frequently present with abnormalities of mood, affect and motivation. Given the disabling nature of these disturbances, accurate clinical assessment is necessary in planning and implementing a comprehensive rehabilitation strategy. It is important to realise at the outset that abnormalities in each domain may occur independently of one another, although a more common clinical picture is one in which all are affected to varying degrees. The importance in making this clinical distinction cannot be overemphasised for distinct abnormalities in mood, affect and motivation each demand a specific treatment. The clinician who fails to tease out these various features of the mental state thus runs the risk of missing potentially treatable conditions that could derail the rehabilitation process and erode the patient's quality of life.

To better understand how such presentations arise in a clinical setting, reference will be made to the neural circuitry underpinning these abnormalities. While there is sound empirical evidence elucidating the neural pathways controlling mood and motivation, the pathogenesis of disturbances in affect, i.e., the display of emotion as distinct from subjective feeling, is less clearly understood. Therefore, only brief reference will be made to it within a clinical perspective in the section dealing with pseudobulbar affect, also termed pathological laughing and crying.

The aim of this chapter is thus to acquaint the reader with a brief summary of the relevant neuroanatomy of mood and motivation, followed by a description of the clinical features, differential diagnosis and treatment of disorders of mood (depression and mania), affect (pathological laughing and crying) and motivation (apathy). Although the role of anxiety disorders in patients with physical illness has been neglected in the literature, the high rate of co-occurrence of anxiety with mood disorders in patients with physical illness necessitates consideration also (Kessler *et al.*, 2005; Popkin & Tucker, 1994). The emphasis of this chapter is clinical and the approach a practical one, for the therapeutic benefits of timely and correct intervention are considerable.

Frontal subcortical circuits and behavior

- Five discrete frontal-subcortical neural circuits associated with specific behavioral difficulties have been identified. Three of these relate to disorders of mood and motivation and are mediated via dysregulation of neurotransmitters such as dopamine and serotonin.
- A dorsolateral prefrontal (DLPF) circuit subserves executive cognitive tasks.
- An orbitofrontal circuit is linked to mood, behavior and personality change.
- An anterior cingulate pathway is associated with motivation.

Cognitive Neurorehabilitation, Second Edition: Evidence and Application, ed. Donald T. Stuss, Gordon Winocur and Ian H. Robertson. Published by Cambridge University Press. © Cambridge University Press 2008.

Five discrete frontal subcortical circuits (Alexander & Crutcher, 1990; Alexander *et al.*, 1986; Tekin & Cummings, 2002) have been delineated. All begin in the frontal lobes and project first to the striatum, then to the globus pallidus and substantia nigra, before synapsing in the thalamus, from where the circuit loops back to the frontal lobes. Two of the five circuits (the motor circuit originating in the supplementary motor area and the oculomotor circuit originating in the frontal eye fields) are involved in motor functions and will not be elaborated upon here. The three remaining circuits originate in separate prefrontal cortical areas, namely dorsolateral prefrontal (DLPF) cortex, lateral orbital cortex and anterior cingulate (AC) cortex.

These three main pathways have subsidiary pathways at various stages throughout their course and send and receive connections to and from related limbic structures. As the circuits progress from cortex to subcortex, the neurons funnel into increasingly smaller areas, all the while maintaining their parallel and distinct anatomical integrity. This "squeezing" of the circuits helps explain how lesions situated at various points along the pathways give rise to differing clinical presentations.

Mechanisms of behavioral change

Each prefrontal circuit is associated with a specific behavioral syndrome (Cummings, 1993). Lesions localised to the DLPF cortex typically produce cognitive (dysexecutive) difficulties, and those in the orbitofrontal cortex are associated with changes in mood, behavior and personality, while anterior cingulate pathology has been implicated in disorders of motivation (Table 12.1). While this schema is conceptually useful, in practice patients rarely present with symptoms that conform to a single, tightly defined neural circuit.

Interruptions to these circuits translate into behavioral abnormalities via a dysregulation of neurotransmitters such as glutamate, dopamine and serotonin amongst others (Robbins, 2005). The

Table 12.1. Syndromes associated with dysfunction of three frontal-subcortical circuits. DLPFC, dorsolateral prefrontal cortex; OFC, orbitofrontal cortex; AC, anterior cingulate cortex.

Circuit	Syndrome
DLPFC	Executive dysfunction
	Poor organisation
	Impaired problem solving
	Poor recall
	Impaired set-shifting
OFC	Disinhibition
	Personality change
	Emotional lability
	Irritability
	Social impropriety
	Obsessive-compulsive behavior
AC	Amotivation
	Apathy, abulia, akinetic mutism
	Psychomotor retardation

relationship between dopamine and the anterior cingulate pathway illustrates the point. Apathy, which stems from dysfunction of this circuit (Adair *et al.*, 1996), may be alleviated by dopaminergic drugs (Bressan & Crippa, 2005; Padala *et al.*, 2005; Ross & Stewart, 1981). An analogous situation pertains to the neurotransmitter serotonin and the orbitofrontal and DLPF circuits. Dysfunction of these circuits may produce behavioral changes such as depression and obsessive-compulsive disorder that respond favorably to drugs that selectively enhance serotonin availability.

Having briefly outlined some basic neuroanatomy, the remainder of the chapter will be devoted to a discussion of the pathogenesis and clinical features of depression, mania, pathological laughing and crying, and impaired motivation.

Depressive disorders

- Clinically significant depression is frequently found in a rehabilitation setting.

- It is associated with cerebral blood flow abnormalities affecting orbitofrontal and DLPF cortex.
- There is also a link with adverse psychosocial stressors.
- Concomitant physical and cognitive abnormalities may obscure the diagnosis.
- Attention to a patient's thought content and interviewing an informant help in establishing the diagnosis.
- Pharmacotherapy is often effective in treating depression, although patients may prove sensitive to adverse side effects. Therefore, selective serotonin reuptake inhibitors (SSRIs) are probably the drugs of choice.

Frequency and pathogenesis

Clinically significant depression, akin to major depression, may be an integral part of many disabling conditions. Robust data from the neurological literature illustrate this point: lifetime prevalence figures approach 50% for Parkinson's disease (Lieberman, 2006; Starkstein & Robinson, 1989) and multiple sclerosis (Patten et al., 2003; Sadovnick et al., 1996), well in excess of the 17% figure reported in general population comorbidity surveys (Kessler et al., 1994, 2005). Similarly, elevated prevalence rates have been reported in stroke (Robinson, 2003; Robinson & Price, 1982), Huntington's disease (Folstein et al., 1983; Paulsen et al., 2005), traumatic brain injury (Jorge & Starkstein, 2005; Robinson & Jorge, 1994) and Alzheimer's disease (Holtzer et al., 2005; Loreck & Folstein, 1993).

The clinician often faces a dilemma in deciding whether depression is etiologically related to the medical disorder or the chance occurrence of an additional illness or an understandable, psychological reaction to physical disability. The complexity in making this distinction is compounded by a bidirectional relationship that appears to exist between depression and certain neurologic disorders such as stroke (Larson et al., 2001), epilepsy (Hesdorffer et al., 2000), and Parkinson's disease (Leentgens et al., 2003). In other words, depression is not only a complication but may also be a risk factor for the development of these neurologic disorders. While on an individual basis it is never possible to be entirely certain on this score, the absence of the usual female preponderance of patients strongly suggests these mood changes are directly attributable to the neurological process (Clayton & Lewis, 1981).

Advances in brain imaging and analysis have unmasked brain-mood correlations. In stroke patients, an association between left (dominant) anterior placed lesions and more serious depressive illness has been reported (Robinson et al., 1983), replicated (Eastwood et al., 1989), and disputed (Carson et al., 2000; Singh et al., 1998). Subcortical pathology, in particular stroke affecting the left basal ganglia, has also been associated with depression, severity of the mood change once again related to more anterior placed lesions (Starkstein et al., 1987). In the case of multiple sclerosis, Pujol et al. (1997) described an association between low mood and lesions in the arcuate fasciculus of the dominant hemisphere. Bakshi et al. (2000) extended these findings by looking beyond the hyperintense lesions noted on proton density and T2 weighted images, reporting a link between depression on the one hand and cerebral atrophy and T1 weighted lesions in frontal and parietal regions on the other. A third study that carefully matched MS depressed and nondepressed patients on all relevant demographic, neurological and psychosocial variables before undertaking a detailed MRI-based regional brain analysis provided the firmest evidence yet that a combination of hyperintense lesions and cerebral atrophy confined to medial inferior frontal areas in the dominant hemisphere were implicated in depression (Feinstein et al., 2004).

The importance of frontal system pathology in the pathogenesis of depression has been confirmed in other neuropsychiatric disorders, using functional brain imaging. Depressed as opposed to nondepressed Parkinson patients have significantly lower metabolic activity in the head of the caudate nucleus and orbitofrontal cortex (Mayberg et al., 1990). In a before- and after-treatment FDG positron emission tomography (PET) study of depressed Parkinson's disease patients, an antidepressant response to fluoxetine was associated with a metabolic increase in dorsal anterior cingulate regional metabolism and a metabolic decrease in ventral anterior cingulate (Mayberg, 2003; Stefurak et al., 2001). Similarly orbitofrontal and inferior prefrontal cortex hypometabolism differentiated depressed from nondepressed Huntington patients (Mayberg et al., 1992). Positron emission tomography findings from both these disorders overlap with neuroimaging data from patients who are depressed, but without concomitant neurological disease (Baxter et al., 1989; Bench et al., 1992; Seminowicz et al., 2004). While there is no direct evidence from any of these studies confirming neuronal loss, hypometabolism in brain areas rich in biogenic amine pathways implicates abnormalities in dopamine and catecholamine transmission in patients who become depressed. This is further supported by Parkinson's patients endorsing more depressive symptomatology when in the "off" state (more bradykinetic) than when motor function improves ("on" state) (Friedenberg & Cummings, 1989), an observation linked to regional cerebral blood changes in the medial frontal gyrus and posterior cingulate cortex (Black et al., 2005).

The assessment of depression

History

It is important to take a thorough psychiatric history from all patients at their initial assessment. Particularly within a rehabilitation setting patients may prove poor historians for a variety of reasons ranging from cognitive impairment to impaired insight and as such an informant who knows the patient well (regular contact over many years) should also be interviewed. Depression may be missed in an aphasic patient, obscured by difficulties they have in expressing their distress. However, it is a frequent concomitant of aphasia and may manifest as grief, catastrophic reactions and suicide (Benson & Ardila, 1993).

The presence of a family history of mental illness and the nature of that illness should be ascertained,

for there is some evidence that mood change, irrespective of an acquired brain insult, remains consistent within families (Schiffer et al., 1988). In addition, the presence of a premorbid psychiatric history may throw light on the subsequent development of mood change. A detailed social history is mandatory to document relevant stressors (financial, residential, occupational, relationship) and supports that are present. The number of drugs implicated in causing a depressive illness is legion and medication lists should therefore be thoroughly checked (Cummings, 1985, p. 185).

Often, it is also difficult to decide what is attributable to depression or the associated physical disorder. This problem frequently occurs with fatigue which is virtually ubiquitous within a rehabilitation population. Vegetative features such as poor sleep, loss of appetite and sexual interest, considered the hallmarks of depression in a psychiatric population may also prove misleading. Patients with acquired brain injuries often display abnormalities in these areas independent of mood variation. While it remains essential to document all these changes plus subjective complaints of low mood, specific attention should be addressed to complaints (or observations of the clinician or caregiver) which may carry greater weight, such as irritability, feelings of hopelessness, frustration and social withdrawal. Anhedonia may be regarded as an equivalent of depressed mood, and it is often fruitful to inquire about activities that formerly gave enjoyment and that could still be pursued. Finally, the duration of symptoms should be noted, wherever possible corroborating this with an informant. Transient lability in mood may be part of adjusting to disability or a new environment. The persistence of a low, nondistractible mood is however a more serious development.

Thoughts of suicide or self-harm should never be overlooked and need to be actively sought as part of the mood assessment. Epidemiological data point to suicide as a significant cause of morbidity in multiple sclerosis, spinal cord injuries and certain subsets of epileptic patients (Carson et al., 2000; Stenager & Stenager, 1992). Nearly a third of patients with MS have thoughts of suicide over their lifetime, an observation linked to presence and severity of major depression, alcohol abuse and social isolation (Feinstein, 2002).

Mental state examination

The mental state assessment in patients with neurological disease presents challenges, e.g., how to differentiate the bradykinesia and masked facies of Parkinson's disease from the psychomotor retardation and blunted affect of depression (Moriarty, 2005). Conversely, low mood may be incorrectly attributed to patients with disorders of prosody associated with nondominant cerebral pathology (George *et al.*, 1996). While speech, language and thought form may prove misleading, thought content characterized by cognitive distortions and somatic preoccupations is often the crucial factor that establishes the diagnosis. Often, the diagnosis may only be reached after combining information from history, mental state assessment and the observations of family informants and allied health workers.

Pseudodementia: "dementia" of depression

Clinicians should be alert to the possibility of depression masquerading as dementia (Caine, 1981). A finding common to many neurological disorders, be it traumatic brain injury (Chamelian & Feinstein, 2006), multiple sclerosis (Benedict *et al.*, 2005) or human immunodeficiency virus (HIV) (Castellon *et al.*, 2006), is that patients who persistently complain of cognitive problems not infrequently turn out to have major depression. The opinion of an informant is often helpful here. In addition, clinical clues suggesting depression as opposed to dementia are a family history of affective disorder, the relatively sudden onset of cognitive problems, and a preserved ability to learn new information. Neuropsychological testing may further help in diagnostic clarification.

Recent studies have, however, painted a more complex relationship between mood and cognition.

Data from depressed patients with and without a neurological disorder suggest that clinically significant depression may lead to impaired cognitive and attentional capacity which may be further refined as deficits in working memory and more specifically, an executive dysfunction (Arnett *et al.*, 1999a, 1999b; Demaree *et al.*, 2003). Thus, in some patients, the deleterious cognitive effects of severe low mood may be attributable to a dysexecutive syndrome. It is, however, important to realize that depression in acquired illnesses irrespective of the disease implicated, is more likely to exacerbate existing problems with executive function rather than cause them per se. These findings nevertheless raise an interesting, clinically relevant question. If depression was successfully treated would there be cognitive improvement as well? To date results from traumatic brain injury (TBI) are encouraging. Should TBI patients have their depression successfully treated with antidepressant medication, concomitant improvements in some of these cognitive deficits follow (Fann *et al.*, 2001). This finding has been replicated in primary depression, i.e., depressed patients without a neurological illness (Gaultieri *et al.*, 2006).

Adjuncts to diagnosis

The diagnosis of a depressive syndrome is essentially a clinical one. In cases of uncertainty, little help can be obtained from adjunctive methods such as the dexamethasone suppression test, where the rate of false positive results as demonstrated in Parkinson's disease is unacceptably high (Frochtengarten *et al.*, 1987). Similarly, rating scales are not a substitute for clinical acumen. They are, however, useful as a research tool and for allowing the patient to subjectively record changes in mood over time. Results need to be interpreted with caution, as many of the better known and most widely used scales are ill suited to a rehabilitation setting because they contain an unacceptably high number of somatic based questions, endorsement of which may give rise to false positive results of depression. Given this potential overlap, rating scales specific for depression in medically ill samples have been developed. The seven-question Beck Fast Screen is one such example (Beck *et al.*, 2000).

Thus far, MRI, fMRI and PET have been largely limited to the research environment. It is anticipated that as the validity of their findings are consolidated, these imaging techniques, including others like diffusion tensor and magnetization transfer imaging, will enter the clinical domain and potentially contribute to diagnosis and monitoring the effects of treatment.

Treatment

There is a paucity of controlled clinical trials for depression within a rehabilitation setting and much of the evidence to date has been anecdotal. Some general principles do, however, apply. When prescribing antidepressant medication, the physician should be alert to possible drug interactions and patient susceptibility to side effects because of compromised cerebral dysfunction. There is a case for using a selective serotonin reuptake inhibitor (SSRI) as a first choice antidepressant because of their lower incidence of troubling side effects, although these drugs are not without their own problems, i.e., insomnia, sexual dysfunction and apathy. It is prudent to start at lower doses than one would in cases of uncomplicated depression (i.e., 10 mg of an SSRI such as citalopram or 18.75 mg of a serotonin noradrenaline reuptake inhibitor (SNRI) like venlafaxine). Though all SSRIs are said to be equally efficacious, citalopram may be favorable for patients with polypharmacy in particular, owing to the minimal effect of this agent on major CYP isoforms (Hemeryck & Belpaire, 2002). The long half-life of citalopram (35 h) also confers less risk of discontinuation syndromes relative to venlafaxine, paroxetine and sertraline. Should patients tolerate the medication well, there is no reason not to use comparable doses to those prescribed for primary depression if clinically indicated. An advantage to some tricyclic antidepressant drugs is the presence of a clear therapeutic window and careful monitoring of plasma levels may allow the physician to gauge the most effective dose. They may also be beneficial in the treatment of neuropathic pain. However, these advantages must be balanced with the lethal hazard of tricyclic agents in intentional overdose and with their troubling anticholinergic side-effect profile. Electroconvulsive therapy should be considered in patients who have not responded well to pharmacotherapy (Greenberg & Kellner, 2005). There are no absolute contraindications to the procedure, although patients with raised intracranial pressure or at risk for an intracerebral bleed demand caution and particularly close monitoring. In patients where the diagnosis of depression versus dementia is unclear, aggressive treatment for depression may provide the answer.

Psychotherapy, particularly cognitive–behavioral therapy, is a useful adjunct to medication. One study found that it was as effective as 50mg of sertraline in alleviating major depression in MS. Both treatments were superior to supportive-expressive group psychotherapy (Mohr *et al.*, 2001). Not surprisingly, the benefits of CBT are receiving additional validation from fMRI studies, where an improvement in mood has been linked to modulation in frontal, cingulate and hippocampal activity (Goldapple *et al.*, 2004)

Bipolar affective disorder

- Bipolar affective disorder may occur as a sequel to an acquired brain injury and symptoms may be difficult to distinguish from a personality change of the disinhibited subtype.
- Manic mood may, however, respond well to mood stabilizers, with benzodiazepine and neuroleptic medication added for sedation and psychotic features respectively.

Secondary mania may follow an acquired brain injury with a frequency that exceeds chance expectation (Schiffer *et al.*, 1986). A constellation of physical overactivity, elevated (or irritable) mood, decreased need for sleep, and grandiose (or persecutory) beliefs should alert the physician to the diagnosis. There may be difficulty in distinguishing mania from a brain disorder causing a personality change of the disinhibited, labile or aggressive subtype (see the section on frontal subcortical circuits).

However, while the latter may show disinhibition and grandiose thinking, the presence of the symptoms mentioned above makes the diagnosis of an affective disorder more likely. Similarly, a positive premorbid and family history of affective disorder helps differentiate the two.

With regard to treatment, mood-stabilizing drugs (lithium, carbamazepine, sodium valproate or the atypical antipsychotics) with a benzodiazepine for sedation are the drugs of choice. Should psychotic symptoms be present, neuroleptic medication will almost certainly be required. The atypical antipsychotics such as risperidone appear to offer significant benefits given their more favorable side-effect profile. Clozapine or quetiapine are the neuroleptics of choice in patients with psychosis and co-existing movement disorders (Miyasaki et al., 2006). As with depression in the context of an acquired brain injury, the likelihood of adverse side effects is increased. This may require keeping serum levels of mood-stabilizing drugs at the lower end of the therapeutic range, which in practical terms may mean a daily dose of lithium of 600 mg as opposed to the 900–1200 mg used more often in a general psychiatry practice. There is however a considerable individual variation in the ability of patients with an acquired brain injury to tolerate side effects, and as such, generalization becomes hazardous. Rather, the clinician should monitor each case according to their individual merits.

Pseudobulbar affect

- Pseudobulbar affect is a less common, but nevertheless disabling complication of cerebral damage that responds well to small doses of an SSRI or dextromethorphan/quinidine.

This condition has been regarded as synonymous with pathological laughing and crying, in which abnormalities of affect do not correspond with subjective alterations in mood (Poeck, 1969). Others have challenged this clean division (Ross & Stewart, 1987), suggesting at least a degree of overlap between outward displays of emotional

dyscontrol and subjective feelings of emotional distress. Although the condition may prove disabling, it is amenable to effective treatment, either with small doses of SSRIs (Iannacone & Ferrini-Strambi, 1996; Lauterbach & Schweri, 1991), amitriptyline (Schiffer et al., 1985), dextromethophan/quinidine (Brooks et al., 2004; Miller, 2006; Panitch et al., 2006), or failing these, levodopa (Wolf et al., 1979).

Anxiety disorders

- While individual symptoms of anxiety are common, the prevalence of anxiety disorders in a rehabilitation sample has yet to be reliably established.
- In some disorders, most notably stroke, the occurrence appears to be a frequent one.

The category "anxiety disorder" is a broad rubric encompassing disorders such as generalized anxiety disorder, obsessive-compulsive disorder and panic disorder. Anxiety disorders in patients with physical illness, unlike their depressive counterparts, have received virtually no attention. Much of this disinterest has been attributed to the high frequency with which symptoms of anxiety occur in this setting (Popkin & Tucker, 1994). A distinction should therefore be made between isolated symptoms of anxiety which are extremely common especially in the context of major depression, and a specific syndrome of anxiety, termed "anxiety disorders due to a general medical condition" by the Diagnostic and Statistical Manual, Fourth Edition (Popkin & Tucker, 1994). Although the prevalence of the latter within a rehabilitation setting has not been accurately ascertained, a review of anxiety syndromes associated with neurological disorders found that it occurred most commonly in patients with cerebral vascular disease, but was also part of the presentation of Huntington's disease, closed head injury, multiple sclerosis, encephalitis and central nervous system tumors, to mention a few of the more common disorders (Hall, 1980). Factors that suggest a causal relationship between the neurological and anxiety disorders are onset after the age of 35 years and an absence of family and personal histories of psychiatric illness. There are no published reports of cerebral correlates for the disorder.

A long list of medications may give rise to anxiety disorders, including steroids, caffeine, bronchodilators, insulin, estrogens, antihistamines, digitalis and L-Dopa.

Disorders of motivation

- Poor motivation (termed apathy) frequently complicates recovery during rehabilitation.
- Apathy may be a primary phenomenon or occur secondary to other disorders such as depression and dementia.
- Reversible causes (biological, psychosocial) should be corrected before resorting to pharmacotherapy as treatment.
- Dopamine augmenting agents may prove an effective treatment in cases of primary apathy or a useful adjunct in secondary cases.

This discussion, while acknowledging a large and important literature from experimental psychology devoted to motivation, will be confined to relevant clinical aspects. The important contributions of Robert Marin (Marin, 1990, 1991, 1996; Marin et al., 1994; Marin & Wilkosz, 2005) in bringing clarity to a loosely defined clinical concept are acknowledged and this chapter follows his approach in assigning the term apathy to denote impaired motivation.

Apathy may exist as a *primary*, independent syndrome, unencumbered by abnormalities of mood, fluctuations in level of consciousness or multiple intellectual deficits. As discussed in the section on frontal-subcortical circuits, an example of such a primary state is frontal lobe injury, particularly damage to the anterior cingulate, where impaired motivation is not accompanied by subjective emotional distress. More commonly, however, apathy may be one symptom comprising part of a larger syndrome and in such cases the disorder of motivation should be regarded as a *secondary* phenomenon. Examples of these syndromes include

delirium, dementia, depression and schizophrenia (Marin, 1991; Marin & Wilkosz, 2005).

Before deciding whether apathy is primary or secondary in origin, the following points should be considered (Marin, 1991, 1996; Marin et al., 2003). Impaired motivation may be: (a) a reflection or exaggeration of premorbid personality traits; (b) part of a numbing of responsiveness and withdrawal induced by overwhelming stress or loss; (c) a response to altered physiological functioning such as loss of any of the primary senses, motor function and coordination. It may also stem from institutional living (Wing & Brown, 1970).

Apathy and depression

Differentiating apathy as a primary disorder from apathy as part of a depressive syndrome is important for they are not synonymous. The assessment of depressed patients as apathetic is based on complaints such as social withdrawal, inability to enjoy activities that formerly gave them pleasure and loss of interest and inactivity with respect to activities of daily living. These changes are unwanted and accompanied by subjective feelings of low mood and a thought content characterised by depressive cognitions such as poor self-esteem, guilt and an expectation of future failure. Attempts at social engagement are actively avoided. In more extreme cases thought and actions may turn to suicide. This contrasts with a primary apathetic syndrome in which patients may bear a superficial behavioral similarity to the above picture, but who do not subjectively experience dysphoria and regard their altered state with emotional indifference (Marin et al., 1994). A final point regarding depression and apathy that must be mentioned is that the existence of an SSRI-induced apathy syndrome can go unrecognised. This adverse effect has been noted to be dose-dependent and reversible, and may occur late in treatment (Barnhart et al., 2004). Thus, apathy occurring in individuals receiving treatment with SSRIs begs the question whether the apathy is due to residual depressive symptoms or due to the treatment itself. In the case of the latter, the effect may subside with a decrease in SSRI dosage (Hoehn-Saric *et al.*, 1990).

Apathy and medical illness

Many neurological disorders are associated with apathy. They share a number of factors that acting individually or in combination produce a reduction in motivation (Marin, 1990). These include cognitive dysfunction hindering the capacity to focus and direct behavior, an altered perception of one's abilities and direct involvement of brain regions that control drive, i.e., frontal lobes. Thus, apathy may be found in dementia, basal ganglia diseases, Korsakoff's syndrome and disorders giving rise to indifference or neglect (e.g., right hemisphere stroke).

Medical conditions such as hyperthyroidism and hypoparathyroidism may also produce apathetic-like states as may drugs ranging from neuroleptics (typical and atypical antipsychotics) and SSRIs to marijuana.

Mention should be made of two related neurological states that represent extreme forms of apathy. Abulia refers to an impairment of will and an inability to initiate behavior. At its most extreme form, patients display akinetic mutism, in which they present as awake, but unresponsive to sensory stimuli except for visual following. There is an absence of noticeable motor findings such as rigidity and dystonia and patients are unable to speak. An interruption in dopaminergic transmission to a cortico-limbic structure such as the anterior cingulate is thought to induce the syndrome (Devinsky *et al.*, 1995; Ross & Stewart, 1981).

Assessment and treatment of apathy

The assessment of a patient's motivation follows on from the points mentioned above. Thus, history taking should include talking to an informant to ascertain the patient's premorbid personality profile and degree of motivation. The informant may also clarify the degree to which motivation is related to environment. A thorough physical and mental state assessment should elucidate whether the loss of motivation is primary or a symptom of another condition. While this distinction appears simple in theory, detecting the various contributory factors frequently presents a considerable clinical challenge. Cognitive, perceptual and sensorimotor impairments should be carefully noted and a complete list of all medications obtained.

A first step to treatment is the removal of reversible psychosocial, medical and pharmacological causes of apathy. When apathy is traced to environmental factors, social interventions are called for while psychotherapy is indicated for patients who feel overwhelmed by their disability and the adjustment to their lives this entails. Correction of sensorimotor impairments such as impaired visual acuity should be attended to and appropriate medical treatment (e.g., thyroid supplementation for hypoparathyroidism) begun. Should apathy be secondary to an existing disorder such as depression, treatment targeted at the latter may successfully alleviate apathy as well. As mentioned, however, SSRIs may themselves be implicated in causing poor motivation so the clinician must remain vigilant (Hoehn-Saric *et al.*, 1990).

The observation that a functional deficiency of dopamine can give rise to apathy suggests possible avenues of pharmacologic intervention. Thus, treatment with psychostimulants (methylphenidate, dextroamphetamine and modafinil), direct dopamine agonists (bromocriptine, pergolide) or indirect dopamine agonists (amantadine) may prove helpful (Marin *et al.*, 1995). Dosages should be adjusted according to individual response and tolerance of side effects. There are reports of patients with profound abulia (Barret, 1991) and akinetic mutism (Ross & Stewart, 1981) responding dramatically to these agents.

Finally, time spent explaining apathy to family members may prevent patients being blamed or criticised for their apparent disinterest and unresponsiveness to well-meaning efforts at their rehabilitation.

Conclusions

Alterations of affect, mood and motivation are frequently found in patients requiring rehabilitation.

This chapter has highlighted certain neural networks associated with these behavioral disturbances and provided a framework for clinical assessment that incorporates biological and psychosocial factors. Treatment targeted at specific disorders may prove singularly effective and should therefore be energetically pursued, all the while remaining cognisant of the patient's enhanced sensitivity to drug side effects and interactions. Improvement in mood and motivation may facilitate other aspects of rehabilitation and contribute significantly to enhancing quality of life.

REFERENCES

Adair, J. C., Williamson, D. J. G., Schwartz, R. L., & Heilman, K. M. (1996). Ventral tegmental area injury and frontal lobe disorder. *Neurology*, **46**, 842–843.

Alexander, G. E., & Crutcher, M. D. (1990). Functional architecture of basal ganglia circuits: neural substrates of parallel processing. *Trends in Neurosciences*, **13**, 266–271.

Alexander, G. E., DeLong, M. R., & Strick, P. L. (1986). Parallel organization of functionally segregated circuits linking basal ganglia and cortex. *Annual Review of Neuroscience*, **9**, 357–381.

Arnett, P. A., Higginson, C. I., Voss, W. D. *et al.* (1999a). Depression in multiple sclerosis: relationship to working memory. *Neuropsychology*, **13**, 546–556.

Arnett, P. A., Higginson, C. I., Voss, W. D. *et al.* (1999b). Depressed mood in multiple sclerosis: relationship to capacity-demanding memory and attentional functioning. *Neuropsychology*, **13**, 434–446.

Bakshi, R., Czarnecki, D., Shaikh, Z. A. *et al.* (2000). Brain MRI lesions and atrophy are related to depression in multiple sclerosis. *NeuroReport*, **11**, 1153–1158.

Barnhart, W. J., Makela, E. H., & Latocha, M. J. (2004). SSRI-induced apathy syndrome: a clinical review. *Journal of Psychiatric Practice*, **10**, 196–199.

Barret, K. (1991). Treating organic abulia with bromocriptine and lisuride: four case studies. *Journal of Neurology, Neurosurgery and Psychiatry*, **56**, 718–721.

Baxter, L. R., Schwartz, J. M., Phelps, M. E. *et al.* (1989). Reduction of prefrontal cortex metabolism common to three types of depression. *Archives of General Psychiatry*, **46**, 243–250.

Beck, A. T., Steer, R. A., & Brown, G. K. (2000). *DI-Fast Screen for Medical Patients*. San Antonio, TX: The Psychological Corporation.

Bench, C. J., Friston, K. J., Brown, R. G. *et al.* (1992). The anatomy of melancholia-focal abnormalities of cerebral blood flow in major depression. *Psychological Medicine*, **22**, 607–615.

Benedict, R. H., Wahlig, E., Bakshi, R. *et al.* (2005). Predicting quality of life in multiple sclerosis: accounting for physical disability, fatigue, cognition, mood disorder, personality, and behavior change. *Journal of Neurological Sciences*, **231**, 29–34.

Benson, D. F., & Ardila, A. (1993). Depression in aphasia. In S. E. Starkstein & R. G. Robinson (Eds.), *Depression in Neurologic Disease* (pp. 152–164). Baltimore, MD: Johns Hopkins Press.

Black, K. J., Hershey, T., Hartlein, J. M., Carl, J. L., & Perl-mutter, J. S. (2005). Levodopa challenge neuroimaging of levodopa-related mood fluctuations in Parkinson's disease. *Neuropsychopharmacology*, **30**, 590–601.

Bressan, R. A., & Crippa, J. A. (2005). The role of dopamine in reward and pleasure behavior: review of data from preclinical research. *Acta Psychiatrica Scandanavia*, **427**, 14–21.

Brooks, B. R., Thisted, R. A., Appel, S. H. *et al.* (2004). Treatment of pseudobulbar affect in ALS with dextromethorphan/quinidine: a randomized trial. *Neurology*, **63**, 1364–1370.

Caine, E. D. (1981). Pseudodementia: current concepts and future directions. *Archives of General Psychiatry*, **38**, 1359–1364.

Carson, A. J., MacHale, S., Allen, K. *et al.* (2000). Depression after stroke and lesion location: a systematic review. *Lancet*, **356**, 122–126.

Castellon, S. A., Hardy, D. J., Hinkin, C. H. *et al.* (2006). Components of depression in HIV-1 infection: their differential relationship to neurocognitive performance. *Journal of Clinical and Experimental Neuropsychology*, **28**, 420–437.

Chamelian, L., & Feinstein, A. (2006). The effect of major depression on subjective and objective cognitive deficits in mild to moderate traumatic brain injury. *Journal of Neuropsychiatry and Clinical Neurosciences*, **18**, 33–38.

Clayton, P. J., & Lewis, C. E. (1981). The significance of secondary depression. *Journal of Affective Disorders*, **3**, 25–35.

Cummings, J. L. (1985). *Clinical Neuropsychiatry*. Orlando, FL: Grune & Stratton.

Cummings, J. L. (1993). Frontal-subcortical circuits and human behaviour. *Archives of Neurology*, **50**, 873–880.

Demaree, H. A., Gaudino, E., & DeLuca, J. (2003). The relationship between depressive symptoms and cognitive dysfunction in multiple sclerosis. *Cognitive Neuropsychiatry*, **8**, 161–171.

Devinsky, O., Morrell, M. J., & Brent, A. V. (1995). Contributions of the anterior cingulate cortex to behaviour. *Brain*, **118**, 279–306.

Eastwood, M. R., Rifat, S. L., Nobbs, H., & Ruderman, J. (1989). Mood disorder following CVA. *British Journal of Psychiatry*, **154**, 195–200.

Fann, J. R., Uomoto, J. M., & Katon, W. J. (2001). Cognitive improvement with treatment of depression following mild traumatic brain injury. *Psychosomatics*, **42**, 48–54.

Feinstein, A. (2002). An examination of suicidal intent in patients with multiple sclerosis. *Neurology*, **59**, 674–678.

Feinstein, A., Roy, P., Lobaugh, N. *et al.* (2004). Structural brain abnormalities in multiple sclerosis patients with major depression. *Neurology*, **62**, 586–590.

Folstein, S. E., Abbott, M. H., Chase, G. A., Jensen, B. A., & Folstein, M. F. (1983). The association of affective disorder with Huntington's disease in a case series and in families. *Psychological Medicine*, **13**, 537–541.

Friedenberg, D. L., & Cummings, J. L. (1989). Parkinson's Disease, depression and the on-off phenomenon. *Psychosomatics*, **30**, 94–99.

Frochtengarten, M. L., Villares, J. C. B., Maluf, E., & Carlini, E. A. (1987). Depressive symptoms and the dexamethasone suppression test in Parkinson patients. *Biological Psychiatry*, **22**, 386–389.

Gaultieri, C. T., Johnson, L. G., & Benedict, K. B. (2006). Neurocognition in depression: patients on and off medication versus healthy comparison subjects. *Journal of Neuropsychiatry and Clinical Neurosciences*, **18**, 217–225.

George, M. S., Parekh, P. I., Rosinsky, N. *et al.* (1996). Understanding emotional prosody activates right hemisphere regions. *Archives of Neurology*, **53**, 665–670.

Goldapple, K., Segal, Z., Garson, C. *et al.* (2004). Modulation of cortical-limbic pathways in major depression: treatment-specific effects of cognitive behavior therapy. *Archives of General Psychiatry*, **61**, 34–41.

Greenberg, R. M., & Kellner, C. H. (2005). Electroconvulsive therapy: a selected review. *American Journal of Geriatric Psychiatry*, **13**, 268–281.

Hall, R. C. W. (1980). Anxiety. In R. C. W. Hall (Ed.), *Psychiatric Presentations of Medical Illness* (pp. 13–32). New York, NY: Spectrum Publications Inc.

Hemeryck, A., & Belpaire, F. M. (2002). Selective serotonin reuptake inhibitors and cytochrome P-450 mediated drug-drug interactions: an update. *Current Drug Metabolism*, **3**, 13–37.

Hesdorffer, D. C., Hauser, W. A., Annegers, J. F., & Cascino, G. (2000). Major depression is a risk factor for seizures in older adults. *Annals of Neurology*, **47**, 246–249.

Hoehn-Saric, R., Lipsey, J. R., & McLeod, D. R. (1990). Apathy and indifference in patients on fluvoxamine and fluoxetine. *Journal of Clinical Psychopharmacology*, **10**, 343–345.

Holtzer, R., Scarmeas, N., Wegesin, D. J. *et al.* (2005). Depressive symptoms in Alzheimer's disease: natural course and temporal relation to function and cognitive status. *Journal of the American Geriatric Society*, **53**, 2083–2089.

Iannaccone, S., & Ferini-Strambi, L. (1996). Pharmacologic treatment of emotional lability. *Clinical Neuropharmacology*, **19**, 532–535.

Jorge, R. E., & Starkstein, S. E. (2005). Pathophysiologic aspects of major depression following traumatic brain injury. *Journal of Head Trauma and Rehabilitation*, **20**, 475–487.

Kessler, R. C., McGonagle, K. A., Zhao, S. *et al.* (1994). Lifetime and 12-month prevalence of DSM-111-R psychiatric disorders in the United States. *Archives of General Psychiatry*, **51**, 8–19.

Kessler, R. C., Chiu, W. T., Demler, O., Merikangas, K. R., & Walters, E. E. (2005). Prevalence, severity, and comorbidity of 12-month DSM-IV disorders in the National Comorbidity Survey Replication. *Archives of General Psychiatry*, **62**, 617–627.

Larson, S. L., Owens, P. L., Ford, D., & Eaton, W. (2001). Depressive disorder, dysthymia and the risk of stroke: Thirteen-year follow-up from the Baltimore Epidemiological Catchment Area Study. *Stroke*, **32**, 1979–1983.

Lauterbach, E. C., & Schweri, M. M. (1991). Amelioration of pseudobulbar affect by fluoxetine: possible alteration of dopamine-related pathophysiology by a selective serotonin reuptake inhibitor. *Journal of Clinical Psychopharmacology*, **11**, 392–393.

Leentgens, A. F. G., Van Der Akker, M., Metsemakers, J. F. M., Lousberg, R., & Verhey, F. R. J. (2003). Higher incidence of depression preceding the onset of Parkinson's disease: a register study. *Movement Disorders*, **18**, 414–418.

Lieberman, A. (2006). Depression in Parkinson's disease: a review. *Acta Neurologica Scandanavia*, **113**, 1–8.

Loreck, D. J., & Folstein, M. F. (1993). Depression in Alzheimer's disease. In S. E. Starkstein & R. G. Robinson (Eds.), *Depression and Neurologic Disease* (pp. 50–62). Baltimore, MD: Johns Hopkins Press.

Marin, R. S. (1990). Differential diagnosis and classification of apathy. *American Journal of Psychiatry*, **147**, 22–30.

Marin, R. S. (1991). Apathy: a neuropsychiatric syndrome. *Journal of Neuropsychiatry and Clinical Neurosciences*, **3**, 243–254.

Marin, R. S. (1996). Apathy: concept, syndrome, neural mechanisms, and treatment. *Seminars in Clinical Neuropsychiatry*, **1**, 304–314.

Marin, R. S., & Wilkosz, P. A. (2005). Disorders of diminished motivation. *Journal of Head Trauma Rehabilitation*, **20**, 377–388.

Marin, R. S., Firinciogullari, S., & Biedrzycki, R. C. (1994). Group differences in the relationship between apathy and depression. *Journal of Nervous and Mental Disease*, **183**, 235–239.

Marin, R. S., Fogel, B. S., Hawkins, J., Duffy, J., & Krupp, B. (1995). Apathy: a treatable syndrome. *Journal of Neuropsychiatry and Clinical Neurosciences*, **7**, 23–30.

Marin, R. S., Butters, M. A., Mulsant, B. H., Pollock, B. G., & Reynolds, C. F. R. (2003). Apathy and executive function in depressed elderly. *Journal of Geriatric Psychiatry and Neurology*, **16**, 112–116.

Mayberg, H. S. (2003). Modulating dysfunctional limbic–cortical circuits in depression: towards development of brain-based algorithms for diagnosis and optimised treatment. *British Medical Bulletin*, **65**, 193–207.

Mayberg, H. S., Starkstein, S. E., Sadzot, B. *et al.* (1990). Selective hypometabolism in the inferior frontal lobe in depressed patients with Parkinson's disease. *Annals of Neurology*, **28**, 57–64.

Mayberg, H. S., Starkstein, S. E., Peyser, C. E. *et al.* (1992). Paralimbic frontal hypometabolism in depression associated with Huntington's Disease. *Neurology*, **42**, 1791–1797.

Miller, A. (2006). Pseudobulbar affect in multiple sclerosis: toward the development of innovative therapeutic strategies. *Journal of Neurological Sciences*, **245**, 153–159.

Miyasaki, J. M., Shannon, K., Voon, V. *et al.* (2006). Practice parameter: Evaluation and treatment of depression, psychosis, and dementia in Parkinson disease (an evidence-based review). Report of the Quality Standards Subcommittee of the American Academy of Neurology. *Neurology*, **66**, 996–1002.

Mohr, D. C., Boudewyn, A. C., Goodkin, D. E., Bostrom, A., & Epstein, L. (2001). Comparative outcomes for individual cognitive-behavior therapy, supportive-expressive group psychotherapy, and sertraline for the treatment of depression in multiple sclerosis. *Journal of Consulting and Clinical Psychology*, **69**, 942–949.

Moriarty, J. (2005). Recognising and evaluating disordered mental states: a guide for neurologists. *Journal of Neurology, Neurosurgery and Psychiatry*, **76**, i39–i44.

Padala, P. R., Petty, F., & Bhatia, S. C. (2005). Methylphenidate may treat apathy independent of depression. *Annals of Pharmacotherapy*, **39**, 1947–1949.

Panitch, H. S., Thisted, R. A., Smith, R. A. *et al.* (2006). Randomized, controlled trial of dextromethorphan/quinidine for pseudobulbar affect in multiple sclerosis. *Annals of Neurology*, **59**, 780–787.

Patten, S. B., Beck, C. A., Williams, J. V., Barbui, C., & Metz, L. M. (2003). Major depression in multiple sclerosis: a population-based perspective. *Neurology*, **61**, 1524–1527.

Paulsen, J. S., Nehl, C., Hoth, K. F. *et al.* (2005). Depression and stages of Huntington's disease. *Journal of Neuropsychiatry and Clinical Neuroscience*, **17**, 496–502.

Poeck, K. (1969). Pathophysiology of emotional disorders associated with brain damage. In P. J. Vinken & G. W. Bruyn (Eds.), *Handbook of Clinical Neurology, Vol. 3* (pp. 343–367). Amsterdam, NL: North Holland Publishing Company.

Popkin, M. K., & Tucker, G. J. (1994). Mental disorders due to a general medical condition. Mood, anxiety, psychotic, catatonic and personality disorders. In T. A. Widiger (Ed.), *DSM-IV Sourcebook, Vol. 1* (pp. 243–276). Washington, DC: American Psychiatric Association.

Pujol, J., Bello, J., Deus, J., Marti-Vilalta, J. L., & Capdevila, A. (1997). Lesions in the left arcuate fasciculus region and depressive symptoms in multiple sclerosis. *Neurology*, **49**, 1105–1110.

Robbins, T. W. (2005). Chemistry of the mind: neurochemical modulation of prefrontal cortical function. *Journal of Comparative Neurology*, **493**, 140–146.

Robinson, R. G. (2003). Poststroke depression: prevalence, diagnosis, treatment and disease progression. *Biological Psychiatry*, **54**, 376–387.

Robinson, R. G., & Price, T. R. (1982). Post stroke depressive disorders: a follow-up study of 103 patients. *Stroke*, **13**, 635–641.

Robinson, R. G., Kubos, K. L., Starr, L. B., Rao, K., & Price, T. R. (1983). Mood changes in stroke patients: relationship to lesion location. *Comprehensive Psychiatry*, **24**, 555–566.

Robinson, R. G., & Jorge, R. E. (1994). Mood disorders. In J. M. Silver, S. C. Yudofsky & R. E. Hales (Eds.),

Neuropsychiatry of Traumatic Brain Injury. Washington, DC: American Psychiatric Press.

Ross, E. D., & Stewart, R. M. (1981). Akinetic mutism from hypothalamic damage: successful treatment with dopamine agonists. *Neurology*, **31**, 1435–1439.

Ross, E. D., & Stewart, R. S. (1987). Pathological display of affect in patients with depression and right frontal brain damage. *Journal of Nervous and Mental Disease*, **175**, 165–172.

Sadovnick, A. D., Remick, R. A., Allen, J. *et al.* (1996). Depression and multiple sclerosis. *Neurology*, **46**, 628–632.

Schiffer, R. B., Herndon, R. M., & Rudick, R. A. (1985). Treatment of pathological laughing and weeping with amitriptyline. *New England Journal of Medicine*, **312**, 1480–1482.

Schiffer, R. B., Wineman, N. M., & Weitkamp, L. R. (1986). Association between bipolar affective disorder and multiple sclerosis. *American Journal of Psychiatry*, **143**, 94–95.

Schiffer, R. B., Weitkamp, L. R., Wineman, N. M., & Guttormsen, S. (1988). Multiple sclerosis and affective disorder: family history, sex, and HLA-DR antigens. *Archives of Neurology*, **45**, 1345–1348.

Seminowicz, D. A., Mayberg, H. S., McIntosh, A. R. *et al.* (2004). Limbic-frontal circuitry in major depression: a path modeling metanalysis. *NeuroImage*, **22**, 409–418.

Singh, A., Herrmann, N., & Black, S. E. (1998). The importance of lesion location in poststroke depression: a critical review. *Canadian Journal of Psychiatry*, **43**, 921–927.

Starkstein, S. E., & Robinson, R. G. (1989). Depression and Parkinson's disease. In R. G. Robinson & P. V. Rabins (Eds.), *Aging and Clinical Practice: Depression and Co-existing Disease* (pp. 213–248). New York, NY: Igaku-Shoi.

Starkstein, S. E., Robinson, R. G., & Price, T. R. (1987). Comparison of cortical and subcortical lesions in the production of post-stroke mood disorders. *Brain*, **110**, 1045–1059.

Stefurak, T. L., New, P., Mahurin, R. K. *et al.* (2001). Response specific regional metabolic changes with fluoxetine treatment in depressed Parkinson's patients. *Movement Disorders*, **16**, S39.

Stenager, E. N., & Stenager, E. (1992). Suicide and patients with neurologic disease. *Archives of Neurology*, **49**, 1296–1303.

Tekin, S., & Cummings, J. L. (2002). Frontal-subcortical neuronal circuits and clinical neuropsychiatry: an update. *Journal of Psychosomatic Research*, **53**, 647–654.

Wing, J. K., & Brown, G. W. (1970). *Institutionalism and Schizophrenia*. Cambridge, UK: Cambridge University Press.

Wolf, J. K., Santana, H. B., & Thorpy, M. (1979). Treatment of emotional incontinence with levodopa. *Neurology*, **29**, 1435–1436.

13

Anosognosia and the process and outcome of neurorehabilitation

George P. Prigatano

Introduction

In the first edition of this book, the chapter on impaired self-awareness (ISA or anosognosia) (Prigatano, 1999a) also included a discussion on how ISA and disturbances of motivation must be addressed in neurorehabilitation. It was noted at that time: "motivation may improve level of performance on specific tasks, without necessarily improving underlying 'capacity' or 'skill.'" (p. 246); "impaired self-awareness can lead to a passive (non-engaging) approach to cognitive rehabilitation and, at times, to clear resistance to such activities" (p. 247); and that "facilitating recovery of impaired self-awareness via a variety of cognitive and interpersonal tasks may aid the process and outcome of neuropsychological rehabilitation, but the data are sparse" (p. 242).

This updated/revised chapter will specifically address in more detail the latter observation/claim. It will also address, in light of further evidence, the notion that improving performance on a specific task (e.g., improving self-monitoring on a behavioral task) may not actually alter the underlying capacity of self-awareness in a person with severe traumatic brain injury (TBI).

The focus of this chapter will be to provide a summary of current information that will potentially aid the practicing clinician in the rehabilitation of patients who show frank anosognosia and/or its residuals several months, and at times years, post brain disease/disorder. This chapter will not discuss the growing literature on anosognosia for dementia of the Alzheimer's type (DAT), or the neuroimaging correlates of anosognosia, denial, repression and self-awareness (e.g., Johnson *et al.*, 2002; Schmitz *et al.*, 2006). Theoretical papers that deal with the nature of consciousness (e.g., Zeman, 2001; see entire issue of *Cortex*, 2005, **41**; Revonsuo, 2006) are beyond the scope of this paper, as are more recent discussions of theoretical concerns as to when anosognosia does or does not appear in a clinical condition (e.g., Cosentino & Stern, 2005). Selected studies in these areas, however, will be referenced when they have relevance for rehabilitation of anosognostic patients.

Anosognosia: clinical and historical observations

- Anosognosia has been reported in a variety of brain disorders.
- Anosognosia appears to negatively impact the process and outcome of neurorehabilitation.

The term "anosognosia" was first used by Babinski (1914, see Critchley, 1953, p. 231) to describe the striking phenomenon of a hemiplegic patient who was apparently not aware of his disability. Since that time, the term has been used to refer "to the clinical phenomenon in which a brain dysfunctional patient does not appear to be aware of impaired neurological or neuropsychological functioning which is obvious to the clinician and other reasonably attentive individuals. The lack of awareness appears specific to individual deficits and cannot be accounted

Cognitive Neurorehabilitation, Second Edition: Evidence and Application, ed. Donald T. Stuss, Gordon Winocur and Ian H. Robertson. Published by Cambridge University Press. © Cambridge University Press 2008.

for by hypoarousal or widespread cognitive impairments" (Prigatano, 1996a, pp. 80–81). Critchley (1953) reminds us that "From a strictly etymological point of view, the term 'anosognosia' indicates a lack of awareness of the existence of *disease*" (p. 231).

While anosognosia was first reported for hemiplegia in patients with cerebrovascular accidents (CVAs), it has been noted in a wide variety of neurological conditions. It has been specifically reported in patients with central (cortical-limbic) blindness (Anton, 1896; see Prigatano & Schachter, 1991), patients with hemianopias and hemi-inattention or "neglect" (Bisiach & Geminiani, 1991), aphasia (Rubens & Garrett, 1991), central (cortical-limbic) hearing loss (Roeser & Daly, 1974), memory disorders (McGlynn & Kaszniak, 1991; Schachter, 1991), disorders of planning and social judgment (i.e., frontal lobe syndromes) (see Prigatano, 1999a), and movement disorders (Leritz *et al.*, 2004).

Frank anosognosia is often observed during the early stages following an abrupt brain disorder (such as CVA), and can rapidly change with the passage of time. This often leads to different impressions regarding the underlying nature of the anosognosia. Also, different syndromes of ISA have been identified after various brain disorders and again, change with time as do aphasic syndromes (Prigatano, 1999b).

The relative importance of ISA/anosognosia for the process and outcome of neurorehabilitation was perhaps first recognised in contemporary times when attempts were made to help post-acute, young adult TBI patients return to work using a holistic and neuropsychological model of rehabilitation (Prigatano *et al.*, 1984, 1986). It was noted that impaired self-awareness in these post-acute patients appeared to be a significant barrier to work re-entry (Prigatano *et al.*, 1984) and that methods of cognitive retraining and psychotherapy were employed conjointly to help facilitate awareness and acceptance of residual neuropsychological impairments. Relatively "accurate" self-awareness after TBI was clinically noted to relate to "successful outcome" (Prigatano, 1991). Since that time, several studies have appeared which both directly and indirectly support this clinical observation (Klonoff *et al.*, 2001; Malec & DeGiorgio, 2002; Prigatano, 2005; Sarajuuri *et al.*, 2005; Schöenberger *et al.*, 2006b; Sherer *et al.*, 1998).

Neurorehabilitation: process and outcome

- Impaired self-awareness impacts rehabilitation outcomes in a variety of ways.
- A number of possible rehabilitation methods may be employed to increase self-awareness following TBI.
- Identifying and addressing the residuals of anosognosia (impaired self-awareness) may enhance the process as well as outcome of neurorehabilitation.

Neurorehabilitation refers to a variety of activities aimed at improving a patient's physical, cognitive, behavioral and emotional-motivational functioning following virtually any injury to the central nervous system (brain, brainstem, spinal cord). Since these activities require the active, as well as passive involvement of the patient (and frequently family), the patient's subjective appraisal of their own clinical condition and the patient's personal view of the usefulness of any given exercise or treatment strategy will clearly influence what happens in neurorehabilitation (i.e., the process). A broader and perhaps more important question is how the patient's self-appraisal of their clinical condition relates to rehabilitation outcome. Does relatively accurate self-awareness regarding one's clinical condition predict return to work and the ability to sustain employment after brain injury? Does it relate to having less psychiatric disability (e.g., anxiety, depression, avoidance of paranoid states) several weeks or months post-injury? Is it predictive of a person's capacity to sustain inter-personal relationships with less distress for the caregivers (which includes family, physician and rehabilitative staff)? Finally, does improving ISA result in less utilization of healthcare resources in the future (Prigatano & Pliskin, 2003)? These are important questions that need to be answered for the justification of paying for neurorehabilitative services that focus, at least in part, on the problems produced or associated with anosognosia.

There is, however, a third question which has direct scientific and ethical implications. Do we have rehabilitation methods that can improve self-awareness after brain injury? Related to this question are several other questions. Under what circumstances should these methods be applied? Who is likely to benefit from "awareness training" and who will likely not benefit? How should we scientifically study the problems that anosognosia pose for neurorehabilitation? If we cannot "treat" ISA, can we learn to manage patients with ISA in a manner that improves outcome? What would be convincing scientific evidence that our methods are indeed effective?

There are also a variety of ethical questions associated with these scientific issues. Can anyone attempt to retrain or manage ISA in brain-dysfunctional patients? Does it require the treating clinician/rehabilitationist to have a specific level of knowledge in neuropsychology and clinical psychology so that problems of ISA can be identified and separated, for example, from problems with denial? What is the role of psychiatry and particularly psychotherapy in the treatment of ISA patients? What type of disclosure statements should treating clinicians make, at least to patients' families, regarding their level of skill and knowledge in this area? Before addressing some of these questions, studies that deal with the impact of anosognosia on neurorehabilitation outcome will be considered.

Anosognosia and neurorehabilitation outcome

- The role of anosognosia in impacting rehabilitation outcome is complex and not well understood.
- Empirical studies presently demonstrate that TBI and stroke patients who are initially anosognostic are less independent and less likely to be employed following neurorehabilitation.

Anosognosia after cerebrovascular accidents (CVAs) has been estimated to occur in about 30% of all patients with motor deficit (Bisiach *et al.*, 1986; Starkstein *et al.*, 1992). In a large population study in Denmark, Pedersen *et al.* (1996) reported "the frequency of anosognosia was 21% on acute admission. The lesion was located in the right hemisphere in 81% of the patients" (p. 243).

The rehabilitation outcome of these patients is only partially understood. Patients with anosognosia or "anosognostic phenomenon" present with significant cognitive and affective disturbances. Sensory loss with visual field deficits are also common (Cutting, 1978). Therefore, the specific contribution of impaired awareness is often difficult to determine, since it occurs in the context of a constellation of other symptoms. This being as it is, Pedersen *et al.* (1996) noted that "the presence of anosognosia per se predicted 11.5 points less in discharge Barthel Index (BI), increased likelihood of death during hospital stay by a factor of 4.4, and reduced the likelihood of discharge to independent living in survivors by 0.43" (p. 243).

Jehkonen *et al.* (2000) followed 57 patients with right hemisphere stroke. Patients were examined during the first 10 days of onset and again at 3 months and 12 months post onset of CVA. None of the patients were unaware of their deficits at 12 month follow-up. Those patients who were initially anosognostic had poorer functional outcome compared with patients who were not initially anosognostic.

Prigatano & Wong (1999) evaluated, among other cognitive skills, the capacity of the patient to accurately predict their memory performance on a screening test (one possible index of self-awareness of memory skills). Ninety-five patients were studied (58 had CVAs or 61.05% of the sample). These investigators demonstrated that the ability of the patient to predict how many of three (3) words they could recall with distraction clearly was related to achieving rehabilitation goals. As Figure 13.1 illustrates, when patients are admitted to a neurorehabilitation unit, they are not generally very accurate in predicting their memory performance. However, those patients who become accurate in predicting their memory performance have a

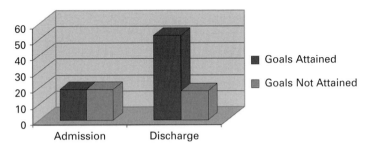

Figure 13.1. Percentage of brain-dysfunctional patients who could accurately predict their verbal memory performance at admission and discharge from acute inpatient neurorehabilitation. At time of discharge, accurate prediction of memory performance (i.e., good awareness) was associated with a greater likelihood of obtaining rehabilitation goals. (Adapted from Prigatano & Wong, 1999 with permission.)

greater likelihood of achieving rehabilitation goals compared with those patients who are not able to accurately predict their memory performance.

Anosognosia and unilateral neglect are frequently related, but have been shown to be separate entities (Bisiach *et al.*, 1986). Perani *et al.* (1993) reported on two patients who also demonstrated neglect following right hemisphere CVA. Both patients had lesions that were demonstrated on computerized tomography (CT) involving the right hemisphere. However, positron emission tomography (PET) studies on both patients revealed hypometabolic activity both in the affected hemisphere (i.e., the right hemisphere) and the so-called nonaffected (left) hemisphere. Interestingly, the patient who recovered from neglect showed increased metabolic activity in the so-called nonaffected hemisphere (i.e., the left hemisphere). The patient who did not recover from neglect showed persistent, chronic hypometabolic activity in both cerebral hemispheres for unexplained reasons. Personal communication with the senior author also indicated that this latter patient continued to show prolonged anosognosia for his hemi-inattention or neglect. These findings suggest that bilateral cerebral dysfunction may be necessary when there is permanent anosognosia, even though CT scans of the brain may only show a unilateral lesion (see Prigatano, 1999b for further discussion of this point). Second, functional outcome in patients who have neglect may be worse if anosognosia is also present.

Gialanella *et al.* (2005) specifically evaluated this latter possibility. Thirty patients with left hemiplegia secondary to stroke were studied. Fifteen patients evidenced neglect (N) only and 15 patients evidenced both neglect and anosognosia (group N+A). Interestingly, at admission patients with N+A had worse performance on the Wechsler Adult Intelligence Scale (WAIS) than the patients with only N. At discharge, that is following rehabilitation, the Functional Independence Measure (FIM) scores were consistently lower for *both* cognitive and motor scores in the N+A group versus the N group. It was argued that rehabilitation prognosis of stroke patients with neglect is worse if anosognosia is also present.

While frank anosognosia for hemiplegia and/or neglect are striking phenomena, and relatively easy to record and measure, the residuals of other forms of anosognosia are not as easily measured. This is especially true in patients who suffer severe traumatic brain injury (TBI) and are rendered unconscious for a prolonged period of time. Upon returning to consciousness (i.e., being able to verbally respond to the environment, showing improved orientation to the environment, etc.) clinicians may mistakenly think that the patient's self-awareness has returned back to normal, particularly as the period of post-traumatic amnesia (PTA) resolves. A few studies suggest that early signs of impaired awareness in TBI patients, even when they do not show frank anosognosia, are

Table 13.1. Anosognosia and rehabilitation outcome

Issue	Reference
The presence of anosognosia results in worse rehabilitation outcome following stroke.	Pedersen *et al.* (1996), Jehkonen *et al.* (2000)
Rehabilitation prognosis of stroke patients with neglect is worse if anosognosia is also present.	Gialanella *et al.* (2005)
Impaired self-awareness (ISA) for traumatic brain injury (TBI) patients is associated with worse rehabilitation outcome when these disturbances exist after the period of post-traumatic amnesia (PTA).	Prigatano *et al.* (1984), Prigatano (1999b), Sherer *et al.* (1998, 2003)

related to poor rehabilitation outcome after PTA resolves. Sherer *et al.* (2003), using the Awareness Questionnaire, studied impaired self-awareness in 129 acute TBI patients who had emerged from PTA. Early impaired self-awareness was predictive of poor employability at time of discharge, accounting for 20% of the variability in employability status.

Sherer *et al.* (1998) also studied the role of impaired awareness after TBI in the post-acute phase, and how it related to employment status. Using a seven-factor model for predicting employability in TBI patients who had undergone a neuropsychological rehabilitation program, measures of impaired self-awareness accounted for 30% of the variability of employment. These observations supported the earlier clinical claims that impaired self-awareness was related to neuropsychological rehabilitation outcome in TBI patients (Prigatano, 1991; Prigatano *et al.*, 1984). These studies suggest that frank anosognosia, as well as subtle forms of impaired awareness during both the acute and post-acute phases following brain injury, relate to rehabilitation outcome. Table 13.1. summarizes these findings.

Anosognosia and the process of neurorehabilitation

- Anosognosia results in poor rehabilitation compliance.
- Anosognosia is negatively associated with the establishment of a working alliance with therapists.
- Strong working alliance is associated with better rehabilitation outcome in patients with TBI.

While studies of anosognosia and rehabilitation outcome after CVA are available, no studies could be located that address the question of whether or not improved self-awareness during rehabilitation of these patients influenced the process of rehabilitation. This is unfortunate, given the Hochstenback *et al.* (2005) finding that patients with CVA underestimate numerous cognitive and behavioral difficulties several weeks and months post stroke. This phenomenon has been reported in TBI patients for a number of years (see Prigatano, 1999b).

Three studies have recently appeared which specifically address the question of whether or not the presence of anosognosia, or impaired self-awareness, influences the process of neurorehabilitation after TBI. These studies, however, approach the problem from different perspectives. Trahan *et al.* (2006) studied the relationship between impaired awareness of deficit (IAD) and treatment adherence in 24 persons with moderate to severe TBI and 16 persons with traumatic spinal cord injury (SCI) admitted to an inpatient neurorehabilitation unit. They replicated the previous observations of Fischer *et al.* (2004), Prigatano (1996b), and Prigatano *et al.* (1990), that TBI patients specifically have difficulties in being aware of their inter-personal, affective and cognitive difficulties. They noted that failure to adequately comply with treatment was related to poor self-awareness in these domains, with the effect being most pronounced for TBI patients. This paper suggests that if one could improve awareness during the acute stages of neurorehabilitation, compliance with treatment might, in fact, improve.

Table 13.2. Anosognosia and rehabilitation process

Issue	Reference
Adherence to rehabilitation or treatment activities is worse in traumatic brain injury (TBI) patients with impaired self-awareness (ISA).	Trahan *et al.* (2006), Schönberger *et al.* (2006a)
Good working alliance relates to better treatment compliance.	Schönberger *et al.* (2006a)
Good working alliance with the treatment team during rehabilitation is associated with better rehabilitation outcome (i.e., increased productivity).	Prigatano *et al.* (1994), Klonoff *et al.* (2001), Schönberger *et al.* (2006b)
ISA is not easily changed during the process of neurorehabilitation.	Schönberger *et al.* (2006b)

Schönberger *et al.* (2006a) evaluated the relationship of working alliance to patient compliance in post-acute TBI and CVA patients who were undergoing a holistic neuropsychological rehabilitation program. They replicated the earlier findings of Prigatano *et al.* (1994) and Klonoff *et al.* (2001) that the working alliance was predictive of higher frequency of employment post rehabilitation. While working alliance and patient compliance to a rehabilitation program are often related, they are dynamic and constantly changing. Schönberger *et al.* (2006a) noted that some patients who did not have a good working alliance with a given therapist, still were compliant with treatment procedures. This is an important observation and suggests that while the two dimensions (working alliance and patient compliance) are related, they are not, in fact, the same thing.

This leads to the question of how is the degree of self-awareness of the patient specifically related to working alliance and compliance during the process of neurorehabilitation? Schönberger *et al.* (2006b) examined the development and interaction of the therapeutic alliance, patient compliance and ISA, during the process of a holistic neuropsychological rehabilitation program. They report that the patients' self-awareness was clearly related to compliance, with greater self-awareness associated with compliance. They noted that the patients' "emotional bond" with the therapist added more to the prediction of the clients' awareness, as did the actual localization of a brain injury (p. 445). While they developed mathematical models for relating

how compliance, awareness and working alliance may be associated, they report one sobering finding. Brain dysfunctional patients' self-awareness scores generally did not change much during the course of a holistic neuropsychological rehabilitation program (see Table 13.2). This observation begs the question of whether or not there are any therapies that are available that can substantially reduce ISA following severe TBI or any other brain disorder.

Treatment studies of impaired self-awareness after TBI

- The treatment and/or management of patients with anosognosia is best achieved by a combination of cognitive rehabilitation and psychotherapeutic treatments.
- Behavioral approaches may help the patients be more vigilant about their errors, but not necessarily improve ISA.

While there is a growing consensus that impaired self-awareness after TBI is related to treatment outcome, especially as it relates to employability after TBI (see Prigatano, 1999b), the questions arise: Can you treat this disorder? Are there methods for improving self-awareness after severe TBI?

Ownsworth *et al.* (2006) recently summarized different models for understanding the phenomenon of self-awareness and self-regulation (including error detection). Using primarily a cognitive neuropsychological model which incorporates the importance of patient motivation and the value of environmental supports and social cues for potentially improving self-awareness, they present a detailed case study of a training program to help improve error detection and self-awareness in a severely injured person with TBI, 4 years post trauma. The awareness and error detection training program focused, in part, on teaching the patient to detect errors in cooking, an area which he showed interest in and was highly motivated to improve. A systematic prompting procedure was used with appropriate reinforcement. They report that such a cognitive–behavioral approach improved performance in the reduction of errors, but did not improve self-awareness in this patient. This is potentially a very important finding and it relates to a point made in the first edition of this chapter. Cognitive–behavioral approaches may help a patient improve their performance in everyday life, but it does not necessarily influence their underlying capacity of self-awareness (i.e., to have an accurate phenomenological experience of one's self). This is a complicated psychological function that may not be easily changed by existing training programs that put an emphasis on behavior only.

Cheng & Man (2006) also attempted to improve self-awareness in patients with TBI using an "Awareness Intervention Programme" or AIP. Patients were randomly assigned to two conditions: AIP versus a conventional rehabilitation program which incorporated many activities of traditional occupational therapy. The AIP included teaching patients about the nature of their brain injuries, helping patients monitor their actual performance on paper and pencil tasks, and compare their performance with what they said they would actually do. It also engaged patients in practical goal-setting exercises. The training was "delivered on an individual basis for two sessions a day, 5 days a week for 4 weeks" (p. 624). While there was evidence that the group that received AIP showed greater self-awareness than the traditionally treated patient at the end of treatment, it was not paralleled with any greater changes in functional outcome. That is, reduction in impaired awareness scores did not translate into higher FIM scores or performance on the Lawton IADL scale. The findings of this study suggest that one may be able to improve self-awareness with appropriate training, but how the patient utilizes this knowledge may greatly impact the degree to which they are functionally more independent.

In both the Cheng & Man (2006) and the Ownsworth et al. (2006) studies, there was no discussion on how the emotional relationship between the therapist and the patient did or did not impact self-awareness and treatment outcomes. It has been argued that both cognitive retraining (for improving self-awareness) and psychotherapy (for improving self-awareness and reducing denial) are both necessary to help the patient obtain a better level of insight into themselves and to make better choices in life (Prigatano, 1999a). Better choices often result in improved rehabilitation outcomes (Prigatano, 1999b). Earlier work of Prigatano et al. (1984) demonstrated that patients showed greater productivity when properly treated within the context of a holistic neuropsychological rehabilitation program that assisted patients in realistically appraising their abilities and accepting limitations. This basic finding was later replicated by Prigatano et al. (1994) and Klonoff et al. (2001). A recent paper from Finland utilising a holistic approach has reported similar findings (Sarajuuri et al., 2005).

When self-awareness improves after various types of brain injury, it appears to be a result of many factors. From a treatment perspective, it appears that a combination of both individual and group exercises aimed at improving self-awareness within the context of a psychotherapeutic environment, seems to provide the best outcome, although no systematic studies have actually been done in this area.

Clinically, it appears that the quality of the working alliance between the patient and therapist is related to the willingness of the patient to utilize compensation techniques and to be guided to make rehabilitation choices that ultimately are in their best interest. Furthermore, it also appears that the "emotional bond" between the therapist and the patient is the basis of the working alliance.

Table 13.3. Treatment studies on impaired self-awareness after traumatic brain injury

Issue	Reference
While you can improve error detection (i.e., increased self-monitoring) after severe traumatic brain injury (TBI) via behavioral methods, it does not appear to translate to overall improved self-awareness in the patient.	Ownsworth *et al.* (2006)
Group exercises for improving self-awareness after TBI may not directly translate into better functional outcomes.	Cheng & Man (2006)
A good working alliance between the patient and the rehabilitation team often results in better choices and at times, improved self-awareness. In turn, these two factors seem to result in better rehabilitation outcome.	No studies have been conducted to date to empirically evaluate this clinical proposition.

While this observation has been repeatedly observed in holistic neuropsychological rehabilitation programs (Prigatano, 1999b), no systematic studies have been conducted to demonstrate this clinical proposition. Table 13.3 summarizes findings of treatment efficacy studies for ISA after TBI.

Treatment considerations with anosognostic patients

- Improved treatments for anosognosia will depend on a better theoretical understanding of the complexity of this phenomenon in different patient groups.
- It is important to differentiate impaired self-awareness from denial of disability.

Improved treatments for anosognostic patients will most likely depend on a better theoretical understanding of this complex phenomenon and its heterogenous features (Bisiach & Geminiani, 1991). While a standardized or uniform method of assessing anosognosia is desirable (Orfei *et al.*, 2007), Bisiach & Geminiani (1991) remind us that "anosognosia deserves assessment tailored to each individual case, comprising faithful records of all relevant spontaneous behavior as well as of that instigated by the examiner's queries, the limits to which are set only by the examiner's inventiveness and the patient's mood and intelligence" (p. 20). Detailed individual case studies provide important sources of information regarding the complexity of the phenomenon and what may be contributing factors to different features of anosognosia (Cutting, 1978). For example, Ramachandran (1994) temporarily reduced anosognosia for left hemiplegia in a 76-year-old woman with a right hemisphere stroke via a left ear caloric stimulation test. Based on the patient's responses to questions he and his colleagues asked both before and after caloric stimulation, he inferred that the patient in fact had some awareness of her paralysis and anosognosia appeared to be a form of denial.

Separating ISA from denial of disability (DD) is indeed an important task, but one that has several difficulties (Prigatano & Klonoff, 1997). Denial implies that some conflict or threatening event is experienced by the individual, but is blocked from reaching conscious awareness. When confronted with information that tends to threaten this defensive system, the individual can become distressed and at times, aggressive and argumentative. Impaired self-awareness implies that there is no conflict that the individual is experiencing, but rather they simply are deprived of a phenomenological representation of their actual functional capacity following brain injury. Impaired self-awareness often is associated with different affective responses than seen in denial (for example, indifference or lack of concern regarding limitations as they are pointed out).

Bilateral cerebral dysfunction may be necessary to produce a "complete" syndrome of ISA, or anosognosia. Case studies by Perani *et al.* (1993) remind us that even when there is only a unilateral lesion detected by structural imaging of the brain, there may well be bilateral cerebral dysfunction as detected by dynamic brain studies such as PET. When the anosognostic patient shows improvement, there is tentative evidence that the so-called unaffected hemisphere may return to normal functioning. It has been argued that this may result in a "partial" syndrome of impaired self-awareness (Prigatano, 1999b).

Partial syndromes of ISA seem to exist in many patients following the acute phase of their brain injury. Patients appear to have partial or limited knowledge as to their disability/impairments. Some of these patients cope with this partial knowledge in a straightforward, nondefensive way. Others may be overwhelmed with their limitations and cope with the partial knowledge in a defensive way. When a defensive manner of coping is utilized, the term "denial" is often applied to describe the patient's condition. This conceptualization suggests that many post-acute brain dysfunctional patients may show a combination of ISA and defensive denial. It is often the responsibility of the clinician to help separate out how these two dimensions interact in a given patient to produce the symptom picture. This can lead to a better understanding of how to approach the patient in the context of neuro-rehabilitation (Prigatano, 1999b). Detailed case studies of patients with partial syndromes of ISA, with and without defensive methods of coping, may well provide guidelines for future treatment in this area.

In addition to these theoretical considerations, Prigatano & Johnson (2003) have suggested that there may be "three vectors of consciousness" that can be disturbed after various forms of brain dysfunction. They argue, following Zeman's (2001) paper, that the term consciousness has been used in three ways. First, it refers to the level of arousal that exists in a patient along the sleep-wake continuum. Second, the term consciousness refers to one's actual phenomenological experience of themselves in the here and now. The third way in which the term consciousness is used refers to the capacity of the individual to be conscious of another person's subjective state. Prigatano & Johnson (2003) argue that these dimensions of consciousness interact and produce different manifestations of ISA which helps account for the great variability that is seen clinically in anosognostic patients.

Treatment suggestions for dealing with each type of impaired awareness are briefly suggested by Prigatano & Johnson (2003). Patients who have a disturbance in the arousal dimension might best be helped by increasing arousal through behavioral and pharmacological methods. Robertson & Halligan (1999) have argued that this approach may be helpful in reducing neglect following CVA.

Disturbances in the second "vector of consciousness," which refers to one's personal experience of one's strengths and limitations in the here and now, may best be treated within the context of holistic neuropsychological rehabilitation program. These programs focus both on cognitive and personality disturbances, and emphasize a psychotherapeutic approach in helping the patients deal with partial knowledge when there are defensive methods of coping with that partial information.

Disturbances of the third "vector of consciousness" are more difficult to understand and to treat. At the present time, there is no clear clinical approach to dealing with this type of ISA. Unfortunately, patients who have severe ISA and who do not improve with time may go on to develop significant psychiatric difficulties including paranoid ideation (Prigatano, 1988).

Measuring ISA in outcome and process neurorehabilitation studies

- Functional magnetic resonance imaging (fMRI) studies which relate dynamic brain changes to behavioral measures of ISA may be a useful source for determining how ISA changes during the rehabilitation process and how it influences rehabilitation outcome.

A major challenge for researchers and clinicians treating patients with ISA is to find an efficient and

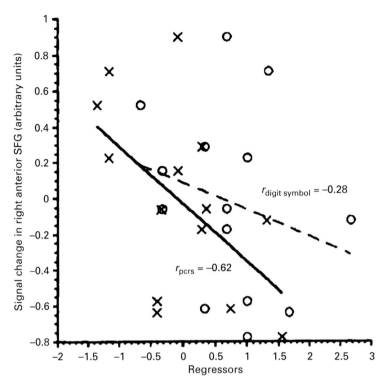

Figure 13.2. Scatter plot of mean-centered regressors (x-axis) against signal change (y-axis) in the right superior frontal gyrus (SFG) cluster. Regressors: (1) PCRS disparity scores (solid regression line; X symbols), (2) digit symbol scaled scores (dashed regression line; O symbols). Reprinted with permission from Schmitz *et al.* (2006).

effective method of evaluating ISA in patients and to relate these measures to outcome and process variables. While the studies reviewed in this chapter provide some interesting examples, a method that has not been utilized is one in which ISA measures are directly related to brain-imaging findings. This could greatly advance the field.

Neuropsychological rehabilitation with patients with moderate to severe TBI resulted in the development of the Patient Competency Rating Scale (PCRS; see Prigatano *et al.*, 1986). It was developed as an adjunct to the clinical interview and allowed for an estimation of the degree to which patients with TBI underestimated various cognitive and behavioral limitations. The method has proven useful in a variety of settings (see Prigatano, 2005).

Recently Schmitz *et al.* (2006) examined 20 TBI patients who were 8–12 weeks post-traumatic brain

injury. Their average admitting Glasgow Coma Scale (GCS) score in the Emergency Room was 10.9 (S.D. = 2.8). Using the PCRS, they identified those patients who showed ISA. They went on to show that poor self-awareness as reflected by PCRS discrepancy scores (i.e., patient vs. relative's ratings of competency) were related to signal change in the right superior frontal gyrus (SFG). Scores on the Digit Symbol subtest of the WAIS-III, which is a marker of severity of neurocognitive changes associated with TBI (Dikmen *et al.*, 1995), did not show a strong relationship with such change (see Figure 13.2). These findings suggest that the fMRI signal changes in the SFG were specifically related to degree of ISA in TBI patients and were not just reflective of degree of neurocognitive impairment.

It would be interesting to determine whether or not changes of ISA, as measured by PCRS discrepancy scores, would also be associated with changes of brain activation in TBI patients before and after neurorehabilitation as well as while they are undergoing neurorehabilitation. Theoretically, those patients who showed reduced ISA might well show quantitative and functional MRI changes not found in individuals who do not show a decrease in ISA. Future studies might wish, therefore, to combine reliable measures of assessing ISA with quantitative and functional MRI brain changes.

A return to some of the unanswered questions

Do we have rehabilitation methods that can substantially improve ISA? Presently there is not strong evidence that existing methods in and of themselves can achieve this goal. Yet, it is well recognized that some patients indeed show reduction of ISA with time and/or treatment. Identifying who those patients are and why certain treatments were seemingly effective is very much needed. What can be said with some clinical confidence is that the quality of the working alliance between the patient and their therapist relates to patients' compliance with treatment during rehabilitation (a process variable). It also appears to relate to rehabilitation outcome (for example, the employment status of the individual). The findings of Klonoff *et al.* (2001), Prigatano *et al.* (1986, 1994), Sarajuuri *et al.* (2005), Schöenberger *et al.* (2006a, 2006b), and Trahan *et al.* (2006) support this conclusion. Thus, while we cannot always "treat" ISA using present methods, there is evidence that we can manage this problem effectively and when this occurs, it leads to better rehabilitation outcomes (Prigatano, 1999b).

Cost-effectiveness studies on neuropsychological rehabilitation programs that specifically address ISA and defensive denial have not been done. This needs to be conducted in order to demonstrate the benefits of appropriately diagnosing and managing ISA following various brain disorders.

Not every clinician has been adequately trained to evaluate ISA and defensive denial and to work with

it effectively. As noted elsewhere (Prigatano, 1999b), the misunderstanding, and therefore the mismanagement, of these disturbances leads to poor rehabilitation outcome. It is crucial, therefore, that clinicians in this field be adequately trained to evaluate and understand these interacting dimensions of disturbances of consciousness. This includes training in neuropsychology and clinical psychology, with an understanding of various concepts and findings in psychiatry and neurology. A thorough understanding of psychodynamic principles (as described by Freud and Jung; see Prigatano, 1999b) is helpful in understanding denial mechanisms and how to manage them.

The most convincing way to demonstrate the cost-effectiveness of neurorehabilitation programs that properly evaluate and manage ISA and defensive denial requires long-term follow-up studies. It is predicted that those individuals who successfully undergo holistic neuropsychological rehabilitation programs of the type described by Prigatano *et al.* (1986) will show a greater percentage of sustained productivity several years post brain injury, less psychiatric morbidity, and report greater meaning to their life than those individuals who have not received such rehabilitation. While these studies require some form of matched-controls, it is doubtful that a truly randomized control study can be conducted. Each patient requires fairly individualised interventions when undergoing psychotherapy after brain injury.

A combination of long-term matched-control follow-up studies with detailed individual case analyses will provide a greater understanding of how anosognosia changes with time, how defensive methods of coping may interact with residuals of impaired awareness, and how various forms of rehabilitation may help the patient understand and manage those disturbances (Prigatano, 2002). Incorporating neuroimaging techniques which help identify unique brain changes associated with anosognosia and its various forms of measurement will obviously be helpful in this venture (see Schmitz *et al.*, 2006).

ACKNOWLEDGMENTS

Funding from the Newsome Foundation to the author provided time to prepare this manuscript. The author would also like to acknowledge Mary Henry for her secretarial skills in preparing this manuscript and Jennifer Gray for her critical review of various drafts of this paper.

REFERENCES

Anton, G. (1896). Blindheit nach beiderseitiger Gehirnerkrankung mit Verlust der Orienterung in Raume. *Mitteil. Vereines Arzte Steirmark*, **33**, 41–46.

Bisiach, E., & Geminiani, G. (1991). Anosognosia related to hemiplegia and hemianopia. In G. P. Prigatano & D. L. Schacter (Eds.), *Awareness of Deficit after Brain Injury: Clinical and Theoretical Issues* (pp. 17–39). New York, NY: Oxford University Press.

Bisiach, E., Vallar, G., Perani, D., Papagno, C., & Berti, A. (1986). Unawareness of disease following lesions of the right hemisphere: anosognosia for hemiplegia and anosognosia for hemianopia. *Neuropsychologia*, **24**, 471–482.

Cheng, S. K. W., & Man, D. W. K. (2006). Management of impaired self-awareness in persons with traumatic brain injury. *Brain Injury*, **20**, 621–628.

Constentino, S., & Stern, Y. (2005). Metacognitive theory and assessment in dementia: do we recognize our areas of weakness? *Journal of the International Neuropsychological Society*, **11**, 910–919.

Critchley, M. (1953). *The Parietal Lobes*. London, UK: Edward Arnold.

Cutting, J. (1978). Study of anosognosia. *Journal of Neurology, Neurosurgery and Psychiatry*, **41**, 548–555.

Dikmen, S., Machamer, J. E., Winn, H. R., & Temkin, N. R. (1995). Neuropsychological outcome at 1-year post head injury. *Neuropsychology*, **9**, 80–90.

Fischer, S., Trexler, L. E., & Gauggel, S. (2004). Awareness of activity limitations and prediction of performance in patients with brain injuries and orthopedic disorders. *Journal of the International Neuropsychological Society*, **10**, 190–199.

Gialanella, B., Monguzzi, V., Santoro, R., & Rocchi, S. (2005). Functional recovery after hemiplegia in patients with neglect: the rehabilitative role of anosognosia. *Stroke*, **36**, 2687–2690.

Hochstenback, J., Prigatano, G. P., & Mulder, T. (2005). Patients' and relatives' reports of disturbances 9 months after stroke: subjective changes in physical functioning, cognition, emotion, and behavior. *Archives of Physical Medicine and Rehabilitation*, **86**, 1587–1593.

Jehkonen, M., Ahonen, J.-P., Dastidar, P., Laippala, P., & Vilkki, J. (2000). Unawareness of deficits after right hemisphere stroke: double-dissociations of anosognosias. *Acta Neurologica Scandinavica*, **102**, 378–384.

Johnson, S. C., Baxter, L. C., Wilder, L. S. *et al.* (2002). Neural correlates of self-reflection. *Brain*, **125**, 1808–1814.

Klonoff, P. S., Lamb, D. G., & Henderson, S. W. (2001). Outcomes from milieu-based neurorehabilitation at up to 11 years post-discharge. *Brain Injury*, **15**, 413–428.

Leritz, E., Loftis, C., Crucian, G., Friedman, W., & Bowers, D. (2004). Self-awareness of deficits in Parkinson disease. *The Clinical Neuropsychologist*, **18**, 352–361.

Malec, J. F., & DeGiorgio, L. (2002). Characteristics of successful and unsuccessful completers of 3 postacute brain injury rehabilitation pathways. *Archives of Physical Medicine and Rehabilitation*, **83**, 1759–1764.

McGlynn, S. M., & Kaszniak, A. W. (1991). Unawareness of deficits in dementia and schizophrenia. In G. P. Prigatano & D. L. Schacter (Eds.), *Awareness of Deficit after Brain Injury: Clinical and Theoretical Issues* (pp. 84–110). New York, NY: Oxford University Press.

Orfei, M. D., Robinson, R. G., Prigatano, G. P. *et al.* (2007). Anosognosia for hemiplegia after stroke is a multifaceted phenomenon: a systematic review of the literature. *Brain*, **130**, 3075–3090.

Ownsworth, T., Fleming, J., Desbois, J., Strong, J., & Kuipers, P. (2006). A metacognitive contextual intervention to enhance error awareness and functional outcome following traumatic brain injury: a single-case experimental design. *Journal of the International Neuropsychological Society*, **12**, 54–63.

Pedersen, P. N., Jorgensen, H. S., Nakayama, H., Raaschou, H. O., & Olsen, T. S. (1996). Frequency, determinants, and consequences of anosognosia in acute stroke. *Journal of Neurologic Rehabilitation*, **10**, 243–250.

Perani, D., Vallar, G., Paulesu, E., Alberoni, M., & Fazio, F. (1993). Left and right hemisphere contribution to recovery from neglect after right hemisphere damage – an {18F} FDG PET study of two cases. *Neuropsychologia*, **31**, 115–125.

Prigatano, G. P. (1988). Anosognosia, delusions, and altered self-awareness after brain injury. *Barrow Quarterly*, **4**, 40–48.

Prigatano, G. P. (1991). Disturbances of self-awareness of deficit after traumatic brain injury. In G. P. Prigatano & D. L. Schachter (Eds.), *Awareness of Deficit after Brain Injury: Clinical and Theoretical Issues* (pp. 111–126). New York, NY: Oxford University Press.

Prigatano, G. P. (1996a). Anosognosia. In J. G. Beaumont, P. M. Kenealy & M. J. L. Rogers (Eds.), *Blackwell Dictionary of Neuropsychology* (pp. 80–84). Oxford, UK: Blackwell Publishers.

Prigatano, G. P. (1996b). Behavioral limitations TBI patients tend to underestimate: a replication and extension to patients with lateralized cerebral dysfunction. *Clinical Neuropsychologist*, **10**, 191–201.

Prigatano, G. P. (1999a). Motivation and awareness in cognitive neurorehabilitation. In D. T. Stuss, G. Winocur & I. H. Robertson (Eds.), *Cognitive Neurorehabilitation* (pp. 240–251). Cambridge, UK: Cambridge University Press.

Prigatano, G. P. (1999b). *Principles of Neuropsychological Rehabilitation*. New York, NY: Oxford University Press.

Prigatano, G. P. (2002). Challenging dogma in neuropsychology and related disciplines. *Archives of Clinical Neuropsychology*, **18**, 811–825.

Prigatano, G. P. (2005). Disturbances of self-awareness and rehabilitation of patients with traumatic brain injury: A 20-year perspective. *Journal of Head Trauma Rehabilitation*, **20**, 19–29.

Prigatano, G. P., & Johnson, S. C. (2003). The three vectors of consciousness and their disturbances after brain injury. *Neuropsychological Rehabilitation*, **13**, 13–29.

Prigatano, G. P., & Klonoff, P. S. (1997). A clinician's rating scale for evaluating impaired self-awareness and denial of disability after brain injury. *Clinical Neuropsychologist*, **11**, 1–12.

Prigatano, G. P., & Pliskin, N. H. (2003). *Clinical Neuropsychology and Cost Outcomes Research: A Beginning*. New York, NY: Psychology Press.

Prigatano, G. P., & Schachter, D. L. (1991). *Awareness of Deficit after Brain Injury: Clinical and Theoretical Issues*. New York, NY: Oxford University Press.

Prigatano, G. P., & Wong, J. L. (1999). Cognitive and affective improvement in brain dysfunctional patients who achieve inpatient rehabilitation goals. *Archives of Physical Medicine and Rehabilitation*, **80**, 77–84.

Prigatano, G. P., Fordyce, D. J., Zeiner, H. K. *et al.* (1984). Neuropsychological rehabilitation after closed head injury in young adults. *Journal of Neurology, Neurosurgery and Psychiatry*, **47**, 505–513.

Prigatano, G. P., Fordyce, D. J., Zeiner, H. K. *et al.* (1986). *Neuropsychological Rehabilitation after Brain Injury*. Baltimore, MD: Johns Hopkins University Press.

Prigatano, G. P., Altman, I. M., & O'Brien, K. P. (1990). Behavioral limitations that traumatic-brain-injured patients tend to underestimate. *Clinical Neuropsychologist*, **4**, 163–176.

Prigatano, G. P., Klonoff, P. S., O'Brien, K. P. *et al.* (1994). Productivity after neuropsychologically oriented, milieu rehabilitation. *Journal of Head Trauma Rehabilitation*, **9**, 91–102.

Ramachandran, V. S. (1994). Phantom limbs, neglect syndromes, repressed memories, and Freudian psychology. *International Review of Neurobiology*, **37**, 291–372.

Revonsuo, A. (2006). *Inner Presence: Consciousness as a Biological Phenomenon*. Cambridge, MA: MIT Press.

Robertson, I. H., & Halligan, P. W. (1999). *Spatial Neglect: a Clinical Handbook for Diagnosis and Treatment*. East Sussex, UK: Psychology Press.

Roeser, R. J., & Daly, D. D. (1974). Auditory cortex disconnection associated with thalamic tumor: a case report. *Neurology*, **24**, 555–559.

Rubens, A. B., & Garrett, M. F. (1991). Anosognosia of linguistic deficits in patients with neurological deficits. In G. P. Prigatano & D. L. Schacter (Eds.), *Awareness of Deficit after Brain Injury: Clinical and Theoretical Issues* (pp. 40–52). New York, NY: Oxford University Press.

Sarajuuri, J. M., Kaipio, M. L., Koskinen, S. K. *et al.* (2005). Outcome of a comprehensive neurorehabilitation program for patients with traumatic brain injury. *Archives of Physical Medicine and Rehabilitation*, **86**, 2296–2302.

Schachter, D. L. (1991). Unawareness of deficit and unawareness of knowledge in patients with memory disorders. In G. P. Prigatano & D. L. Schacter (Eds.), *Awareness of Deficit after Brain Injury: Clinical and Theoretical Issues* (pp. 127–151). New York, NY: Oxford University Press.

Schmitz, T. W., Rowley, H. A., Kawahara, T. N., & Johnston, S. C. (2006). Neural correlates of self-evaluative accuracy after traumatic brain injury. *Neuropsychologia*, **44**, 762–773.

Schönberger, M., Humle, F., & Teasdale, T. W. (2006a). The development of the therapeutic working alliance, patients' awareness and their compliance during the process of brain injury rehabilitation. *Brain Injury*, **20**, 445–454.

Schönberger, M., Humle, F., Zeeman, P., & Teasdale, T. W. (2006b). Working alliance and patient compliance in brain injury rehabilitation and their relation to psychosocial outcome. *Neuropsychological Rehabilitation*, **16**, 298–314.

Sherer, M., Bergloff, P., Levin, E. *et al.* (1998). Impaired awareness and employment outcome after traumatic brain injury. *Journal of Head Trauma Rehabilitation*, **13**, 52–61.

Sherer, M., Hart, T., Nick, T. G. *et al.* (2003). Early impaired self-awareness after traumatic brain injury. *Archives of Physical Medicine and Rehabilitation*, **84**, 168–176.

Starkstein, S. E., Fedoroff, J. P., Price, T. R., Leiguarda, R., & Robinson, R. G. (1992). Anosognosia in patients with cerebrovascular lesions: a study of causative factors. *Stroke*, **23**, 1446–1453.

Trahan, E., Pépin, M., & Hopps, S. (2006). Impaired awareness of deficits and treatment adherence among people with traumatic brain injury or spinal cord injury. *Journal of Head Trauma Rehabilitation*, **21**, 226–235.

Zeman, A. (2001). Invited Review. Consciousness. *Brain*, **124**, 1263–1289.

14

Psychosocial considerations in cognitive rehabilitation

Deirdre R. Dawson and Gordon Winocur

Introduction

The ultimate goal of cognitive rehabilitation is that its recipients achieve satisfying and successful participation in a range of personally meaningful daily activities including working, leisure, relationships and so on. One of the objectives of this book is to identify ways that this can be achieved. In this chapter, we discuss the substantive role that psychosocial factors play in achieving these outcomes in people with cognitive impairments related to aging, stroke and/or traumatic brain injury. Each of these conditions produces cognitive changes and changes in day-to-day function. However, the relationship between the two (cognitive impairment and day-to-day function) is neither linear nor inevitable. These psychosocial, non-neurological, person factors have been considered as mediators, moderators and/or determinants of this relationship. Thus, in this chapter we consider the following questions:

- What are the important personal psychosocial factors to consider in relation to outcome and in relation to rehabilitation?
- How have these factors been addressed in rehabilitation (i.e., the literature on intervention)?
- What principles can we derive from the literature to guide clinical practice and future research?

It is important to be clear at the outset that we are not discussing psychosocial factors with psychosocial adjustment as the endpoint of interest. Rather, we are pursuing the notion that the psychosocial antecedents and response to cognitive impairment play a fundamental role in determining a range of functioning in day-to-day life. We believe that, to be most effective, personal psychosocial factors (e.g., coping behaviors) must be explicitly considered in the rehabilitation process to enable people to solve real-life problems and to function in their real-life roles and responsibilities. Environmental psychosocial factors that take the form of social support are also critical. However, the topic of social support is beyond the scope of this chapter and we refer the reader elsewhere for reviews of this material (Driver, 2005; Salter et al., 2006; Ylvisaker et al., 2003).

The idea of addressing personal psychosocial factors in cognitive rehabilitation is neither new nor unique (see, for example, Ben-Yishay, 1996) but only recently is it being widely discussed and utilized in the academic neuropsychological rehabilitation literature (e.g., Mateer et al., 2005; Ownsworth et al., 2006a; Rath et al., 2003; Rutterford & Wood, 2006; Yates, 2003). Some of this recent work suggests that greater progress could be made in understanding how psychosocial factors impact outcomes, if studies investigating outcomes following stroke and traumatic brain injury (TBI) were theoretically guided. The same could be argued for studies of well-being in aging in the presence of cognitive change. Thus, this

Cognitive Neurorehabilitation, Second Edition: Evidence and Application, ed. Donald T. Stuss, Gordon Winocur and Ian H. Robertson. Published by Cambridge University Press. © Cambridge University Press 2008.

chapter begins with a discussion of the models that inform us regarding the psychosocial factors of interest.

Theories and models for understanding the influence of psychosocial factors on outcomes

Numerous theoretical frameworks and models have attempted to identify the active ingredients in successful rehabilitation for people with cognitive impairments (see Walker *et al.*, 2004 for review). Some fall directly within a biomedical classification. Put simply, these are models that assume a direct relationship between brain dysfunction and behavior. Although these models have yielded considerable valuable knowledge, it is now widely accepted that participation outcomes also depend on "extra"-biological factors. As a starting point, we review the most widely used theory for understanding the psychological response to injury, aging and stroke – Lazarus and Folkman's cognitive-phenomenological theory of stress and adjustment (1984) – and consider how it has informed model development and research into the rehabilitation of people with cognitive impairments.

- Lazarus and Folkman's cognitive-phenomenological theory of stress and adjustment has been the most influential model for the investigation of psychosocial factors in cognitive rehabilitation.
- Based on this model, others have hypothesized that suboptimal outcomes, initially related to cognitive impairment, become even worse due to resultant self-limiting cognitive beliefs. In turn, these contribute to the selection of poor coping strategies.
- Whether these factors are mediators, moderators or direct determinants of outcome is unknown but it is clear their influence is significant.

Central to Lazarus and Folkman's (1984) theory is a relational view of stress stated as follows: "Psychological stress is a particular relationship between the person and the environment that is appraised by the person as taxing or exceeding his

or her resources and endangering his or her well-being" (p. 19). There are a number of key components to this theory that require explication. First, the theory has been modeled such that personal factors, environmental resources and situational factors are antecedents to psychosocial adjustment. Cognitive appraisal and coping are the two key processes that mediate the relationship between the antecedents and outcome. Cognitive appraisal refers to the evaluative process used to determine if an encounter or situation is irrelevant, benign-positive or stressful, and secondarily to evaluate what can be done about it. The coping process refers to efforts (cognitive and behavioral) directed at managing the internal or external demands appraised as exceeding or taxing the resources of the person. Severe illness and other more predictable losses associated with aging can be viewed as environmental situations antecedent to psychosocial adjustment.

This theoretical framework has been utilized and built upon in rehabilitation research related to many health conditions including stroke (Boynton De Sepulveda & Chang, 1994; Donnellan *et al.*, 2006), aging (Aldwin *et al.*, 1996; de Raedt & Ponjaert-Kirstoffersen, 2006), and TBI (Kendall & Terry, 1996). In the TBI literature, Kendall & Terry and Moore & Stambrook (1995) have developed more comprehensive models that draw on the work of Lazarus and Folkman. Kendall & Terry posited several modifications that include the necessity of considering premorbid psychosocial functioning and links between neurological factors and psychosocial adjustment. Further, they suggested that individuals' locus of control and self-efficacy beliefs, in particular, play an important role in their appraisal of difficulties and ability to cope with them. Moore & Stambrook based their model on the hypothesis that individuals who had sustained TBIs were at risk for developing self-limiting cognitive belief systems as they appraised the changes that resulted from the TBI. They further hypothesized that these self-limiting belief systems were characterized by an externalized locus of control, a helpless/hopeless attributional style and a poor choice of coping strategies. The similarities between the models are clear – both emphasize the appraisal and coping process and both maintain that locus of control is an important part of that appraisal. Further, Moore & Stambrook see externalized locus of control and a helpless/hopeless attributional style as overlapping with and contributing to lowered self-esteem and self-efficacy. Suboptimal outcomes following TBI are seen through the filter of these self-limiting cognitive beliefs that in turn contribute to the selection of poor coping strategies. They also contribute to additional suboptimal outcomes and the cycle continues in a downward direction.

As suggested above, an important question is whether such factors are independent predictors, mediators or moderators of outcome. If independent predictors, they make a unique contribution to the variance found in the dependent measure. If mediators, they are a driving force in the causal pathway between the brain injury and the outcome of interest and affect everyone in a similar way. Mediators explain how or why the relationship exists. If a true mediator is included in a model the relationship between the variables previously included in the model is attenuated. If moderators, they have a differential effect, with individuals being affected in different ways. In modeling, a significant interaction term between two variables signifies the moderating effect of one on the other. Baron & Kenny (1986) provide a full discussion of the distinction between mediators and moderators. Does this distinction matter? The short answer is yes, as the nature of their relationship to outcome can inform our rehabilitation interventions. Bisconti & Bergeman (1999) provide an excellent example of this in their study of social control as a mediator of the relationship between social support and depression. The association between social support and depression is well established but when social control was included as a variable, the relationship virtually disappeared. In a rehabilitation setting one would clearly want to direct efforts towards improving social control rather than social support.

Unfortunately, these terms are often interchangeably and rigorous investigations of the factors associated with mediators or moderators are rare. Kendall & Terry discuss these factors as mediators of outcome whereas Moore & Stambrook discuss them as moderators. To the best of our knowledge, only one group of investigators has undertaken empirical work to validate one of the models (Kendall & Terry's) (Rutterford & Wood, 2006; Wood & Rutterford, 2006). Many others (including ourselves) have investigated these factors as direct determinants of outcome (e.g., Dawson *et al.*, 2006, 2007). Thus, at this point, our knowledge is extremely limited about whether these factors are mediators, moderators or direct determinants of outcome, and how these relationships alter depending on the factor and outcome under investigation. It is highly probable that the same factor(s) can act in all three ways.

Finally, it is important to acknowledge that these psychosocial factors are also impacted by the same events that cause cognitive impairments. For example, the diffuse axonal injury that occurs with traumatic brain injury must have some impact on the neurological structures subserving these factors as well as cognitive processes. Thus, it follows that executive dysfunction is associated with the maladaptive appraisal of stressful situations and impairments in that both these functions may share neural substrates (see Krpan *et al.*, 2007). At the moment, little is known about the possible biological mechanisms that underlie the associations between cognition, coping behaviors and other psychosocial factors and well-being. This will undoubtedly change over the next 10 years, particularly with the advent, in 2006, of two new journals dedicated to reporting the increasing amounts of research in this area (*Social Cognitive Neuroscience* and *Social Neuroscience*).

Psychosocial factors as related to participation outcomes

This section discusses four psychosocial factors of particular interest: coping, self-efficacy, locus of control and optimism. These are not the only important psychosocial factors but they are the most widely discussed in the literature. Indeed, each of these constructs has an enormous literature in its own right. Yet, relatively little has been written about them, particularly optimism, in relation to the cognitive changes following stroke, TBI and aging. As Mateer *et al.* (2005) noted, there is a critical gap in explicating (and undoubtedly implementing) treatment interventions that not only acknowledge but mesh cognitive, emotional and motivational interventions. As a start to addressing this gap, we define each of these factors, and provide a summary of what is known about them in relation to cognitive function, recovery and outcome (following stroke and TBI and success in aging). The section concludes with a summary of the inter-relationships between these four factors.

The psychosocial factors most widely discussed in relation to the rehabilitation of people with cognitive impairment are coping, locus of control, self-efficacy and optimism.

- Brain impairment has a negative effect on psychosocial resources and poor psychosocial adjustment worsens outcome.
- Problem-focused coping, internal locus of control and positive self-efficacy are associated with more positive outcomes.
- Optimism, as a psychosocial construct predicting cognitive recovery in cognitively impaired populations, warrants further study.

Coping

The move to investigate coping in relation to the cognitive changes associated with stroke, TBI and aging is readily understandable as cognitive change is easily understood as a stressor. Two primary hypotheses direct research in this area: (1) TBI, stroke and aging all reduce the capacity of individuals to cope adaptively and (2) being unable to cope adaptively with the changes wrought by TBI, stroke and/or aging worsens outcomes (Smith, 2003). The connecting link is that reduced capacity for adaptive coping in and of itself results in a maladaptive response that in turn increases the stress on the individual who will "cope" with this increased stress in a maladaptive manner.

In general, coping strategies (the specific behavioral and cognitive efforts put in place to manage stressors) have been classified as problem-solving (e.g., change something so things would turn out all right) or emotion-focused (e.g., take it out on other people) (Folkman & Lazarus, 1980) or as avoidance-oriented (e.g., wishing the problem would go away) and approach-oriented (e.g., positive reinterpretation of stressful situation) (Finset & Andersson, 2000). Although some coping behaviors may be adaptive in one situation and maladaptive in another, it is possible to classify others as primarily maladaptive (e.g., escape-avoidance strategies such as "wishing the problem would go away" or "drinking too much").

Given the nature of coping behaviors it is not surprising that some associations with cognitive function have been reported. However, investigations of these associations are in their infancy. The few available studies confirm the association and provide directions for further research. One can hypothesize that the use of problem-solving coping behaviors is associated with higher levels of cognitive function. Curran *et al.* (2000) found a positive association between problem-solving coping behaviors and overall cognitive function. More specifically, Krpan *et al.* (2007) found a positive association between the use of problem-solving coping behaviors and better performance on neuropsychological tests of executive function, and conversely an increase in the use of escape-avoidance coping in those with worse executive function performance.

Available data on the relation between coping behaviors and other psychosocial factors on the one hand, and participation outcomes and the nature of the relationships on the other hand, is quite consistent among people with TBI, stroke and older adults. Avoidance coping has been associated with negative outcomes and with worse psychosocial functioning (Dawson *et al.*, 2007; Harvey & Bryant, 1998; King *et al.*, 2002; Malia *et al.*, 1995; Moos *et al.*, 2006) whereas the use of positive reappraisal or problem-solving coping techniques has been associated with better psychosocial outcome and higher levels of productivity (Curran *et al.*, 2000; Moore & Stambrook, 1992; Rochette & Desrosiers, 2002; Sinyor *et al.*, 1986). We have also found that persons with TBI with higher scores on the escape-avoidance coping scale had poorer psychosocial outcome and were less likely to have returned to productive activity (Dawson *et al.*, 2007).

Although the choice of coping behaviors appears to be altered in the first 6 months following a TBI (Dawson *et al.*, 2006), in contrast, after a stroke, coping behaviors are reasonably stable (Donnellan *et al.*, 2006). Coping behaviors have not been found to be associated with severity of TBI (Anson & Ponsford, 2006a; Dawson *et al.*, 2007). There are contradictory reports as to whether the pattern of coping behaviors is different in people with neurological pathology compared with normal controls (Curran *et al.*, 2000; Dawson *et al.*, 2007; Tomberg *et al.*, 2005). Age, premorbid personality and IQ levels have been shown to be associated with coping style among survivors of TBI and older adults (Aldwin *et al.*, 1996; Anson & Ponsford, 2006b; Dawson *et al.*, 2006; Krpan *et al.*, 2007) but not among survivors of stroke (Rochette & Desrosiers, 2002). Some of the age-related differences in coping behaviors may be related to the type of stressor. For example, age-related changes in social roles (e.g., worker) influence the type of coping behaviors reported (Aldwin *et al.*, 1996).

The question as to whether direct rehabilitation efforts can alter people's coping behaviors is addressed later in this chapter.

Locus of control

Rotter's (1966) seminal work on locus of control, asserted that people who believe that *their* actions and achievement of a goal were related have an internal locus of control; people who do not believe this have an external locus of control. Thus, individuals with a more internalized locus of control have a greater sense of being in control of what happens in their life. People with a more internalized locus of control are more likely to appraise situations in a manner that leads them to choose active coping

behaviors. As one would expect, internal locus of control is associated with higher levels of cognition, health and overall well-being.

We have known for a long time that locus of control is related to cognitive function in the elderly (e.g., Brown & Granick, 1983; Winocur & Moscovitch, 1990). In one of several prospective, longitudinal studies reporting on locus of control and cognitive function in relation to aging, Wight *et al.* (2003) found that for men with some high school education, higher levels of internal locus of control were associated with higher levels of cognitive function. Thus, an internal locus of control seemed to provide some protective effect from cognitive decline although this was moderated by education. van den Heuvel *et al.* (1996) also reported a protective effect of internal locus of control. They found that women with general cognitive impairment were less likely to be depressed if their internal locus of control was strong. Similar studies do not appear to have been conducted with adults with TBI or stroke.

A more internal locus of control is generally associated with a variety of more positive daily life outcomes among older adults and those with TBI or stroke. Older adults report better self-health and overall functioning if they have a more internalized locus of control (Brown & Granick, 1983). There are reports that, following TBI, people with a higher external locus of control are less likely to return to pre-injury levels of employment, less likely to be working, and more likely to have poorer psychosocial outcome (Dawson *et al.*, 2007; Moore & Stambrook, 1992; Lubosko *et al.*, 1994). Similar findings have been reported in the stroke population where higher levels of internal locus of control are associated with higher scores of independence in daily living, less psychosocial distress, and overall quality of life (Kobayashi *et al.*, 2000; Morrison *et al.*, 2000). Interestingly, locus of control seems to be quite stable over time following TBI.

Locus of control is an important factor in relation to rehabilitation both because it is associated with outcomes and also because it is associated with progress in rehabilitation (Norman & Norman, 1991). Although reports of adults with TBI show locus of control to be relatively stable (Dawson *et al.*, 2004; Malia *et al.*, 1995), there is some literature that suggests this is something that can be altered (e.g., Anson & Ponsford, 2006b). This is reviewed later in this chapter.

Self-efficacy

Self-efficacy is an individual's assessment of his/her ability to perform successfully specific behaviors in specific situations. Bandura has argued that behaviors are cognitively mediated by the strength of one's self-efficacy beliefs. When self-efficacy is high with regards to one's abilities in a particular situation, coping is more adaptive and one has a greater sense of control. Individuals with higher levels of self-efficacy engage in broader ranges of activities, direct more energy towards these and persevere more (Bandura, 1982). In turn, at least in the aging population, engaging in more challenging and demanding activities has been shown to have positive associations with higher cognitive function (Singh-Manoux *et al.*, 2003).

The relationship between self-efficacy beliefs and functioning in daily life seems quite intuitive (and will be discussed in more detail shortly). But, can the belief that one has good cognitive function make it so? Likely not. However, in older adults, stronger self-efficacy beliefs have been reported as being associated with better real and perceived memory performance (Evers *et al.*, 1998; McDougall, 2004). General measures of self-efficacy are predictive of better cognitive functioning as people age (Albert, 1995). Also, in cognitively intact older adults, stronger self-efficacy beliefs have been related to higher levels of memory performance and greater use of external memory aids (McDougall, 1996). This latter finding suggests that older adults who believe that they will accomplish their daily activities without forgetting what they have to do are more likely to make use of devices that will help them achieve this. This is highly adaptive behavior. A similar line of reasoning might be used in relation to Albert *et al.*'s study (1995). Older adults who believe they have the resources to participate in their daily living tasks are

more likely to do so. In turn this engagement may protect against cognitive deterioration.

Work done with TBI individuals leads to similar conclusions. Wood & Rutterford (2006), in a rigorous analysis, reported that self-efficacy mediates the relationship between working memory and the outcomes of satisfaction with life and depression. As this is one of the few studies that carefully investigates the nature of the relationships (i.e., determinant, mediator or moderator) we provide some detail about the study. Participants in this study were 131 individuals at least 10 years post-injury in order to focus on later stages of adjustment and recovery. Injury severity details were obtained from health records and data on neuropsychological, community integration, and psychosocial status from testing and self-report questionnaires. Self-efficacy, coping and locus of control were measured in this study and evaluated as possible mediators of the relationship between injury severity and cognitive status and community integration outcomes. They found that self-efficacy mediated the relationship between working memory and life satisfaction and the relationship between working memory and depression. They suggested that those with ongoing problems in working memory appear to have weak self-efficacy beliefs which, in turn, lead to poor life satisfaction and depression. They also noted that they found little evidence of coping or locus of control acting as mediators of the relationship between cognition and outcome. Thus, the psychosocial factors did not consistently act as mediators on outcome. Interestingly, a similar conclusion was reached in a study investigating self-regulation as a mediator of the relationship between cognition and outcomes in children with TBI (Ganesalingam *et al.*, 2007).

To date, no-one has investigated specifically how poor self-awareness, a major cognitive problem particularly associated with TBI, might impact on the trajectory between poor cognition and outcome that is mediated by self-efficacy. When there is reduced awareness, people tend to over-estimate their abilities (Abreu *et al.*, 2001). Thus, they perform poorly on tasks they expect to do well.

Presumably, over time, this could ultimately lead to both reduced self-efficacy and reduced task performance such as appears to be the case for poor working memory. It may also be that self-efficacy and self-awareness share neural substrates. These are rich areas for future investigation.

Although much has been written about self-efficacy and daily life outcomes, there have been relatively few reports on this in relation to cognition. However, as previously stated, available evidence confirms that stronger self-efficacy beliefs are associated with better outcomes. Among people with TBI, self-efficacy has been found to predict social participation and overall community integration status (Dumont *et al.*, 2005; Wood & Rutterford, 2006). Similarly, stronger self-efficacy beliefs in adults with stroke are predictive of greater independence in activities of daily living (Hellstrom *et al.*, 2003; Robinson-Smith *et al.*, 2000). The same relationship has been found in older adults both in cross-sectional studies and in prospective studies. For example, Mendes de Leon *et al.* (1996) reported that high self-efficacy was associated with less functional decline in community dwelling elders.

Stronger self-efficacy beliefs have also been associated with more adaptive coping strategies and higher ratings on measures of control. So we return to our question – can self-efficacy beliefs be altered through intervention in a manner that will improve outcomes? This question is addressed later in the chapter.

Optimism

Although optimism has been of interest to psychologists for many years it has been revitalized with the recent emergence of the field of positive psychology (Shogren *et al.*, 2006). There are two primary views of optimism. The first, dispositional optimism, is defined as "looking forward to many desirable events and being very confident that these will take place" (Reker, 1997, p. 710). This form of optimism involves a global expectation of many good things and a future orientation (Giltay *et al.*, 2006; Peterson, 2000). A second view of optimism relates

to a person's characteristic explanatory style of specific events. A person with an optimistic explanatory style understands bad events to be unstable (they won't last long), having an external source, and being related to a specific, rather than pervasive, aspect of function (Moore & Stambrook, 1995; Peterson, 2000). This view of optimism emerged from earlier work on attributional style (Abramson *et al.*, 1978), a construct included as one of the important moderators of outcome following TBI (see the model proposed by Moore & Stambrook and discussed in the early part of this chapter). Investigation of the relationship between these two forms of optimism is limited but it does seem that they may be different constructs (Isaacowitz & Seligman, 2002).

Although there is considerable literature showing that optimism is associated with many desirable characteristics including happiness, achievement and health (Kubzansky *et al.*, 2001; Peterson, 2000), optimism as a construct is not well explored in its relation to impaired cognition in adults and older adults. Winocur & Moscovitch found that optimism was related to higher levels of cognitive function in both institutionalized and community-dwelling elderly (cited in Dawson *et al.*, 1999; see also Isaacowitz, 2005). Along the same lines, Ylvisaker & Feeney (2002) found that optimism is significantly associated with executive function in children and adults with TBI. Intuitively, this makes sense as dispositional optimism could be seen to be important in motivating goal-directed action.

The work done by Winocur & Moscovitch (described in Dawson *et al.*, 1999) is particularly interesting because it is longitudinal work and provides us with some further opportunity to reflect on the nature of the relationship between optimism and outcome. The participants in this study were community-dwelling or institutional-dwelling older adults who were assessed three times over a period of about 2 years on measures of cognitive status, psychosocial status (locus of control, optimism, life attitude) and daily function. Although these data were not subjected to analyses that would determine the mediating role of the psychosocial factors, the results allow us to hypothesize. First, living situation had a significant relationship with cognitive status. Specifically, people living in the community had higher levels of cognitive function. Second, improvements or declines in psychosocial function were mirrored by improvements or declines in cognitive function. Third, cognitive function was associated with activity levels. We do not know whether the relationship between cognitive function and activity level would be attenuated by the inclusion of psychosocial variables in a regression model but we hypothesize that we would see this consistent relationship between cognition and psychosocial factors.

Dispositional optimism has been related to higher levels of psychosocial function, reduced mortality, and other positive health-related and daily life outcomes. Tomberg *et al.* (2005) reported that an optimistic life orientation was significantly associated with resuming work and health-related quality of life in a group of adults with moderate-severe TBI. In the elderly, optimism appears to have a protective effect against depression (Giltay *et al.*, 2006) and conversely is predictive of increased odds of recovery following a variety of health-related events including stroke (Ostir *et al.*, 2002).

Optimism seems to be a construct more widely explored in the pediatric brain injury literature, perhaps emerging from the interest in this area shown in literature on children with developmental delay (Ylvisaker & Feeney, 2002). It is time to begin exploring this construct more fully in terms of how it is affected by brain injury and conversely how it affects outcome in the presence of cognitive decline.

Summary

Coping, locus of control, self-efficacy and optimism can explain significant variance in real world outcomes such as returning to work, community integration, and health-related quality of life. Yet many questions remain. At a theoretical level, there is still a debate as to whether these constructs are states, traits or both (Carifio & Rhodes, 2002). As well, it is not entirely clear that they represent separate constructs. Some have argued that there may be fundamental underlying processes that explain the close relationship between some of these factors (Judge *et al.*, 2002). Further, we are only beginning to reflect on the nature of the relationship of these factors to outcome. Work by Winocur & Moscovitch (in Dawson *et al.*, 1999) in older adults suggests a mediating relationship. More recent studies by Wood & Rutterford (2006) and Ganesalingam *et al.* (2007) provide more conclusive data showing that particular psychosocial factors (i.e., self-efficacy and self-regulation) act as mediators in some but not all situations. Clearly, considerably more work is needed in this area including perhaps some rethinking of data we have already collected. Do these factors truly mediate outcomes?

Are they direct determinants? Do they moderate outcomes? Do they act in different ways in different instances and/or populations? Are they, in fact, separate constructs or is the overlap such that there may be some more fundamental underlying process? At this point we also have relatively little information about the neural and other physiological mechanisms that underlie these processes.

Although many basic questions remain, clinical practice demands that rehabilitation interventions occur. A number of investigators (including ourselves) have explicitly incorporated these factors into their rehabilitation interventions (e.g., Rath *et al.*, 2003; Winocur *et al.*, 2007). The nature of these programs and their efficacy is discussed forthwith.

Psychosocial factors considered in the rehabilitation literature for adults with cognitive impairments

Psychosocial issues are clearly important in relation to cognitive status and to outcomes following stroke and TBI, as well as to successful aging. This section reviews the rehabilitation literature that has (1) explicitly incorporated psychosocial factors in the intervention and (2) reported effects on the day-to-day functioning of cognitively impaired adults and older adults. The review is circumscribed by the populations (stroke, TBI, older adults experiencing cognitive decline), the intervention and real-world outcomes. We have organized our review by type of intervention: comprehensive day-treatment (holistic-milieu) programs, community-based interventions, tele-rehabilitation, and interventions targeting specific psychosocial factors.

- Comprehensive day treatment programs can be effective but require major commitments of time and resources.
- Community-based interventions are cost-efficient programs that have focused on community living skills.
- Tele-rehabilitation is a new approach that warrants further investigation.
- Specific intervention programs are multifaceted and favored in outpatient rehabilitation centers.

Comprehensive day treatment programs (CDTPs)

The first comprehensive day treatment program (also known as comprehensive neurorehabilitation and/or milieu-based neurorehabilitation programs) was established by Yehuda Ben-Yishay in the mid-1970s for adults with TBI (Ben-Yishay, 1996). Ben-Yishay believed that multidimensional, holistic, therapeutic milieu programs were the necessary way to proceed to achieve effective rehabilitation following severe brain injury. Subsequently, a number of similar programs were developed (Hashimoto *et al.*, 2006; Klonoff *et al.*, 2001; Malec, 2001; Prigatano, 1999; Salazar *et al.*, 2000; Sarajuuri *et al.*, 2005; Scherzer, 1986). The programs have seven key elements: establishment of a therapeutic milieu, establishment of a working alliance between staff, clients and family, cognitive rehabilitation, psychotherapy, involvement of family members, a protected work trial and a high staff:client ratio. Programs typically require a commitment of 4–5 days each week and run for 6 weeks (Sarajuuri *et al.*, 2005) to 1 year (Ben-Yishay *et al.*, 1987).

The stated aims of these programs include developing self-reflection, building self-esteem, and teaching participants how to cope with the changes they face. Although initially developed for the rehabilitation of people with severe TBIs published reports indicate that about 20% of participants sustained stroke (Klonoff *et al.*, 2001; Malec, 2001; Teasdale *et al.*, 1993).

Most outcome studies of these programs entail comparison of performance before and after intervention. As most people entering these programs are long-term post-TBI, to some extent, people entering these programs can serve as their own controls. For example, Scherzer (1986) reported that, of 32 participants in their program, 10 were working in some form (seven of these requiring weekly or bi-weekly support), and another nine had moved into private apartments. In an 11-year follow-up study, Klonoff *et al.* (2001) reported that over 80% of the graduates from their programs were productive in some capacity (competitive employment, school, volunteer work) and these numbers were generally maintained. One of the primary predictors of better long-term productivity status was the working alliance between family, patients and staff rated during the intervention and at time of discharge.

More recently, several case-control studies have evaluated CDTPs. Cicerone *et al.* (2004) found a significant treatment effect for their CDTP relative to their standard program on a measure of community integration. However, in that study, the CDTP group was significantly longer post-injury, which may have affected the outcomes in the desired direction. Hashimoto *et al.* (2006) also reported a positive treatment effect on community integration but also had the problem of a non-matched control group. In a study with a more carefully matched control group, Sarajuuri *et al.* (2005) reported 89% of the treatment group relative to 55% of the control group being involved in productive activity at 2-year follow-up. In this study participants were considered productive if they were working, at school, in a work-trial and/or doing volunteer work. The proportion involved in paid work was 4/19 in the treatment and 8/20 in the nontreatment group, a nonstatistically significant difference.

The evidence to date led Cicerone and colleagues (2005) to recommend CDTPs as a practice guideline[1] for post-acute rehabilitation for moderate to severe TBI. At this time, it is not possible to determine whether all components of such programs are necessary to achieve the stated goals. It is reasonable to conclude that, to be effective, rehabilitation must integrate interventions directed at cognitive, behavioral, functional and psychosocial effects of stroke and TBI.

Community based interventions

Community-based rehabilitation (CBR) is defined here as rehabilitation that is delivered in the clients' community. Typically this involves one or more professionals going to the person's home. Rehabilitation delivered in individuals' communities may have positive effects at least in part because it reduces the demands for generalization (people with cognitive impairment have tremendous difficulty generalising learning from one situation to another). Taking into account the costs of therapy delivered in an institution versus in the community, this type of rehabilitation makes sense.

We are particularly interested in community-based interventions that have explicitly identified psychosocial factors as being included in the intervention. Unfortunately, very few papers in this area provide comprehensive descriptions of the intervention. For the most part, they specify the disciplines involved in delivering service but the content of the intervention is described only in very general terms.

Community-based rehabilitation has been investigated most thoroughly in stroke patients relative to TBI and older adult populations. However, randomized control trials (RCTs) have been undertaken in all three groups and have shown positive effects of community-based rehabilitation on community living skills. Barnes (2003) notes that the value of early discharge to home with care post-stroke is reasonably well established. A Cochrane review of home-based rehabilitation for people with stroke shows increased independence in activities of daily living among the treated patients (Outpatient Service Trialists, 2003). There is also preliminary evidence for the efficacy of community-based rehabilitation for adults with stroke who are not admitted to hospital (Walker *et al.*, 1999). Similar results are found in the TBI literature. For example, in a CBR intervention that involved healthcare professionals developing written contracts outlining the individualized goals and intervention plans they developed with their TBI patients, the CBR group improved on psychosocial and community integration measures relative to a group receiving only education (Powell *et al.*, 2002).

Among older adults, community-based services can be effective in promoting well-being and community participation in the well-elderly (Clark *et al.*, 1997), in maintaining older people at home, and maintaining functional status in older adults at risk for decline following acute illness and/or hospitalization (Tinetti *et al.*, 2002). Clark *et al.* (1997) compared a planned, individualized intervention with an education-only group. Tinetti *et al.* (2002) compared usual home care services with what they termed restorative care. Restorative care included four key characteristics: (1) training of all home care staff in issues relevant to rehabilitation, geriatrics and goal attainment; (2) organization of all staff into an integrated team; (3) reorientation of the team's focus from "taking care of" to working with the patient to optimize function and comfort; and (4) working with the staff, patient and family to establish goals and agreeing on a process to reach them. Neither study was specifically directed at older adults with cognitive impairments, but 20% of the participants in the Tinetti study were documented as having mild to moderate cognitive impairment.

---

[1] Practice guidelines are defined as recommendations based on one or more randomized control trials with some methodological limitations *or* on well-designed prospective cohort studies and nonrandomized studies with controls.

Although more research is needed, studies to date support the efficacy of community-based rehabilitation. The work done by Tinetti *et al.* (2002) is of particular interest because they compared two CBR approaches and found the restorative care approach to be superior. We also believe that the use of goal-planning, explicitly mentioned in some studies, may be important. Involving patients in setting their own goals could be considered a technique for building self-efficacy. Further, it is not unreasonable to assume that CBR delivered by occupational therapists (as described by Clark *et al.*, 1997) would have included this as involving clients in their goal-setting is a central tenet of their practice (Townsend *et al.*, 1997). Thus, we cautiously conclude that the evidence from these studies supports the use of multifaceted therapy and goal planning.

Tele-rehabilitation

The use of distance technology in healthcare is of growing interest for its potential for cost-effective healthcare delivery, for its ability to transcend geography, and for its apparent success (e.g., Weinberger *et al.*, 1993). To date, there have been several tele-rehabilitation studies published in the stroke and TBI literature that fit our criteria (i.e., explicitly incorporate psychosocial factors in the intervention; report effects on day-to-day functioning of cognitively impaired adults and older adults). Findings from two randomized controlled studies in the TBI literature suggest that telephone interventions may be at least as good as inpatient rehabilitation in relation to 1-year return to work rates and better than routine follow-up for overall functional status (Bell *et al.*, 2005; Salazar *et al.*, 2000; Warden *et al.*, 2000). Both telephone interventions used highly trained counselors who explicitly worked to foster self-direction, support adjustment to TBI including monitoring anxiety and depression and enhance self-efficacy. Bell *et al.* (2005) focused their efforts on the first year post-injury. Initial telephone contact was made within 2 weeks of discharge with subsequent contacts 2 weeks later and then at months 2, 3, 5, 7 and 9. Telephone calls

lasted 30 to 45 minutes and were supplemented by mailed resources specific to the call as well as a brief written summary of the call with an action list. The intervention by Salazar *et al.* occurred over a much shorter time-frame. Telephone calls were made weekly over an 8-week period. Lai *et al.* (2004) used another form of distance support. They developed an 8-week stroke intervention delivered by videoconference to community seniors' centers. The 1.5 hour intervention included education, exercise, discussion of psychosocial impact and community support. Significant improvement among participants was noted across a wide range of areas including physical and social functioning.

Whether the key ingredients of the positive findings were the highly individualized nature of the intervention, the explicit psychosocial mandate and/or the fact that people were in their own context talking about real-life issues, the preliminary evidence establishes this as a valuable avenue for future research.

Specific interventions

This last part of this section reviews studies that have either explicitly targeted one of the psychosocial factors addressed in this chapter or have addressed these factors as part of a cognitive rehabilitation intervention. The interventions described are typically outpatient programs of rehabilitation centers. Although multifaceted programs have incorporated psychosocial interventions, there are few studies that have targeted specifically the psychosocial factors we have been discussing. For example, Anson & Ponsford (2006a) reported on a coping skills group intervention for adults with TBI. The aim was to provide participants with the necessary resources to cope more effectively with injury-related changes and thereby decrease emotional distress. Thirty-one participants completed the 10-session program (90 minutes, twice/week). Following training, there was a significant increase in self-reported adaptive coping that declined at 5-weeks post-intervention, but was seen again at longer term follow-up (6–24 months) supported by positive feedback from the participants. Although no significant changes were noted on measures of depression, self-esteem or other psychosocial dysfunction this study illustrates the possibility of changing coping behaviors through an explicit intervention.

Coping was also the target of a workbook intervention (Frank *et al.*, 2000). Adults discharged from acute care following stroke were randomly allocated to receive the intervention or to a wait-list control. The workbook was designed to enhance perceptions of control, enhance coping resources and provide a place to rehearse planning and problem-solving skills. After two introductory sessions, stroke survivors and their caregivers worked independently on the exercises. Both groups showed comparable improvement at the post-test on measures of function and psychosocial distress. Following a somewhat different approach, Man *et al.* (2006) investigated the effects of different trainer-trainee interaction patterns on self-efficacy related to problem-solving in adults with brain injury. They reported that human-administered training is beneficial relative to computer-assisted training in building self-efficacy, although there were no differences on improvements in actual problem-solving skills.

More common is the inclusion of psychotherapy or psychosocial interventions along with cognitive remediation techniques. However, most of the research involving this approach has been conducted on TBI patients. In a RCT, Tiersky *et al.* (2005) evaluated the results of a program in which participants received thrice weekly individual psychotherapy and thrice weekly individual cognitive remediation. The treatment group showed reduced distress and improved attention but was no different than the control group on measures of community integration. Ownsworth *et al.* (2000) combined cognitive rehabilitation, cognitive–behavioral therapy and social skills training in a 16-week program (90 minutes/week) to improve self-awareness and psychosocial distress. The program incorporated discussion of difficulties experienced in day-to-day life and strategies to overcome

these. Participants reported significant improvements on self-regulation skills and broad improvements in how psychosocial distress manifest in their daily lives. Relatives also reported significant improvement on a head injury behavior scale. In another approach, Rath *et al.* (2003) compared "conventional" rehabilitation with an innovative intervention. Both groups received 48 hours of group therapy. For the "conventional" group this consisted of 24 hours of cognitive remediation that focused on awareness, attention, using feedback, and social skills, as well as 24 hours of psychosocial group therapy that focused on coping with emotional reactions and changes post-injury. The "innovative" group was split between sessions that focused on emotional self-regulation and sessions that focused on learning a step-by-step model of cognitive-behavioral problem-solving skills. Results showed that people in the innovative group improved more on measures of executive function and in self-appraisal of their problem-solving abilities, improvements that were maintained at 6 months post-treatment. In the conventional group, there was very little improvement shown on measures of problem solving but significant others reported less severe cognitive and somatic symptoms. Rath *et al.* suggest that the improvements noted by the significant others may be attributable to the psychosocial component of the conventional group.

A recently developed cognitive rehabilitation program, developed by our group, also incorporated a psychosocial component. We randomized 49 older adults to a treatment group or wait-list control (Stuss *et al.*, 2007). All participants were living independently in the community but had expressed concerns about their memory or related cognitive function. The intervention protocol included 12, 3-hour weekly sessions. Included in this were four sessions each on memory training, modified goal management training and psychosocial training (Craik *et al.*, 2007; Levine *et al.*, 2007; Winocur *et al.*, 2007). The psychosocial training focused on educating participants about the constructs discussed in this chapter and asking them to apply them to their own daily life experiences and to particular tasks. Overall, the results of this protocol were positive. Participants improved on measures of cognitive function and several measures of psychosocial function with gains maintained at 6-month follow-up.

Summary

The preceding review highlighted several important points. First, the inclusion of psychosocial interventions in many comprehensive and community-based rehabilitation programs speaks to the widespread belief that therapy directed at these factors is important and necessary. Second, the inclusion of a real-life focus seems important for making real-life changes. More generally, improvements are related to where therapy is directed. Third, studies investigating the value of targeting the psychosocial factors discussed in this chapter are almost nonexistent. Future research should be directed at determining whether these factors must be explicitly addressed in rehabilitation for people with cognitive impairments to achieve maximum gain.

Conclusion

We began this chapter with three key questions. What are the important personal psychosocial factors to consider in relation to outcome and in relation to rehabilitation? How have these factors been addressed in rehabilitation? What principles can we derive from the literature to guide clinical practice and future research? Using Folkman and Lazarus's theoretical work as a jumping off-point we elaborated four key psychosocial factors that have been shown to be significantly associated with real-world outcomes. Coping, locus of control and self-efficacy have been widely discussed in the literature. Optimism has provided a lesser focus for researchers but work to date shows that it is also an important factor. This, by no means, is a comprehensive list. Other factors that should be considered in concert with these are self-regulation, life

attitude, self-esteem and sense of coherence to name only a few (Dawson *et al.*, 2007; Schnyder *et al.*, 1999; Ylvisaker & Feeney, 2002). Part of future investigations must address the relationships between these constructs, as well as the relationships between the psychological and cognitive.

As we and other contributors to this volume have discussed, improving real-world outcomes for individuals with cognitive impairment is a complex undertaking. A broad range of approaches has been used to achieve this worthy goal. Although improvements were seen in each class of interventions we believe some principles have emerged.

- To achieve positive real-world outcomes, psychosocial factors must be explicitly incorporated into rehabilitation interventions.
- Addressing only psychosocial factors has specific positive effects but generalization to real-world changes has not been reported.
- Involving patients in goal setting may have a positive effect on achieving outcomes.
- Attention must be paid to real-world concerns and goals if changes are to be made in this realm.

At the end of our discussion we are left with another question – where to from here? There are many avenues of exploration that will enable us to further our knowledge regarding how to address psychosocial factors in relation to cognitive rehabilitation. We suggest a few for which preliminary exploration is underway. The first is represented by the work of Anson & Ponsford (2006a). It is important that we target these psychosocial factors explicitly and individually to determine whether changes can be made. This work will almost certainly be experimental in nature as the evidence supporting multifaceted work is very convincing. Nevertheless it will enable us to understand these constructs more thoroughly and determine whether underlying processes can be remediated or whether teaching compensatory strategies is a more worthwhile endeavour. A second avenue is represented in the social cognitive neuroscience literature. Work in this field will enable us to identify the neural pathways and mechanisms responsible for social phenomena, to understand the shared and discrete pathways for cognitive and psychological behaviors. For example, recent work suggests that social exclusion interferes with the executive control of attention (Campbell *et al.*, 2006). This work may help us address the effects of social isolation that is common following TBI and stroke. A third avenue is to further refine multifaceted approaches that explicitly attend to the psychosocial and cognitive. An example of this might be a clinical trial currently underway, called Executive Plus (www.clinicaltrials.gov/ct/show/NCT00233129). The protocol states that there is a focus on executive function deficits and emotional self-regulation. A fourth avenue might be to focus attention entirely in the real-world, that is to undertake rehabilitation in a contextual fashion. A recent study by Ownsworth *et al.* (2006b) is on a meta-cognitive, contextual intervention that was developed from a model that illustrates an individual's deficits arising from the interaction between neurocognitive, psychological and socio-environmental factors. We are undertaking similar work although not specifically focused on self-awareness (Dawson *et al.*, 2007).

How the pieces of the puzzle will come together is not entirely clear. However, current research efforts show promise for our ultimate goal of improving well-being and quality of life for people with cognitive impairments.

ACKNOWLEDGMENTS

The authors acknowledge the JSF McDonnell Foundation for its support of much of the authors' research in the area of cognitive rehabilitation and in the preparation of this chapter. The excellent technical support provided by Marie-Ève Couture and Karen Lau is also gratefully acknowledged.

REFERENCES

Abramson, L. Y., Seligman, M. E. P., & Teasdale, J. D. (1978). Learned helplessness in humans: critique and reformulation. *Journal of Abnormal Psychology*, **87**, 49–74.

Abreu, B. C., Seale, G., Scheibel, R. S., *et al.* (2001). Levels of self-awareness after acute brain injury: how patients' and rehabilitation specialists' perceptions compare. *Archives of Physical Medicine and Rehabilitation*, **82**, 49–56.

Albert, M. S. (1995). How does education affect cognitive function? *Annals of Epidemiology*, **5**, 76–78.

Albert, M. S., Savage, C. R., Blazer, D., *et al.* (1995). Predictors of cognitive change in older persons: MacArthur studies of successful aging. *Psychology and Aging*, **10**, 578–589.

Aldwin, C. M., Sutton, K. J., Chiara, G., & Spiro, A., III (1996). Age differences in stress, coping, and appraisal: findings from the normative aging study. *Journals of Gerontology*, **51**B, 179–188.

Anson, K., & Ponsford, J. (2006a). Who benefits? Outcome following a coping skills group intervention for traumatically brain injured individuals. *Brain Injury*, **20**, 1–13.

Anson, K., & Ponsford, J. (2006b). Evaluation of a coping skills group following traumatic brain injury. *Brain Injury*, **20**, 167–178.

Bandura, A. (1982). Self-efficacy mechanism in human agency. *American Psychologist*, **37**, 122–147.

Barnes, M. P. (2003). Principles of neurological rehabilitation. *Journal of Neurology, Neurosurgery and Psychiatry*, **74**, iv3–iv7.

Baron, R. M., & Kenny, D. A. (1986). The moderator-mediator variable distinction I social psychological research: conceptual, strategic, and statistical considerations. *Journal of Personality and Social Psychology*, **51**, 1173–1182.

Bell, K. R., Temkin, N. R., Esselman, P. C. *et al.* (2005). The effect of a scheduled telephone intervention on outcome after moderate to severe traumatic brain injury: a randomized trial. *Archives of Physical Medicine and Rehabilitation*, **86**, 851–856.

Ben-Yishay, Y. (1996). Reflections on the evolution of the therapeutic milieu concept. *Neuropsychological Rehabilitation*, **6**, 327–343.

Ben-Yishay, Y., Silver, S. M., Piasetsky, E., & Rattok, J. (1987). Relationship between employability and vocational outcome after intensive holistic cognitive rehabilitation. *Journal of Head Trauma Rehabilitation*, **2**, 35–48.

Bisconti, T. L., & Bergeman, C. S. (1999). Perceived social control as a mediator of the relationships among social support, psychological well-being, and perceived health. *The Gerontologist*, **39**, 94–102.

Boynton De Sepulveda, L. I., & Chang, B. (1994). Effective coping with stroke disability in a community setting: the development of a causal model. *Journal of Neuroscience Nursing*, **26**, 193–203.

Brown, B. R., & Granick, S. (1983). Cognitive and psychosocial differences between I-locus and E-locus of control aged persons. *Experimental Aging Research*, **9**, 107–110.

Campbell, W. K., Krusemark, E. A., Dyckman, K. A. *et al.* (2006). A magnetoencephalography investigation of neural correlates for social exclusion and self-control. *Social Neuroscience*, **1**, 124–134.

Carifio, J., & Rhodes, L. (2002). Construct validities and the empirical relationships between optimism, hope, self-efficacy, and locus of control. *Work: A Journal of Prevention, Assessment & Rehabilitation*, **19**, 125–136.

Cicerone, K. D., Mott, T., Azulay, J., & Friel, J. C. (2004). Community integration and satisfaction with functioning after intensive cognitive rehabilitation for traumatic brain injury. *Archives of Physical Medicine and Rehabilitation*, **85**, 943–950.

Cicerone, K. D., Dahlberg, C., Malec, J. F., *et al.* (2005). Evidence-based cognitive rehabilitation: updated review of the literature from 1998 through 2002. *Archives of Physical Medicine and Rehabilitation*, **86**, 1681–1692.

Clark, F., Azen, S. P., Zemke, R. *et al.* (1997). Occupational therapy for independent-living older adults: a randomized controlled trial. *Journal of the American Medical Association*, **278**, 1321–1326.

Craik, F. I. M., Winocur, G., Palmer, H. *et al.* (2007). Cognitive rehabilitation in the elderly: effects on memory. *Journal of the International Neuropsychological Society*, **13**, 132–142.

Curran, C. A., Ponsford, J. L., & Crowe, S. (2000). Coping strategies and emotional outcome following traumatic brain injury: a comparison with orthopedic patients. *Journal of Head Trauma Rehabilitation*, **15**, 1256–1274.

Dawson, D., Winocur, G., & Moscovitch, M. (1999). The psychosocial environment and cognitive rehabilitation in the elderly. In D. T. Stuss, G. Winocur, & I. H. Robertson (Eds.), *Cognitive Neurorehabilitation* (pp. 94–108). New York, NY: Cambridge University Press.

Dawson, D. R., Levine, B., Schwartz, M. L., & Stuss, D. T. (2004). Acute predictors of real-world outcomes following traumatic brain injury: a prospective study. *Brain Injury*, **18**, 221–238.

Dawson, D. R., Cantanzaro, A. M., Firestone, J., Schwartz, M., & Stuss, D. T. (2006). Changes in coping style following traumatic brain injury and their relationship to productivity status. *Brain and Cognition*, **60**, 214–216.

Dawson, D., Polatajko, H., & Levine, B. (Published online 08 Mar 2007). Naturalistic rehabilitation for executive

dysfunction. *Journal of the International Neuropsychological Society*, **13**, *Suppl. 1*, 120, DOI: 0.1017/S1355617707079969, www.journals.cambridge.org/action/displayJournal?jid=INS.

Dawson, D. R., Schwartz, M. L., Winocur, G., & Stuss, D. T. (2007). Return to productivity following traumatic brain injury: cognitive, psychological, physical, spiritual and environmental correlates. *Disability and Rehabilitation*, **29**, 301–313.

de Raedt, R., & Ponjaert-Kirstoffersen, I. (2006). Self-serving appraisal as a cognitive coping strategy to deal with age-related limitations: an empirical study with elderly adults in a real-life stressful situation. *Aging and Mental Health*, **10**, 195–203.

Donnellan, C., Hevey, D., Hickey, A., & O'Neill, D. (2006). Defining and quantifying coping strategies after stroke: a review. *Journal of Neurology, Neurosurgery and Psychiatry*, **77**, 1208–1218.

Driver, S. (2005). Social support and the physical activity behaviours of people with a brain injury. *Brain Injury*, **19**, 1067–1075.

Dumont, C., Gervais, M., Fougeyrollas, P., & Bertrand, R. (2005). Perceived self-efficacy as a factor associated with the social participation of adults who have sustained a traumatic brain injury. *Canadian Journal of Occupational Therapy*, **72**, 222–233.

Evers, S., Stevens, F. C. J., Diederiks, J. P. M. *et al.* (1998). Age-related differences in cognition. *European Journal of Public Health*, **8**, 133–139.

Finset, A., & Andersson, S. (2000). Coping strategies in patients with acquired brain injury: relationships between coping, apathy, depression and lesion location. *Brain Injury*, **14**, 887–905.

Folkman, S., & Lazarus, R. S. (1980). An analysis of coping in a middle-aged community sample. *Journal of Health and Social Behavior*, **21**, 219–239.

Frank, G., Johnston, M., Morrison, V., Pollard, B., & MacWalter, R. (2000). Perceived control and recovery from functional limitations: preliminary evaluation of a workbook-based intervention for discharged stroke patients. *British Journal of Health Psychology*, **5**, 413–420.

Ganesalingam, K., Sanson, A., Anderson, V., & Yeates, K. O. (2007). Self-regulation as a mediator of the effects of childhood traumatic brain injury on social and behavioural functioning. *Journal of the International Neuropsychological Society*, **13**, 298–311.

Giltay, E. J., Kamphuis, M. H., Kalmijn, S., Zitman, F. G., & Kromhout, D. (2006). Dispositional optimism and the risk of cardiovascular death: the Zutphen Elderly Study. *Archives of Internal Medicine*, **166**, 431–436.

Harvey, A. G., & Bryant, R. A. (1998). The effect of attempted thought suppression in acute stress disorder. *Behaviour Research and Therapy*, **36**, 583–590.

Hashimoto, K., Okamoto, T., Watanabe, S., & Ohashi, M. (2006). Effectiveness of a comprehensive day treatment program for rehabilitation of patients with acquired brain injury in Japan. *Journal of Rehabilitation Medicine*, **38**, 20–25.

Hellstrom, K., Lindmark, B., Wahlberg, B., & Fugl-Meyer, A. R. (2003). Self-efficacy in relation to impairments and activities of daily living disability in elderly patients with stroke: a prospective investigation. *Journal of Rehabilitation Medicine*, **35**, 202–207.

Isaacowitz, D. M. (2005). Correlates of well-being in adulthood and old age: a tale of two optimisms. *Journal of Research in Personality*, **39**, 224–244.

Isaacowitz, D. M., & Seligman, M. E. P. (2002). Cognitive style predictors of affect change in older adults. *International Journal of Aging and Human Development*, **54**, 233–253.

Judge, T. A., Erez, A., Bono, J. E., & Thoresen, C. J. (2002). Are measures of self-esteem, neuroticism, locus of control, and generalized self-efficacy indicators of a common core construct? *Journal of Personality and Social Psychology*, **83**, 693–710.

Kendall, E., & Terry, D. J. (1996). Psychosocial adjustment following closed head injury: a model for understanding individual differences and predicting outcome. *Neuropsychological Rehabilitation*, **6**, 101–132.

King, R. B., Shde-Zeldow, Y., Carlson, C. E., Feldman, J. L., & Philip, M. (2002). Adaptation to stroke: a longitudinal study of depressive symptoms, physical health, and coping process. *Topics in Stroke Rehabilitation*, **9**, 46–66.

Klonoff, P. S., Lamb, D. G., & Henderson, S. W. (2001). Outcomes from milieu-based neurorehabilitation at up to 11 years post-discharge. *Brain Injury*, **15**, 413–428.

Kobayashi, R., Kai, N., Hosoda, M. *et al.* (2000). The locus of control of Japanese senior citizens with hemiplegia. *Journal of Physical Therapy Science*, **12**, 13–17.

Krpan, K. M., Levine, B., Stuss, D. T., & Dawson, D. R. (2007). Executive function and coping at one-year post traumatic brain injury. *Journal of Clinical and Experimental Neuropsychology*, **29**, 36–46.

Kubzansky, L. D., Sparrow, D., Vokonas, P., & Kawachi, I. (2001). Is the glass half empty or half full? A prospective study of optimism and coronary heart disease in the normative aging study. *Psychosomatic Medicine*, **63**, 910–916.

Lai, J. C. K., Woo, J., Hui, E., & Chan, W. M. (2004). Telerehabilitation – a new model for community-based stroke rehabilitation. *Journal of Telemedicine and Telecare*, **10**, 199–205.

Lazarus, R. S., & Folkman, S. (1984). *Stress, Appraisal and Coping*. New York, NY: Springer.

Levine, B., Stuss, D. T., Winocur, G. *et al.* (2007). Cognitive rehabilitation in the elderly: effects on strategic behavior in relation to goal management. *Journal of the International Neuropsychological Society*, **13**, 143–152.

Lubosko, A. A., Moore, A. D., Stambrook, M., & Gill, D. (1994). Cognitive beliefs following severe traumatic brain injury. *Brain Injury*, **8**, 65–70.

Malec, J. F. (2001). Impact of comprehensive day treatment on societal participation for persons with acquired brain injury. *Archives of Physical Medicine and Rehabilitation*, **82**, 885 895.

Malia, K., Powell, G., & Torode, S. (1995). Coping and psychosocial function after brain injury. *Brain Injury*, **9**, 607–618.

Man, D. W. K., Soong, W. Y. L., Tam, S. F., & Hui-Chan, C. W. Y. (2006). Self-efficacy outcomes of people with brain injury in cognitive skill training using different types of trainer-trainee interaction. *Brain Injury*, **20**, 959–970.

Mateer, C. A., Sira, C. S., & O'Connell, M. E. (2005). Putting Humpty Dumpty together again: the importance of integrating cognitive and emotional interventions. *Journal of Head Trauma Rehabilitation*, **20**, 62–75.

McDougall, G. J. (1996). Predictors of the use of memory improvement strategies by older adults. *Rehabilitation Nursing*, **21**, 202–209.

McDougall, G. J. (2004). Memory self-efficacy and memory performance among black and white elders. *Nursing Research*, **53**, 323–331.

Mendes de Leon, C. F., Seeman, T. E., Baker, D. I., Richardson, E. D., & Tinetti, M. E. (1996). Self-efficacy, physical decline, and change in functioning in community-living elders: a prospective study. *Journals of Gerontology*, **51**B, 183–189.

Moore, A. D., & Stambrook, M. (1992). Coping strategies and locus of control following traumatic brain injury: relationship to long-term outcome. *Brain Injury*, **6**, 89–94.

Moore, A. D., & Stambrook, M. (1995). Cognitive moderators of outcome following traumatic brain injury: a conceptual model and implications for rehabilitation. *Brain Injury*, **9**, 109–130.

Moos, R. H., Brennan, P. L., Schutte, K. K., & Moos, B. S. (2006). Older adults' coping with negative life events:

common processes of managing health, interpersonal, and financial/work stressors. *International Journal of Aging and Human Development*, **62**, 39–59.

Morrison, V., Johnston, M., & Walter, R. M. (2000). Predictors of distress following an acute stroke: disability, control cognitions, and satisfaction with care. *Psychology and Health*, **15**, 395–407.

Norman, E. J., & Norman, V. L. (1991). Relationships of patients' health locus of control beliefs to progress in rehabilitation. *Journal of Rehabilitation*, **57**, 27–30.

Ostir, G. V., Goodwin, J. S., Markides, K. S. *et al.* (2002). Differential effects of premorbid physical and emotional health on recovery from acute events. *Journal of the American Geriatric Society*, **50**, 713–718.

Outpatient Service Trialists (2003). Therapy-based rehabilitation services for stroke patients at home. *Cochrane Database of Systematic Reviews*, **1**, Rev. No.: CD002925. DOI: 10.1002/14651858.CD002925.

Ownsworth, T. L., McFarland, K., & Young, R. M. (2000). Self-awareness and psychosocial functioning following acquired brain injury: an evaluation of a group support programme. *Neuropsychological Rehabilitation*, **10**, 465–484.

Ownsworth, T., Clare, L., & Morris, R. (2006a). An integrated biopsychosocial approach to understanding awareness deficits in Alzheimer's disease and brain injury. *Neuropsychological Rehabilitation*, **16**, 415–438.

Ownsworth, T., Fleming, J., Desbois, J., Strong, J., & Kuipers, P. (2006b). A metacognitive contextual intervention to enhance error awareness and functional outcome following traumatic brain injury: a single-case experimental design. *Journal of the International Neuropsychological Society*, **12**, 54–63.

Peterson, C. (2000). The future of optimism. *American Psychologist*, **55**, 44–55.

Powell, J., Heslin, J., & Greenwood, R. (2002). Community-based rehabilitation after severe traumatic brain injury: a randomised controlled trial. *Journal of Neurology, Neurosurgery and Psychiatry*, **72**, 193–202.

Prigatano, G. P. (1999). *Principles of Neuropsychological Rehabilitation*. New York, NY: Oxford University Press.

Rath, J. F., Simon, D., Langenbahnm, D. M., Sherr, R. L., & Diller, L. (2003). Group treatment of problem-solving deficits in outpatients with traumatic brain injury: a randomised outcome study. *Neuropsychological Rehabilitation*, **13**, 461–488.

Reker, G. T. (1997). Personal meaning, optimism, and choice: existential predictors of depression in community and institutional elderly. *The Gerontologist*, **37**, 709–716.

Robinson-Smith, G., Johnston, M. V., & Allen, J. (2000). Self-care self-efficacy, quality of life, and depression after stroke. *Archives of Physical Medicine and Rehabilitation*, **81**, 460–464.

Rochette, A., & Desrosiers, J. (2002). Coping with the consequences of stroke. *International Journal of Rehabilitation Research*, **25**, 17–24.

Rotter, J. B. (1966). Generalized expectancies for internal versus external control of reinforcement. *Psychological Monographs*, **80**, 1–28.

Rutterford, N. A., & Wood, R. L. (2006). Evaluating a theory of stress and adjustment when predicting long-term psychological outcome after brain injury. *Journal of the International Neuropsychological Society*, **12**, 359–367.

Salazar, A. M., Warden, D. L., Schwab, K. *et al.* (2000). Cognitive rehabilitation for traumatic brain injury: a randomized trial. *Journal of the American Medical Association*, **283**, 3075–3081.

Salter, K., Teasell, R., Bhogal, S., Foley, N., & Speechley, M. (2006). *Evidence-based review of stroke rehabilitation: Community integration* (9th Edition). www.ebrsr.com/index_home.html (also available on CD-ROM).

Sarajuuri, J. M., Kaipio, M. L., Koskinen, S. K. *et al.* (2005). Outcome of a comprehensive neurorehabilitation program for patients with traumatic brain injury. *Archives of Physical Medicine and Rehabilitation*, **86**, 2296–2302.

Scherzer, B. P. (1986). Rehabilitation following severe head trauma: results of a three-year program. *Archives of Physical Medicine and Rehabilitation*, **67**, 366–374.

Schnyder, U., Büchi, S., Mörgeli, H., Sensky, T., & Klaghofer, R. (1999). Sense of coherence – a mediator between disability and handicap? *Psychotherapy and Psychosomatics*, **68**, 102–110.

Shogren, K. A., Lopez, S. J., Wehmeyer, M. L., Little, T. D., & Pressgrove, C. L. (2006). The role of positive psychology constructs in predicting life satisfaction in adolescents with and without cognitive disabilities: an exploratory study. *Journal of Positive Psychology*, **1**, 37–52.

Singh-Manoux, A., Richards, M., & Marmot, M. (2003). Leisure activities and cognitive function in middle age: evidence from the Whitehall II study. *Journal of Epidemiology and Community Health*, **57**, 907–912.

Sinyor, D., Amato, P., Kaloupek, D. G. *et al.* (1986). Post-stroke depression: relationships to functional impairment, coping strategies, and rehabilitation outcome. *Stroke*, **17**, 1102–1107.

Smith, J. (2003). Stress and aging: theoretical and empirical challenges for interdisciplinary research. *Neurobiology of Aging*, **24**, S77–S80.

Stuss, D. T., Robertson, I., Craik, F. I. M. *et al.* (2007). Cognitive rehabilitation in the elderly: a randomized trial to evaluate a new protocol. *Journal of the International Neuropsychological Society*, **13**, 120–131.

Teasdale, T. W., Christensen, A. L., & Pinner, E. M. (1993). Psychosocial rehabilitation of cranial trauma and stroke patients. *Brain Injury*, **7**, 535–542.

Tiersky, L. A., Anselmi, V., Johnston, M. V. *et al.* (2005). A trial of neuropsychological rehabilitation in mild-spectrum traumatic brain injury. *Archives of Physical Medicine and Rehabilitation*, **86**, 1565–1574.

Tinetti, M. E., Baker, D., Gallo, W. T. *et al.* (2002). Evaluation of restorative care vs usual care for older adults receiving an acute episode of home care. *Journal of the American Medical Association*, **287**, 2098–2010.

Tomberg, T., Toomela, A., Pulver, A., & Tikk, A. (2005). Coping strategies, social support, life orientation and health-related quality of life following traumatic brain injury. *Brain Injury*, **19**, 1181–1190.

Townsend, E., Stanton, S., Law, M. *et al.* (1997). *Enabling Occupation: An Occupational Therapy Perspective.* Ottawa, CA: CAOT Pub.

van den Heuvel, N., Smits, C. H., Deeg, D. J., & Beekman, A. T. (1996). Personality: a moderator of the relation between cognitive functioning and depression in adults aged 55–85? *Journal of Affective Disorders*, **41**, 229–240.

Walker, J. G., Jackson, H. I., & Littlejohn, G. O. (2004). Models of adjustment to chronic illness: using the example of rheumatoid arthritis. *Clinical Psychology Review*, **24**, 461–488.

Walker, M. F., Gladman, J. R., Lincoln, N. B., Siemonsma, P., & Whiteley, T. (1999). Occupational therapy for stroke patients not admitted to hospital: a randomised controlled trial. *Lancet*, **354**, 278–280.

Warden, D. L., Salazar, A., Martin, E. *et al.* (2000). A home program of rehabilitation for moderately severe traumatic brain injury patients. *Journal of Head Trauma Rehabilitation*, **15**, 1092–1102.

Weinberger, M., Tierney, W., Cowper, P., Katz, B., & Booher, P. (1993). Cost-effectiveness of increased telephone contact for patients with osteoarthritis: a randomized controlled trial. *Arthritis and Rheumatism*, **36**, 243–246.

Wight, R. G., Aneshensel, C. S., Seeman, M., & Seeman, T. E. (2003). Late life cognition among men: a life course perspective on psychosocial experience. *Archives of Gerontology and Geriatrics*, **37**, 173–193.

Winocur, G., & Moscovitch, M. (1990). A comparison of cognitive function in community-dwelling and institutionalized old people of normal intelligence. *Canadian Journal of Psychology*, **44**, 435–444.

Winocur, G., Craik, F. I. M., Levine, B. *et al.* (2007). Cognitive rehabilitation in the elderly: overview and future directions. *Journal of the International Neuropsychological Society*, **13**, 166–171.

Wood, R. L., & Rutterford, N. A. (2006). Demographic and cognitive predictors of long-term psychosocial outcome following traumatic brain injury. *Journal of the International Neuropsychological Society*, **12**, 350–358.

Yates, P. J. (2003). Psychological adjustment, social enablement and community integration following acquired brain injury. *Neuropsychological Rehabilitation*, **13**, 291–306.

Ylvisaker, M., & Feeney, T. (2002). Executive functions, self-regulation, and learned optimism in paediatric rehabilitation: a review and implications for intervention. *Pediatric Rehabilitation*, **5**, 51–70.

Ylvisaker, M., Jacobs, H. E., & Feeney, T. (2003). Positive supports for people who experience behavioral and cognitive disability after brain injury: a review. *Journal of Head Trauma Rehabilitation*, **18**, 7–32.

15

Exercise, cognition and dementia

Erik Scherder and Laura Eggermont

Introduction

- Although there is a strong association between physical activity and cognition, there is a paucity in clinical intervention studies investigating the effects of exercise on cognition in older people with dementia.
- Results from clinical studies on the effects of cognition in people with dementia have been inconsistent.
- The effects of physical activity on cognition may have been mitigated by vascular disease, often present in dementia.
- Vascular disease can lead to cerebral hypoperfusion and white matter lesions, which may result in executive dysfunction and gait disturbances, decreasing the level of physical activity.
- Disturbances in executive functioning and gait are present in Alzheimer's disease (AD), vascular dementia (VaD), and frontotemporal dementia (FTD), already in an early stage.
- Disturbances in executive functions and gait may be the cause of a physical activity program to be ineffective.
- In future studies concerning the effects of physical activity on cognition in patients with dementia, cardiovascular risk factors should be controlled for and special attention should be paid to subtle changes in gait and executive function.
- To be most effective, physical activity programs should be offered to people with dementia as early as possible.

Epidemiological studies show a positive relationship between the level of physical activity and cognitive functioning (Fratiglioni *et al.*, 2004; Laurin *et al.*, 2001; Rovio *et al.*, 2005; van Gelder *et al.*, 2004). In one prospective cohort study, in which participants were tested with a time interval of 5 years, it was observed that physical activity of a high intensity reduced the risk of cognitive impairment (Laurin *et al.*, 2001). These findings were particularly observed in women. A 10-year follow-up study with elderly men showed that the longer and the more intense the physical activity, the less cognitive function declined (van Gelder *et al.*, 2004). In another study, participants were tested twice with a mean time-interval of 21 years (Rovio *et al.*, 2005). The first moment of measurement (baseline) took place at midlife. A questionnaire was used to measure leisure-time physical activity. People who performed physical activity twice a week or more were classified as "active people"; sedentary subjects were those who were active less than two times a week. The results of this prospective epidemiological study show that an active lifestyle is associated with a considerable reduction in the risk for Alzheimer's disease (AD).

However, epidemiological studies are not able to indicate a *causal* relationship (Fratiglioni *et al.*, 2004). A more causal relationship, i.e., that physical activity really improves cognition, has been observed in randomized controlled trials on the effects of, for example, walking on cognition in older persons with a normal mental status or with mild cognitive impairment (MCI). These effects are described by Kramer, Erickson and McAuley in Chapter 24 of this

Cognitive Neurorehabilitation, Second Edition: Evidence and Application, ed. Donald T. Stuss, Gordon Winocur and Ian H. Robertson. Published by Cambridge University Press. © Cambridge University Press 2008.

volume. An important finding of those studies is that walking improves executive functions in particular and not cognition in general. Executive functions play a major role in one's autonomy (Cahn-Weiner *et al.*, 2000); in other words, physical activity (e.g., walking) has a beneficial influence on the subject's autonomy. The effects of exercise on cognition in normal aging will be addressed in Chapter 24.

In contrast to normal aging, a very limited number of *intervention* studies examined the effects of physical activity such as walking on cognition in patients with dementia. In discussing those studies in this chapter, a distinction will be made between the three main subtypes of dementia: Alzheimer's disease (AD), vascular dementia (VaD) and frontotemporal dementia (FTD). We will also discuss studies that included "older people with dementia," living in a nursing home without further specifying the subtype. When nursing home residents are described, studies with participants showing a mean score of less than 23/24 on the Mini Mental State Examination (MMSE) (Folstein *et al.*, 1975) are included as this is the standard cut-off point for cognitive impairment (Grut *et al.*, 1993). Another distinction that will be made is between studies that examined the influence of *exclusively* physical activity on cognition in older persons with dementia and studies that examined the effects of physical activity *in combination with* another type of intervention, for example, music, on cognition in this population. The results of these clinical studies will be discussed first.

It is noteworthy that the above-mentioned studies report both positive and negative findings. These negative findings may be related to the *intensity* of the exercise. As will be addressed in this chapter, the more intense the physical activity, the greater the cerebral perfusion, and is therefore an important factor in attaining a beneficial effect on cognition (Kramer *et al.*, 1999). However, the intensity of physical activity may be lowered by vascular disease to such an extent that participation in a physical activity program may be insufficient to increase the level of physical activity enough to improve cognition. In other words, vascular disease may be a crucial factor in weakening a positive effect of exercise on

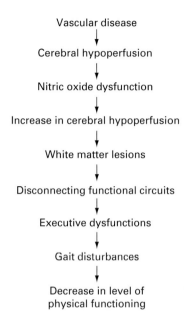

Vascular disease
↓
Cerebral hypoperfusion
↓
Nitric oxide dysfunction
↓
Increase in cerebral hypoperfusion
↓
White matter lesions
↓
Disconnecting functional circuits
↓
Executive dysfunctions
↓
Gait disturbances
↓
Decrease in level of
physical functioning

Figure 15.1. A cascade of events, initiated by vascular disease.

cognition. Therefore, we will indicate in each clinical study if vascular disease was controlled for.

We further argue that vascular disease, a neuropathological hallmark of the most prevalent subtypes of dementia, i.e., AD, VaD and FTD (Fernando & Ince, 2004; Nichol *et al.*, 2001; Pugh & Lipsitz, 2002), may initiate a cascade of events (Figure 15.1). In this cascade, vascular disease, through cerebral hypoperfusion, white matter lesions (WMLs), executive dysfunctions and gait disturbances will eventually lead to a decrease in patients' level of physical functioning. This cascade will be discussed in more detail in this chapter. Finally, clinically relevant suggestions about the application of a physical activity program in older persons with dementia will be presented.

Physical activity and cognition: intervention studies

- In patients with AD or "dementia," studies of physical activity on cognition report both positive and negative findings (Table 15.1).

- No studies were performed that specifically included patients with VaD or FTD.
- Most studies show serious methodological flaws.
- In studies that combine two types of intervention it remains debatable which type of stimulation was (most) effective.
- Differences in design or severity of dementia may explain some of the inconsistencies in the findings.
- Only a few studies excluded patients with cardiovascular disease, the presence of which may have attenuated the effects of physical activity on cognition.

Alzheimer's disease

- Four studies on the effects of physical activity on cognition in AD patients have shown positive results, two noted a maintenance of function and two reported no positive effects.
- Only three of the eight studies specifically excluded patients with cardiovascular disease.

Exclusively physical activity

One study used a single exercise session in AD patients to examine the effects of physical activity on cognition. One 20-minute session of walking or arm and leg extensions, was not found to lead to statistical differences in language ability, word retrieval or verbal recognition in a group of 25 AD patients (Sobel, 2001). No information was provided about the presence of cardiovascular risk factors in these participants. One explanation for the lack of improvement might be that some of the participants were physically less active and one might wonder whether they could perform the exercises intensively enough to improve cognition.

A few studies have implemented exercise programs of a longer period in which AD patients participated. In one study, 15 males diagnosed with possible AD exercised on a cycle ergometer for more than 20 minutes a day, 3 days a week, for 3 months (Palleschi *et al.*, 1996). The AD patients

showed an improvement in their performance on three tests of attention and short-term memory and the MMSE. Electrocardiography performed at rest and during physical activity did not show any abnormalities in the patients. A group of 23 moderate to severe AD patients also showed significantly improved performance on the MMSE after a program of endurance exercise that consisted of walking and riding an exercise bicycle for a mean of 7 weeks (5–12 weeks) (Rolland *et al.*, 2000). Patients with cardiac disease were excluded from participation. It should be noted however that a control group was lacking in both of these studies. Another flaw of the latter study was that the time the patients participated in the daily activity program varied from 10–80 minutes. Finally, one study reports positive effects of exercise (somatic exercises and relaxation exercises) during a period of 8 weeks on cognitive functioning, without further specifying the nature of the cognitive abilities (Lindenmuth & Moose, 1990). Of note is that the participants were allowed to choose whether they preferred to be in the experimental group or control group. Moreover, participation in the exercise group was irregular, and the control group did not take part in any alternative activity. Information about the cardiovascular condition of these patients was not provided.

In sum, three out of four studies report an improvement in global cognitive functioning in AD patients, after participation in an exercise program. Nevertheless, these results should be considered with caution, in view of serious methodological flaws.

Physical activity combined with another type of intervention

Two studies that examined the effects of walking in combination with talking on communication in AD patients have found inconsistent results. Friedman & Tappen (1991) reported on 30 moderate to severe AD patients who were randomly assigned to two groups: the experimental group received a 30-minute walking and conversation program and a control group received a 30-minute conversation-only

Table 15.1. Characteristics of intervention studies examining the effects of physical activity on cognition in patients with dementia. ADL = Activities of Daily Living; M = mean; MMSE = Mini-Mental State Examination; ROM = Range of Motion; SD = standard deviation.

Study	n	Age	Stage of AD	Design	Type of physical intervention	Results	Comorbidity
Exclusively physical activity; AD patients							
Palleschi et al. (1996)	15	M=74.0 (SD=1.5)	MMSE: M=19.4 (18–21) GDS stage 4 or 5	Pre-post measurement. No control group	Exercise on a cycloergometer	Improvement in MMSE score and attention	Controlled for cardiovascular disease: not present
Rolland et al. (2000)	23	M=78 (71–92)	MMSE: M=16.3 (1–25)	Individual physical activity program. No control group	Endurance or resistance exercise, warming-up exercise, balance	Improvement in MMSE score	Patients with cardiac disease were excluded
Sobel (2001)	50	M=82 (62–99)	MMSE: M=14.08 (8–25)	One single session; pre-post measurement. No control group	Walking or arm/leg extensions	No effects on a naming task and a word recognition task	Not indicated
Lindenmuth & Moose (1990)	43	M=82.8 (65–98)	Not indicated	Experimental and control group; pre-post measurement	Exp. group: isometric and relaxation exercises. Control group: no intervention	Improvement in cognition, not further specified	Not indicated
Physical activity in combination; AD patients							
Friedman & Tappen (1991)	30	M = 72.8 (60–87)	MMSE: Exp. group M=6.5 Control group M=6.4	Experimental and control group; pre-post measurement	Exp. group: walking and talking Control group: talking	Improved communication	Patients with a history of stroke were excluded. Medical conditions including diabetes, hypertension and congestive heart failure were present
Cott et al. (2002)	54	M=82 (SD=8)	MMSE: Exp group I M=6.2 Exp group II M=5.4 Control group M=6.3	Two treatment groups and one control group; pre-post measurement	Exp. group I: walking and talking. Exp. group II: Conversation. Control group: No study-provided intervention	No change in communication	Patients that showed contraindications to participate were excluded. Not further specified
Arkin (2001)	11	M=79 (59–86)	MMSE: M=23 (15–29)	Pre-post measurement. No control group	Physical fitness training, consisting of aerobic and weight training activities	Performance on several cognitive tasks was maintained	Not indicated
Arkin (2003)	24	M=78.8 (SD=8)	MMSE (15–29)	Pre-post measurement. No control group	As for Arkin (2001), plus 10 recreational sessions	Cognitive decline was slowed. Not further specified	Before exercising, it was assessed whether resting pulse was below 100

Table 15.1. (*cont.*)

Study	n	Age	Stage of AD	Design	Type of physical intervention	Results	Comorbidity
Exclusively physical activity; people with dementia/nursing home residents							
Diesfeldt & Diesfeldt-Groenendijk (1977)	40	M=82	Serious difficulty in performing ADL and many had memory problems and were disoriented	Experimental group/control group; pre-post measurement	Exp. group: bending/stretching, playing a game consisting of throwing and kicking a ball and knocking down skittles Control group: No study-provided intervention	Improved memory performance	"Acute illness" formed a criterion for exclusion. Not further specified
Powell (1974)	30	M= 69.3 (59–89)	Not indicated	Two treatment groups/one control group; pre-post measurement	Exp. group: mild exercise: brisk walking, callisthenics, rhythmical movements Control group: social interaction and music	Increased memory	Patients with hypertension and a history of heart trouble for which drugs were administered were excluded from participation. Electrocardiograms were given prior to the intervention
de Carvalho Bastone & Filho (2004)	37	Exp. group M=76.8 Control group M=80.3 (60–99)	MMSE: Exp. group M=19.2 Control group M=20.9	Experimental and control group; pre-post measurement	Exp. group: exercise program including mobility exercises, strengthening exercises and walking	Maintenance of MMSE score compared with the control group	People identified with any condition that precluded participation in exercise such as symptomatic coronary insufficiency, congestive heart failure and hypertension were excluded from participation
Baum et al. (2003)	20	M=88 (75–99)	MMSE: Exp. group M=21 Control group M=22 (10–29)	Experimental and control group; pre-post measurement	Exp. group: exercise program containing seated strength and range of motion exercises Control group: recreational therapy	Increased MMSE score	People with unstable acute illness or chronic illness (e.g., uncompensated congestive heart failure) were excluded from participation

Study	N	Mean age	Cognitive measure	Design	Intervention	Outcome	Medical condition / exclusion
Mulrow et al. (1994)	189	Exp. group M = 79.7 (SD=8.5) Control group M=81.4 (SD=8.5)	MMSE: M=21	Experimental and control group; pre-post measurement	Exp. group: physical therapy: ROM exercises, resistance exercises, endurance activities and gait training. Control group: social visits	Performance on the MMSE did not improve	People with terminal illness or active medical condition that in the judgment of the physician precluded participation were excluded from the study. Not further specified
Scherder et al. (2005)	43	Exp. group I: M=84 Exp. group II: M=89 Control group: M=86 (76–94)	MMSE (short version): 7–12 indicative for mild/cognitive deterioration	Two treatment groups/one control group; repeated measures	Exp. group I: self-paced slow walking with an aid. Exp. group II: carrying out hand movements and facial expressions. Control group: social visits or continuance of normal social activities	Improvement in tasks appealing to executive functioning	Congestive heart failure, hypertension and diabetes was present in the participants

Physical activity in combination; people with dementia/nursing home residents

Study	N	Mean age	Cognitive measure	Design	Intervention	Outcome	Medical condition / exclusion
McMurdo & Rennie (1994)	65	M=83 (67–98)	MMSE: Exp. group M=15.7 Control group M=15.2	Experimental and control group; pre-post measurement	Exp. group: seated exercises to music. Control group: reminiscence therapy	No improved reaction time. No improved performance on the MMSE	No participants were excluded on the basis of any specific pre-existing medical condition
Hopman-Rock et al. (1999)	92	Exp. group M=83.8 (SD=5.8) Control group M=84.2 (SD=5.6)	Cognitive screening test-14 Exp. group: M=5.1 Control group: M=6.1	Experimental and control group; pre-post measurement	Exp. group: psychomotor activation program (PAP) which consists of sporting activities, games and hobby activities. Control group: No study-provided intervention	Stabilisation of cognition	Not indicated
van de Winckel et al. (2004)	25	Exp. group M=81.33 (SD=4.2) Control group M=81.9 (SD=4.2)	MMSE: Exp. group M=12.9 Control group M=10.8	Experimental and control group; pre-post measurement	Exp: seated exercises supported by music, consisting of extremities strengthening, trunk movements and balance/flexibility training. Control group: conversation	Improved score on the MMSE and a verbal fluency task	Physicians gave medical clearance for participation in the study

program, for 10 weeks. It is noteworthy that people with a history of stroke were excluded from the study. Medical conditions including diabetes, hypertension and congestive heart failure however were present. After the treatment period, communication improved only in the group with combined walking and conversation. These results were not confirmed in another study, in which 90 AD patients were divided at random into three groups: a walk-and-talk group (walking and talking in pairs), a talk-only group (talking in pairs) and a nonintervention group (Cott *et al.*, 2002). The interventions were performed for 30 minutes, 5 days a week, for 16 weeks. Patients were excluded if the physician identified contraindications; the nature of these contraindications was not further specified. Social communication skills and communication of basic needs were not found to change after the intervention period in the walk-and-talk group compared with the other two groups. However, the participants in this study demonstrated large differences in level of cognitive impairment at study onset, though most were severely cognitively impaired; this might explain the lack of improvement.

In a small study by Arkin (2001), 11 patients with mild to moderate AD followed a twice-weekly physical fitness training course, containing a variety of exercises such as aerobic and weight resistance activities, for 10 weeks. Seven out of the 11 elderly participants also received specific memory and language stimulation exercises; for example, they played word games and were asked their advice and opinion on various issues. It was claimed that the exercise prevented a significant cognitive decline, irrespective of whether memory and language training was given. A limitation of this study was the small sample size. In a longitudinal follow-up study, a comparable exercise program with an additional 10 recreational activity sessions was followed by 24 patients with early to early-moderate AD (MMSE scores 15–29) during a period of 1 to 4 years (Arkin, 2003). The author reports the slowing of cognitive decline. Unfortunately, no details of the cognitive benefits were given. Moreover, in both studies a control group was lacking. In the latter

study, before exercise was started, patients were checked whether their pulse was below 100.

In sum, results of studies in AD patients examining a combination of physical activity and another type of stimulation have been both positive and negative. Differences in study design or the severity of dementia might explain the inconsistency. In addition, when combined with another type of activity, positive effects can not be purely explained by the exercise performed.

Vascular dementia and frontotemporal dementia

- There are no clinical intervention studies on the effects of physical activity on cognition in patients with VaD or FTD.

As far as the authors know, studies examining the effects of exclusively physical activity and the effects of physical activity combined with another type of intervention on cognition have not been performed with respect to VaD and FTD.

Older persons with "dementia" or living in a long-term care facility

- Studies on the effects of physical activity on cognitive functioning in older people with "dementia" have shown inconsistent results.
- In only one third of the studies, patients with cardiovascular risk factors were specifically excluded from participation.
- Whether all participants in the reviewed studies were cognitively impaired remains obscure.

Exclusively physical activity

In one study evaluating treatment effects after a single session, 20 psychogeriatric patients underwent an acute bout of exercise for 40 minutes and showed a significant improvement in memory performance compared with a control group (Diesfeldt & Diesfeldt-Groenendijk, 1977). "Acute illness" formed an exclusion criterion of the study. Some studies have been described in which older people with dementia or people living in a nursing home showing cognitive impairment as a group were given exercise for a longer period. In a randomized controlled study, 30 older psychiatric patients were divided into two treatment groups; one group received conventional social therapy and one received exercise therapy. Also a control group was included (Powell, 1974). Patients with hypertension and a history of heart disease with prescriptive medication were not included in the study. Both treatment groups met for 1 hour, 5 days per week. After 12 weeks of treatment the exercise group showed improved logical reasoning and memory performance compared with the other groups. In a more recent study (de Carvalho Bastone & Filho, 2004) 40 people living in a nursing home participated. All participants were medically screened and people with symptomatic coronary insufficiency, uncontrolled chronic disease-diabetes, congestive heart failure and hypertension were excluded from participation. People were assigned to either an exercise group or a control group. The exercise program was performed twice weekly for 1 hour and the control group did not attend to any alternative activity. After 6 months, performance on the MMSE was maintained in the exercise group, but the performance on the MMSE deteriorated significantly in the control group. In another study (Baum et al., 2003) that used the MMSE as an outcome measure, 20 frail assisted living and nursing home residents participated. Participants were randomly divided into two groups: one group received an exercise program for 1 hour 3 times per week and the other group received recreational therapy in the same frequency. People with unstable acute illness or chronic illness, such as uncompensated congestive heart failure were excluded from participation. The exercise program contained seated range of motion (ROM) exercises and strength training. After 6 months, performance on the MMSE improved significantly. In contrast, in a study in which 189 frail nursing home residents participated (Mulrow et al., 1994), performance on the MMSE was not found to be improved after 4 months of physical therapy. In this study, persons were randomly assigned to physical therapy

sessions or friendly visits for 3 times a week. People with terminal illness or an active medical condition that precluded participation were not included in the study. Physical therapy included ROM exercises, resistance exercises, endurance activities and gait training. A recent pilot study (Scherder et al., 2005) included 43 older individuals with mild cognitive impairment – a transitional stage to AD (Petersen et al., 1999) – living in a nursing home. Among these individuals, congestive heart failure, hypertension and diabetes were present. Persons were randomly divided into three groups: a walking group, a group carrying out hand and face exercises and a control group that received social visits. Treatment was provided for 30 minutes, 3 days a week for 6 weeks. Performance on tasks that measure executive functioning and verbal fluency, improved in both the walking group and the hand/face exercise group.

Taken together, the effects on cognition in studies offering exercise programmes in nursing home residents have been inconsistent. It is of note, however, that in the above mentioned studies except for the last one reviewed, people were living in a nursing home and generally appeared to be cognitively impaired, but it remains uncertain if *all* people were cognitively impaired.

Physical activity combined with another type of intervention

A study examining the effects of the combination of exercise and music included 65 older persons living in a nursing home (McMurdo & Rennie, 1994). People were randomly allocated to either an exercise group or a reminiscence group. Irrespective of pre-existing medical conditions, people could participate in the study. The people in the exercise group participated in a twice-weekly group session for 45 minutes during which they exercised to music while sitting on a chair. The reminiscence group received reminiscence therapy in the same frequency. After 6 months both groups did not show improved reaction time (recognition movement time and response time) nor improved MMSE score (McMurdo & Rennie, 1994). Another randomized controlled study in which a similar intervention was performed did show positive results (van de Winckel *et al.*, 2004). Fifteen women with dementia participated in a 3-month exercise program which consisted of daily seated exercises supported by music. The control group that consisted of 10 patients received daily conversation in the same frequency. After the intervention period the exercise group showed a significant improvement on the MMSE and a verbal fluency measure compared with the control group. Participation of the patients was approved by a physician; specific contraindications were not mentioned in the study (van de Winckel *et al.*, 2004).

The effects of a twice weekly psychomotor activation program (PAP) were examined in people with dementia in a randomized controlled study (Hopman-Rock *et al.*, 1999). The program consists of sporting activities, games and hobby activities to stimulate both cognitive and psychosocial function. Forty-five older persons with dementia completed the study period of 6 months and 47 older individuals with dementia functioned as the control group and engaged in the regular activities provided by the nursing home. Results show maintenance in global cognitive function (Hopman-Rock *et al.*, 1999). Comorbidity of the participants was not reported.

In sum, studies in older people living in long-term care facilities examining a combination of physical activity with another type of stimulation have shown inconsistent results. Differences in intervention frequency or the presence or absence of dementia in the participants might explain the inconsistent findings.

Summary

Four out of 17 studies reviewed here reported that physical activity applied exclusively or in combination with another type of stimulation, did not improve cognition in patients with dementia (Cott *et al.*, 2002; McMurdo & Rennie, 1994; Mulrow *et al.*, 1994; Sobel, 2001). Three other studies reported that the observed maintenance of cognitive performance and a slowing of the cognitive decline should

be considered positive treatment effects (Arkin, 2001, 2003; de Carvalho Bastone & Filho, 2004) but in the latter two studies a control group was lacking (Arkin, 2001, 2003). Except for the study of de Carvalho Bastone & Filho (2004), it is remarkable that in the other six studies, cardiovascular disease was not controlled for. Although we will argue in this chapter that vascular disease may weaken or even prevent a beneficial effect of physical activity on cognition, the presence of vascular disease does not exclude a positive effect. Two of the studies discussed here found positive effects of physical activity on cognition in people with dementia, among whom were patients with vascular disease. The question whether the effects would have been stronger in the absence of vascular disease remains unanswered.

Another striking finding is that most studies do not differentiate between subtypes of dementia. Only a few studies focused specifically on AD patients, and we could not find studies that included patients with VaD and FTD.

Negative findings, the intensity of physical activity and cerebral blood flow

- Positive effects of physical activity on cognition seem to depend on the intensity of physical activity.
- Aerobic physical activity (and hence physical energy expenditure) declines with age and is even lower in AD patients.
- Low levels of physical energy expenditure are most pronounced in patients with vascular disease.

A crucial finding in the study of Kramer and colleagues (1999) (see also Chapter 24 of this volume) in which older persons without dementia participated is that an increase in aerobic power, expressed in VO_2max (the highest rate of oxygen, which can be taken up and utilized by the body during exercise), is a prerequisite for exercise to improve cognitive functioning; stretching exercises did not exert a beneficial influence on cognition. Indeed, observational studies show that, for healthy older people (both men and women), the intensity of physical activity and the consequent level of physical energy expenditure is positively correlated with the level of cognitive functioning (van Gelder et al., 2004; Weuve et al., 2004).

A biological basis for these findings emerges from a recent study of cognitively intact older people; this study showed that higher levels of aerobic fitness (expressed in VO$_2$max) are associated with lower levels of age-related decline in tissue density in the frontal, parietal and temporal lobes (Colcombe et al., 2003). Indeed, dynamic activities such as rowing (Pott et al., 1997) and cycling (Hellström et al., 1996) increases the velocity of the cerebral blood flow (CBF) in healthy participants; CBF was even enhanced by submaximal cycling (Jørgensen et al., 1992). Dynamic activities increase the heart rate and mean arterial blood pressure, and consequently, enhance the CBF in various cortical and subcortical areas in healthy volunteers (Critchley et al., 2000). Interestingly, CBF appeared to be dependent on the extent of increase in heart rate and mean arterial blood pressure. A mild increase in mean arterial blood pressure enhanced the CBF in, for example, the hippocampus and the medial temporal gyrus, whereas a strong increase in mean arterial blood pressure enhanced the CBF in the anterior cingulate cortex, cerebellar vermis and brain stem (Critchley et al., 2000). Indeed, an increase in CBF is frequently used as a global measure for neural activity in brain imaging studies (Iadecola, 2004; Wolf et al., 2001).

Concerning the negative findings in some studies in which the effects of physical activity on cognition in older persons with dementia were examined, it is important to note that in normal aging, aerobic physical activity progressively declines, regardless of whether older people are endurance-trained or sedentary (Schilke, 1991; Wilson et al., 2000). The reduction in aerobic physical activity among older people is reflected in a decrease of energy expenditure in physical activity (Westerterp, 2000; Wilson & Morley, 2003). Compared with older persons without dementia, the level of aerobic physical activity (and hence of physical energy expenditure) is even lower among AD patients (Pettersson et al., 2002; Poehlman et al., 1997; Wang et al., 2004). The

finding that the lowest levels of physical energy expenditure can be observed among elderly individuals with vascular disease such as hypertension and diabetes (Weuve et al., 2004), together with the fact that such individuals also report difficulties in more than one Activity of Daily Living and Instrumental Activity of Daily Living (Podewils et al., 2005), has important implications for subcortical ischemic vascular dementia (SIVD), the most prevalent subtype of vascular dementia (Román et al., 2002). Vascular disease (e.g., hypertension) forms the pathophysiological basis for SIVD (Román et al., 2002), but may also play a role in AD (Newman et al., 2005).

In sum, as well as AD patients, SIVD patients may also experience decreased physical energy expenditure, which may coincide with impairments in cognitive functioning. Studies examining the relationship between FTD and physical energy expenditure could not be found.

Taken together, a decrease in the level of aerobic physical activity, and hence in the level of physical activity energy expenditure, shows a close relationship with vascular disease. Vascular disease initiates a cascade of events that, at the end, will cause a decrease in the level of physical activity. We will elaborate on this cascade of events in the next sections.

Vascular disease, level of physical activity and cognition in dementia: a cascade of events

- Vascular disease may lower cerebral perfusion and disturb nitric oxide (NO) metabolism.
- Exercise leads to increased cerebral perfusion and may attenuate NO dysfunction.
- Cerebral hypoperfusion negatively affects several cognitive functions in AD, VaD and FTD.
- Hypoperfusion can cause white matter lesions and may disrupt functional circuits in the brain.
- Disruptions of fronto-cortical and fronto-subcortical circuits lead to disturbances in executive function and gait, which reduce physical activity.

A cascade of events, initiated by vascular disease, will be addressed (see Figure 15.1) with respect to three main subtypes of dementia: AD, VaD and FTD. In this cascade, vascular disease exerts a negative effect on the level of physical activity, and consequently on cognitive functioning, through cerebral hypoperfusion in relationship with a disturbance in nitric oxide (NO), and white matter lesions.

Vascular disease and cerebral hypoperfusion

- In AD, vascular pathology like cerebral amyloid angiopathy and cerebral infarcts are common and cause hypoperfusion.
- VaD is characterized by vascular disease, and by infarctions of the white matter and in the basal forebrain, cerebral perfusion is reduced.
- In FTD, hypoperfusion has been reported in several areas of the anterior brain regions.

As described above, vascular disease like hypertension and diabetes mellitus lowers cerebral perfusion in several ways, for example by lowering the level of aerobic physical activity (Weuve *et al.*, 2004), or by causing cerebrovascular pathology (Eggermont *et al.*, 2006). Cerebrovascular disease is responsible for ischemic hypoperfusion (Román, 2004), a neuropathological hallmark of AD (Miklossy, 2003), vascular dementia (Román, 2004) and frontotemporal dementia (Osawa *et al.*, 2004).

Alzheimer's disease

Results from a recent study show that the majority of the Alzheimer patients that participated in the study suffered from vascular pathology in the brain (Fernando & Ince, 2004). Cerebrovascular disease in AD is responsible for hypoperfusion (de la Torre, 2002). Vascular problems in AD may be expressed as cerebral amyloid angiopathy (CAA) which could be viewed as a combination of pathology typical for AD (amyloid) and vascular pathology (angiopathy). Cerebral amyloid angiopathy concerns the deposition of protein in the blood vessel walls of the brain (Castellani *et al.*, 2004), among which is the amyloid β-precursor protein. The involvement of the

amyloid β-precursor protein in CAA underscores a relationship between CAA and Alzheimer's disease (Castellani *et al.*, 2004). Of note is that CAA causes ischemia and hemorrhage (Castellani *et al.*, 2004). Cerebral ischemia initiates the degeneration and death of neurons (Koistinaho & Koistinaho, 2005). A consequence might be that the cognitive decline in AD with CAA is much more severe than AD without CAA (Castellani *et al.*, 2004). Of note is that a considerable number of Alzheimer patients show evidence of cerebral infarcts and that the presence of cerebrovascular disease aggravates the course of AD. One of the underlying mechanisms might be that brain ischemia may enhance inflammatory processes by inducing pro-inflammatory mediators (Koistinaho & Koistinaho, 2005); their release is enhanced on the basis of, among others, oxygen deprivation. The reverse is also possible: the presence of Alzheimer neuropathology may increase the risk for cerebrovascular disease (Koistinaho & Koistinaho, 2005). Alzheimer's disease patients may later develop a stroke.

Vascular dementia

Patients with hypertension have an increased risk of developing SIVD (Pugh & Lipsitz, 2002), which is the most prevalent subtype of vascular dementia (Román *et al.*, 2002). The pathological sequence of events underlying subcortical ischemic vascular dementia is as follows: hypertension causes a disease of the small vessels (arteriolosclerosis) which subsequently causes either an occlusion or a hypoperfusion. An occlusion leads to a complete infarction, also called a lacunar infarction ("lacunar state"); hypoperfusion creates an incomplete infarction which damages the white matter, a disease entity called "Binswanger's disease" (Román *et al.*, 2002).

Small arteries, most vulnerable for hypertension, penetrate areas of the cholinergic basal forebrain, among which is the septum (Román, 2004). Patients with vascular dementia also show infarctions of the basal forebrain nucleus basalis of Meynert (Román & Kalaria, 2006). The cholinergic system, originating from among others the nucleus basalis of Meynert, activates a vasodilatory system, resulting in an increase in cerebral blood flow (Román, 2004). This relationship appears to be reciprocal: the cerebral blood flow also influences the functioning of the cerebral cholinergic neurons (Román & Kalaria, 2006). In other words, damage to one system may thus have a negative effect on the other. A decline in cerebral blood flow is reflected in a decrease in, for example, glucose metabolism (Román & Kalaria, 2006).

Frontotemporal dementia

A change in the perfusion of the anterior brain regions has been observed in FTD (Mariani *et al.*, 2006). More specifically, hypoperfusion has been observed in the left superior frontal cortex, the right middle and inferior frontal region (Osawa *et al.*, 2004), the right anterior cingulate, the right ventrolateral prefrontal cortex, and the right orbitofrontal cortex (Varrone *et al.*, 2002). Moreover, in that study a decrease in rCBF was also found in the right anterior temporal lobe. A related finding is a decline in the glucose metabolism in the frontal lobe, due to a deficit in the serotonergic neurotransmitter system (Franchesi *et al.*, 2005). The involvement of the serotonergic system in this disorder has been confirmed by others (Yang & Schmitt, 2001).

Cerebral hypoperfusion and nitric oxide

- Nitric oxide (NO) plays a pivotal role in cerebral perfusion.
- In AD, and possibly VaD, NO metabolism is affected and causes hypoperfusion.
- High homocysteine levels inhibit NO production and form a risk factor for cardiovascular disease.
- Exercise leads to an increase of NO and subsequent vasodilatation.

Nitric oxide (NO) is derived from vascular endothelial nitric oxide synthase (eNOS) and plays a crucial role in the cerebral perfusion by influencing vascular tone, blood pressure and vascular homeostasis (Huang *et al.*, 1995; Kubes & Granger, 1992). Nitric oxide mediates cerebral autoregulation

(White *et al.*, 2000). Moreover, NO reduces the risk for atherosclerosis and thrombosis and improves blood flow by lowering stress on the blood vessel wall. In this way, NO protects endothelial cell function (Maxwell, 2002). A dysfunction of NO metabolism will be discussed in relationship with cerebral hypoperfusion with respect to AD and VaD; NO has not been studied concerning FTD, as far as the authors know.

Alzheimer's disease

A key factor associated with cerebral hypoperfusion in AD is a dysfunction of NO metabolism (Churchill *et al.*, 2002; Selley, 2003). In AD, hypoperfusion may disturb basal NO levels, causing alterations in the endothelium and inducing vascular injury (Cooke & Dzau, 1997). More specifically, it is argued that when the cerebral perfusion decreases below a certain critical level, eNOS tries to maintain vascular homeostasis by upregulating NO (de la Torre, 2002). In failing to do so, NO becomes deregulated, damages the endothelial cells and impairs glucose transport to the brain (Chen *et al.*, 1999). This vicious circle is presented in Figure 15.2. It is noteworthy that inhibition of NO production also results from increased levels of homocysteine in the blood of AD patients (Selley, 2003). A high level of homocysteine is a risk factor for cardiovascular disease (Herrmann, 2001).

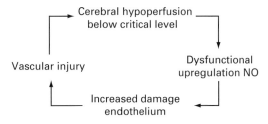

Figure 15.2. A vicious circle characteristic for cerebral hypoperfusion in Alzheimer's disease. Below a critical level, cerebral hypoperfusion causes a dysfunctional upregulation of nitric oxide (NO), enhancing vascular injury and, consequently, aggravating cerebral hypoperfusion.

Vascular dementia

Results from a recent study suggest that homocysteine levels of VaD patients were increased and coincided with a decrease in plasma NO levels (Folin *et al.*, 2005).

In sum, recent findings show that NO plays an essential role in cerebral hypoperfusion, particularly in AD patients and possibly also in VaD patients. The role of NO in cerebral perfusion is even more interesting since studies have examined the relationship between NO and exercise.

Nitric oxide and exercise

A positive relationship between nitric oxide, cardio- and cerebrovascular functioning, and exercise has been observed in animal experimental studies (Endres *et al.*, 2003). Running provoked an upregulation of eNOS, together with vasodilatation and a significant reduction in the size of the lesion, brain swelling, and sensory-motor deficits, in mice with cerebral ischemia due to an occlusion of the middle cerebral artery (Endres *et al.*, 2003). Irrespective of the nature of the running, i.e., voluntary or trained, the increase in rCBF showed high values in the hippocampus (Endres *et al.*, 2003). Of note is that serotoninergic dysfunction resulting in a hyposerotoninergic condition, causes a supersensitivity to NO (Srikiatkhachorn *et al.*, 2000), implying that even mild physical activity could result in beneficial effects. Serotoninergic dysfunction is characteristic for AD (Meltzer *et al.*, 1998), VaD (Court & Perry, 2003), and FTD (Huey *et al.*, 2006). The serotoninergic system is, however, not the only neurotransmitter system that responds to exercise. Animal experimental studies show some support for a relationship between exercise and the cholinergic system, i.e., walking significantly increased release of acetylcholine in conscious rats (Kurosawa *et al.*, 1993). Interestingly, the higher the walking speed, the higher the cholinergic-induced increase in CBF in the hippocampus (Nakajima *et al.*, 2003). The cholinergic system is affected in AD (Wenk, 2006), VaD (Court & Perry, 2003), and relatively preserved in FTD (Huey *et al.*, 2006).

Finally, the NO dysfunction caused by high levels of homocysteine may be attenuated by exercise (Hayward *et al.*, 2003). This effect may be dependent on the duration and the intensity of exercise. For example, strenuous exercise may even lead to a homocysteine increase in recreational endurance athletes (Herrmann *et al.*, 2003), damaging the NO function.

Cerebral hypoperfusion and cognition

- Cerebral hypoperfusion in AD, VaD and FTD is associated with impaired global cognitive functioning, memory, and visuoconstructive and visuospatial abilities.

Alzheimer's disease

In AD, significant correlations were found between MMSE scores and hypoperfusion in frontal, parietal and temporal cortex (Jagust *et al.*, 1997; Tsolaki *et al.*, 2001; Ushijima *et al.*, 2002). Items appealing to attention/calculation were related to a decline in the CBF in the frontal cortex; all other items covering, for example, orientation and recall, were related to a decreased CBF in the posterior brain regions (Ushijima *et al.*, 2002). Concerning more specific neurocognitive functioning, the scores on the Cambridge Cognitive Examination (CAMCOG) (Roth *et al.*, 1986) appeared to be significantly associated with hypoperfusion (Tsolaki *et al.*, 2001). In another study, left posterior temporal regional CBF (rCBF) was a predictor of performance on the clock drawing test (Ueda *et al.*, 2002). A decline in working memory, semantic memory and episodic memory was associated with hypoperfusion in the left superior and right middle and inferior frontal region, in the bilateral angular, temporal, occipital and precentral regions, hippocampi, thalami and periclallosal regions and in the left lenticular nucleus (Osawa *et al.*, 2004). Furthermore, AD patients who progressively decline show a reduction in the rCBF in the right posterodorsal anterior and superior prefrontal cortex and the inferior parietal cortex (Nagahama *et al.*, 2003).

Vascular dementia

Measured by a three-dimensional stereotaxic regions of interest template method (3DSRT), hypoperfusion was observed in the left superior and right middle and inferior frontal region, in the bilateral angular, temporal, occipital and precentral regions, hippocampi, thalami and pericallosal regions and in the left lenticular nucleus (Osawa *et al.*, 2004). These patients showed lower scores on the MMSE, on tests appealing to working and episodic memory, as well as on the score of the Raven's Progressive Matrices (Osawa *et al.*, 2004). In another study, using among others single photon emission computed tomography (SPECT) (Cohen *et al.*, 2001), a strong relationship was observed between total cerebral perfusion and the performance on tests appealing to episodic memory, and verbal and visuospatial capacities.

Frontotemporal dementia

In FTD patients, hypoperfusion was observed in the left superior and right middle and inferior frontal region (Osawa *et al.*, 2004). These patients showed a decline in the performance on working memory and episodic memory (Osawa *et al.*, 2004).

Taken the three subtypes of dementia together, cerebral hypoperfusion negatively influences global cognitive functioning, working memory, episodic memory, semantic memory, visuoconstructive and visuospatial capacities. It is of note that cerebral hypoperfusion specifically affects white matter, which degeneration has a profound effect on executive functions and gait; executive dysfunctions and gait disturbances further impair patients' level of physical activity.

Hypoperfusion, white matter lesions, executive dysfunctions and gait in various subtypes of dementia

- Degeneration of periventricular white matter by ischemic hypoperfusion damages functional fronto-cortical and fronto-subcortical circuits which may lead to executive dysfunction and gait disturbances.

By affecting particularly periventricular white matter, ischemic hypoperfusion damages functional neural circuits by disconnecting brain areas such as the hippocampus, the basal ganglia and the frontal lobe (Román, 2004). Since these functional circuits play an essential role in executive functions and gait, periventricular white matter and related brain areas will be discussed first.

Degeneration of the periventricular white matter disturbs the functioning of fronto-cortical circuits, among which the fronto-hippocampal circuit and fronto-subcortical circuits, for example the fronto-striatal system (Pugh & Lipsitz, 2002). A dysfunction of the fronto-hippocampal circuit by hippocampal degeneration (van de Pol *et al.*, 2006) might explain why AD patients show an impairment in executive functions (Diaz *et al.*, 2004). A disconnection of the fronto-striatal system is responsible for executive dysfunctions in VaD patients (Duke & Kaszniak, 2000; Pugh & Lipsitz, 2002). In FTD, the fronto-striatal system is strongly affected (Panegyres, 2004) by, for example, degeneration of the dopaminergic nigrostriatal system (Rinne *et al.*, 2002).

The role of the hippocampus in gait is less well known than in cognition. However, based on the involvement of the hippocampus in space representation and navigation (Kaske *et al.*, 2006; Shapiro, 2001), it is argued that its degeneration in AD (van de Pol *et al.*, 2006), VaD (Bowler, 2002), and FTD (Franchesi *et al.*, 2005), contributes to a gait disturbance. Support for this suggestion emerges from animal experimental studies that show that the hippocampus plays a key role in a vicious circle in which internally and externally generated sensory information is integrated into voluntary motor activity (Bland & Oddie, 2001). Internally and externally motor-related sensory information is related to head direction, necessary for spatial orientation and navigation (Wiener *et al.*, 2002).

In contrast to the hippocampus, the basal ganglia and functional related areas are known for their role in gait. It has been suggested that gait disturbances in AD might be provoked by, among others, neuronal loss in the substantia nigra (Burns *et al.*, 2005), in VaD by lacunar infarcts in the striatum (Kim *et al.*, 1981) and in FTD by degeneration of the dopaminergic nigrostriatal system (Rinne *et al.*, 2002).

In sum, neuropathology in fronto-cortical and fronto-subcortical circuits, disrupting the functional relationship between the basal ganglia, the hippocampus and the frontal lobe, causes a co-existence of executive dysfunctions and gait disturbances in the various subtypes of dementia. Characteristics of the disturbances in executive functions and gait concerning AD, VaD and FTD will be discussed in the next sections.

Executive dysfunctions in various subtypes of dementia

- In AD, executive functions such as volition, planning and attention are impaired. Considering attention, particularly dual tasking that requires divided attention seems to be problematic.
- As a result of the fronto-striatal system disruption, VaD patients show executive dysfunctioning that involves a reduction in psychomotor speed, working memory impairment, attentional problems and apathy.
- Frontotemporal dementia is characterized by executive dysfunction as well as disturbances in behavior and personality.
- The impairment in executive functioning may lead to gait disturbances and a decrease in activities of daily life.

It is known that executive functions are not a unitary concept. We use here the classification of Lezak (1995): volition (e.g., initiation of activity, motivation, self-awareness), planning and attention, purposive action (self-regulation, productivity and flexibility), and effective performance (Duke & Kaszniak, 2000).

Executive dysfunctions in AD

Disturbances in executive functions are manifest in AD (Duke & Kaszniak, 2000). Alzheimer's disease patients with a disturbance in volition show apathy

and passivity. Apathy implies neuropathology in the basal ganglia (Duke & Kaszniak, 2000). Furthermore, AD patients show problems in planning, attention and purposive action. Concerning purposive action, an impairment in, for example, cognitive flexibility implies that one is less able to divide attention (Duke & Kaszniak, 2000). Indeed, in AD patients it has been observed that distraction during walking increased unsteadiness, resulting in stride time variability (Sheridan *et al.*, 2003). The distraction required that the patient read aloud a number of digits. Similar findings were observed in another recent study, in which AD patients showed a decrease in communication when walking was combined with talking (Cott *et al.*, 2002). To perform a dual task, the patient has to divide attention, a cognitive function that heavily depends on executive functions. These findings suggest that in AD, executive dysfunction, expressed in an impaired performance of dual-tasks, has a close association with physical activities such as walking. Finally, AD patients are less able to monitor their own behavior (Duke & Kaszniak, 2000).

Executive dysfunctions in VaD

As mentioned earlier, due to a disruption of the fronto-striatal systems, VaD patients primarily show a decline in executive functions (Pugh & Lipsitz, 2002). The consequence is, among other things, a reduction in psychomotor speed with which information is processed, an impairment in working memory and in attention (Román *et al.*, 2002). Furthermore, a disruption of the fronto-striatal circuit is responsible for behavioral disturbances related to executive functions such as a lack of motivation, resulting in apathy (Román *et al.*, 2002).

Executive dysfunctions in FTD

Three out of the four executive functions (Lezak, 1995), i.e., "volition" (taking initiatives, goal setting and motivation), purposive action and self-regulation, and effective performance are impaired in frontal frontotemporal dementia (Duke & Kaszniak, 2000). There is some empirical evidence for an impairment in "planning" and for an impairment in executing motor activity in the appropriate sequence (Duke & Kaszniak, 2000). Disturbances in behavior and personality are also prominent clinical symptoms of frontal frontotemporal dementia (Duke & Kaszniak, 2000). One of the behavioral symptoms that might negatively influence patients' level of physical activity is apathy (Hodges, 2001). As described earlier, this latter symptom might be due to an impairment in "volition".

Taken together, in patients with AD, VaD and FTD, executive dysfunctions are prominent clinical symptoms and may have serious functional consequences, reflected in, among others, a disturbance in gait and a decrease in (instrumental) activities of daily life (Kiosses & Alexopoulos, 2005; Wang *et al.*, 2002).

Gait disturbances in the various subtypes of dementia

- "Cautious gait" is typical for a mild stage of AD, while a "frontal" gait disorder is more frequently shown in a later stage of the disease.
- In persons with (some type of) VaD, several gait disturbances have been observed.
- Some patients in FTD show involuntary trunk movements, which may negatively affect balance and stability during walking.

- In all three types of dementia, gait disturbances are present in a relatively early stage of the disease.

A comparison of gait disturbances between the various subtypes of dementia may give the impression that the *nature* of the disturbed motor activity is comparable between the various disorders. Nonetheless, studies that examine the precise nature and characteristics of gait disturbances in dementia are still lacking (Kurlan *et al.*, 2000).

Gait disturbances in AD

A gait disorder that is characteristic for a mild stage of AD is called "cautious gait" (Table 15.2) (O'Keeffe *et al.*, 1996; Prehogan & Cohen, 2004). Cautious gait is composed of a decrease in gait velocity and step length, and postural instability, reflected in an impairment in static and dynamic balance and a widened base (Alexander *et al.*, 1995; Goldman *et al.*, 1999; Nakamura *et al.*, 1997; O'Keeffe *et al.*, 1996; Pettersson *et al.*, 2002; Prehogan & Cohen, 2004; Sheridan *et al.*, 2003; Tanaka *et al.*, 1995; Visser, 1983). Hesitation and freezing are also part of cautious gait (Prehogan & Cohen, 2004). A "frontal" gait disorder has been observed in a more advanced stage of AD, characterized by additional symptoms such as shuffling and hesitation in starting and turning (Table 15.2) (O'Keeffe *et al.*, 1996; Prehogan & Cohen, 2004).

Table 15.2. Subtypes of dementia in relation to disturbances in gait. AD: Alzheimer's disease; SIVD: Subcortical ischemic vascular dementia; FTD: frontotemporal dementia; FTLD: frontotemporal lobe degeneration. +: present; [cg]: "cautious gait"; [fg]: "frontal gait".

	Wide base	Decreased velocity	Decreased step length	Gait apraxia	Static instability	Dynamic instability	Hesitation freezing	Shuffling gait	Involuntary trunk movements
Early AD[cg]		+	+	+	+	+	+		
Mid stage AD[fg]		+	+	+	+	+	+	+	
SIVD	+	+	+	+	+	+	+		
FTD (FTLD)									+

Gait disturbances in VaD

As mentioned before, SIVD is considered the main cause of vascular cognitive deterioration and dementia (Andin *et al.*, 2005; Román *et al.*, 2002). Subcortical ischemic vascular dementia (SIVD) shows a wide range of symptoms such as gait with a wide-base and gait apraxia, decreased step length, disturbance in initiation of gait, static and dynamic instability, and freezing (Table 15.2) (Pohjasvaara *et al.*, 2003; Román *et al.* 2002). Also a decrease in velocity has been observed in patients with vascular dementia (Tanaka *et al.*, 1995). However, in that study the diagnosis of vascular dementia was not further specified.

Gait disturbances in FTD

In a recent study, a subgroup of patients in a relatively early stage of probably the "frontal variant" of FTD showed involuntary trunk movements (Table 15.2) (Mendez *et al.*, 2005). One could argue that involuntary trunk movements may negatively influence trunk sway during walking; trunk sway is highly associated with balance stability during walking (Gill *et al.*, 2001). The stereotypical trunk movements that have also been observed in patients with "frontotemporal lobe degeneration" (FTLD), i.e., a collection of the frontal variant of FTD, semantic dementia and progressive nonfluent aphasia (Rosen *et al.*, 2002), indicate an involvement of the fronto-striatal system (Mendez *et al.*, 2005; Rosen *et al.*, 2002).

Taken together, in AD, VaD and "frontal" FTD gait disturbances are already present in a relatively early stage of the disease.

Conclusions

Despite the fact that epidemiological studies show a strong relationship between physical activity and cognition in people with dementia, for example, physical activity decreases the risk for dementia (Rovio *et al.*, 2005), and despite the fact that a *causal*

relationship between physical activity and cognition has been observed in older persons without dementia (Kramer *et al.*, 1999), there is a striking lack of randomized clinical trials examining the effects of physical activity on cognition in people *with dementia*. The few studies that have been performed show both positive and negative findings. We provided in this chapter theory-driven evidence that these negative findings are due to vascular disease. Of note is that in the clinical studies reviewed here that showed negative findings, vascular disease was not specifically controlled for (Arkin, 2001; Cott *et al.* 2002; McMurdo & Rennie, 1994; Mulrow *et al.*, 1994; Sobel, 2001). It is emphasized that controlling for vascular risk factors is a prerequisite for future studies that are focused on the relationship between physical activity and cognition in persons with dementia.

Vascular disease initiates a cascade of events which, through cerebral hypoperfusion, WMLs, executive dysfunctions, and gait disturbances, leads to a decrease in the level of physical activity. Of note is that this cascade of events is applicable to all three subtypes of dementia. From a preventive point of view, it would be worthwhile to examine if this cascade of events (or parts of it) is also applicable to a preclinical stage of dementia. Bottom-up, there are indeed some indications that in patients with mild cognitive impairment (MCI), vascular cognitive impairment no dementia (vCIND), and frontotemporal mild cognitive impairment (FT-MCI), transitional states between normal aging and dementia (de Mendonça *et al.*, 2004; Grundman *et al.*, 2004; Nyenhuis *et al.*, 2004), gait disturbances occur. More specifically, impaired balance has been observed in patients with MCI and vCIND, whereas patients with FT-MCI show problems in initiating motor activity (de Mendonça *et al.*, 2004; Franssen *et al.*, 1999; Geroldi *et al.*, 2003). In addition, executive dysfunctions and WMLs have been observed in patients with MCI (Bäckman *et al.*, 2004; Saka *et al.*, 2007) and with vCIND (Inzitari & Basile, 2003; Jellinger, 2005). In other words, those who are working with these patients should be continuously on the alert for detecting even the most subtle changes in gait and executive functions (e.g., a modest decline in taking initiatives). This is important since these changes may imply the onset of a decrease in physical activity and, consequently, a further decline in cognitive function. Equally important, an early diagnosis of subtle changes in gait and executive functions allows for an *early* application of a physical activity program, optimizing its effect on cognitive function in patients with dementia.

ACKNOWLEDGMENTS

We are most grateful to Frédérique Scherder for her valuable assistance in preparing this chapter.

REFERENCES

Alexander, N. B., Mollo, J. M., Giordani, B. *et al.* (1995). Maintenance of balance, gait patterns, and obstacle clearance in Alzheimer's disease. *Neurology*, **45**, 908–914.

Andin, U., Gustafson, L., Passant, U., & Brun, A. (2005). A clinico-pathological study of heart and brain lesions in vascular dementia. *Dementia and Geriatric Cognitive Disorders*, **19**, 222–228.

Arkin, S. M. (2001). Alzheimer rehabilitation by students: interventions and outcomes. *Neuropsychological Rehabilitation*, **11**, 273–317.

Arkin, S. M. (2003). Student-led exercise sessions yield significant fitness gains for Alzheimer's patients. *American Journal of Alzheimer's Disease and Other Dementias*, **18**, 159–170.

Bäckman, L., Jones, S., Berger, A.-K., Laukka, E. J., & Small, B. J. (2004). Multiple cognitive deficits during the transition to Alzheimer's disease. *Journal of Internal Medicine*, **256**, 195–204.

Baum, E. E., Jarjoura, D., Polen, A. E., Faur, D., & Rutecki, G. (2003). Effectiveness of a group exercise program in a long-term care facility: a randomized pilot trial. *Journal of the American Medical Directors Association*, **4**, 74–80.

Bland, B. H., & Oddie, S. D. (2001). Theta band oscillation and synchrony in the hippocampal formation and associated structures: the case for its role in sensorimotor integration. *Behavioural Brain Research*, **127**, 119–136.

Bowler, J. V. (2002). The concept of vascular cognitive impairment. *Journal of the Neurological Sciences*, **203–204**, 11–15.

Burns, J. M., Galvin, J. E., Roe, C. M., Morris, J. C., & McKeel, D. W. (2005). The pathology of the substantia nigra in Alzheimer disease with extrapyramidal signs. *Neurology*, **64**, 1397–1403.

Cahn-Weiner, D. A., Malloy, P. F., Boyle, P. A., Marran, M., & Salloway, S. (2000). Prediction of functional status from neuropsychological tests in community-dwelling elderly individuals. *Clinical Neuropsychologist*, **14**, 187–195.

Castellani, R. J., Smith, M. A., Perry, G., & Friedland, R. P. (2004). Cerebral amyloid angiopathy: major contributor or decorative response to Alzheimer's disease pathogenesis. *Neurobiology of Aging*, **25**, 599–602.

Chen, Y., McCarron, R. M., Bembry, J. *et al.* (1999). Nitric oxide modulates endothelin 1-induced Ca^{2+} mobilization and cytoskeletal F-actin filaments in human cerebromicrovascular endothelial cells. *Journal of Cerebral Blood Flow and Metabolism*, **19**, 133–138.

Churchill, J. D., Galvez, R., Colcombe, S. *et al.* (2002). Exercise, experience and the aging brain. *Neurobiology of Aging*, **23**, 941–955.

Cohen, R. A., Paul, R. H., Zawacki, T. M. *et al.* (2001). Single photon emission computed tomography, magnetic resonance imaging hyperintensity, and cognitive impairments in patients with vascular dementia. *Journal of Neuroimaging*, **11**, 253–260.

Colcombe, S. J., Erickson, K. I., Raz, N. *et al.* (2003). Aerobic fitness reduces brain tissue loss in aging humans. *Journals of Gerontology: Medical Sciences*, **58**, 176–180.

Cooke, J. P., & Dzau, V. J. (1997). Nitric oxide synthase: role in the genesis of vascular disease. *Annual Review of Medicine*, **48**, 489–509.

Cott, C. A., Dawson, P., Sidani, S., & Wells, D. (2002). The effects of a walking/talking program on communication, ambulation, and functional status in residents with Alzheimer disease. *Alzheimer Disease and Associated Disorders*, **16**, 81–87.

Court, J. A., & Perry, E. K. (2003). Neurotransmitter abnormalities in vascular dementia. *International Psychogeriatrics*, **15**, 81–87.

Critchley, H. D., Corfield, D. R., Chandler, M. P., Mathias, C. J., & Dolan, R. J. (2000). Cerebral correlates of autonomic cardiovascular arousal: a functional neuroimaging investigation in humans. *Journal of Physiology*, **523**, 259–270.

de Carvalho Bastone, A., & Filho, W. J. (2004). Effect of an exercise program on functional performance of institutionalized elderly. *Journal of Rehabilitation Research and Development*, **41**, 659–668.

de la Torre, J. C. (2002). Vascular basis of Alzheimer's pathogenesis. *Annals of the New York Academy of Sciences*, **977**, 196–215.

de Mendonça, A., Ribeiro, G., Guerreiro, M., & Garcia, C. (2004). Frontotemporal mild cognitive impairment. *Journal of Alzheimer's Disease*, **6**, 1–9.

Diaz, M., Sailor, K., Cheung, D., & Kuslansky, G. (2004). Category size effects in semantic and letter fluency in Alzheimer's patients. *Brain and Language*, **89**, 108–114.

Diesfeldt, H. F., & Diesfeldt-Groenendijk, H. (1977). Improving cognitive performance in psychogeriatric patients: the influence of physical exercise. *Age and Ageing*, **6**.

Duke, L. M., & Kaszniak, A. W. (2000). Executive control functions in degenerative dementias: a comparative review. *Neuropsychology Review*, **10**, 75–99.

Eggermont, L., Swaab, D., Luiten, P., & Scherder, E. (2006). Exercise, cognition and Alzheimer's disease: more is not necessarily better. *Neuroscience and Biobehavioral Reviews*, **30**, 562–575.

Endres, M., Gertz, K., Lindauer, U. *et al.* (2003). Mechanisms of stroke protection by physical activity. *Annals of Neurology*, **54**, 582–590.

Fernando, M. S., & Ince, P. G. (2004). Vascular pathologies and cognition in a population-based cohort of elderly people. *Journal of the Neurological Sciences*, **226**, 13–17.

Folin, M., Baiguera, S., Gallucci, M. *et al.* (2005). A cross-sectional study of homocysteine-, NO-levels, and CT-findings in Alzheimer dementia, vascular dementia and controls. *Biogerontology*, **6**, 255–260.

Folstein, M. F., Folstein, S. E., & McHugh, P. R. (1975). "Mini-Mental State": a practical method for grading the cognitive state of patients for the clinician. *Journal of Psychiatric Research*, **12**,

Franchesi, M., Anchisi, D., Pelati, O. *et al.* (2005). Glucose metabolism and serotonin receptors in the frontotemporal lobe degeneration. *Annals of Neurology*, **57**, 216–225.

Franssen, E. H., Souren, L. E. M., Torossian, C. L., & Reisberg, B. (1999). Equilibrium and limb coordination in mild cognitive impairment and mild Alzheimer's disease. *Journal of the American Geriatrics Society*, **47**, 463–469.

Fratiglioni, L., Paillard-Borg, S., & Winblad, B. (2004). An active and socially integrated lifestyle in late life might protect against dementia. *Lancet Neurology*, **3**, 343–353.

Friedman, R., & Tappen, R. M. (1991). The effect of planned walking on communication in Alzheimer's disease. *Journal of the American Geriatrics Society*, **39**, 650–654.

Geroldi, C., Ferrucci, L., Bandinelli, S. *et al.* (2003). Mild cognitive deterioration with subcortical features: prevalence, clinical characteristics, and association with cardiovascular risk factors in community-dwelling older persons (The inCHIANTI Study). *Journal of the American Geriatrics Society*, **51**, 1064–1071.

Gill, J., Allum, J. H. J., Carpenter, M. G. *et al.* (2001). Trunk sway measures of postural stability during clinical balance tests: effects of age. *Journals of Gerontology; Series A; Biological Sciences and Medical Sciences*, **56**, M438–M447.

Goldman, W. P., Baty, J. D., Buckles, V. D., Sahrmann, S., & Morris, J. C. (1999). Motor dysfunction in mildly demented AD individuals without extrapyramidal signs. *Neurology*, **53**, 956–962.

Grundman, M., Petersen, R. C., Ferris, S. H. *et al.* (2004). Mild cognitive impairment can be distinguished from Alzheimer disease and normal aging for clinical trials. *Archives of Neurology*, **61**, 59–66.

Grut, M., Fratiglioni, L., Viitanen, M., & Winblad, B. (1993). Accuracy of the Mini-Mental Status Examination as a screening test for dementia in a Swedish elderly population. *Acta Neurologica Scandinavica*, **87**, 312–317.

Hayward, R., Ruangthai, R., Karnilaw, P. *et al.* (2003). Attenuation of homocysteine-induced endothelial dysfunction by exercise training. *Pathophysiology*, **9**, 207–214.

Hellström, G., Fischer-Colbrie, W., Wahlgren, N. G., & Hogestrand, T. (1996). Carotid artery blood flow and middle cerebral artery blood flow velocity during physical exercise. *Journal of Applied Physiology*, **81**, 413–418.

Herrmann, M., Schorr, H., Obeid, R. *et al.* (2003). Homocysteine increases during endurance exercise. *Clinical Chemistry and Laboratory Medicine*, **41**, 1518–1524.

Herrmann, W. (2001). The importance of hyperhomocysteinemia as a risk factor for diseases: an overview. *Clinical Chemistry and Laboratory Medicine*, **39**, 666–674.

Hodges, J. R. (2001). Frontotemporal dementia (Pick's disease): clinical features and assessment. *Neurology*, **56**, S6–S10.

Hopman-Rock, M., Staats, P. G. M., Tak, E. C. P. M., & Dröes, R.-M. (1999). The effects of a psychomotor activation programme for use in groups of cognitively impaired people in homes for the elderly. *International Journal of Geriatric Psychiatry*, **14**, 633–642.

Huang, P. L., Huang, S., Mashimo, H. *et al.* (1995). Hypertension in mice lacking the gene for endothelial nitric oxide synthase. *Nature*, **377**, 239–242.

Huey, E. D., Putnam, K. T., & Grafman, J. (2006). A systematic review of neurotransmitter deficits and treatments in frontotemporal dementia. *Neurology*, **66**, 17–22.

Iadecola, C. (2004). Neurovascular regulation in the normal brain and in Alzheimer's disease. *Nature Reviews Neuroscience*, **5**, 347–360.

Inzitari, D., & Basile, A. M. (2003). Activities of daily living and global functioning. *International Psychogeriatrics*, **15** S1, 225–229.

Jagust, W. J., Eberling, J. L., Reed, B. R., Mathis, C. A., & Budinger, T. F. (1997). Clinical studies of cerebral blood flow in Alzheimer's disease. *Annals of the New York Academy of Sciences*, **826**, 254–262.

Jellinger, K. A. (2005). Understanding the pathology of vascular cognitive impairment. *Journal of the Neurological Sciences*, **229–230**, 57–60.

Jørgensen, L. G., Perko, G., & Secher, N. H. (1992). Regional cerebral artery mean flow velocity and blood flow during dynamic exercise in humans. *Journal of Applied Physiology*, **73**, 1825–1830.

Kaske, A., Winber, G., & Cöster, J. (2006). Motor-maps, navigation and implicit space representation in the hippocampus. *Biological Cybernetics*, **94**, 46–57.

Kim, R. C., Ramachandran, T., Parisi, J. E., & Collins, G. H. (1981). Pallidonigral pigmentation and spheroid formation with multiple striatal lacumar infarcts. *Neurology*, **31**, 774–777.

Kiosses, D. N., & Alexopoulos, G. S. (2005). IADL functions, cognitive deficits, and severity of depression. *American Journal of Geriatric Psychiatry*, **13**, 244–249.

Koistinaho, M., & Koistinaho, J. (2005). Interactions between Alzheimer's disease and cerebral ischemia – focus on inflammation. *Brain Research Reviews*, **48**, 240–250.

Kramer, A. F., Hahn, S., Cohen, N. J. *et al.* (1999). Ageing, fitness and neurocognitive function. *Nature*, **400**, 418–419.

Kubes, P., & Granger, D. N. (1992). Nitric oxide modulates microvascular permeability. *American Journal of Physiology*, **262**, H611–H615.

Kurlan, R., Richard, I. H., Papka, M., & Marshall, F. (2000). Movement disorders in Alzheimer's disease: more rigidity of definitions is needed. *Movement Disorders*, **15**, 24–29.

Kurosawa, M., Okada, K., Sato, A., & Uchida, S. (1993). Extracellular release of acetylcholine, noradrenaline and serotonin increases in the cerebral-cortex during walking in conscious rats. *Neuroscience Letters*, **161**, 73–76.

Laurin, D., Verreault, R., Lindsay, J., MacPherson, K., & Rockwood, K. (2001). Physical activity and risk of cognitive impairment and dementia in elderly persons. *Archives of Neurology*, **58**, 498–504.

Lezak, M. (1995). *Neuropsychological Assessment*. New York: Oxford University Press.

Lindenmuth, G. F., & Moose, B. (1990). Improving cognitive abilities of elderly Alzheimer's patients with intense exercise therapy. *American Journal of Alzheimer's Disease and Other Dementias*, **5**(1), 31–33.

Mariani, C., Defendi, S., Mailland, E., & Pomati, S. (2006). Frontotemporal dementia. *Neurological Sciences*, **27**, S35–S36.

Maxwell, A. J. (2002). Mechanisms of dysfunction of the nitric oxide pathway in vascular diseases. *Nitric Oxide*, **6**, 101–124.

McMurdo, M. E., & Rennie, L. M. (1994). Improvements in quadriceps strength with regular seated exercise in the institutionalized elderly. *Archives of Physical Medicine and Rehabilitation*, **75**, 600–603.

Meltzer, C. C., Smith, G., DeKosky, S. T. *et al.* (1998). Serotonin in aging, late-life depression, and Alzheimer's disease: the emerging role of functional imaging. *Neuropsychopharmacology*, **18**, 407–430.

Mendez, M. F., Shapira, J. S., & Miller, B. L. (2005). Stereotypical movements and frontotemporal dementia. *Movement Disorders*, **20**, 742–745.

Miklossy, J. (2003). Cerebral hypoperfusion induces cortical watershed microinfarcts which may further aggravate cognitive decline in Alzheimer's disease. *Neurological Research*, **25**, 605–610.

Mulrow, C. D., Gerety, M. B., Kanten, D. *et al.* (1994). A randomized trial of physical rehabilitation for very frail nursing-home residents. *Journal of the American Medical Association*, **271**, 519–524.

Nagahama, Y., Nabatame, H., Okina, T. *et al.* (2003). Cerebral correlates of the progression rate of the cognitive decline in probable Alzheimer's disease. *European Neurology*, **50**, 1–9.

Nakajima, K., Uchida, S., Suzuki, A., Hotto, H., & Aikawa, Y. (2003). The effect of walking on regional blood flow and acetylcholine in the hippocampus in conscious rats. *Autonomic Neuroscience: Basic and Clinical*, **103**, 83–92.

Nakamura, T., Meguro, K., Yamazaki, H. *et al.* (1997). Postural and gait disturbance correlated with decreased frontal cerebral blood flow in Alzheimer disease. *Alzheimer Disease and Associated Disorders*, **11**, 132–139.

Newman, A. B., Fitzpatrick, A. L., Lopez, O. *et al.* (2005). Dementia and Alzheimer's disease incidence in relationship to cardiovascular disease in the Cardiovascular Health Study cohort. *Journal of the American Geriatrics Society*, **53**, 1101–1107.

Nichol, K. E., Kim, R., & Cotman, C. W. (2001). Bcl-2 family protein behavior in frontotemporal dementia implies vascular involvement. *Neurology*, **56**, S35–S40.

Nyenhuis, D. L., Gorelick, P. B., Geenen, E. J. *et al.* (2004). The pattern of neuropsychological deficits in Vascular Cognitive Impairment-No Dementia (Vascular CIND). *Clinical Neuropsychology*, **18**, 41–49.

O'Keeffe, S. T., Kazeem, H., Philpott, R. M. *et al.* (1996). Gait disturbance in Alzheimer's disease: a clinical study. *Age and Ageing*, **25**, 313–316.

Osawa, A., Maeshima, S., Shimamoto, Y. *et al.* (2004). Relationship between cognitive function and regional cerebral blood flow in different types of dementia. *Disability and Rehabilitation*, **26**, 739–745.

Palleschi, L., Vetta, F., De Gennaro, E. *et al.* (1996). Effect of aerobic training on the cognitive performance of elderly patients with senile dementia of Alzheimer type. *Archives of Gerontology and Geriatrics, Suppl. 5*, 47–50.

Panegyres, P. K. (2004). The contribution of the study of neurodegenerative disorders to the understanding of human memory. *Quarterly Journal of Medicine*, **97**, 555–567.

Petersen, R. C., Smith, G. E., Waring, S. C. *et al.* (1999). Mild cognitive impairment: clinical characterization and outcome. *Archives of Neurology*, **56**, 303–308.

Pettersson, A. F., Engardt, M., & Wahlund, L. O. (2002). Activity level and balance in subjects with mild Alzheimer's disease. *Dementia and Geriatric Cognitive Disorders*, **13**, 213–216.

Podewils, L. J., Guallar, E., Kuller, L. H. *et al.* (2005). Physical activity, APOE genotype, and dementia risk: findings from the Cardiovascular Health Cognition Study. *American Journal of Epidemiology*, **161**, 639–651.

Poehlman, E. T., Toth, M. J., Goran, M. I. *et al.* (1997). Daily energy expenditure in free-living non-institutionalized Alzheimer's patients: a doubly labeled water study. *Neurology*, **48**, 997–1002.

Pohjasvaara, T., Mantyla, R., Ylikoski, R., Kaste, M., & Erkinjuntti, T. (2003). Clinical features of MRI-defined subcortical vascular disease. *Alzheimer Disease and Associated Disorders*, **17**, 236–242.

Pott, F., Knudsen, L., Nowak, M., Nielsen, H. B., Hanel, B., & Secher, N. H. (1997). Middle cerebral artery blood velocity during rowing. *Acta Physiologica Scandinavica*, **160**, 251–255.

Powell, R. R. (1974). Psychological effects of exercise therapy upon institutionalized geriatric mental patients. *Journal of Gerontology*, **29**, 157–164.

Prehogan, A., & Cohen, C. I. (2004). Motor dysfunction in dementias. *Geriatrics*, **59**, 53–54.

Pugh, K. G., & Lipsitz, L. A. (2002). The microvascular frontal-subcortical syndrome of aging. *Neurobiology of Aging*, **23**, 421–431.

Rinne, J. O., Laine, M., Kaasinen, V. *et al.* (2002). Striatal dopamine transporter and extrapyramidal symptoms in frontotemporal dementia. *Neurology*, **58**, 1489–1493.

Rolland, Y., Rival, L., Pillard, F. *et al.* (2000). Feasibility of regular physical exercise for patients with moderate to severe Alzheimer's disease. *Journal of Nutrition, Health and Aging*, **4**, 109–113.

Román, G. C. (2004). Brain hypoperfusion: A critical factor in vascular dementia. *Neurological Research*, **26**, 454–458.

Román, G. C., & Kalaria, R. N. (2006). Vascular determinants of cholinergic deficits in Alzheimer disease and vascular dementia. *Neurobiology of Aging*, **27**, 1769–1785.

Román, G. C., Erkinjuntti, T., Wallin, A., Pantoni, L., & Chui, H. C. (2002). Subcortical ischaemic vascular dementia. *Lancet Neurology*, **1**, 426–436.

Rosen, H. J., Hartikainen, K. M., Jagust, W. *et al.* (2002). Utility of clinical criteria in differentiating frontotemporal lobar degeneration (FTLD) from AD. *Neurology*, **58**, 1608–1615.

Roth, M., Tym, E., Mountjoy, C. Q. *et al.* (1986). Camdex-A standardized instrument for the diagnosis of mental disorder in the elderly with special reference to the early detection of dementia. *British Journal of Psychiatry*, **149**, 698–709.

Rovio, S., Kåreholt, I., Helkala, E.-L. *et al.* (2005). Leisure-time physical activity at midlife and the risk of dementia and Alzheimer's disease. *Lancet Neurology*, **4**, 705–711.

Saka, E., Dogan, E. A., Topcuoglu, M. A., Senol, U., & Balkan, S. (2007). Linear measures of temporal lobe atrophy on brain magnetic resonance imaging (MRI) but not visual rating of white matter changes can help discrimination of mild cognitive impairment (MCI) and Alzheimer's disease (AD). *Archives of Gerontology and Geriatrics*, **44**, 141–151.

Scherder, E. J. A., Van Paasschen, J., Deijen, J.-B. *et al.* (2005). Physical activity and executive functions in the elderly with mild cognitive impairment. *Aging and Mental Health*, **9**, 272–280.

Schilke, J. M. (1991). Slowing the aging process with physical activity. *Journal of Gerontological Nursing*, **17**, 4–8.

Selley, M. L. (2003). Increased concentrations of homocysteine and asymmetric dimethylarginine and decreased concentrations of nitric oxide in the plasma of patients with Alzheimer's disease. *Neurobiology of Aging*, **24**, 903–907.

Shapiro, M. (2001). Plasticity, hippocampal place cells, and cognitive maps. *Archives of Neurology*, **58**, 874–881.

Sheridan, P. L., Solomont, J., Kowall, N., & Hausdorff, J. M. (2003). Influence of executive function on locomotor function: divided attention increases gait variability in Alzheimer's disease. *Journal of the American Geriatrics Society*, **51**, 1633–1637.

Sobel, B. P. (2001). Bingo vs. physical intervention in stimulating short-term cognition in Alzheimer's disease patients. *American Journal of Alzheimer's Disease and Other Dementias*, **16**, 115–120.

Srikiatkhachorn, A., Anuntasethakul, T., Maneesri, S. *et al.* (2000). Hyposerotonin-induced nitric oxide supersensitivity in the cerebral microcirculation. *Headache*, **40**, 267–275.

Tanaka, A., Okuzumi, H., Kobayashi, I., Murai, N., & Meguro, K. (1995). Gait disturbance of patients with vascular and Alzheimer-type dementias. *Perceptual and Motor Skills*, **80**, 735–738.

Tsolaki, M., Sakka, V., Gerasimou, G. *et al.* (2001). Correlation of rCBF (SPECT), CSF tau, and cognitive function in patients with dementia of the Alzheimer's type, other types of dementia, and control subjects. *American Journal of Alzheimer's Disease and Other Dementias*, **16**, 21–31.

Ueda, H., Kitabayashi, Y., Narumoto, J. *et al.* (2002). Relationship between clock drawing test performance and regional cerebral blood flow in Alzheimer's disease: a single photon emission computed tomography study. *Psychiatry and Clinical Neurosciences*, **56**, 25–29.

Ushijima, Y., Okuyama, C., Mori, S. *et al.* (2002). Relationship between cognitive function and regional cerebral blood flow in Alzheimer's disease. *Nuclear Medicine Communications*, **23**, 779–784.

van de Pol, A. L., Hensel, A., van der Flier, W. M. *et al.* (2006). Hippocampal atrophy on MRI in frontotemporal lobar degeneration and Alzheimer's disease. *Journal of Neurology, Neurosurgery, and Psychiatry*, **77**, 439–442.

van de Winckel, A., Feys, H., De Weerdt, W., & Dom, R. (2004). Cognitive and behavioural effects of music-based exercises in patients with dementia. *Clinical Rehabilitation*, **18**, 253–260.

van Gelder, B. M., Tijhuis, M. A. R., Kalmijn, S. *et al.* (2004). Physical activity in relation to cognitive decline in elderly men: the FINE study. *Neurology*, **63**, 2316–2321.

Varrone, A., Pappatà, S., Caracò, C. *et al.* (2002). Voxel-based comparison of rCBF SPET images in frontotemporal dementia and Alzheimer's disease highlights the involvement of different cortical networks. *European Journal of Nuclear Medicine and Molecular Imaging*, **29**, 1447–1454.

Visser, H. (1983). Gait and balance in senile dementia of Alzheimer's type. *Age and Ageing*, **12**, 296–301.

Wang, L., van Belle, G., Kukull, W. B., & Larson, E. B. (2002). Predictors of functional change: a longtudinal study of nondemented people aged 65 and older. *Journal of the American Geriatrics Society*, **50**, 1525–1534.

Wang, P., Yang, C., Lin, K. *et al.* (2004). Weight loss, nutritional status and physical activity in patients with Alzheimer's disease: a controlled study. *Journal of Neurology* **251**, 314–320.

Wenk, G. L. (2006). Neuropathologic changes in Alzheimer's disease: potential targets for treatment. *Journal of Clinical Psychiatry*, **67**, Suppl. 3, 3–7.

Westerterp, K. R. (2000). Daily physical activity and ageing. *Current Opinion in Clinical Nutrition and Metabolic Care*, **3**, 485–488.

Weuve, J., Kang, J. H., Manson, J. E. *et al.* (2004). Physical activity, including walking, and cognitive function in older women. *Journal of the American Medical Association*, **292**, 1454–1461.

White, R. P., Vallance, P., & Markus, H. S. (2000). Effect of inhibition of nitric oxide synthase on dynamic cerebral autoregulation in humans. *Clinical Science*, **99**, 555–560.

Wiener, S. I., Berthoz, A., & Zugaro, M. B. (2002). Multisensory processing in the elaboration of place and head direction responses by limbic system neurons. *Cognitive Brain Research*, **14**, 75–90.

Wilson, M.-M. G., & Morley, J. E. (2003). Invited review: Aging and energy balance. *Journal of Applied Physiology*, **95**, 1728–1736.

Wilson, R. S., Bennett, D. A., Gilley, D. W. *et al.* (2000). Progression of parkinsonian signs in Alzheimer's disease. *Neurology*, **54**, 1284–1289.

Wolf, R. L., Alsop, D. C., Levy-Reis, I. *et al.* (2001). Detection of mesial temporal lobe hypoperfusion in patients with temporal lobe epilepsy by use of arterial spin labeled perfusion MR imaging. *American Journal of Neuroradiology*, **22**, 1334–1341.

Yang, Y., & Schmitt, H. P. (2001). Frontotemporal dementia: evidence for impairment of ascending serotoninergic but not noradrenergic innervation. Immunocytochemical and quantitative study using a graph method. *Acta Neuropathologica (Berlin)*, **101**, 256–270.

16

Is there a role for diet in cognitive rehabilitation?

Matthew Parrott and Carol Greenwood

Introduction

The body of knowledge linking diet and nutrition with incidence of chronic disease, health promotion and optimal physiological functioning is large and compelling. Until recently, however, this link had been recognized to apply only in the broadest sense to brain health and the support of cognitive function. In this chapter, both chronic diet, a person's usual pattern of eating and drinking, and acute diet, the consumption of a single food or meal, will be examined for their ability to influence those biological processes underlying the functional benefits associated with cognitive rehabilitation. Only inferences can be made; nevertheless, results from cellular, animal and population-based studies provide support for diet's ability to influence neuronal survival and growth, pathological neurodegeneration, and molecular and biochemical processes involved in neuronal communication and memory formation. To apply this information to rehabilitation, our underlying assumption is that for cognitive gain to occur, new neuronal networks must be established. To support these new networks, synaptogensis and potentially neurogenesis will be required and consequently diet- or health-induced processes that facilitate or enhance synaptic plasticity, the potential for neurogenesis, or overall neuronal health and metabolism will associate with superior rehabilitation outcome.

Thus the underlying hypotheses to be explored are that:

- Chronic diet, through its ability to modulate overall neuronal health, can facilitate or interfere with the establishment of new networks essential for cognitive gain.
- Acute diet, by providing essential substrates and energy to support neuronal metabolism, facilitates biochemical processes needed for memory formation occurring during rehabilitation training.

Role of chronic diet

This section explores evidence showing that:

- Consumption of poor quality diets, especially those high in fat and low in fruits, vegetables and cereals, interfere with numerous physiologic processes necessary to support memory formation, establishment of new neuronal networks and neuronal survival.
- This is mediated by disturbances in brain insulin signaling, enhancement of neuroinflammation, and increases in oxidative damage.
- By contrast, diets containing fatty fish, such as salmon, and fruits and vegetables, because of their high quality fat and antioxidant contents, protect the brain from the aforementioned events thereby allowing for a more conducive environment needed for physiologic responses to cognitive rehabilitation.

Numerous cross-sectional and prospective epidemiologic studies demonstrate associations between diet quality and retention of cognitive abilities with aging. In general, older individuals consuming diets high in fat and low in fruits, vegetables and cereals perform worse on cognitive tasks relative to

Cognitive Neurorehabilitation, Second Edition: Evidence and Application, ed. Donald T. Stuss, Gordon Winocur and Ian H. Robertson. Published by Cambridge University Press. © Cambridge University Press 2008.

age-matched individuals with better-quality diets even after adjustment for other lifestyle characteristics (Barberger-Gateau *et al.*, 2002; Luchsinger & Mayeux, 2004; Ortega *et al.*, 1997; Panza *et al.*, 2004). A variety of nutrients, including fat quality and content, antioxidants and vitamins such as folate and B12 are implicated. Both brain-specific mechanisms and the fact that inappropriate intake of these nutrients concomitantly elevate risk for chronic diseases, such as cardiovascular disease (CVD), hypertension (Newman *et al.*, 2005) and type 2 diabetes mellitus (T2DM) (Arvanitakis *et al.*, 2004; Luchsinger *et al.*, 2004; Ott *et al.*, 1999; Peila *et al.*, 2002), which are themselves independent risk factors for cognitive decline, likely explain their influence.

There is no question that diet is a major risk factor for cerebrovascular disorders, including stroke, due to its ability to modulate blood pressure and blood lipid levels. Nevertheless, given the known contribution of vascular disorders to dementia risk (Honig *et al.*, 2003), it will be assumed that screening and if warranted, medical management including diet change and medications, will have been implemented in those entering rehabilitation programs. Rather than concentrate on diet's recognized role in maintaining vascular health, we will argue that the presence of diet-induced insulin resistance (IR) or overt T2DM, because of their adverse brain effects particularly as they relate to impaired insulin signaling and its downstream consequences, have the potential to interfere with physiologic processes of rehabilitation and that if uncorrected, could be a major modifiable factor contributing to rehabilitation failure. By contrast, a healthy diet including fish, fruits and vegetables, is linked to preservation and/or protection against many adverse processes which need to be minimized to maintain neuronal health – a prerequisite to establishing new networks.

Neuropathologic events associated with disruptions to brain insulin, insulin-mediated cell signaling, inflammation and oxidative stress

It is increasingly recognized that disruptions in brain insulin mediated cell signaling, apparent in those with IR or T2DM, result in brain insults leading to cognitive decline and neuropathologic progression of Alzheimer's disease (AD) (Craft, 2005; Craft & Watson, 2004; Zhao & Alkon, 2001). This section will briefly review data demonstrating that:

- Insulin signaling is intimately involved in memory processing.
- Its disruption is associated with development of neuropathologic hallmarks of Alzheimer's disease, including accumulation of amyloid-beta peptide (Aβ) involved in plaque formation and production of hyperphosphorylated tau proteins involved in neurofibrillary tangle formation.
- Loss of insulin signaling can interfere with the action of other neurotrophins, and facilitate neuroinflammatory processes which collectively impede synaptic plasticity and contribute to neuronal death.
- Dietary components, especially dietary fat, can lead to loss of insulin signaling and promotion of inflammation which may contribute to less effective rehabilitation.

The importance of understanding the potential adverse consequences of IR and T2DM can not be understated. Given that half of all adults over 60 years of age have some degree of IR (Kahn *et al.*, 2005), it should be assumed that many in rehabilitation programs are experiencing these adverse events to varying degrees and that, if uncorrected, poorer outcome would be anticipated as injured and dying neurons would be unlikely to have the resources to establish new networks. This is compounded by the fact that the brain insult or injury leading to the need for rehabilitation likely involved neuronal death or dysfunction, thereby minimizing the protection normally afforded by redundancy.

Role of insulin signaling in memory processing

Evidence demonstrating the essentiality of brain insulin signaling for memory processing is compelling (see Table 16.1 for synopsis of this evidence). These effects are in addition to the more traditional role of insulin in stimulating cerebral glucose metabolism in specific brain areas versus total

Table 16.1. Evidence linking brain insulin signaling to memory processing.

Localization of the insulin receptor (IRc) to key brain regions including the frontal and cerebral cortices, hippocampus and medial temporal lobe	(Craft & Watson, 2004; Zhao *et al.*, 1999; Zhao & Alkon, 2001)
In situ brain insulin synthesis	(Devaskar *et al.*, 1994; Rulifson *et al.*, 2002; Schechter *et al.*, 1988)
Presence of the major signaling pathways including phosphotidylinositol-3 kinase (PI3K) and its downstream effector Akt and the cytoplasmic intermediate protein Shc and their convergence on mitogen-activated protein kinase (MAPK) activation	(Foulstone *et al.*, 1999; Orban *et al.*, 1999; Ryu *et al.*, 1999; Yang & Raizada, 1999; Zhao *et al.*, 1999)
Insulin and IRc stimulated synthesis of those proteins necessary and sufficient for long-term memory formation	(Alkon *et al.*, 2005; Kahn *et al.*, 1993; Zhao & Alkon, 2001)
Enhancement of insulin signaling pathways when animals are exposed to learning paradigms	(Bank *et al.*, 1988; Olds *et al.*, 1989; Zhao *et al.*, 1999)
Ability of insulin signaling to modulate long-term potentiation (LTP) – a molecular model of memory – by regulation of the pre- and postsynaptic synthesis and activity of neurotransmitters including acetylcholine, GABA, serotonin, dopamine and NMDA	(Devaskar *et al.*, 1994; Havrankova *et al.*, 1978; Zhao & Alkon, 2001)

brain glucose uptake – in this sense brain remains an insulin-insensitive organ. Overlapping distributions of insulin, insulin receptors (IRc), and insulin-sensitive glucose transporters in the hippocampus provide a platform for insulin-stimulated glucose uptake which is known to improve a wide range of memory functions (Craft & Watson, 2004; Korol & Gold, 1998). Consistent with this molecular role are studies indicating that acute insulin elevations facilitate memory function when given at optimal doses to rodents (Park *et al.*, 2000) and humans, provided there is adequate glucose availability (Craft *et al.*, 1999; Reger *et al.*, 2006).

Brain insulin signaling becomes increasingly impaired with IR and T2DM since chronic elevations in plasma insulin downregulate brain insulin transport and IRc expression, such that the brain experiences an insulin-deficient state (Baura *et al.*, 1996; Wallum *et al.*, 1987), placing individuals at increased risk for cognitive decline (Awad *et al.*, 2004). Indeed, cognitive deficits are already apparent in those with IR. For example, we report decrements in delayed verbal memory that associate with measures of IR (Kaplan *et al.*, 2000) and glycemic

control (Greenwood *et al.*, 2003; Papanikoloau *et al.*, 2006), as well as impaired long-term memory and indication of disrupted brain insulin signaling in genetically obese and insulin-resistant Zucker rats (Winocur *et al.*, 2005). Many patients with AD show evidence of deficient brain insulin signaling, including lower cerebrospinal fluid (CSF) insulin levels, and resistance to insulin-mediated memory facilitation, compared with healthy controls (Craft *et al.*, 1998, 2003), and progressive loss of insulin and IRc expression accompanied by loss of downstream signaling through PI3K/Akt (Frolich *et al.*, 1998; Rivera *et al.*, 2005). Thus, progressive loss of brain insulin signaling occurs in tandem with cognitive decline throughout the spectrum of age-associated memory loss to AD, with many arguing a cause and effect relationship.

Loss of insulin signaling and neuropathologic events

While loss of insulin signaling in and of itself could interfere with rehabilitation success due to impaired memory processing, other pathologic events associated with brain insulin deficiency could have more serious consequences as they relate to neuronal plasticity and survival. Specifically, brain insulin deficiency leads to increased brain accumulation of Aβ – accumulation of which is thought to be an initiating event in AD pathogenesis (Oddo *et al.*, 2003) – and neuronal death by a variety of mechanisms. Both decreases in brain insulin levels per se and disturbances in insulin-mediated cell signaling play a role as the former primarily impairs the brain's ability to degrade and export Aβ while the latter primarily increases its production. This accumulation, in turn, leads to disruptions in other aspects of cell signaling, including those involved in long-term potentiation (LTP). Loss of insulin-mediated cell signaling may also contribute to the formation of neurofibrillary tangles, another hallmark of AD highly correlated with cognitive deterioration (Arriagada *et al.*, 1992), since this signaling pathway suppresses enzymes involved in tau hyperphosphorylation (see Table 16.2 for synopsis of this evidence).

Table 16.2. Evidence linking negative and positive attributes of chronic diet to neuronal characteristics essential for successful neurorehabilitation.

Potential mechanisms for proposed adverse effect of a high-fat diet containing mostly saturated fatty acids and few servings of fruits or vegetables	
Promotion of insulin resistance and peripheral hyperinsulinemia which in turn can lead to:	
Decreased brain insulin, which in turn associates with brain Aβ accumulation by:	(Baura *et al.*, 1996; Wallum *et al.*, 1987)
Decreasing brain Aβ degradation	(Authier *et al.*, 1996; Craft & Watson, 2004; Farris *et al.*, 2003, 2004; Vekrellis *et al.*, 2000)
Impairing brain Aβ export	(Carro *et al.*, 2002; Gasparini & Xu, 2003; Nestler *et al.*, 1990; Stein & Johnson, 2002)
Decreased transport and expression of Aβ carrier proteins	(Carro *et al.*, 2002; Gasparini & Xu, 2003; Nestler *et al.*, 1990; Stein & Johnson, 2002)
Inhibited peripheral and brain Aβ degradation by insulin degrading enzyme	(Authier *et al.*, 1996; Craft & Watson, 2004; Farris *et al.*, 2003, 2004; Vekrellis *et al.*, 2000)
Loss of brain insulin mediated PI3K/Akt signaling also enhances Aβ accumulation by:	(Frolich *et al.*, 1998; Rivera *et al.*, 2005)
Increasing caspase-3 activity which	
Contributes to apoptotic cell death	(Yuan & Yankner, 2000)
Results in production of short cytoplasmic APP fragments which in turn may increase Aβ generation	(Dumanchin-Njock *et al.*, 2001; Galvan *et al.*, 2002; Gervais *et al.*, 1999; Lu *et al.*, 2000; Marin *et al.*, 2000; Su *et al.*, 2002; Tesco *et al.*, 2003; Uetsuki *et al.*, 1999)
Aβ accumulation then:	
Disrupts LTP and neurotransmission due to its cytotoxic properties	(Kar *et al.*, 2004; Oddo *et al.*, 2003)
Further enhance caspases allowing for escalation of Aβ accumulation	(Marin *et al.*, 2000; Uetsuki *et al.*, 1999)
Loss of brain insulin mediated PI3K/Akt signaling may also contribution to the formation of neurofibrillary tangles through:	(Hong & Lee, 1997; Schechter *et al.*, 2005a, 2005b)
Disinhibition of glycogen-synthase kinase-3	(Hong & Lee, 1997; Schechter *et al.*, 2005b)
Increased inflammation and oxidative stress	(Dimopoulos *et al.*, 2006; Fishel *et al.*, 2005)
Decreased neurotrophin levels and activity can lead to:	(Duan *et al.*, 2003; Yu *et al.*, 2006)

Table 16.2. (*cont.*)

Disrupted LTP, and decreased neuronal survival, and brain plasticity	(Mattson *et al.*, 2004)
Decreased neurogenesis and cell survival	(Yuan & Yankner, 2000)

Potential mechanisms for proposed beneficial effect of a low-fat diet enriched in omega-3 fatty acids that includes 10 servings of fruits or vegetables, and limits saturated fat intake

Maintained or improved DHA levels and overall fatty acid profile	(Bourre, 2004)
Maintained or improved peripheral insulin levels and sensitivity, which in turn could protect against events described above	(Storlien *et al.*, 1987; Taouis *et al.*, 2002)
Stimulation and protection of insulin signaling including PI3K/Akt	(Akbar *et al.*, 2005; Joseph *et al.*, 2003; Mandel *et al.*, 2005; Taouis *et al.*, 2002; Weinreb *et al.*, 2004)
Inhibited Aβ production	(Lim *et al.*, 2001, 2005; Yang *et al.*, 2005)
Maintenance of synaptic plasticity	(Calderon & Kim, 2004; Calon *et al.*, 2004)
Increased neuroprotectin D1 leading to increased anti-apoptotic and neuroprotective, anti-inflammatory gene-expression programs	(Lukiw *et al.*, 2005; Marcheselli *et al.*, 2003)
Decreased inflammation and oxidative stress	(Cao *et al.*, 2005; Joseph *et al.*, 2005; Lau *et al.*, 2005; Lim *et al.*, 2001; Maher *et al.*, 2004; Yang *et al.*, 2005)
Maintained or improved neurotrophin levels and activity	(Casadesus *et al.*, 2004)
Maintained or improved neurogenesis and cell survival	(Calderon & Kim, 2004)

Insulin resistance, type 2 diabetes mellitus, inflammation and oxidative stress

Insulin resistance increases inflammatory responses and oxidative stress. Recent observational studies have implicated serum levels of pro-inflammatory cytokines with lower cognitive status, lower nerve conduction velocity and greater cognitive decline among senior citizens (Di Iorio *et al.*, 2006; Weaver *et al.*, 2002; Wright *et al.*, 2006), even after adjustments for a wide variety of socio-demographic variables. Low-grade, systemic inflammation, as often found in insulin-resistant individuals, is associated with decline and early cognitive deterioration (Dimopoulos *et al.*, 2006). Our own studies in adults with T2DM suggest that those individuals carrying a single nucleotide polymorphism (SNP) which reduces the expression of tumor necrosis factor-alpha have better delayed verbal memories and show less loss of its function over 48 weeks compared with those not carrying the SNP (Chui *et al.*, 2007). Indeed not only do individuals diagnosed with metabolic syndrome, a condition characterized by IR, exhibit greater cognitive impairment than healthy controls, but within the metabolic syndrome group, those participants with the greatest inflammation exhibited the greatest impairment (Yaffe *et al.*, 2004). The role of peripheral hyperinsulinemia to produce systemic inflammation is well known (Caballero, 2003), and can translate into increased markers of central nervous system (CNS) inflammation (Fishel *et al.*, 2005).

Interestingly, increased CNS inflammation was positively correlated with changes in Aβ suggesting that synchronous hyperinsulinemia-induced increases in Aβ and inflammation may represent an important pathway through which IR promotes both cognitive deterioration and AD pathology. This is compounded by the facts that Aβ cytotoxicity, through its pro-oxidant properties (Behl *et al.*, 1994), may feedback to promote further production (Misonou *et al.*, 2000) and that inflammatory cytokines downregulate brain expression of Aβ scavengers possibly leading to increased deposition. Increased pro-inflammatory cytokine levels can downregulate PI3K/Akt in aged rat brains leading to subsequent caspase activation (Maher *et al.*, 2004) suggesting that insulin-related signaling is negatively affected by inflammation ultimately leading to increased neuronal death.

Insulin resistance and neurotrophins

The interplay between insulin levels and neurotrophins represents another way in which IR can negatively impact on brain function. Traditional neurotrophins, including brain-derived neurotrophic factor (BDNF), like insulin, use tyrosine kinase signal transduction to activate downstream targets including PI3K/Akt (Mattson *et al.*, 2004). Obese and typically insulin-resistant mice exhibit reduced BDNF levels (Duan *et al.*, 2003) which can adversely affect LTP, neuronal survival and brain plasticity, and consequently memory and learning (Mattson *et al.*, 2004). Conversely, treatment of neurons with BDNF promotes PI3K/Akt signaling, and reduces caspase activity, highlighting the possible importance of neurotrophins in the regulation of insulin signaling and vice-versa (Lesne *et al.*, 2005). Plasma hyperinsulinemia also downregulates the transport of insulin-like growth factor-1 (IGF-1) across the blood–brain barrier from the periphery where it is synthesized (Yu *et al.*, 2006). Although not a traditional neurotrophin, IGF-1 rapidly and significantly stimulates the process of membrane assembly at the axonal growth cone through direct stimulation of the PI3K/Akt pathway – an effect not shared with BDNF (Laurino *et al.*, 2005; Pfenninger *et al.*, 2003) and increases neurite sprouting and outgrowth (Aizenman & de Vellis, 1987; Caroni & Grandes, 1990). The high degree of amino acid homology between IGF-1 and insulin allows for cross-reactivity between their respective membrane receptors, making their signaling cascades almost indistinguishable (Dupont & LeRoith, 2001; Pandini *et al.*, 2002). Furthermore, like insulin, IGF-1 activity can be reduced by pro-inflammatory cytokines (Hansen *et al.*, 1999; Maher *et al.*, 2006). Thus, IR

can negatively impact on the processes of neuronal growth, plasticity and survival through its ability to reduce brain levels of neurotrophins like IGF-1 and BDNF. Given recent findings that learning may be accompanied by hippocampal neurogenesis in adult rodent brains (Winocur *et al.*, 2006), and the reliance of neurogenesis on similar biologic signals, like IGF-1 and BDNF (Mattson *et al.*, 2004), this negative pathway has the potential to impair a number of processes recruited during learning and presumably rehabilitation ultimately leading to worse cognitive outcomes.

Diet as a contributor to insulin resistance

There is no question that most cases of IR are mediated by inappropriate lifestyle, including diet. Excess dietary fat, particularly saturated fat, worsens IR in humans while animal studies indicate that dietary saturated fat intake can actually induce IR (Riccardi *et al.*, 2004; Storlien *et al.*, 1991). Corroborating this assertion are our studies of high saturated fat feeding that consistently link both the level and type of fat to cognitive deficits in young adult rats. These deficits are widespread, influencing a number of cognitive domains, with hippocampally mediated memory functions being the most adversely affected (reviewed in Winocur & Greenwood, 2005). High fat feeding also contributes to AD pathology by inducing even higher levels of Aβ in Tg$_{2576}$ mice (Ho *et al.*, 2004), and increasing brain inflammation and decreasing BDNF levels (Duan *et al.*, 2003; Molteni *et al.*, 2004; Zhang *et al.*, 2005).

Collectively, studies indicate that consumption of high-fat diets adversely influences many biological parameters including neuronal signaling cascades involved in memory, neurotransmission, neuronal growth and survival, AD pathology, and neurotrophin activity – either directly or through promotion of IR – ultimately leading to impairments in behavioral function. Importantly, in most instances, animal-based diets were modeled to provide dietary fat levels consistent with upper limits of typical North American diets and epidemiologic data demonstrate relationships between high-fat diets and poorer cognitive function (Morris *et al.*, 2003a). Without assessing, and where necessary recommending dietary change, the continued consumption of a diet high in saturated fat would not be supportive, and perhaps even harmful, to neuronal processes required for successful cognitive rehabilitation. Importantly, clinical studies demonstrating improvements in cognitive function in adults with T2DM who improve their glycemic control by reducing saturated fat intake and consuming more dietary fibre (Gradman *et al.*, 1993; Meneilly *et al.*, 1993; Naor *et al.*, 1997; Ryan *et al.*, 2006) suggest that some of the adverse effects of diabetes are reversible, meaning that it is never "too late" to implement change.

The preceding discussion focused on negative effects of diet on brain integrity and function. By contrast, healthier diets lower the risk of developing IR or T2DM and help protect the brain from their deleterious effects. Indeed, there is especially compelling evidence that two nutrients – omega-3 fatty acids and plant-based antioxidants – are especially beneficial.

Omega-3 fatty acids and fish oils

The omega-3 (ω-3) family of fatty acids, especially those found in fish oils, have the capacity to modulate a wide variety of cellular processes through their ability to modulate membrane composition and function, suppress adverse inflammatory events and directly or indirectly modulate gene expression. This family of fatty acids is characterized by their relatively long chain length and large number of double bonds between carbons causing a U-shaped or "kinked" molecular conformation. In contrast, saturated fatty acids typically contain fewer carbon atoms, lack double bonds, and have a straight chain conformation. In this section we will briefly present evidence that:

- Omega-3 fatty acids are necessary dietary components that are highly enriched in nervous tissues and participate in a wide variety of functions including long-term potentiation, membrane function and neurotransmitter release.

- Reduced ω-3 fatty acid availability decreases levels in the brain and insulin signaling resulting in compromised cognitive function in aging animals and explaining strong epidemiological relationships in humans.
- Reduced dietary ω-3 fatty acids promotes AD-related neuropathology.
- Omega-3 fatty acids modulate production of neurotrophins and neuroinflammatory markers.

Although dietary ω-3 fatty acids appear protective against AD and cognitive decline in large, prospective studies, this effect is somewhat specific to docosahexaenoic acid (DHA) (Barberger-Gateau *et al.*, 2002; Morris *et al.*, 2003b, 2005). Docosahexaenoic acid is a long-chain (22 carbons, 6 double bonds) ω-3 fatty acid found in especially high amounts in fish oil. Intake changes even in late-life alter brain fatty acid profiles and behavioral outcomes (Bourre, 2004; Winocur & Greenwood, 2005). Historically, it is thought humans evolved consuming a diet containing up to 15 times the proportion of ω-3 fatty acids found in the present North American diet (Simopoulos, 1991, 1999), making many argue that our current diet is relatively deficient in ω-3 and that this may contribute to a number of brain-related disorders (Young & Conquer, 2005). Since mammals cannot directly synthesise DHA, it must be obtained preformed from the diet or from other dietary ω-3 fatty acids that are inefficiently converted to DHA (1–6%) through a series of enzymatic steps, setting the stage for inadequate brain supply of DHA just as local turnover increases and conversion decreases with aging (Bourre, 2004; Young & Conquer, 2005).

Docosahexaenoic acid is highly enriched in the brain, where it is synthesized from precursors in astrocytes and then transported and concentrated in neurons (Moore, 1993; Moore *et al.*, 1991). The structural predominance of DHA in the brain is linked to its functional importance since changes in availability and content influence neural membrane-bound enzyme and ion channel activities, membrane fluidity, LTP, and neurotransmitter release (Horrocks & Farooqui, 2004; Young & Conquer, 2005). While there is considerable evidence indicating a developmental role for ω-3 fats, dietary deficiency, or reduction, even in old and adult animals impairs learning and readily depletes neuronal membrane content (Barcelo-Coblijn et al., 2003; Catalan et al., 2002). Furthermore, dietary supplementation with DHA readily improves membrane content and neurotransmitter receptors that were adversely affected by dietary depletion (Bourre, 2004; Dyall et al., 2006). In the Tg_{2576} mouse model of AD, reductions in dietary DHA led to decreased brain levels and adversely impacted on Aβ deposition, plaque load, dendritic spine formation, synaptic loss, neurotransmitter receptors, and protein oxidation (Calon et al., 2004, 2005; Lim et al., 2005). In the one study addressing functional outcomes, impaired performance in the Morris Water Maze following DHA depletion was prevented by a DHA replete diet (Calon et al., 2004).

These, and other studies (Akbar et al., 2005), consistently link loss of brain DHA with reduced PI3K/Akt activity resulting in downstream caspase activation and neuronal apoptosis in both wildtype and AD-engineered animals. A link between neuronal survival and DHA is further supported by its ability to promote neurite growth in culture (Calderon & Kim, 2004).

Furthermore, DHA induces anti-apoptotic and neuroprotective, anti-inflammatory gene-expression programs in the brain through conversion to neuroprotectin D1. This less well-known role for DHA was subsequently shown to protect neurons from Aβ-induced neurotoxicity which is highly dependent on promotion of oxidative stress/inflammation (Lukiw et al., 2005; Marcheselli et al., 2003). Dietary ω-3 fatty acid enrichment also attenuates inflammatory responses by shifting production of local inflammatory mediators in the brain such as prostaglandins from pro- to anti-inflammatory forms (Cao et al., 2005), and suppresses adverse age-related changes in cortical interleukin and PI3K activity (Maher et al., 2004).

Taken together, studies indicate that DHA deficiency and IR can work through shared mechanisms to impair neuronal health and survival by interfering with PI3K/Akt signaling and promoting oxidative stress and neuroinflammation. Importantly dietary DHA repletion can improve IRc signaling in insulin-resistant individuals (Taouis et al., 2002), and prevent the development of IR by high-fat feeding in animals (Storlien et al., 1987). These mechanisms work in concert with DHA effects on general membrane function, neurotransmitters and neuronal survival and growth.

Dietary antioxidants of plant origin

Dietary antioxidants scavenge the reactive oxygen species (ROS) responsible for oxidative damage and inflammation. The following section will briefly advance a role for plant-based antioxidants in:

- Improving markers of oxidative stress and inflammation.
- Supporting brain insulin signaling and other cell survival pathways.
- Improving cognitive function in aged and AD-engineered animals.

Epidemiological evidence indicates that serum levels of dietary antioxidants and consumption of food-based antioxidants decreases risk of AD and cognitive decline (Engelhart et al., 2002; Hu et al., 2006; in't Veld et al., 2001; Morris et al., 2002; Stewart et al., 1997; Zandi et al., 2002, 2004). The most abundant dietary antioxidants are a large class of compounds commonly found in plants called polyphenols. Their total dietary intake could be as high as 1 g/day which is substantively higher than that of all other classes of known antioxidants. Although ubiquitous in most plant foods, their main sources are darkly or brightly colored fruits, vegetables and plant-derived beverages such as tea (Scalbert et al., 2005).

Polyphenols not only improve the status of different oxidative stress biomarkers (Williamson & Manach, 2005), but may also directly modulate enzymes involved in signal transduction resulting in modification of redox status of the cell, and activation of survival pathways (Scalbert et al., 2005). For example, green tea polyphenols directly influence many signaling pathways including PI3K/Akt (Mandel et al., 2005; Weinreb et al., 2004) independent of their antioxidant roles, resulting in reduced Aβ fibril formation, soluble Aβ release, and potent radical-scavenging/anti-inflammatory properties. Similarly, blueberry polyphenols exert high antioxidant capacity, and blueberry-polyphenol enriched rodent diets consistently prevent age-related deficits in learning and memory by decreasing brain ROS levels and altering neuronal signaling (Joseph *et al.*, 2005; Lau *et al.*, 2005).

Greater cognitive benefits associate with consumption of foods with higher antioxidant capacity, such as blueberries, compared with those with lower levels of antioxidants, including spinach and strawberry. Blueberry extract prevented cognitive decline in Tg$_{APP/PS1}$ treated mice and increased ERK and PKC activity – both of which are also regulated by insulin and downstream of PI3K (Joseph *et al.*, 2003). In normal, aged rats blueberry polyphenols increased IGF-1 protein levels which associated with reduced memory errors (Casadesus *et al.*, 2004). Comparable studies in Tg$_{2576}$ mice supplemented with spice-polyphenol curcumin demonstrated potent reductions in Aβ, plaque formation, Aβ fibril formation, oxidative stress, and many pro-inflammatory markers including IL-1β even when administered in aged mice that already possess significant AD pathology (Lim *et al.*, 2001; Yang *et al.*, 2005). Thus, plant-based dietary antioxidants have an important role to play in controlling brain inflammation, influencing beneficial neuronal signaling and behavior, as well as having positive impacts on limiting pathological neurodegeneration. The mechanisms employed by polyphenols, once again, indicate the degree of convergence between diet, inflammation and insulin-related signaling on cognitive function and brain health.

Summary and recommendations related to chronic diet

In summary, chronic diet has important impacts on biologic systems intimately involved in neuronal growth, survival and function which are important to maintaining cognitive function. While a large number of systems, involving IR, inflammatory responses, oxidative stress, and changes to membrane structure and function, are implicated, these systems converge at two critical points: (1) sustainability of insulin and insulin-related cell signaling and (2) limiting inflammation. The dietary components discussed all share the ability to influence these processes, and indeed, can beneficially and adversely influence each other. Thus, common clinical trials which focus on only one nutrient or nutrient class are unlikely to be successful as other adverse consequences of a poor quality diet would minimise effectiveness, arguing for a more global change. That is, a "mixed" approach in dietary interventions allows for protection of these two critical points by simultaneously recruiting multiple systems associated with their protection. Although not well researched, one recent study indicated that a low-fat diet enriched with both DHA and polyphenol extract improved learning in old rats compared with a diet high in saturated fat. Importantly, benefits were only seen in old rats with the combined use of DHA and polyphenols, but not when either component was separately provided (Shirai & Suzuki, 2004).

Human food consumption patterns indicate that diets high in saturated fat usually contain lower amounts of plant matter, and place individuals at increased obesity risk (Davis *et al.*, 2006; Nelson & Tucker, 1996). Since saturated fat and obesity are key promoters of IR and many chronic diseases associated with cognitive dysfunction and AD – including stroke (Honig *et al.*, 2003), diabetes (Arvanitakis *et al.*, 2004; Ott *et al.*, 1999), heart disease (Newman *et al.*, 2005) – these and other studies highlight the importance of maintaining a diet that supports good peripheral health given its close relationship with brain health.

The increased demands imposed by rehabilitation reinforce the importance of making appropriate dietary changes as a prudent and inherently sensible contribution to brain recovery. Based on available evidence, these changes could easily be achieved by consuming an overall healthy diet as defined by many federal guidelines including Canada's Food Guide (Health Canada, 2005), that includes one serving of fresh, fatty fish per week (salmon, mackerel, tuna), 5–10 servings of darkly or brightly colored fruits and vegetables per day – or as many servings as possible – and limits intake of saturated fat as much as possible (fatty meats and processed foods). For a diet likely to minimize IR that also meets the goals of including fish and plant matter, guidelines of the American Diabetes Association (American Diabetes Association, 2006) should be considered.

Although diet is an important aspect of lifestyle, adequate physical activity is another factor known to be greatly beneficial for cognitive function and supporting neuronal health, and the reader is referred to Chapter 24 by Kramer, Erickson and McAuley in this volume for a good review. Importantly, mechanisms implicated with physical activity, including improved brain oxygen delivery and expression of neurotrophins, including BDNF (Cotman & Berchtold, 2002; McAuley *et al.*, 2004; Vaynman & Gómez-Pinilla, 2005), could function synergistically with diet to support processes essential to the formation of new neural networks, and augment cognitive approaches currently used in rehabilitation.

Role of acute diet

While chronic diet modulates major processes involved in neuronal signaling and synaptic plasticity, thereby setting the tone, or local environment, in which physiologic processes associated with cognitive rehabilitation occur, recently consumed food or meals provide brain with substrates, including glucose, needed to support immediate biochemical pathways involved in neuronal communication. A large body of literature exists demonstrating the benefits of food and/or glucose ingestion, on cognitive performance; unfortunately, the application of this information to rehabilitation programs has not been tested.

In this section, we will make the arguments that:

- The fed/fasted state of an individual is an important contributor to cognitive function – particularly tasks involving the hippocampus.

- Cognitive benefits of food ingestion may result from overlapping influences on blood glucose, insulin, gut hormones and sensory afferents.
- Unlike healthy people, cognitive function in individuals with T2DM is negatively affected by foods that rapidly raise blood glucose, possibly due to greater post-ingestive oxidative stress.
- Ensuring that an individual is in the fed state may be a way to boost performance during rehabilitation sessions, potentially contributing to longer-term outcome.

Many original studies investigating the role of food ingestion on cognition lay in the evaluation of school breakfast programs, where school performance was the most common outcome measure. While these studies generally reported benefits associated with the breakfast programs, results were confounded by the fact that concurrent improvements in other parameters, including school attendance, made it difficult to attribute the benefits to the nutrition intervention alone (Pollitt & Mathews, 1998). Numerous, subsequent studies using placebo-controlled cross-over designs have shown benefits on various measures of cognitive performance following ingestion of a single meal or nutrient across a much broader age-span (Kanarek, 1997). These benefits are likely attributed to both eating per se and the provision of energy, or calories, as well as attributes of individual nutrients, notably glucose.

Importantly, an individual's underlying health status, particularly the presence of T2DM, is an important predictor of the response to ingestion of glucose or carbohydrate-rich foods (Greenwood *et al.*, 2003; Papanikoloau *et al.*, 2006), with a focus on high-quality, low glycemic index carbohydrate foods being particularly important for those with T2DM. The fact that most studies were conducted in the early morning and compared a fasting versus fed (nutrient intervention) condition, attests to the importance of breakfast consumption (Greenwood *et al.*, 2003; Kanarek, 1997). However, at least one study found greater glucose-induced enhancement in cognitive performance among older adults who were tested in the afternoon compared with the

Table 16.3. Evidence associated with memory-enhancing benefits of glucose ingestion.

Intake of moderate (50–75 g), but not high, levels of glucose are associated with improvements in cognitive performance	(Parsons & Gold, 1992)
Subjects with poorer overall levels of cognition, including older adults and those with dementia show greater sensitivity to the benefits of glucose ingestion, compared with age-matched subjects with higher baseline levels of performance	(Craft et al., 1992, 1993, 1994, Hall et al., 1989; Manning et al., 1997; Messier et al., 2003)
Not all cognitive domains are sensitive to glucose administration, with functions associated with the hippocampus and medial temporal lobes, such as delayed verbal memory, showing greater sensitivity	(Manning et al., 1993; Parsons & Gold, 1992)
While both acquisition and retrieval of verbal information are augmented, more robust benefits are attributed to encoding processes	(Manning et al., 1998)
Individuals with poorer overall measures of gluco-regulatory status, including IR, show both lower baseline cognitive performance and greater benefits of glucose ingestion. Thus there is a somewhat paradoxical effect of glucose, such that those with decreased abilities to clear blood glucose after ingestion are the very individuals who benefit most from its ingestion	(Craft et al., 1994; Kaplan et al., 2000; Messier et al., 1999)
The benefits of glucose ingestion are no longer evident, and induce memory deficits, when an individual has transitioned from glucose intolerance or IR to overt T2DM	(Greenwood et al., 2003; Papanikoloau et al., 2006)

morning (Greenwood & Winocur, 2005) – a time of day when older individuals are at a circadian nadir in performance (Hasher et al., 1999).

Specifically, the outcome of many studies administering glucose to humans and rats, reviewed in detail elsewhere (Gold, 2005; Korol & Gold, 1998; Messier, 2004), shows benefits associated with glucose ingestion, particularly in tasks associated with the function of the hippocampus and medial temporal lobes and in those with poor underlying memories (for synopsis of evidence see Table 16.3).

Much work has been conducted to understand glucose's mechanism of action. Research demonstrating transient decreases in rat hippocampal, extraneuronal glucose levels during memory-demanding cognitive tasks and its replenishment with glucose administration (McNay et al., 2000) suggests that under conditions of increased neuronal activity local neuronal glucose supply may become limiting. Since glucose supplies energy and also serves as a substrate for synthesis of neurotransmitters such as acetylcholine, glutamate and GABA (Messier, 2004), local glucose depletion may be detrimental to actively firing neurons.

Interestingly, the level of hippocampal glucose depletion and improvement in a memory-demanding task was greater in aged animals relative to young adult rats (McNay & Gold, 2001). Since intra-cerebro-ventricular glucose injection produces comparable cognitive benefits to peripherally administered glucose (Lee et al., 1988), results point to a brain-specific benefit of glucose.

Yet, not all benefits of glucose ingestion can be attributed to a localized brain-specific mechanism. For example, administration of fructose, which does not cross the blood–brain barrier, also enhances memory function (Messier & White, 1987; Rodriguez et al., 1994). This fructose-induced improvement in brain function has been attributed to stimulation of afferent vagal fibres. Similarly, others have suggested that eating, in and of itself, through the release of gut peptides, such as cholecystokinin (CCK), can enhance cognitive function either through vagal receptors or blood–brain barrier uptake (Flood et al., 1987; Morley, 1987).

An important confound in many studies of glucose administration is the inability to distinguish between a potential cognitive-enhancing role of glucose versus that of insulin since glucose administration stimulates pancreatic insulin secretion such that concomitant increases in blood levels of both are observed. Indeed, others have attributed a glucose effect to be mediated via insulin and not glucose per se. For example, glucose-induced enhancement of delayed verbal memory in older adults with AD could be abolished by the co-administration of somatostatin – a compound which suppresses insulin secretion (Craft *et al.*, 1999).

Thus, while it is clear that glucose consumption, mediated either via glucose or an event occurring in tandem with glucose consumption, may enhance memory function in those with poor memories and poor gluco-regulatory status, the question becomes how to translate this experimental approach to humans who consume food and not glucose. The vast majority of dietary glucose is consumed as high carbohydrate-containing foods. Not surprisingly, when older adults consume carbohydrate foods which are rapidly absorbed such as mashed potatoes, producing a similar blood glucose profile to that observed with glucose ingestion (high glycemic index (GI) foods), the same profile of cognitive benefits to that observed with glucose are apparent (Kaplan *et al.*, 2000). Interestingly, however, the consumption of more complex carbohydrate foods, such as barley, which have a minimal impact on blood glucose levels (low GI foods), also enhance verbal declarative memory to the same extent as glucose and high GI foods (Kaplan *et al.*, 2000). Thus it would appear that raising blood glucose levels into an optimal range for cognitive function (Benton *et al.*, 1996; Manning *et al.*, 1993; Parsons & Gold, 1992) is not needed to observe benefits associated with the ingestion of high carbohydrate foods – indeed, the ingestion of healthier, low GI, foods have the same benefit.

The comparable cognitive-enhancing attributes of lower GI carbohydrate foods are important, since consumption of high GI foods, such as white bread and bagels, can have deleterious cognitive effects in those with T2DM (Greenwood *et al.*, 2003; Papanikoloau *et al.*, 2006). The post-ingestive cognitive deficits, especially delayed verbal recall,

observed in the T2DM population is highly associated with food-induced increases in blood glucose levels and can be prevented by switching the carbohydrate food from a high GI to a low GI food such as pasta (Papanikoloau *et al.*, 2006). While the mechanisms surrounding the deleterious effects of high GI foods and extreme elevations in blood glucose levels post consumption in those with T2DM are under investigation, results from one study in which a deficit following ingestion of a meal high in fat and simple carbohydrates was prevented by the co-consumption of the antioxidant vitamins C and E suggest that food-induced oxidative stress may underlie some of the negative effects (Chui & Greenwood, in press).

A weakness of many glucose studies relates to the fact that the control treatment was an artificially sweetened beverage such that the impact of consuming energy in and of itself was not controlled for. Consequently, the specificity of glucose's effect could not be evaluated. When we provided older adults with drinks containing equal energy as protein, fat, or glucose, all three macronutrients led to an initial, robust improvement on delayed paragraph recall; however, only glucose ingestion trended toward a sustained improvement on this task (Kaplan *et al.*, 2001), weakly arguing for glucose specificity on measures of verbal memory. Nevertheless, lack of nutrient specificity was apparent in tests of attention and executive function (e.g., Trails Part B) where improvements were observed with all three macronutrients relative to water and better sustained attention, as measured by the elevator task, was observed in adults with T2DM irrespective of whether or not they experienced a hyperglycemia-associated decrement in verbal memory performance following consumption of carbohydrate foods (Papanikoloau *et al.*, 2006).

Collectively, results suggest that cognitive functions associated with the hippocampus and medial temporal lobes likely show a degree of specificity to glucose ingestion, however, other cognitive functions, especially measures of sustained attention and executive function appear more sensitive to the fed-fasted state of the individual.

Summary and recommendations for acute diet

While chronic diet influences processes involved in the longer-term health of neurons, acute diet, or recently ingested food, provide substrates and biologic signals emanating from vagal afferent innervation, that support neurons in their actively firing state. Numerous studies point to the benefits of food ingestion, making it essential to ensure that individuals are not in the fasted state when commencing a rehabilitation session so as to help maximise their performance during the session. Indeed, if sessions are long, it would be prudent to ensure that snacks are consumed periodically to help sustain neuronal needs. While carbohydrate-rich foods have the benefit of providing both energy and glucose, they should have a low glycemic-index to help offset potential decrements in performance that may be apparent in those with T2DM.

Conclusions

While attention has not previously been paid to the potential benefit of diet in cognitive rehabilitation programs, this chapter draws inferences on its importance. Both chronic diet, through its ability to influence neuronal health and survival, and acute diet, through its ability to support actively firing neurons, require attention. It is essential that individuals avoid diets which promote the development of IR, or if present, take aggressive dietary steps to improve their gluco-regulatory status – otherwise the impact of IR, especially if progressed to T2DM, would be predicted to impair synaptogenesis, neurogenesis and overall neuronal survival, thereby limiting the brain's ability to launch physiologic processes needed for cognitive gain. Equally important is that individuals not participate in rehabilitation sessions in the fasted state as neurons would not be bathed in substrate needed to support neuronal activity. Indeed, if sessions are long, planned snacks should be provided to ensure that the brain is adequately nourished throughout cognitive training.

ACKNOWLEDGMENTS

The authors gratefully acknowledge support from the Natural Sciences and Engineering Research Council of Canada for work emanating from their laboratory.

REFERENCES

Aizenman, Y., & de Vellis, J. (1987). Brain neurons develop in a serum and glial free environment: effects of transferrin, insulin-like growth factor-I and thyroid hormone on neuronal survival, growth and differentiation. *Brain Research*, **406**, 32–42.

Akbar, M., Calderon, F., Wen, Z., & Kim, H. Y. (2005). Docosahexaenoic acid: a positive modulator of Akt signaling in neuronal survival. *Proceedings of the National Academy of Sciences of the United States of America*, **102**, 10858–10863.

Alkon, D. L., Epstein, H., Kuzirian, A., Bennett, M. C., & Nelson, T. J. (2005). Protein synthesis required for long-term memory is induced by PKC activation on days before associative learning. *Proceedings of the National Academy of Sciences of the United States of America*, **102**, 16432–16437.

American Diabetes Association (2006). http://www.diabetes.org/nutrition-and-recipes/nutrition/overview.jsp.

Arriagada, P. V., Growdon, J. H., Hedley-Whyte, E. T., & Hyman, B. T. (1992). Neurofibrillary tangles but not senile plaques parallel duration and severity of Alzheimer's disease. *Neurology*, **42**, 631–639.

Arvanitakis, Z., Wilson, R. S., Bienias, J. L., Evans, D. A., & Bennett, D. A. (2004). Diabetes mellitus and risk of Alzheimer disease and decline in cognitive function. *Archives of Neurology*, **61**, 661–666.

Authier, F., Posner, B. I., & Bergeron, J. J. (1996). Insulin-degrading enzyme. *Clinical and Investigative Medicine*, **19**, 149–160.

Awad, N., Gagnon, M., & Messier, C. (2004). The relationship between impaired glucose tolerance, type 2 diabetes, and cognitive function. *Journal of Clinical and Experimental Neuropsychology*, **26**, 1044–1080.

Bank, B., Deweer, A., Kuzirian, A. M., Rasmussen, H., & Alkon, D. L. (1988). Classical conditioning induces long-term translocation of protein kinase C in rabbit hippocampal CA1 cells. *Proceedings of the National Academy of Sciences of the United States of America*, **85**, 1988–1992.

Barberger-Gateau, P., Letenneur, L., Deschamps, V. et al. (2002). Fish, meat, and risk of dementia: cohort study. British Medical Journal, 325, 932–933.

Barcelo-Coblijn, G., Hogyes, E., Kitajka, K. et al. (2003). Modification by docosahexaenoic acid of age-induced alterations in gene expression and molecular composition of rat brain phospholipids. Proceedings of the National Academy of Sciences of the United States of America, 100, 11321–11326.

Baura, G. D., Foster, D. M., Kaiyala, K. et al. (1996). Insulin transport from plasma into the central nervous system is inhibited by dexamethasone in dogs. Diabetes, 45, 86–90.

Behl, C., Davis, J. B., Lesley, R., & Schubert, D. (1994). Hydrogen peroxide mediates amyloid beta protein toxicity. Cell, 77, 817–827.

Benton, D., Parker, P. Y., & Donohoe, R. T. (1996). The supply of glucose to the brain and cognitive functioning. Journal of Biosocial Science, 28, 463–479.

Bourre, J. M. (2004). Roles of unsaturated fatty acids (especially omega-3 fatty acids) in the brain at various ages and during ageing. Journal of Nutrition, Health and Aging, 8, 163–174.

Caballero, A. E. (2003). Endothelial dysfunction in obesity and insulin resistance: a road to diabetes and heart disease. Obesity Research, 11, 1278–1289.

Calderon, F., & Kim, H. Y. (2004). Docosahexaenoic acid promotes neurite growth in hippocampal neurons. Journal of Neurochemistry, 90, 979–988.

Calon, F., Lim, G. P., Yang, F. et al. (2004). Docosahexaenoic acid protects from dendritic pathology in an Alzheimer's disease mouse model. Neuron, 43, 633–645.

Calon, F., Lim, G. P., Morihara, T. et al. (2005). Dietary n-3 polyunsaturated fatty acid depletion activates caspases and decreases NMDA receptors in the brain of a transgenic mouse model of Alzheimer's disease. European Journal of Neuroscience, 22, 617–626.

Cao, D., Zhou, C., Sun, L. et al. (2005). Chronic administration of ethyl docosahexaenoate reduces gerbil brain eicosanoid productions following ischemia and reperfusion. Journal of Nutritional Biochemistry, 17, 234–241.

Caroni, P., & Grandes, P. (1990). Nerve sprouting in innervated adult skeletal muscle induced by exposure to elevated levels of insulin-like growth factors. Journal of Cell Biology, 110, 1307–1317.

Carro, E., Trejo, J. L., Gomez-Isla, T., LeRoith, D., & Torres-Aleman, I. (2002). Serum insulin-like growth factor I regulates brain amyloid-beta levels. Nature Medicine, 8, 1390–1397.

Casadesus, G., Shukitt-Hale, B., Stellwagen, H. M. et al. (2004). Modulation of hippocampal plasticity and cognitive behavior by short-term blueberry supplementation in aged rats. Nutritional Neuroscience, 7, 309–316.

Catalan, J., Moriguchi, T., Slotnick, B. et al. (2002). Cognitive deficits in docosahexaenoic acid-deficient rats. Behavioral Neuroscience, 116, 1022–1031.

Chui, M. H., & Greenwood, C. E. (in press). Antioxidant vitamins reduce acute meal-induced memory deficits in adults with type-2 diabetes. Nutrition Research.

Chui, M. H., Papanikoloau, Y., Fontaine-Bisson, B. et al. (2007). The TNF-α-238G > A single nucleotide polymorphism protects against memory decline in older adults with type 2 diabetes. Behavioral Neuroscience, 121, 619–624.

Cotman, C. W., & Berchtold, N. C. (2002). Exercise: a behavioral intervention to enhance brain health and plasticity. Trends in Neurosciences, 25, 295–301.

Craft, S. (2005). Insulin resistance syndrome and Alzheimer's disease: age- and obesity-related effects on memory, amyloid, and inflammation. Neurobiology of Aging, 26, 65–69.

Craft, S., & Watson, G. S. (2004). Insulin and neurodegenerative disease: shared and specific mechanisms. Lancet Neurology, 3, 169–178.

Craft, S., Zallen, G., & Baker, L. D. (1992). Glucose and memory in mild senile dementia of the Alzheimer type. Journal of Clinical and Experimental Neuropsychology, 14, 253–267.

Craft, S., Dagogo-Jack, S. E., Wiethop, B. V. et al. (1993). Effects of hyperglycemia on memory and hormone levels in dementia of the Alzheimer type: a longitudinal study. Behavioral Neuroscience, 107, 926–940.

Craft, S., Murphy, C., & Wemstrom, J. (1994). Glucose effects on complex memory and nonmemory tasks: the influence of age, sex, and glucoregulatory response. Psychobiology, 22, 95–105.

Craft, S., Peskind, E., Schwartz, M. W. et al. (1998). Cerebrospinal fluid and plasma insulin levels in Alzheimer's disease: relationship to severity of dementia and apolipoprotein E genotype. Neurology, 50, 164–168.

Craft, S., Asthana, S., Newcomer, J. W. et al. (1999). Enhancement of memory in Alzheimer's disease with insulin and somatostatin, but not glucose. Archives of General Psychiatry, 56, 1135–1140.

Craft, S., Asthana, S., Cook, D. G. et al. (2003). Insulin dose-response effects on memory and plasma amyloid precursor protein in Alzheimer's disease: interactions with apolipoprotein E genotype. *Psychoneuroendocrinology*, **28**, 809–822.

Davis, J. N., Hodges, V. A., & Gillham, M. B. (2006). Normal-weight adults consume more fiber and fruit than their age- and height-matched overweight/obese counterparts. *Journal of the American Dietetic Association*, **106**, 833–840.

Devaskar, S. U., Giddings, S. J., Rajakumar, P. A. *et al.* (1994). Insulin gene expression and insulin synthesis in mammalian neuronal cells. *Journal of Biological Chemistry*, **269**, 8445–8454.

Di Iorio, A., Cherubini, A., Volpatos, S. *et al.* (2006). Markers of inflammation, vitamin E and peripheral nervous system function: the InCHIANTI study. *Neurobiology of Aging*, **27**, 1280–1288.

Dimopoulos, N., Piperi, C., Salonicioti, A. *et al.* (2006). Indices of low-grade chronic inflammation correlate with early cognitive deterioration in an elderly Greek population. *Neuroscience Letters*, **398**, 118–123.

Duan, W., Guo, Z., Jiang, H., Ware, M., & Mattson, M. P. (2003). Reversal of behavioral and metabolic abnormalities, and insulin resistance syndrome, by dietary restriction in mice deficient in brain-derived neurotrophic factor. *Endocrinology*, **144**, 2446–2453.

Dumanchin-Njock, C., Alves da Costa, C. A., Mercken, L., Pradier, L., & Checler, F. (2001). The caspase-derived C-terminal fragment of betaAPP induces caspase-independent toxicity and triggers selective increase of Abeta42 in mammalian cells. *Journal of Neurochemistry*, **78**, 1153–1161.

Dupont, J., & LeRoith, D. (2001). Insulin and insulin-like growth factor I receptors: similarities and differences in signal transduction. *Hormone Research*, **55**, *Suppl. 2*, 22–26.

Dyall, S. C., Michael, G. J., Whelpton, R., Scott, A. G., & Michael-Titus, A. T. (2006). Dietary enrichment with omega-3 polyunsaturated fatty acids reverses age-related decreases in the GluR2 and NR2B glutamate receptor subunits in rat forebrain. *Neurobiology of Aging*, **28**, 424–439.

Engelhart, M. J., Geerlings, M. I., Ruitenberg, A. *et al.* (2002). Dietary intake of antioxidants and risk of Alzheimer disease. *Journal of the American Medical Association*, **287**, 3223–3229.

Farris, W., Mansourian, S., Chang, Y. *et al.* (2003). Insulin-degrading enzyme regulates the levels of insulin, amyloid beta-protein, and the beta-amyloid precursor protein intracellular domain in vivo. *Proceedings of the National Academy of Sciences of the United States of America*, **100**, 4162–4167.

Farris, W., Mansourian, S., Leissring, M. A. *et al.* (2004). Partial loss-of-function mutations in insulin-degrading enzyme that induce diabetes also impair degradation of amyloid beta-protein. *American Journal of Pathology*, **164**, 1425–1434.

Fishel, M. A., Watson, G. S., Montine, T. J. *et al.* (2005). Hyperinsulinemia provokes synchronous increases in central inflammation and beta-amyloid in normal adults. *Archives of Neurology*, **62**, 1539–1544.

Flood, J. F., Smith, G. E., & Morley, J. E. (1987). Modulation of memory processing by cholecystokinin: dependence on the vagus nerve. *Science*, **236**, 832–834.

Foulstone, E. J., Tavare, J. M., & Gunn-Moore, F. J. (1999). Sustained phosphorylation and activation of protein kinase B correlates with brain-derived neurotrophic factor and insulin stimulated survival of cerebellar granule cells. *Neuroscience Letters*, **264**, 125–128.

Frolich, L., Blum-Degen, D., Bernstein, H. G. *et al.* (1998). Brain insulin and insulin receptors in aging and sporadic Alzheimer's disease. *Journal of Neural Transmission*, **105**, 423–438.

Galvan, V., Chen, S., Lu, D. *et al.* (2002). Caspase cleavage of members of the amyloid precursor family of proteins. *Journal of Neurochemistry*, **82**, 283–294.

Gasparini, L., & Xu, H. (2003). Potential roles of insulin and IFG-1 in Alzheimer's disease. *Trends in Neurosciences*, **26**, 404–406.

Gervais, F. G., Xu, D., Robertson, G. S. *et al.* (1999). Involvement of caspases in proteolytic cleavage of Alzheimer's amyloid-beta precursor protein and amyloidogenic A beta peptide formation. *Cell*, **97**, 395–406.

Gold, P. E. (2005). Glucose and age-related changes in memory. *Neurobiology of Aging*, **26**, *Suppl. 1*, 60–64.

Gradman, T. J., Laws, A., Thompson, L. W., & Reaven, G. M. (1993). Verbal learning and/or memory improves with glycemic control in older subjects with non-insulin-dependent diabetes mellitus. *Journal of the American Geriatrics Society*, **41**, 1305–1312.

Greenwood, C. E., & Winocur, G. (2005). High-fat diets, insulin resistance and declining cognitive function. *Neurobiology of Aging*, **61**, S68–S74.

Greenwood, C. E., Kaplan, R. J., Hebblethwaite, S., & Jenkins, D. J. (2003). Carbohydrate-induced memory impairment in adults with type 2 diabetes. *Diabetes Care*, **26**, 1961–1966.

Hall, J. L., Gonder-Frederick, L. A., Chewning, W. W., Silveira, J., & Gold, P. E. (1989). Glucose enhancement of performance on memory tests in young and aged humans. *Neuropsychologia*, **27**, 1129–1138.

Hansen, L. L., Ikeda, Y., Olsen, G. S., Busch, A. K., & Mosthaf, L. (1999). Insulin signaling is inhibited by micromolar concentrations of H_2O_2. Evidence for a role of H_2O_2 in tumor necrosis factor alpha-mediated insulin resistance. *Journal of Biological Chemistry*, **274**, 25078–25084.

Hasher, L., Zacks, R., & May, C. (1999). Inhibitory control, circadian arousal, and age. In D. Gopher & A. Koriat (Eds.), *Attention & Performance, XVII, Cognitive Regulation of Performance: Interaction of Theory and Application* (pp. 653-675). Cambridge, MA: MIT Press.

Havrankova, J., Schmechel, D., Roth, J., & Brownstein, M. (1978). Identification of insulin in rat brain. *Proceedings of the National Academy of Sciences of the United States of America*, **75**, 5737–5741.

Health and Canada (2005). http://www.hc-sc.gc.ca/fn-an/food-guide-aliment/fg_rainbow-arc_en_ciel_ga_e.html.

Ho, L., Qin, W., Pompl, P. N. *et al.* (2004). Diet-induced insulin resistance promotes amyloidosis in a transgenic mouse model of Alzheimer's disease. *FASEB Journal*, **18**, 902–904.

Hong, M., & Lee, V. M. (1997). Insulin and insulin-like growth factor-1 regulate tau phosphorylation in cultured human neurons. *Journal of Biological Chemistry*, **272**, 19547–19553.

Honig, L. S., Tang, M. X., Albert, S. *et al.* (2003). Stroke and the risk of Alzheimer disease. *Archives of Neurology*, **60**, 1707–1712.

Horrocks, L. A., & Farooqui, A. A. (2004). Docosahexaenoic acid in the diet: its importance in maintenance and restoration of neural membrane function. *Prostaglandins, Leukotrienes, and Essential Fatty Acids*, **70**, 361–372.

Hu, P., Bretsky, P., Crimmins, E. M. *et al.* (2006). Association between serum beta-carotene levels and decline of cognitive function in high-functioning older persons with or without apolipoprotein E 4 alleles: MacArthur studies of successful aging. *Journals of Gerontology, Series A: Biological Sciences and Medical Sciences*, **61**, 616–620.

in't Veld, B. A., Ruitenberg, A., Hofman, A. *et al.* (2001). Nonsteroidal antiinflammatory drugs and the risk of Alzheimer's disease. *New England Journal of Medicine*, **345**, 1515–1521.

Joseph, J. A., Denisova, N. A., Arendash, G. *et al.* (2003). Blueberry supplementation enhances signaling and prevents behavioral deficits in an Alzheimer disease model. *Nutritional Neuroscience*, **6**, 153–162.

Joseph, J. A., Shukitt-Hale, B., & Casadesus, G. (2005). Reversing the deleterious effects of aging on neuronal communication and behavior: beneficial properties of fruit polyphenolic compounds. *American Journal of Clinical Nutrition*, **81**, 313S–316S.

Kahn, C. R., White, M. F., Shoelson, S. E. *et al.* (1993). The insulin receptor and its substrate: molecular determinants of early events in insulin action. *Recent Progress in Hormone Research*, **48**, 291–339.

Kahn, R., Buse, J., Ferrannini, E., & Stern, M. (2005). The metabolic syndrome: time for a critical appraisal. Joint statement from the American Diabetes Association and the European Association for the Study of Diabetes. *Diabetes Care*, **28**, 2289–2304.

Kanarek, R. (1997). Psychological effects of snacks and altered meal frequency. *British Journal of Nutrition*, **77**, Suppl. 1, S105–S118.

Kaplan, R. J., Greenwood, C. E., Winocur, G., & Wolever, T. M. (2000). Cognitive performance is associated with glucose regulation in healthy elderly persons and can be enhanced with glucose and dietary carbohydrates. *American Journal of Clinical Nutrition*, **72**, 825–836.

Kaplan, R. J., Greenwood, C. E., Winocur, G., & Wolever, T. M. (2001). Dietary protein, carbohydrate, and fat enhance memory performance in the healthy elderly. *American Journal of Clinical Nutrition*, **74**, 687–693.

Kar, S., Slowikowski, S. P., Westaway, D., & Mount, H. T. (2004). Interactions between beta-amyloid and central cholinergic neurons: implications for Alzheimer's disease. *Journal of Psychiatry and Neuroscience*, **29**, 427–441.

Korol, D. L., & Gold, P. E. (1998). Glucose, memory, and aging. *American Journal of Clinical Nutrition*, **67**, 764S–771S.

Lau, F. C., Shukitt-Hale, B., & Joseph, J. A. (2005). The beneficial effects of fruit polyphenols on brain aging. *Neurobiology of Aging*, **26**, 128–132.

Laurino, L., Wang, X. X., de la Houssaye, B. A. *et al.* (2005). PI3K activation by IGF-1 is essential for the regulation of membrane expansion at the nerve growth cone. *Journal of Cell Science*, **118**, 3653–3662.

Lee, M. K., Graham, S. N., & Gold, P. E. (1988). Memory enhancement with posttraining intraventricular glucose injections in rats. *Behavioral Neuroscience*, **102**, 591–595.

Lesne, S., Gabriel, C., Nelson, D. A. *et al.* (2005). Akt-dependent expression of NAIP-1 protects neurons against amyloid-{beta} toxicity. *Journal of Biological Chemistry*, **280**, 24941–24947.

Lim, G. P., Chu, T., Yang, F. *et al.* (2001). The curry spice curcumin reduces oxidative damage and amyloid pathology in an Alzheimer transgenic mouse. *Journal of Neuroscience*, **21**, 8370–8377.

Lim, G. P., Calon, F., Morihara, T. *et al.* (2005). A diet enriched with the omega-3 fatty acid docosahexaenoic acid reduces amyloid burden in an aged Alzheimer mouse model. *Journal of Neuroscience*, **25**, 3032–3040.

Lu, D. C., Rabizadeh, S., Chandra, S. *et al.* (2000). A second cytotoxic proteolytic peptide derived from amyloid beta-protein precursor. *Nature Medicine*, **6**, 397–404.

Luchsinger, J. A., & Mayeux, R. (2004). Dietary factors and Alzheimer's disease. *Lancet Neurology*, **3**, 579–587.

Luchsinger, J. A., Tang, M. X., Shea, S., & Mayeux, R. (2004). Hyperinsulinemia and risk of Alzheimer disease. *Neurology*, **63**, 1187–1192.

Lukiw, W. J., Cui, J. G., Marcheselli, V. L. *et al.* (2005). A role for docosahexaenoic acid-derived neuroprotectin D1 in neural cell survival and Alzheimer disease. *Journal of Clinical Investigation*, **115**, 2774–2783.

Maher, F. O., Martin, D. S., & Lynch, M. A. (2004). Increased IL-1beta in cortex of aged rats is accompanied by downregulation of ERK and PI-3 kinase. *Neurobiology of Aging*, **25**, 795–806.

Maher, F. O., Clarke, R. M., Kelly, A., Nally, R. E., & Lynch, M. A. (2006). Interaction between interferon gamma and insulin-like growth factor-1 in hippocampus impacts on the ability of rats to sustain long-term potentiation. *Journal of Neurochemistry*, **96**, 1560–1571.

Mandel, S. A., Avramovich-Tirosh, Y., Reznichenko, L. *et al.* (2005). Multifunctional activities of green tea catechins in neuroprotection. Modulation of cell survival genes, iron-dependent oxidative stress and PKC signaling pathway. *Neurosignals*, **14**, 46–60.

Manning, C. A., Ragozzino, M. E., & Gold, P. E. (1993). Glucose enhancement of memory in patients with probable senile dementia of the Alzheimer's type. *Neurobiology of Aging*, **14**, 523–528.

Manning, C., Parsons, M., Cotter, E., & Gold, P. E. (1997). Glucose effects on declarative and nondeclarative memory in healthy elderly and young adults. *Psychobiology*, **25**, 103–108.

Manning, C. A., Stone, W. S., Korol, D. L., & Gold, P. E. (1998). Glucose enhancement of 24-h memory retrieval in healthy elderly humans. *Behavioural Brain Research*, **93**, 71–76.

Marcheselli, V. L., Hong, S., Lukiw, W. J. *et al.* (2003). Novel docosanoids inhibit brain ischemia-reperfusion-mediated leukocyte infiltration and pro-inflammatory gene expression. *Journal of Biological Chemistry*, **278**, 43807–43817.

Marin, N., Romero, B., Bosch-Morell, F. *et al.* (2000). Beta-amyloid-induced activation of caspase-3 in primary cultures of rat neurons. *Mechanisms of Ageing and Development*, **119**, 63–67.

Mattson, M. P., Maudsley, S., & Martin, B. (2004). BDNF and 5-HT: a dynamic duo in age-related neuronal plasticity and neurodegenerative disorders. *Trends in Neurosciences*, **27**, 589–594.

McAuley, E., Kramer, A. F., & Colcombe, S. J. (2004). Cardiovascular fitness and neurocognitive function in older adults: a brief review. *Brain, Behavior and Immunity*, **18**, 214–220.

McNay, E. C., & Gold, P. E. (2001). Age-related differences in hippocampal extracellular fluid glucose concentration during behavioral testing and following systemic glucose administration. *Journals of Gerontology, Series A: Biological Sciences and Medical Sciences*, **56**, 66–71.

McNay, E. C., Fries, T. M., & Gold, P. E. (2000). Decreases in rat extracellular hippocampal glucose concentration associated with cognitive demand during a spatial task. *Proceedings of the National Academy of Sciences of the United States of America*, **97**, 2881–2885.

McNay, E. C., McCarty, R. C., & Gold, P. E. (2001). Fluctuations in brain glucose concentration during behavioral testing: dissociations between brain areas and between brain and blood. *Neurobiology of Learning and Memory*, **75**, 325–337.

Meneilly, G. S., Cheung, E., Tessier, D., Yakura, C., & Tuokko, H. (1993). The effect of improved glycemic control on cognitive functions in the elderly patient with diabetes. *Journal of Gerontology*, **48**, M117–M121.

Messier, C. (2004). Glucose improvement of memory: a review. *European Journal of Pharmacology*, **490**, 33–57.

Messier, C., & White, N. M. (1987). Memory improvement by glucose, fructose, and two glucose analogs: a possible effect on peripheral glucose transport. *Behavioral and Neural Biology*, **48**, 104–127.

Messier, C., Desrochers, A., & Gagnon, M. (1999). Effect of glucose, glucose regulation, and word imagery value on human memory. *Behavioral Neuroscience*, **113**, 431–438.

Messier, C., Tsiakas, M., Gagnon, M., Desrochers, A., & Awad, N. (2003). Effect of age and glucoregulation on cognitive performance. *Neurobiology of Aging*, **24**, 985–1003.

Misonou, H., Morishima-Kawashima, M., & Ihara, Y. (2000). Oxidative stress induces intracellular accumulation of amyloid beta-protein (Aβ) in human neuroblastoma cells. *Biochemistry*, **39**, 6951–6959.

Molteni, R., Wu, A., Vaynman, S. *et al.* (2004). Exercise reverses the harmful effects of consumption of a high-fat diet on synaptic and behavioral plasticity associated to the action of brain-derived neurotrophic factor. *Neuroscience*, **123**, 429–440.

Moore, S. A. (1993). Cerebral endothelium and astrocytes cooperate in supplying docosahexaenoic acid to neurons. *Advances in Experimental Medicine and Biology*, **331**, 229–233.

Moore, S. A., Yoder, E., Murphy, S., Dutton, G. R., & Spector, A. A. (1991). Astrocytes, not neurons, produce docosahexaenoic acid (22:6 omega-3) and arachidonic acid (20:4 omega-6). *Journal of Neurochemistry*, **56**, 518–524.

Morley, J. E. (1987). Neuropeptide regulation of appetite and weight. *Endocrine Reviews*, **8**, 256–287.

Morris, M. C., Evans, D. A., Bienias, J. L. *et al.* (2002). Dietary intake of antioxidant nutrients and the risk of incident Alzheimer disease in a biracial community study. *Journal of the American Medical Association*, **287**, 3230–3237.

Morris, M. C., Evans, D. A., Bienias, J. L. *et al.* (2003a). Dietary fats and the risk of incident Alzheimer disease. *Archives of Neurology*, **60**, 194–200.

Morris, M. C., Evans, D. A., Bienias, J. L. *et al.* (2003b). Consumption of fish and n-3 fatty acids and risk of incident Alzheimer disease. *Archives of Neurology*, **60**, 940–946.

Morris, M. C., Evans, D. A., Tangney, C. C., Bienias, J. L., & Wilson, R. S. (2005). Fish consumption and cognitive decline with age in a large community study. *Archives of Neurology*, **62**, 1849–1853.

Naor, M., Steingruber, H. J., Westhoff, K., Schottenfeld-Naor, Y., & Gries, A. F. (1997). Cognitive function in elderly non-insulin-dependent diabetic patients before and after inpatient treatment for metabolic control. *Journal of Diabetes and its Complications*, **11**, 40–46.

Nelson, L. H., & Tucker, L. A. (1996). Diet composition related to body fat in a multivariate study of 203 men. *Journal of the American Dietetic Association*, **96**, 771–777.

Nestler, J. E., Barlascini, C. O., Tetrault, G. A. *et al.* (1990). Increased transcapillary escape rate of albumin in non-diabetic men in response to hyperinsulinemia. *Diabetes*, **39**, 1212–1217.

Newman, A. B., Fitzpatrick, A. L., Lopez, O. *et al.* (2005). Dementia and Alzheimer's disease incidence in relationship to cardiovascular disease in the Cardiovascular Health Study cohort. *Journal of the American Geriatrics Society*, **53**, 1101–1107.

Oddo, S., Caccamo, A., Shepherd, J. D. *et al.* (2003). Triple-transgenic model of Alzheimer's disease with plaques and tangles: intracellular Aβ and synaptic dysfunction. *Neuron*, **39**, 409–421.

Olds, J. L., Anderson, M. L., McPhie, D. L., Staten, L. D., & Alkon, D. L. (1989). Imaging of memory-specific changes in the distribution of protein kinase C in the hippocampus. *Science*, **245**, 866–869.

Orban, P. C., Chapman, P. F., & Brambilla, R. (1999). Is the Ras-MAPK signalling pathway necessary for long-term memory formation? *Trends in Neurosciences*, **22**, 38–44.

Ortega, R. M., Requejo, A. M., Andres, P. *et al.* (1997). Dietary intake and cognitive function in a group of elderly people. *American Journal of Clinical Nutrition*, **66**, 803–809.

Ott, A., Stolk, R. P., van Harskamp, F. *et al.* (1999). Diabetes mellitus and the risk of dementia: the Rotterdam Study. *Neurology*, **53**, 1937–1942.

Pandini, G., Frasca, F., Mineo, R., Sciacca, L., Vigneri, R., & Belfiore, A. (2002). Insulin/insulin-like growth factor I hybrid receptors have different biological characteristics depending on the insulin receptor isoform involved. *Journal of Biological Chemistry*, **277**, 29684–29695.

Panza, F., Solfrizzi, V., Colacicco, A. M. *et al.* (2004). Mediterranean diet and cognitive decline. *Public Health Nutrition*, **7**, 959–963.

Papanikoloau, Y., Palmer, H., Binns, M. A., Jenkins, D. J., & Greenwood, C. E. (2006). Better cognitive performance following a low-glycaemic-index compared with a high-glycaemic-index carbohydrate meal in adults with type 2 diabetes. *Diabetologia*, **49**, 855–862.

Park, C. R., Seeley, R. J., Craft, S., & Woods, S. C. (2000). Intracerebroventricular insulin enhances memory in a passive-avoidance task. *Physiology and Behavior*, **68**, 509–514.

Parsons, M. W., & Gold, P. E. (1992). Glucose enhancement of memory in elderly humans: an inverted-U dose-response curve. *Neurobiology of Aging*, **13**, 401–404.

Peila, R., Rodriguez, B. L., & Launer, L. J. (2002). Type 2 diabetes, APOE gene, and the risk for dementia and related pathologies: the Honolulu-Asia Aging Study. *Diabetes*, **51**, 1256–1262.

Pfenninger, K. H., Laurino, L., Peretti, D. *et al.* (2003). Regulation of membrane expansion at the nerve growth cone. *Journal of Cell Science*, **116**, 1209–1217.

Pollitt, E., & Mathews, R. (1998). Breakfast and cognition: an integrative summary. *American Journal of Clinical Nutrition*, **67**, 804S–813S.

Reger, M. A., Watson, G. S., Frey, W. H. n. *et al.* (2006). Effects of intranasal insulin on cognition in memory-impaired older adults: modulation by APOE genotype. *Neurobiology of Aging*, **27**, 451–458.

Riccardi, G., Giacco, R., & Rivellese, A. A. (2004). Dietary fat, insulin sensitivity and the metabolic syndrome. *Clinical Nutrition*, **23**, 447–456.

Rivera, E. J., Goldin, A., Fulmer, N. *et al.* (2005). Insulin and insulin-like growth factor expression and function deteriorate with progression of Alzheimer's disease: link to brain reductions in acetylcholine. *Journal of Alzheimer's Disease*, **8**, 247–268.

Rodriguez, W. A., Horne, C. A., Mondragon, A. N., & Phelps, D. D. (1994). Comparable dose-response functions for the effects of glucose and fructose on memory. *Behavioral and Neural Biology*, **61**, 162–169.

Rulifson, E. J., Kim, S. K., & Nusse, R. (2002). Ablation of insulin-producing neurons in flies: growth and diabetic phenotypes. *Science*, **296**, 1118–1120.

Ryan, C., Freed, M., Rood, J. *et al.* (2006). Improving metabolic control leads to better working memory in adults with type 2 diabetes. *Diabetes Care*, **29**, 345–351.

Ryu, B. R., Ko, H. W., Jou, I., Noh, J. S., & Gwag, B. J. (1999). Phosphatidylinositol 3-kinase-mediated regulation of neuronal apoptosis and necrosis by insulin and IGF-I. *Journal of Neurobiology*, **39**, 536–546.

Scalbert, A., Johnson, I. T., & Saltmarsh, M. (2005). Polyphenols: antioxidants and beyond. *American Journal of Clinical Nutrition*, **81**, 215S–217S.

Schechter, R., Holtzclaw, L., Sadiq, F., Kahn, A., & Devaskar, S. (1988). Insulin synthesis by isolated rabbit neurons. *Endocrinology*, **123**, 505–513.

Schechter, R., Beju, D., & Miller, K. E. (2005a). Insulin deficiency induces neuron cell death in knock-out mice by hyperphosphorylation of JNK. *Society for Neuroscience, Abstract No. 252.2*. Washington, DC.

Schechter, R., Beju, D., & Miller, K. E. (2005b). The effect of insulin deficiency on tau and neurofilament in the insulin knockout mouse. *Biochemical and Biophysical Research Communications*, **334**, 979–986.

Shirai, N., & Suzuki, H. (2004). Effect of dietary docosahexaenoic acid and catechins on maze behavior in mice. *Annals of Nutrition and Metabolism*, **48**, 51–58.

Simopoulos, A. P. (1991). Omega-3 fatty acids in health and disease and in growth and development. *American Journal of Clinical Nutrition*, **54**, 438–463.

Simopoulos, A. P. (1999). Essential fatty acids in health and chronic disease. *American Journal of Clinical Nutrition*, **70**, 560S–569S.

Stein, T. D., & Johnson, J. A. (2002). Lack of neurodegeneration in transgenic mice overexpressing mutant amyloid precursor protein is associated with increased levels of transthyretin and the activation of cell survival pathways. *Journal of Neuroscience*, **22**, 7380–7388.

Stewart, W. F., Kawas, C., Corrada, M., & Metter, E. J. (1997). Risk of Alzheimer's disease and duration of NSAID use. *Neurology*, **48**, 626–632.

Storlien, L. H., Kraegen, E. W., Chisholm, D. J. *et al.* (1987). Fish oil prevents insulin resistance induced by high-fat feeding in rats. *Science*, **237**, 885–888.

Storlien, L. H., Jenkins, A. B., Chisholm, D. J. *et al.* (1991). Influence of dietary fat composition on development of insulin resistance in rats. Relationship to muscle triglyceride and omega-3 fatty acids in muscle phospholipid. *Diabetes*, **40**, 280–289.

Su, J. H., Kesslak, J. P., Head, E., & Cotman, C. W. (2002). Caspase-cleaved amyloid precursor protein and activated caspase-3 are co-localized in the granules of granulovacuolar degeneration in Alzheimer's disease and Down's syndrome brain. *Acta Neuropathologica (Berlin)*, **104**, 1–6.

Taouis, M., Dagou, C., Ster, C. *et al.* (2002). N-3 polyunsaturated fatty acids prevent the defect of insulin receptor signaling in muscle. *American Journal of Physiology, Endocrinology and Metabolism*, **282**, E664–671.

Tesco, G., Koh, Y. H., & Tanzi, R. E. (2003). Caspase activation increases beta-amyloid generation independently of caspase cleavage of the beta-amyloid precursor protein (APP). *Journal of Biological Chemistry*, **278**, 46074–46080.

Uetsuki, T., Takemoto, K., Nishimura, I. *et al.* (1999). Activation of neuronal caspase-3 by intracellular accumulation of wild-type Alzheimer amyloid precursor protein. *Journal of Neuroscience*, **19**, 6955–6964.

Vaynman, S., & Gómez-Pinilla, F. (2005). License to run: exercise impacts functional plasticity in the intact and injured central nervous system by using neurotrophins. *Neurorehabilitation and Neural Repair*, **19**, 283–295.

Vekrellis, K., Ye, Z., Qiu, W. Q. *et al.* (2000). Neurons regulate extracellular levels of amyloid beta-protein via proteolysis by insulin-degrading enzyme. *Journal of Neuroscience*, **20**, 1657–1665.

Wallum, B. J., Taborsky, G. J. J., Porte, D. J. *et al.* (1987). Cerebrospinal fluid insulin levels increase during intravenous insulin infusions in man. *Journal of Clinical Endocrinology and Metabolism*, **64**, 190–194.

Weaver, J. D., Huang, M. H., Albert, M. *et al.* (2002). Interleukin-6 and risk of cognitive decline: MacArthur studies of successful aging. *Neurology*, **59**, 371–378.

Weinreb, O., Mandel, S., Amit, T., & Youdim, M. B. (2004). Neurological mechanisms of green tea polyphenols in Alzheimer's and Parkinson's diseases. *Journal of Nutritional Biochemistry*, **15**, 506–516.

Williamson, G., & Manach, C. (2005). Bioavailability and bioefficacy of polyphenols in humans. II. Review of 93 intervention studies. *American Journal of Clinical Nutrition*, **81**, 243S–255S.

Winocur, G., & Greenwood, C. E. (2005). Studies of the effects of high fat diets on cognitive function in a rat model. *Neurobiology of Aging*, **26**, 46–49.

Winocur, G., Greenwood, C. E., Piroli, G. G. *et al.* (2005). Memory impairment in obese Zucker rats: an investigation of cognitive function in an animal model of insulin resistance and obesity. *Behavioral Neuroscience*, **119**, 1389–1395.

Winocur, G., Wojtowicz, J. M., Sekeres, M., Snyder, J. S., & Wang, S. (2006). Inhibition of neurogenesis interferes with hippocampus-dependent memory function. *Hippocampus*, **16**, 296–304.

Wright, C. B., Sacco, R. L., Rundek, T. R. *et al.* (2006). Interleukin-6 is associated with cognitive function: the Northern Manhattan Study. *Journal of Stroke and Cerebrovascular Diseases*, **15**, 34–38.

Yaffe, K., Kanaya, A., Lindquist, K. *et al.* (2004). The metabolic syndrome, inflammation, and risk of cognitive decline. *Journal of the American Medical Association*, **292**, 2237–2242.

Yang, F., Lim, G. P., Begum, A. N. *et al.* (2005). Curcumin inhibits formation of amyloid beta oligomers and fibrils, binds plaques, and reduces amyloid in vivo. *Journal of Biological Chemistry*, **280**, 5892–5901.

Yang, H., & Raizada, M. K. (1999). Role of phosphatidyl-inosital 3-kinase in angiotensin II regulation of nor-epinephrine neuromodulation in brain neurons of the spontaneously hypertensive rat. *Journal of Neuroscience*, **19**, 2413–2423.

Young, G., & Conquer, J. (2005). Omega-3 fatty acids and neuropsychiatric disorders. *Reproduction, Nutrition, Development*, **45**, 1–28.

Yu, Y., Kastin, A. J., & Pan, W. (2006). Reciprocal interactions of insulin and insulin-like growth factor I in receptor-mediated transport across the blood–brain barrier. *Endocrinology*, **147**, 2611–2615.

Yuan, J., & Yankner, B. A. (2000). Apoptosis in the nervous system. *Nature*, **407**, 802–809.

Zandi, P. P., Anthony, J. C., Hayden, K. M. *et al.* (2002). Reduced incidence of AD with NSAID but not H2 receptor antagonists: the Cache County Study. *Neurology*, **59**, 880–886.

Zandi, P. P., Anthony, J. C., Khachaturian, A. S. *et al.* (2004). Reduced risk of Alzheimer disease in users of antioxidant vitamin supplements: the Cache County Study. *Archives of Neurology*, **61**, 82–88.

Zhang, X., Dong, F., Ren, J., Driscoll, M. J., & Culver, B. (2005). High dietary fat induces NADPH oxidase-associated oxidative stress and inflammation in rat cerebral cortex. *Experimental Neurology*, **191**, 318–325.

Zhao, W., Chen, H., Xu, H. *et al.* (1999). Brain insulin receptors and spatial memory. Correlated changes in gene expression, tyrosine phosphorylation, and signaling molecules in the hippocampus of water maze trained rats. *Journal of Biological Chemistry*, **274**, 34893–34902.

Zhao, W. Q., & Alkon, D. L. (2001). Role of insulin and insulin receptor in learning and memory. *Molecular and Cellular Endocrinology*, **177**, 125–134.

Pharmacologic and biological approaches

Introduction to Section 4

Gordon Winocur

One of the objectives of the second edition was to update progress in pharmacological interventions and other forms of biological treatment of cognitive disorders. Accordingly, the first three chapters in this section address the use of medications in treating cognitive impairment resulting from various etiologies. Other chapters provide timely reviews of developments in stem cell therapy, techniques for promoting neurogenesis as a mediator of hippocampus-based memory loss, and the link between small vessel disease and cognitive impairment.

McAllister and Arnsten begin the section with a thorough review of the animal and human literatures that link various neurotransmitter systems (e.g., cholinergic, noradrenergic, catecholaminergic) to specific forms of cognitive impairment (e.g., memory, attention, executive function). These discoveries have led to four distinct pharmacological intervention strategies that target primary prevention, secondary prevention, recovery of brain function and enhancement of cognitive skills. For example, with respect to secondary prevention, because cognitive impairment can result from numerous secondary mechanisms, the authors provide an informative discussion of excitotoxic, inflammatory and apoptosis cascades that are part of the evolution of neural damage and cognitive deficits. In considering mechanisms that can be exploited for purposes of inducing brain recovery and, in line with other chapters in this section, McAllister and Arnsten note the potential for pharmacologically promoting neurogenesis, synaptic organization, and successful cell replacement

strategies. The chapter ends on a cautionary note. Notwithstanding advances in our understanding of relationships between biochemical processes and cognitive function, we are still a long way from effectively treating specific deficits that characterize different types of brain damage. At the same time, there is much progress on which to build and the clear message is that the future appears brighter than it does bleak.

Whyte's chapter also is concerned with pharmacological treatment, especially as it applies to traumatic brain injury (TBI). At the outset, he makes the important point that, because TBI is so variable, no single drug has proven effective for all forms of resultant cognitive impairment. And, as McAllister and Arnsten point out in their chapter, progress in treating deficits in specific cognitive domains is limited, although Whyte is encouraged by results with certain drugs that have specific neurotransmitter targets. The chapter includes an interesting section on controversial single-subject experimental methods which, Whyte believes, have a role in evaluating treatment outcome, particularly in real-world situations. Whyte also provides an overview of methodological problems that have plagued studies of long-term outcome following drug treatment (e.g., failure to account for spontaneous recovery, inappropriate measures, small sample sizes, and inadequate randomization). He also evaluates the strengths and weaknesses of commonly used designs to assess drug effects, and discusses the dilemma facing clinicians who must treat cognitively impaired patients (e.g., memory loss) whose

Cognitive Neurorehabilitation, Second Edition: Evidence and Application, ed. Donald T. Stuss, Gordon Winocur and Ian H. Robertson. Published by Cambridge University Press. © Cambridge University Press 2008.

clinical circumstances are not consistent with any drug trials (e.g., donepezil). This is a comprehensive review that covers a wide range of academic and practical issues and provides clear direction for making progress in treating TBI-induced cognitive impairment.

Ringman and Cummings extend coverage of pharmacological treatment to dementias associated with progressive neurological disorders including, in particular, Alzheimer's disease (AD). Following an account of the neuropathology associated with various diseases, the authors review progress in developing medications aimed at reducing cognitive impairment. They note that dementia is a multidimensional illness that can also affect the individual's psychiatric state, activities of daily living and overall quality of life. As a result, the specific target symptoms of an intervention need to be defined to properly assess outcome. Progress generally has been limited but it is encouraging that, in AD, at least three anticholinesterase inhibitors (AChEI) have undergone extensive testing and are in common usage. Ringman and Cummings make the interesting observation that, despite the reported benefits of such drugs, clinical observations do not always support the results of clinical trials. This could be due to the different types of measurements but it could also be due to inherent flaws in the trials. AChEIs have also been studied as a treatment for memory loss in other disease (e.g., Parkinson's, Lewy Body), with moderately encouraging results. Ringman and Cummings conclude that the statistical superiority of medications over placebo in various trials is encouraging. However, in a clinical sense, the practical benefits are relatively small and the tremendous effort that is currently going into the development of new drugs must be reinforced.

Stickland, Weiss and Kolb's chapter deals with the exciting potential of stem cell therapy as a form of rehabilitation treatment. Stickland *et al.* discuss various ways that stem cells may be recruited endogenously by manipulating factors that promote neurogenesis (e.g., enriched environments, physical exercise, new learning). Unfortunately, many patients are unable to engage in such activities

and, in such cases, exogenous stimulation (e.g., epidermal or fibroblast growth factors) may be the best strategy for promoting neurogenesis (see also Wojtowicz's chapter). Increasingly, direct stem cell transplantation is becoming an option which, although invasive, does allow stem cells to locate optimally. When combined with an infusion of growth factors, this procedure has produced promising results in terms of cell survival and differentiation. The authors acknowledge that there is much to be learned about promoting cell replacement and functionally integrating stem cells into existing circuitry. There is hope that advances in genetics will allow for cells, with specific trophic factors, to be delivered to appropriate locations where they can assist in disease recovery. Already, this approach has enjoyed some success in developing and monitoring dopaminergic neurons in animal models and human trials. It is not yet clear if stem cell therapy will ever become a standard form of cognitive therapy but early indications demand that the possibilities be fully explored.

Now that it is an established fact that the adult mammalian brain can produce new neural cells (neurogenesis), the implications of this phenomenon for cognitive recovery in old age and following brain damage has generated tremendous interest. Neurogenesis is most widely studied in the hippocampus but, in his enlightening chapter, Wojtowicz suggests that it may also occur in other brain areas. Because the focus has been on the hippocampus, not surprisingly, the link between neurogenesis and memory has been the subject of considerable research. Wojtowicz asks the critical question as to how neurogenesis might be harnessed for the purpose of treating memory and related cognitive deficits. As Stickland *et al.* point out in their chapter, there are numerous ways to promote neurogenesis but, to derive full benefits from the production of new cells, they must be guided to the site of injury where the necessary "neural infrastructure" must exist to ensure their survival and functional integration. Neurogenesis in humans and nonhuman primates is poorly understood but there is evidence that it does occur in higher species. Interestingly, neurogenesis accompanies recovery from stroke, anoxia and ischemia, and Wojtowicz suggests that neurogenesis-promoting treatments that are known to be effective in animals could be applied to humans. With progress in creating the proper tissue environment in the human brain, it may well be possible to entertain trials to evaluate benefits of promoting neurogenesis as part of the rehabilitation of cognitive deficits resulting from brain injury.

The chapter by Vinters and Carmichael is concerned with the various forms of small vessel damage that result from ischemic vascular disease (IVD) and its impact on cognitive function. Such investigations are complicated by the fact that autopsy studies are typically conducted on elderly individuals who have been ill for some time and who often show signs of progressive neurodegenerative disease (e.g., AD), which are also associated with vascular morbidity. Because lesions associated with IVD are extremely variable in terms of size, distribution and number, the pathological and reparative responses have received little study. On the other hand, it is well established that hippocampal damage is a common neuropathological finding in IVD and that is undoubtedly a factor in IVD-related memory loss. Vinters and Carmichael suggest that cerebral amyloid angiopathy, resulting from amyloid-Beta protein deposits or a mutation in the cystatin (gamma trace) gene, is an under-appreciated feature of IVD that may also contribute to cognitive impairment. At this point, the cognitive sequelae resulting from small vessel disease are not well understood and any attempt at cognitive intervention must necessarily follow the leads of treatments designed for related diseases. Vinters and Carmichael have provided a valuable service in highlighting the pathological conditions that give rise to cognitive impairment related to small vessel disease.

17

Pharmacologic approaches to cognitive rehabilitation

Thomas W. McAllister and Amy F. T. Arnsten

Introduction

Neurological injuries and disorders are the cause of the majority of severe acquired disabilities (Wade, 1996). Andlin-Sobocki *et al.* (2005) suggest that neurological disorders comprise about one third of the burden of all disease in Europe. Estimates of the US prevalence of several of the more common disorders suggest that over 10 million individuals are living with the sequelae of traumatic brain injury, stroke, multiple sclerosis and brain tumors (American Brain Tumor Association website, www.abta.org; www.stroke.org; Langlois *et al.*, 2004; National MS Society website, www.nationalmssociety.org). For these individuals and their family/caregivers, neurobehavioral disorders, especially problems with cognition, are of greatest concern (Ben-Yishay & Diller, 1993; Cicerone, 2002; Whyte *et al.*, 1996).

Each neurological disorder has its own neuropathological process and profile of central nervous system (CNS) damage. However, many of these processes share common features. For example, downstream effects of both traumatic brain injury (TBI) and stroke include the triggering of excitotoxic injury cascades, inflammation and immune responses. Regardless of etiology, pathological processes that affect regions important in memory circuitry, attention, and executive functions will typically be associated with complaints and measurable deficits in these domains. These commonalities allow for the delineation of guiding principles in the pharmacologic management of cognitive impairment. Much of our current understanding of this area comes from animal and human studies of ischemia and trauma. Thus much of our discussion will be drawn from these disorders.

Overview of the neural substrate and neurochemistry of key cognitive domains

- The neural substrate of memory involves numerous brain regions including mesial temporal structures, basal forebrain nuclei, mamillary bodies and anterior thalamic nuclei for episodic memory, and prefrontal cortex, parietal cortex, cingulate and cerebellum for working memory.
- The neural substrate of attention involves three overlapping networks that modulate alerting, orienting and executive control.
- The neural substrate of executive functions includes several frontal-striatal-thalamo-cortical circuits.
- Cholinergic and catecholaminergic systems, particularly the dopaminergic and alpha-adrenergic systems play fundamental roles in modulation of memory, attention and executive functions.

From a practical standpoint, the pharmacologic treatment of cognitive deficits centers on memory, attention and executive functions. It is helpful to outline relevant components of the neural substrate and neurochemistry of these domains to set the stage for a rational approach to pharmacologic intervention. This brief review is intended to focus

Cognitive Neurorehabilitation, Second Edition: Evidence and Application, ed. Donald T. Stuss, Gordon Winocur and Ian H. Robertson. Published by Cambridge University Press. © Cambridge University Press 2008.

on areas that influence clinical practice, and is not an exhaustive treatment of the topic.

Memory

There are a variety of different types of memory such as episodic, procedural, semantic and working. Thus the neuroanatomy of memory is complex and involves overlapping circuitry in widely distributed areas of the brain (Budson & Price, 2005). This accounts for the ubiquitous nature of memory complaints in individuals with diverse brain disorders. However, episodic and working memory appear to be particularly vulnerable to brain disease and have received much attention.

Episodic memory

This term is generally used to describe the who, what, when, and where of memory. A wide variety of disorders impair episodic memory including Alzheimer's disease, frontotemporal dementias, multiple sclerosis and traumatic brain injury. Patients commonly report difficulty with recent as opposed to remote memory, implying difficulty with encoding and/or retrieval processes. Mesial temporal structures including the hippocampus, basal forebrain nuclei with related cholinergic projections, mamillary body, anterior thalamic nuclei, the fornix and prefrontal cortex play key roles in episodic memory (Budson & Price, 2005).

Working memory

Working memory facilitates the ability to hold information in mind while processing additional information. Impairment of working memory is also seen in a wide array of neuropsychiatric disorders. The substrate of working memory involves large areas of prefrontal cortex bilaterally (particularly the middle frontal gyri), bilateral posterior parietal cortex, the cingulate gyrus and the cerebellum.

Several neurotransmitter systems modulate different components of memory. The cholinergic system plays a key role in episodic memory and modulation of attention, particularly divided attention. Catecholaminergic mechanisms, particularly through dopaminergic and alpha-2 adrenergic systems, also play important roles in attention and memory function, especially in the prefrontal cortical area (see below). Furthermore, cholinergic cells in the basal forebrain receive important catecholaminergic modulation from noradrenergic afferents arising in the brain stem.

Attention

Attention is not a unitary construct and there have been a variety of schemes proposed to describe related component processes and functions (see Raz & Buhle, 2006 for review). More recently three broad, overlapping, attentional networks have been described; alerting, orienting and executive control (Fan *et al.*, 2005; Raz, 2004). These components have different regional nodal points and differ somewhat in terms of the predominant neurotransmitter systems that modulate their function. The alerting system includes elements related to arousal and preparation of the system for reception of incoming stimuli. Imaging studies suggest strong activation of thalamic, parietal and frontal cortices in paradigms comparing attentional tasks with and without alerting cues. This system (sometimes referred to as the "bottom up" system) has prominent catecholaminergic and cholinergic involvement. The second component is the orienting system. This component facilitates the selection of particular stimuli amidst many competing incoming stimuli. Imaging studies suggest involvement of bilateral superior parietal and temporo-parietal junction cortices, and regions in and around the frontal eye fields (Fan *et al.*, 2005). Cholinergic input, arising from cells in the basal forebrain nuclei, is considered critical to this system. The third attentional network facilitates the allocation of attentional resources, particularly under conditions of significant mental effort or competing task demands. Imaging studies consistently demonstrate involvement of the anterior cingulate and bilateral dorsolateral frontal cortices.

This component also receives input from a drive and motivational network with prominent catecholaminergic input, particularly the mesocortical dopaminergic system (Fan *et al.*, 2005; Raz, 2004). Attention can be domain specific (as in "visual attention") or domain independent (arousal, allocation of attentional network resources).

Executive functions

Although often referred to as "frontal-executive" functions, the neural substrate of executive function is more properly viewed as a series of frontal-striatal-thalamo-cortical circuits (Tekin & Cummings, 2002). Each of these circuits is named for its site of origin in the frontal cortex (e.g., the dorsolateral frontal-subcortical circuit, the orbitofrontal-subcortical circuit, and the anterior cingulate-subcortical circuit). Each circuit follows a similar path starting from the site of origin in the frontal cortex and subsequently projecting to the striatum, the globus pallidus, the thalamus and then back to the frontal cortex. Although not completely closed circuits, it is helpful to view each one as having major roles in different cognitive domains. For example, damage to the dorsolateral prefrontal cortex and its circuitry impairs executive functions such as decision making, problem solving and mental flexibility. Damage to the orbitofrontal cortex and related nodal points impairs intuitive, reflexive, social behaviors as well as the capacity to self-monitor and self-correct in real time within a social context. Damage to anterior cingulate and related circuitry impairs motivated and reward-related behaviors.

The neurochemistry of the frontal-subcortical circuits is complex and at best one can make simplistic generalizations with respect to the primary neurochemical modulators of the key nodal points in the circuits (Arciniegas *et al.*, 2007). This is a finely balanced system with dopaminergic, glutamatergic, GABA-ergic and serotonergic systems all playing roles in the proper functioning of these circuits. In the diseased or injured state, it is difficult to predict the net effect of altered central tone of any of the involved neurotransmitters.

The role that the prefrontal cortex (PFC) plays in memory, attention, and related executive functions, suggests that understanding the role of certain neurotransmitter systems in modulating PFC can inform pharmacologic approaches to enhancing these cognitive domains.

Role of dopamine

Both the D1 and D2 receptor families play a role in memory and executive functions in the PFC. For example, deficits in spatial working memory can be produced by infusion of a D1 receptor antagonist (Sawaguchi & Goldman-Rakic, 1991). Arnsten *et al.* (1994) showed that in monkeys, a D1 antagonist produced spatial working memory deficits in young but not aged monkeys (who presumably were DA depleted) and these deficits could be reversed by a D1 agonist. A partial D1 agonist improved performance in the aged monkeys; a full D1 agonist improved performance in young monkeys. The improvement could be blocked with a D1 antagonist (Arnsten *et al.*, 1994). Selective D1, but not D2 antagonists impair performance on an oculomotor delay task in monkeys (Sawaguchi & Goldman-Rakic, 1991). This effect is dose dependent, as small doses may actually enhance performance (Williams & Goldman-Rakic, 1995). The facilitative effects of D1 agonists also appear to be dose dependent, showing an inverted "U" shaped dose response relationship (Arnsten, 1998; Arnsten *et al.*, 1994; Cai & Arnsten, 1997). This same inverted U can be seen at the cellular level, where low doses of D1 agonist enhance spatially tuned delay-related firing by reducing firing to nonpreferred spatial directions, while high doses erode spatial tuning by suppressing firing to all directions (Vijayraghavan *et al.*, 2007).

Human studies suffer from the lack of a selective D1 agonist available for human use. However several lines of evidence suggest an important role of frontal dopaminergic systems in human cognition, both in normals and individuals with disorders such as TBI (Elliot *et al.*, 1997; Luciana & Collins, 1997; Luciana *et al.*, 1992; McDowell *et al.*, 1998).

Role of noradrenergic function

In animal studies, there is evidence that alpha-2-adrenergic (A2A) mechanisms also play a prominent role in the activation and modulation of executive functions (see Arnsten *et al.*, 1988 for review; Arnsten & Goldman-Rakic, 1985; Arnsten & Li, 2005; Carlson *et al.*, 1992; Franowicz & Arnsten, 1998; Rama *et al.*, 1996). Infusion of A2A antagonists produces spatial working memory impairment in both monkeys and rats (Steere & Arnsten, 1997; Tanila *et al.*, 1996). Adrenergic enhancement has been shown to be relatively specific to manipulation of the alpha-2 receptors, in that alpha-1 and beta-adrenergic antagonists had no effect on working memory performance (Li & Mei, 1994). However, A1A *agonists* can impair working memory, suggesting that (1) different adrenergic receptors have opposing effects on cognitive function (Arnsten, 1998; Birnbaum *et al.*, 1999) and (2) norepinephrine (NE) has a higher affinity for A2A receptors than A1A receptors, thus broad-spectrum adrenergic agents, or agents that increase the endogenous release of norepinephrine such as methylphenidate, may have opposing effects on working memory function at low vs. high doses.

Alpha-2-adrenergic receptors can be found either presynaptically on NE neurons, or postsynaptically on nonNE neurons. Norepinephrine neuronal cell bodies arise in the brain stem within the locus ceruleus (LC) and project throughout most of the central nervous system. Thus LC activity is capable of altering a wide array of CNS functions. It is noteworthy that the LC receives much of its "intelligent" input from the prefrontal cortex (PFC). Much of the classical research on A2 actions focused on the presynaptic effects of drugs like clonidine and their powerful ability to inhibit the firing of LC neurons and inhibit NE release from NE terminals. It is clinically relevant that guanfacine is 10 times weaker than clonidine in assays of presynaptic function, and this may explain in part why clonidine is more sedating than guanfacine (clonidine also likely has more potent effects on A2B receptors in thalamus which have powerful effects on arousal). However,

the majority of A2A receptors in the brain are actually localized postsynaptic to NE neurons, and these are of particular relevance to working memory. Alpha-2-adrenergic agonists enhance working memory through actions at postsynaptic A2A receptors on PFC neurons (Arnsten & Li, 2005). Alpha-2-adrenergic receptors are localized on the dendritic spines of PFC neurons, as well as at sites removed from traditional synapses. These receptors are especially dense in the superficial layers of PFC that contain the cortical-cortical networks essential for working memory. Alpha-2-adrenergic receptors are co-localized with HCN channels (hyperpolarization-activated cyclic nucleotide-gated cation channels) on the dendritic spines of PFC neurons. When HCN channels are opened by cAMP, they make the membrane "leaky," and weaken the efficacy of inputs onto the dendritic spines. As these are the synapses where PFC networks interconnect, opening of HCN channels reduces network connectivity and impairs working memory. Recent research shows that A2A agonists like guanfacine improve working memory by inhibiting the production of cAMP (Ramos *et al.*, 2006), closing HCN channels and strengthening PFC network connectivity. Thus guanfacine improves working memory at the cellular and behavioral levels (Wang *et al.*, 2007). Low doses of methylphenidate increase endogenous NE release, and to a lesser degree, DA release in the PFC (Berridge *et al.*, 2006), and improve working memory through enhanced endogenous stimulation of A2 and D1 receptors (Arnsten & Li, 2005). Thus, stimulant medications likely have their therapeutic effects through these mechanisms.

In contrast to the beneficial effects of A2A receptor stimulation, high levels of NE released in the PFC during stress exposure engage lower affinity A1 receptors which impair PFC function. Stimulation of A1 receptors in PFC suppresses delay-related cell firing and impairs working memory through activation of phosphotidyl inositol intracellular signaling pathways, which release calcium from internal stores (Birnbaum *et al.*, 2004). Norepinephrine may also engage low affinity beta1 receptors, increasing cAMP and impairing working memory (Ramos *et al.*, 2005). These detrimental actions are likely exacerbated with chronic stress or after brain injury. Evidence suggests that NE axons in the PFC increase their synthesis of NE in response to chronic stress (Miner *et al.*, 2006). Of particular relevance to the current topic, it has recently been found that there is a hypercatecholaminergic state in the PFC in response to brain injury (Kobori & Dash, 2006). Under these conditions, A2A agonists such as guanfacine may be helpful via both presynaptic and postsynaptic drug actions, reducing excessive catecholamine release, and strengthening the functional connectivity of surviving networks, respectively.

Overview of pharmacological interventions

- The therapeutic approach depends on whether the cognitive deficits occur in the context of a neurological disorder that is progressive, reversible or static.

It is important to note that the pharmacologic treatment of cognitive deficits is directed at three broad clinical groups. The first group includes individuals with progressive neurological disorders (e.g., some individuals with multiple sclerosis, Alzheimer's disease and other neurodegenerative dementias). The second group includes individuals with delirium or dementing disorders that are reversible with appropriate treatment (e.g., dementia secondary to depression). The third group consists of individuals with relatively static brain insults that effect cognitive function (e.g., individuals with traumatic brain injury or stroke). The prognosis and goals of treatment vary across groups. There are currently few if any disease-altering treatments for progressive neurodegenerative disorders. In other potentially progressive disorders such as multiple sclerosis, there are some disease altering treatments but none that unequivocally halt disease progression. Thus, in these patients the treatment goal is to delay progression of the symptoms of the illness, and to prolong cognitive quality of life. In the second group, those with delirium or "reversible" dementia

syndromes, prognosis is generally excellent providing the proper diagnosis is made and appropriate treatment provided. Thus, here the treatment goal is actually a "cure." In the group with static brain insults affecting cognitive function (traumatic brain injury, "chemo brain," stroke), or those with a fluctuating course of illness (e.g., relapsing and remitting multiple sclerosis) the prognosis is variable and the goal is improved quality of life and elimination or mitigation of cognitive deficits as a primary source of excess disability.

Categories of intervention

- Pharmacologic and other interventions can be used to prevent injury, to minimize the extent of injury, to enhance recovery from injury or to augment residual function.

There are four contexts in which pharmacological interventions (and other strategies) are used; primary prevention, secondary prevention, enhancement of recovery and augmentation of residual cognitive skills. The goals of treatment, the treatment strategies and the time course of intervention vary as a function of these contexts, as outlined below.

Primary prevention

If injury or illness can be prevented, then the need for rehabilitation is obviated. Two of the four leading causes of neurological injury/disorder, stroke and TBI, can be prevented or at least the risk greatly reduced (see Elkind, 2005; Elovic & Zafonte, 2005; Goldstein & Hanley, 2006). For example, lowering of systolic blood pressure with antihypertensives, reduction of serum lipids with statins, and use of aspirin and anticoagulants in certain populations, significantly reduce the risk of stroke (Elkind, 2005; Goldstein & Hanley, 2006; Sanossian & Oybiagele, 2006). Use of seat belts and related motor vehicle safety devices, fall and violence prevention efforts, and use of appropriate protective gear during at-risk recreational activities have measurable effects on brain injury rates (Elovic & Zafonte, 2005). The link between substance abuse and brain injury is clear (see Miller & Adams, 2005) and pharmacologic treatments that reduce risk of relapse in individuals with substance abuse are reasonably viewed as primary preventive measures with respect to TBI.

Secondary prevention

- There are several well-described injury mechanisms that evolve over time following an initial insult.
- Based on the pathophysiology of these mechanisms, numerous attempts have been made to alter or reduce the extent of this "secondary injury."
- Most of these trials are effective in small animal models of neurotrauma, but have shown disappointing results in human studies.

Functional cognitive impairment from neurological illness/injury results from damage that occurs through a variety of mechanisms over a variable period of time. For example damage from TBI is often categorized into *primary* injury and *secondary* injury. The former occurs as a result of the contact and acceleration/deceleration forces acting on the brain at the time of the injury event and includes focal injuries such as contusions and diffuse injuries such as diffuse axonal injury (DAI). Secondary injury results from events that follow from these initial forces and includes the effects of cerebral edema, increased intracranial pressure, ischemia, hypo- or hypertension, and the triggering of excitotoxic injury cascades, active cell death pathways (apoptosis), and disruption of cellular energy regulation. These secondary injury mechanisms evolve over variable periods of time ranging from minutes to weeks following the traumatic event, thus providing an opportunity for pharmacologic intervention to minimize the long-term effects of the primary injury (see Gennarelli & Graham, 2005; Povlishock & Katz, 2005; Shimizu et al., 2005).

These same excitotoxic, inflammatory, immune, necrosis and apoptosis cascades play important roles in the evolution of neural damage from other disorders such as cerebrovascular disease, MS and

neurodegenerative disorders (for example, see Smith, 2004 for discussion of pathophysiology of ischemia). Delineation of these mechanisms has resulted in the development of pharmacologic strategies to minimize the extent of damage from the primary underlying process (e.g., initial neurotrauma or stroke). Much of this work, both experimental and clinical, has been in stroke and TBI, and is geared towards developing effective neuroprotective strategies. Reviews of neuroprotective trials in both stroke (Gladstone et al., 2002; Wahlgren & Ahmed, 2004) and TBI (Narayan et al., 2002; Shimizu et al., 2005; Tobias & Bullock, 2004) have been recently published and the reader is referred to these papers for further details. However, it is worth briefly outlining the rationale and principles underlying these approaches. Although the sequence and timing of these overlapping processes differ across disorder/injury conditions, the results are quite similar and have led to similar neuroprotective or secondary prevention efforts in human studies.

Excitatory amino acid (EAA) neurotoxicity

Both TBI and ischemia prompt the release of large amounts of the EAA neurotransmitters glutamate and aspartate, resulting in stimulation of EAA receptors including ionotropic (kainate [KA] and alpha-amino-3hydroxy-5-methyl-4-isoxazole propionate [AMPA]) receptors found in glia and neurons, and N-methyl-D-aspartate (NMDA) receptors found primarily in neurons. Stimulation of the AMPA and KA receptors is associated with an influx of Na^+ and K^+ into the cell. This in turn causes sufficient membrane depolarization to overcome a voltage-dependent Mg^{2+} blockade of the NMDA receptor ionophore. Removal of the Mg^{2+} blockade facilitates a large influx of Ca^{2+} into the neuron with a variety of subsequent downstream effects (see below). There are several factors which point to the important role that dysregulation of EAA transmission may play in cognitive dysfunction in brain disorders/injury. In animal models of TBI, the extent of cognitive deficits correlates with the degree of reduced NMDA receptor binding in the hippocampus

(Miller *et al.*, 1990). Of interest is that EAA receptors are not uniformly distributed throughout the brain. The apparent heightened vulnerability of the hippocampus to traumatic and ischemic injury may result from the increased density of EAA receptors found in this structure (Monaghan & Cotman, 1986; Nakanishi, 1992). Thus strategies that target the release of EAAs, alter EAA receptor function (competitive and noncompetitive antagonists, alteration of glycine and polyamine sites) and restore Mg^{2+} (as a means of blocking Ca^{2+} influx) have been hypothesized to reduce neurotoxicity associated with excessive EAA neurotransmission.

Effects of increased intracellular Ca^{2+}

A direct result of excessive EAA activity is the influx of Ca^{2+} into the cell. Excess intracellular Ca^{2+} in turn triggers at least four pivotal events that can lead to cell damage and death (Smith, 2004). The first is activation of two families of proteases involved in cell death – caspases and calpains. Both play important roles in mediating excitotoxic and inflammatory cell damage. Caspases are cysteine-dependent proteases that play a role in apoptotic cell death (see below), often related to fragmentation of cellular DNA or interference with repair of DNA (DeKosky *et al.*, 1998; Friedlander, 2003). The calpains are also cysteine-dependent proteases that can degrade elements of the cytoskeleton such as microfilaments and microtubules (DeKosky *et al.*, 1998), structural elements critical to ongoing cell function.

The second Ca^{2+} initiated event is the activation of several phospholipase enzymes that alter critical elements of the cell membrane, resulting in further influx of extracellular cations. Third, Ca^{2+} increases nitric oxide synthase activity with resultant production of harmful free radical species. Fourth, mitochondrial attempts to sequester the excess Ca^{2+} can result in damage to mitochondrial membrane function, swelling, and release of a variety of agents that in turn trigger the initial stages of the apoptosis pathway.

Apoptosis and necrosis

The above-described EAA activity and related increases in intracellular Ca^{2+} initiate two broad pathways to cell death: necrosis and apoptosis. These processes differ with respect to time course (acute vs. longer-term), modulators of activity, primary enzymes involved (proteases), and energy dependency (necrosis is passive, does not require energy input, while apoptosis is active, and requires energy). However, the cascades overlap at several points and cells can die from a combination of these processes (see Artal-Sanz & Tavernarakis, 2005, for recent review). Factors that seem to determine the predominant pathway of cell death include cellular energy access, severity of insult and time course of exposure to the toxic event.

Secondary prevention or neuroprotection trials

Based on an understanding of the cell death mechanisms described above, there have been efforts to reduce extent of injury/disease and thus improve outcomes (Gladstone *et al.*, 2002; Narayan *et al.*, 2002; Shimizu *et al.*, 2005; Tobias & Bullock, 2004; Wahlgren & Ahmed, 2004).

Modulation of EAA effects

Since many of the cascades start with the effects of excessive EAA release, a variety of strategies have been developed to mitigate these effects. These include competitive and noncompetitive NMDA and AMPA receptor blockers, as well as modulators of NMDA receptor function through manipulation of the Mg^{2+} gated channel, the polyamine site and the glycine site. One of the most consistent findings is that in animal studies, whether it be in models of ischemia or trauma, most interventions that effectively dampen EAA activity at the level of the receptors reduce histopathological indicators of injury extent, and often reduce functional deficits (assessed in terms of motor function or performance on cognitive tasks such as the Morris water maze in rodents). Unfortunately, these results have not been as impressive in human trials, and at this time there is no established agent for the treatment EAA activity in the context of acute stroke or TBI. Several reasons may account for the failure of the animal work to generalize to humans and they have been nicely outlined in both the stroke (Wahlgren & Ahmed, 2004) and TBI contexts (Narayan *et al.*, 2002).

Modulation of Ca^{2+} effects

As noted, the influx of Ca^{2+} into the cell plays a critical role in initiating a variety of harmful effects. In an experimental model of brain trauma, Hovda and colleagues (Hovda *et al.*, 1991) observed a regional increase in calcium for at least 48 hours following injury, suggesting that a significant window exists for therapeutic intervention. In a similar model of brain trauma, Okiyama *et al.* (1992) demonstrated that (S)-emopamil, a phenylalkylamine calcium channel/5-HT2 antagonist reduced regional cerebral edema formation, dramatically improved neurologic motor outcome, and attenuated cognitive dysfunction. Although the effects of Ca^{2+} channel blockers were effective in animal models of injury they have proved disappointing in human trials. A trial of (S)-emopamil in humans found no benefit (Gentile *et al.*, 1993), and the calcium channel antagonist nimodipine showed no beneficial effects in individuals with TBI (Teasdale, 1991). A similar story has emerged in stroke (Wahlgren & Ahmed, 2004). A review of some 27 trials involving over 7000 patients with stroke suggested no strong evidence for the use of Ca^{2+} antagonists in the management of acute stroke (Horn & Limburg, 2000).

Modulation of free radical/reactive oxygen species

One of the major pathways of the injury cascades is the production of free radical species that participate in the peroxidation of critical structural cellular elements and metabolic processes. Polyunsaturated fatty acids contained in cell membranes are particularly vulnerable to attack (Gutteridge & Halliwell, 1990). Endogenous defense mechanisms have been identified that use antioxidants or free radical scavengers to neutralize free radical-generated lipid peroxidation. Following injury to the central nervous system, the concentration of these endogenous antioxidants has been shown to be severely depleted, suggesting that this endogenous defense mechanism may become overwhelmed, permitting uncontrolled progression of peroxidative damage to cellular membranes (Hall *et al.*, 1989). Based on these observations investigators began to explore the use of nonglucocorticoid steroid analogues of methylprednisolone, referred to as 21-aminosteroids or lazeroids, particularly Tirilazad or Freedox. Hall *et al.* (1988) and Sanada *et al.* (1993) showed improved motor strength in rodent models of TBI. McIntosh *et al.* (1992) also showed reduced cerebral edema and mortality. Unfortunately, large-scale trials in humans failed to show significant efficacy (Shimizu *et al.*, 2005). A variety of other approaches designed to minimize the effects of free radical damage including iron chelators, antioxidants (e.g., SOD), and anti-inflammatory agents (COX and COX-2 inhibitors) have been tried with similar disappointing results (Shimizu *et al.*, 2005). A similar picture emerges in the treatment of stroke, with encouraging preclinical studies but very little consistent efficacy demonstrated in human studies (Wahlgren & Ahmed, 2004).

Modulators of protease activity

The role that caspases and calpains play in the necrotic and apoptotic cell death pathways has led to the suggestion that protease inhibitors may be neuroprotective following brain injury. Cerebrolysin, that appears to inhibit both caspase and calpain activity, has been shown to improve memory and motor outcome following TBI in rats (Saatman *et al.*, 1996), and reduce indicators of infarct size in experimental stroke models. In one relatively small human trial, it was associated with improved motor function (Ladurner *et al.*, 2005). Other experimental approaches under development include modulation of pro- and anti-apoptotic gene expression, and approaches to interfere with the various steps involved in activating and modulating various members of the caspase and calpain family of enzymes. These approaches are promising theoretically but not available for human trials at this time (Shimizu *et al.*, 2005; Wahlgren & Ahmed, 2004).

Enhancement of repair and recovery

- Once the injury or disease process is fully evolved and established, and perhaps even before this is the case, strategies to encourage repair of neural function can be important and will become more so in the future.
- The general strategies available include promotion of new neurons (neurogenesis), promotion of new synaptic connections (plasticity), transplantation of neural tissue or stem cells into damaged areas, and modulation of central tone of certain neurotransmitters.
- These strategies are not fully developed but are likely to become more critical in the near future.

The first two categories of pharmacologic intervention for cognitive impairment have focused on the prevention of neural damage either before it occurs (primary prevention, e.g., stroke prophylaxis in high-risk patients) or limitation of evolving damage following an initial insult (secondary prevention). The third category of intervention targets the speed and extent of neurological recovery. Repair, regeneration and plasticity of the central nervous system can, to a certain extent, reverse the functional effects of neural injury. There are several component processes worth considering; neurogenesis, adaptive synaptic organization, cell replacement strategies and modulation of central neurotransmitter tone.

Neurogenesis

It has only been accepted in the last 15 years that neurogenesis occurs in the adult human brain (see Kempermann *et al.*, 2002; Schaffer & Gage, 2004 for reviews). The hippocampus, particularly the dentate gyrus, is the primary site of neurogenesis.

Furthermore, a variety of mediators of this process have been identified (see Kempermann *et al.*, 2002 for review). Fibroblast growth factor-2 (FGF-2), epidermal growth factor (EGF), sonic hedgehog (Shh), central serotonergic tone, environmental enrichment and exercise, all appear to play roles in facilitating neurogenesis by promoting progenitor cell proliferation in the hippocampus. A variety of mediators influence the differentiation of the progenitors into neurons or glial cells. These mediators include bone morphogenetic proteins (BMPs), noggin, and brain-derived neurotrophic factor (BDNF) among others (Schaffer & Gage, 2004). A variety of factors counteract these effects including NMDA agonists, stress (probably through glucocorticoid receptors), and environmental factors (Schaffer & Gage, 2004). Manipulation of the mediators of neurogenesis is an important and exciting line of investigation; however, as yet there are no agents available for human trials.

Synaptic organization and adaptation (neurotrophins)

In addition to growth of new neurons, both new and surviving neurons are capable of synaptic reorganization. Plasticity is essentially the alteration of neuronal structure and function in response to changes in activity pattern and density. The two primary indicators of activity-dependent change are long-term potentiation and dendritic spine density. Critical to the success of this process are a family of neurotrophic factors known as the neurotrophins (see Chao, 2003; Lang *et al.*, 2004; Lim *et al.*, 2003 for reviews). There are four broad families of neurotrophins: (1) the nerve growth factor family; (2) the glial derived factor family; (3) the neurokine family; and (4) the non-neuronal growth factor family (Lang *et al.*, 2004). Each of these families include several compounds which in theory could be relevant to recovery from neurotrauma. The best, albeit limited, evidence suggests roles for the nerve growth factor family and the glial derived factor family in the response to neurotrauma (Hicks *et al.*, 1997; Oyesiku *et al.*, 1999; Ray *et al.*, 2002). Within the nerve growth factor family (sometimes called super-family) there are four major neurotrophins: nerve growth factor (NGF); brain-derived neurotrophic factor (BDNF); neurotrophin 3 (NT3); and neuro-trophin 4 (NT4). There is some evidence that NGF and BDNF influence the response and recovery of the CNS to trauma. For example, expression of NGF has been shown to be increased shortly after TBI in a rodent model (DeKosky *et al.*, 1994). Intraparenchy-mal administration of NGF has reduced hippocam-pal cell loss and improved cognitive outcomes in similar models (Dixon *et al.*, 1997). Furthermore, neural progenitor cells transfected to produce NGF and transplanted into peri-injury sites have reduced hippocampal CA3 cell loss and improved both motor and cognitive function (Philips *et al.*, 2001). Brain-derived neurotrophic factor mRNA is also elevated in hippocampus within one hour of trauma and remains elevated for several days (Hicks *et al.*, 1997, 1998).

Another neurotrophin family of interest is the glial cell line-derived neurotrophic factors or GDNF. These neurotrophins are known to play a role in the protection, maintenance and signaling of dop-aminergic neurons (particularly in the midbrain) (Granholm *et al.*, 2000; Sariola & Saarma, 2003), and have been the focus of some efforts in the develop-ment of novel treatments for Parkinson's disease. There is some evidence to suggest elevation of GDNF levels after TBI in a rodent model (Shimizu *et al.*, 2002, 2005). Furthermore, GDNF has been shown to reduce hippocampal cell loss when infused shortly after injury (Kim *et al.*, 2001) and to reduce lesion volume (Hermann *et al.*, 2001).

Other peptide growth factors including basic fibro-blast growth factor and insulin-like growth factor may also play important roles in the response to neuro-trauma and are undergoing evaluation as potential interventions after injury (McDermott *et al.*, 1997; Wahlgren & Ahmed, 2004; Shimizu *et al.*, 2005).

Transplantation strategies

In addition to strategies that enhance neurogenesis and neural plasticity, cell replacement strategies are being explored. Much of the initial work was done in the context of exploring treatment strategies for dis-orders with relatively well described and localized neuropathology such as Parkinson's and Hunting-ton's diseases. More recently these approaches have been considered for stroke and TBI (Royo *et al.*, 2003). A variety of cell types have been used in animal models including fetal stem cells, terminally differentiated postmitotic neurons derived from human embryonal teratocarcinoma cell lines, and multipotential immortalized stem and progenitor cell lines (see Royo *et al.*, 2003). A variety of techni-cal and ethical challenges remain before these tech-niques will be effective in human disorders. Factors such as the source of the transplanted tissue, the timing of the transplantation, the immune status of the host and the use of various neurotrophins in conjunction with transplantation strategies need to be further clarified. However, progress is being made on these fronts and it is likely that these strat-egies will become part of the therapeutic armamen-tarium in the future.

Modulation of central neurotransmitter tone

Several lines of evidence suggest that the extent and rate of repair of neural injury of various etiologies can be affected by manipulation of the neurochem-ical milieu. Much of this evidence comes from the TBI literature and is briefly summarized below.

Role of central catecholaminergic tone in injury and recovery

There is evidence of dysfunction of catecholaminer-gic systems associated with TBI (see McIntosh, 1994; McIntosh *et al.*, 1998 for review) and other CNS disorders. For example, animal studies suggest that alterations and elevations in dopamine (DA), NE, and epinephrine can be prolonged after TBI, may be associated with alterations in catecholami-nergic receptors in damaged cortical areas, and can impair catecholaminergic function after trauma (Goldstein, 2003; McIntosh, 1994; Prasad *et al.*, 1993). Aquilani *et al.* (2003) found reduced levels of plasma tyrosine (an amino acid precursor for catecholamine synthesis) in TBI patients at both time of admission to acute rehabilitation units (44 days after injury) and at time of discharge (110 days after injury). Similar findings were reported for a group of individuals with ischemic stroke (Aquilani *et al.*, 2004).

Augmentation of catecholaminergic tone may enhance recovery from neural injury. In certain animal models of brain injury, administration of amphetamine (which enhances both DA and NE systems) can facilitate recovery of some functions (Feeney *et al.*, 1981; Feeney & Hovda, 1983; Feeney & Sutton, 1987). Subsequent work has suggested that a single dose of NE can enhance recovery of motor function in rats (Boyeson & Feeney, 1984). Single doses of amphetamine were also effective in a weight-drop model of TBI in rats, but interestingly only after milder injuries (Feeney *et al.*, 1981). Zhu *et al.* (2000) administered L-deprenyl, a selective and irreversible MAO-B inhibitor to rats subjected to combined fluid percussion TBI and entorhinal cortical lesions and found significantly reduced cognitive impairment (Morris water maze performance) compared with the rats treated with vehicle only. Amphetamine has also been shown to be effective in enhancing recovery in a fluid percussion model of brain injury in rats (Romhanyi *et al.*, 1990; Tandian *et al.*, 1990), and to improve recovery of motor function and stereoscopic vision in cats (Hovda *et al.*, 1984, 1989; Sutton *et al.*, 1989). Furthermore, catecholaminergic *antagonists* can slow rate of recovery from certain types of brain injury (Sutton & Feeney, 1992). Amphetamines also appear to enhance recovery from stroke (see Martinsson & Eksborg, 2004 for review), perhaps through enhancing sprouting and synaptogenesis in areas around the infarct and in the contralateral cortex (Stroemer *et al.*, 1998).

Catecholaminergic augmentation can improve recovery in humans as well. In individuals with TBI, methylphenidate, which augments both the dopaminergic and adrenergic systems, is effective in ameliorating certain cognitive deficits (Whyte *et al.*, 2002). Significant improvement in executive function tasks with another dopamine agonist,

bromocriptine, has also been shown (McDowell *et al.*, 1998). A variety of pilot studies suggest that amphetamines may improve recovery from a variety of deficits including aphasia (Walker-Batson *et al.*, 2001) and motor function (Martinsson & Wahlgren, 2003). However, the results are not consistent. A recent well-designed study found little additional benefit with amphetamine compared to physiotherapy alone in patients with severe motor deficits (Gladstone *et al.*, 2006) although there was some benefit in the group with more modest deficits. Drug effect has been most consistently found when paired with some form of learning or practice such as speech/language therapy or physiotherapy. Coupled with the observation that amphetamines and other catecholamine agonists facilitate long-term potentiation, these results suggest that one of the mechanisms through which catecholamines work is by facilitating practice and learning of compensatory strategies. Other mechanisms including facilitation of synaptogenesis and normalization of ischemia-induced hypometabolism have also been suggested (Martinsson & Eksborg, 2004).

Role of central cholinergic tone in injury and recovery

Cerebral cholinergic neurons and their ascending projections are vulnerable to trauma (Arciniegas, 2003). Acutely, cholinergic neurons release large amounts of acetylcholine, which is then followed by long-term reductions in cerebral acetylcholine levels (Dixon *et al.*, 1995). Sudden release of acetylcholine at the time of injury may contribute to the extent of injury through facilitation of the excitotoxic cascades described earlier. Conversely, cholinergic antagonists can be neuroprotective in models of TBI (see Arciniegas, 2003 for review). Several studies have shown damage to the nucleus basalis of Meynert, as well as reduced levels of choline acetyl transferase (a marker of cholinergic afferents) in brain regions vulnerable to trauma including temporal cortex, cingulate and posterior parietal regions in humans (Arciniegas, 2003; Dewar & Graham, 1996; Murdoch *et al.*, 1998, 2002). Postsynaptic muscarinic and nicotinic receptors remained intact (Dewar & Graham, 1996; Murdoch *et al.*, 1998, 2002), suggesting cholinergic agonists as a potential point of intervention for cognitive deficits (Arciniegas, 2003).

Role of central GABA tone in injury and repair

Central gamma-aminobutyric acid (GABA) is the primary inhibitory neurotransmitter in the CNS. Gamma-aminobutyric acid is found predominantly in interneurons modulating local circuitry, and GABA tone is important both in the acute response to neural injury and in recovery (see Schwartz-Bloom & Sah, 2001 for review). The effects of GABA dysregulation vary according to several factors including injury to assessment interval (i.e., acute effects vs. chronic effects), brain region and injury etiology. In most ischemia models, extracellular GABA accumulates acutely, related to Ca^{2+} dependent release from synaptic vesicles, reversal of GABA transporters (not Ca^{2+} dependent), and/or leakage from damaged neurons (Schwartz-Bloom & Sah, 2001). Depending on the brain region considered, the increased extracellular GABA confers either increased or decreased sensitivity to ischemic injury (Schwartz-Bloom & Sah, 2001). Over time the increase in GABA results in a complex set of interactions with the GABAa receptor that can reduce receptor function (downregulation), production and expression (Schwartz-Bloom & Sah, 2001). In addition, there are complex interactions between GABA and many of the intracellular events precipitated by the influx of Ca^{2+} into the cell. For example, Ca^{2+} induced production of arachidonic acid and reactive oxygen species can interfere with GABAa receptor binding and GABAa induced responses (Samochocki & Strosznaider, 1993; Schwartz-Bloom *et al.*, 1996; Schwartz-Bloom & Sah, 2001). A variety of GABA-ergic agents have shown promise as neuroprotective agents in both global and focal ischemia models in gerbils, rats and other species (see Gilby *et al.*, 2005; Schwartz-Bloom & Sah, 2001) The above suggests that there is a delicate choreography to the injury cascades and more work is needed to define the optimal injury-to-treatment windows, as well as interactions with injury profile.

This complexity is reflected in the clinical literature to date. Wahlgren *et al.* (1999) reported on the results of clomethiazole in acute stroke (CLASS study) which found no significant difference between placebo- and drug-treated groups on functional independence 3 months after stroke. However, in a subgroup of individuals with large anterior circulation strokes there was a significant increase in the number of those with functional independence in those treated with clomethiazole. Subsequent studies were unable to replicate this finding (Lyden *et al.*, 2001, 2002). Lodder *et al.* (2006) recently reported on the results of the early GABA-ergic activation study in stroke trial (EGASIS), a randomized placebo-controlled clinical trial of the GABA-ergic drug diazepam (a benzodiazepine) started within 12 hours of a stroke. Both functional independence and complete recovery, measured 3 months after stroke, occurred more frequently in the diazepam-treated group although the difference was not statistically significant. A planned subgroup analysis breaking out participants by stroke subtype did show a significant diazepam effect in the cardio-embolic group. This group is more likely to have greater degrees of re-perfusion of the affected territory, thus allowing for the diazepam to reach the injured area.

Role of central serotonin in injury and repair

Serotonergic neurons are richly represented in both hippocampal and cortical regions, and appear to play important roles in cognition. In addition, stimulation of one of the better-characterized serotonin receptors, the 5-HT1a receptor, can result in hyperpolarization of neuronal membranes and reduced release of glutamate. In theory, both of these actions could attenuate excitotoxicity. In fact, alterations in central serotonergic function appear to influence response to injury and repair. Mauler *et al.* (2001) demonstrated that a 5-HT1a receptor agonist, BAY x 3702 (repinotan), reduced potassium-induced glutamate release in vitro in rat hippocampal slices and this effect was blocked by a selective 5-HT1a receptor antagonist. Using microdialysis techniques, they showed up to a 50% reduction of cortical glutamate release following middle cerebral artery occlusion. Schaper *et al.* (2000) also showed reduction of hippocampal damage associated with repinotan following temporary ischemia in rats. Furthermore, there was evidence of reduced DNA degradation 4 days after the insult suggesting a potential neuroprotective effect on the apoptotic pathway. A similar role has been shown in animal models of both TBI and ischemia. Kline *et al.* (2002) showed reduced CA1 and CA3 cell loss and reduced cortical damage 4 weeks after controlled cortical impact (CCI) injury in rats using repinotan. This was associated with attenuation of injury-related deficits in a water maze task. This same group also used 8-hydroxy-2-(di-n-propylamino) tetralin (8-OH DPAT), another 5-HT1a receptor agonist in a controlled cortical impact model in rodents with similar results (Kline *et al.*, 2002). Mauler & Horvath (2005) replicated these neuroprotective effects in rat models of permanent middle cerebral artery occlusion, temporary middle cerebral artery occlusion and subdural hematoma. Based on these and related preclinical results, phase I and phase II clinical trials were conducted with repinotan in acute ischemic stroke. Teal *et al.* (2005) reported a trend for improved outcome in the repinotan group (treated within 6 hours of symptom onset) in a multi-center study of 240 patients, particularly in those with moderate to severe strokes. Ohman *et al.* (2001) reported on a randomized placebo controlled trial of 60 individuals with TBI using the Glasgow Outcome Scale as the primary outcome measure. There was a trend for better outcomes in the repinotan-treated group.

Role of opiate peptide modulation in injury and repair

Changes in endogenous opiate peptide modulation have also been implicated in the pathophysiology of secondary injury (Faden *et al.*, 1981; Flamm *et al.*, 1982; Young *et al.*, 1981). In experimental models of brain trauma in the cat and the rat, a nonselective opiate receptor blocker, naloxone, reversed posttraumatic hypotension and increased brain perfusion pressure (Hayes *et al.*, 1983; McIntosh *et al.*, 1991; Robinson *et al.*, 1987). In addition, kappa

receptor antagonists showed promise in animal models of neural injury from both ischemia and trauma (McIntosh *et al.*, 1987; Vink *et al.*, 1990; Wahlgren & Ahmed, 2004). Unfortunately, clinical trials of the kappa receptor antagonist nalmefene showed no benefit in a trial of stroke patients (Clark *et al.*, 2000). More work on this system is needed to clarify potential therapeutic avenues for future use.

Enhancement of cognitive function

- The approach to static deficits in cognitive function should take into account several general principles such as clearly defining the target symptoms, eliminating exacerbating factors and conditions, identifying the context in which the deficits are most apparent and modifying the environment accordingly.
- The pharmacological approach to prominent episodic memory and learning deficits usually starts with the use of pro-cholinergic agents.
- The approach to prominent deficits in arousal, attention and working memory usually starts with CNS stimulants and/or pro-catecholaminergic agents.
- The approach to executive deficits depends on the predominant profile of deficits and complaints.

The fourth category of intervention is the use of pharmacologic agents to enhance cognitive function impaired by neural injury/disease. It is helpful to consider certain principles when formulating pharmacological treatment interventions.

General principles

One must first determine whether the problem is subjective (cognitive complaints), objective (cognitive impairment), or both. This requires a careful history as well as collateral information from other reliable observers. The time course of the problem must be carefully outlined. Did the problem develop acutely or show a more insidious course? Has the decline shown a continuous or interrupted trajectory? This will help to inform whether one is dealing with a static or progressive problem, and in the case of the latter, give important clues as to the etiology.

It is necessary to define the spectrum of target behaviors. Do the problems fall primarily within the domain of memory, attention, executive functions, speech/language, or some combination of the above? This sheds light on the likely underlying etiology and will also help to inform initial treatment attempts. Obtaining this information will necessitate a careful history, "bedside" cognitive testing, and quite likely more systematic neurocognitive and neurodiagnostic assessment.

It is important to consider that individuals may have more than one cause of cognitive impairment. Serum laboratory assessments for common reversible causes of cognitive impairment (i.e., vitamin B12 and thyroid stimulating hormone) is recommended; when justified by the clinical history, other serum (e.g., HIV, RPR, ANA, liver function tests, electrolytes, complete blood count, etc.) and urine (e.g., urinalysis, urine toxicology) assessments may be appropriate. When epilepsy or delirium is suspected, electroencephalography (EEG) can be helpful. Baseline structural brain imaging is strongly recommended in the evaluation of all patients with cognitive impairment, and particularly among those in whom there is a change or decline in the level of cognitive function.

A variety of conditions can produce or exacerbate cognitive impairments. Among the most common are depression, anxiety, substance use disorders, sleep disorders, and physical discomfort or pain. Medications used to treat many medical, neurological, and psychiatric conditions are also common causes of cognitive impairment. A thorough assessment of these issues is imperative before prescribing medications for cognition. Optimizing treatment of comorbid conditions and reducing or eliminating medications with adverse effects on cognition are important steps.

Prior to initiating pharmacologic interventions, several strategies can be effective in minimizing the functional consequences of cognitive impairments and will improve the efficacy of medications used to improve cognition.

Time for performance

One of the core deficits associated with many neurological disorders is reduced speed of information processing. Absolute function or task-accuracy may be reasonably normal if the patient is afforded sufficient time to perform. Simple interventions such as waiting longer for verbal responses (i.e., teaching others not to respond or perform immediately for the individual) and allowing longer intervals to accomplish tasks, whether in the context of activities of daily living, educational endeavors, or in vocational settings, may permit the individual to maximize his or her "real-world" functional performance.

Environmental accommodation

Stimulating environments may tax the ability of persons to select and sustain attention appropriately, to process information at the speed demanded by the environment, and to develop flexible and adaptive responses to environmental demands. Such environments may produce cognitive failures and precipitate otherwise avoidable and unwanted affective and behavioral responses. Identifying environmental antecedents to cognitive failures and the affective/behavioral problems they produce may facilitate improvements in functional cognition, reduce disability and alleviate patient and caregiver distress.

Tailor demands to peak capacity

Individuals with cognitive impairment and neurological disorders often struggle with physical and cognitive fatigue. Performance on tasks otherwise within the functional abilities of such individuals may decline significantly as they fatigue. It is helpful to outline daily events and challenges and schedule them to coincide with periods when the individual is well rested and refreshed.

Approaches to specific cognitive syndromes

Attention

Although there are several Food and Drug Administration (FDA) approved treatments for attentional impairments among persons with attention deficit hyperactivity disorder (ADHD) (Biederman *et al.*,

2004; Jadad *et al.*, 1999), there are no FDA-approved treatments for impaired attention due to other neuropsychiatric or neurological conditions. The neurochemistry of attention as reviewed above, predicts that augmentation of cerebral catecholaminergic and cholinergic function may be useful. Several small-scale, randomized, double-blind, placebo-controlled studies of methylphenidate (Whyte *et al.*, 2002) and donepezil (Arciniegas & Silver, 2006) suggest that these agents are effective and safe for the treatment of impaired attention following traumatic brain injury. Donepezil may be similarly effective for the treatment of impaired attention due to multiple sclerosis (Greene *et al.*, 2000). There remains insufficient evidence on which to base the use of these agents for impaired attention in other conditions, but they are often used for this purpose nonetheless.

In clinical practice, we generally begin pharmacotherapy of attention and processing speed impairments with methylphenidate. Treatment with methylphenidate usually begins with doses of 5 mg twice daily and is gradually increased in increments of 5 mg twice daily until either beneficial effect or medication intolerance is achieved. Most studies suggest that optimal doses of methylphenidate are in the range of 20–40 mg twice daily (i.e., 0.15–0.3 mg/kg twice daily). This medication generally takes effect quickly (within 0.5–1 hour following administration), although this effect may wane after only a few hours. Therefore, the first issue in the administration of this agent is determining optimal dose and dosing frequency. Individuals requiring relatively high and frequent doses of methylphenidate may benefit from use of longer-acting preparations of this medication. Mild increases in heart rate or blood pressure may occur during treatment with methylphenidate, but are only rarely of sufficient magnitude to require treatment discontinuation. Serious adverse reactions to these medications are most often related to increases in central dopamine, and to a lesser extent central norepinephrine, activity; when these occur, they may include paranoia, dysphoria, anxiety, agitation and irritability. However, these adverse effects are in practice very uncommon at doses typically used to treat attention and speed of processing impairments.

When methylphenidate fails to improve attention, or does so incompletely, use of a cholinesterase inhibitor is recommended. Donepezil is prescribed most commonly when a cholinesterase inhibitor is used; treatment with this agent begins with 5 mg daily. If this dose is tolerated but does not produce improvements in attention after approximately 4 weeks of treatment, titration to 10 mg daily is generally undertaken. Slower dose titration may limit the development of treatment-emergent side effects, which are gastrointestinal in nature. Rivastigmine and galantamine, other cholinesterase inhibitors, have shorter half-lives, and require twice daily dosing. Rivastigmine is generally started at 1.5 mg BID and increased in 1.5 mg BID increments every 4 weeks until maximal benefits are attained or treatment intolerance develops. Galantamine is generally started at 4 mg BID and increased in 4 mg BID increments until maximal benefits are attained or treatment intolerance develops. An extended-release once-daily preparation of galantamine is also available; treatment with this agent is generally started at 8 mg daily and increased to 16 mg daily after 4 weeks. A further increase to 24 mg daily after 4 weeks at 16 mg daily may be considered if maximal benefits are not achieved at the lower dose.

Memory

There are no FDA-approved treatments for memory impairments. Although several agents (i.e., donepezil, rivastigmine, galantamine, memantine) are indicated for the treatment of dementia due to Alzheimer's disease, the FDA indications for the use of these agents does not extend to memory specifically. The neurochemistry of memory predicts that augmentation of cholinergic, stabilization of glutamatergic, and augmentation of catecholaminergic function may be useful targets for the treatment of memory impairments. Multiple case reports, open-label trials and small-scale, double-blind, placebo-controlled trials of cholinesterase inhibitors suggest that these agents may be safe and effective for the treatment of impairments in new learning and retrieval across many neurological conditions (Devi & Silver, 2000).

When working memory impairments are the focus of clinical concern, catecholaminergic augmentation may improve working memory impairments (Barch, 2004; McAllister *et al.*, 2004). Methylphenidate is the most commonly prescribed agent for this purpose; recommendations for the use of this agent are described in the section on the pharmacologic treatment of attention (see above).

We recommend donepezil as a first-line agent for the treatment of declarative memory impairment due to a neurological condition. This agent may also be useful for the treatment of working memory impairments (Barch & Carter, 2005). Use of donepezil and other cholinesterase inhibitors is described above.

In the absence of a robust response to cholinesterase inhibitors we generally attempt to augment these agents using memantine. Memantine is an uncompetitive NMDA receptor antagonist that may secondarily improve dopaminergic function in frontal-subcortical circuits. Treatment with memantine begins with 5 mg daily, and is increased by 5 mg daily at intervals of 1 week until a dose of 10 mg twice daily is reached or treatment-intolerance emerges. Memantine is generally well-tolerated, although confusion may develop during treatment initiation or dose titration. Temporary dose reduction may mitigate this adverse effect of treatment.

Executive functions
There are currently no FDA-approved treatments for executive dysfunction. The neurochemistry of executive functions predicts that augmentation of cerebral catecholaminergic and cholinergic function, as well as augmentation or stabilization of glutamatergic function, may be useful targets for the treatment of executive dysfunction. The current evidence regarding pharmacotherapy for executive dysfunction is comprised of case reports, case series, small-scale open-label studies, and a few double-blind placebo-controlled trials.

Based on these reports, we recommend methylphenidate for the treatment of executive function when accompanied by impairments in arousal, attention, and/or processing speed. When executive dysfunction is comorbid with impairments in memory (new learning and/or retrieval), we recommend cholinesterase inhibitors as our first-line pharmacologic intervention. Use of donepezil and related cholinesterase inhibitors is described above. Some patients will respond to stimulants alone, some to cholinesterase inhibitors alone, some to either or both classes of medication, and some to neither. In all cases, treatment of executive dysfunction remains a matter of empiric trial.

Summary

Each neurological disorder has its own neuropathological process but many of these processes share common features. Regardless of etiology, pathological processes that effect regions important in memory circuitry, attention and executive functions will typically be associated with complaints and measurable deficits in these domains. These commonalities allow for the delineation of guiding principles in the pharmacologic management of cognitive impairment.

Designing appropriate pharmacological interventions follows from an understanding of the neural circuitry and neurochemistry of memory, attention and executive functions, as well as an appreciation of the pathophysiology of the disease process responsible for the cognitive deficits.

Processes affecting the integrity of frontal cortex, mesial temporal structures, thalamus and basal ganglia, cerebellum and parietal cortex are commonly associated with subjective and objective problems in memory, attention and executive functions. The complex integrated circuitry of these cognitive domains makes them vulnerable to a large array of neuropathological processes. Our understanding of the neurochemistry of these cognitive domains is incomplete; however, it is clear that cholinergic, catecholaminergic and glutamatergic systems play critical roles in all of these domains with additional contributions from many other neurotransmitter systems. At this time pharmacologic interventions are often targeted towards altering central cholinergic and/or catecholaminergic tone.

There are four contexts in which pharmacologic interventions (and other strategies) are used; primary prevention, secondary prevention, enhancement of recovery and augmentation of residual cognitive skills. Most efforts have targeted the latter three categories. The goals of treatment, the treatment strategies and the time course of intervention vary as a function of these contexts. With respect to secondary prevention or neuroprotective efforts, there has been enormous progress made in defining the underlying pathophysiology of various disease pathways such as apoptosis, necrosis and excitotoxic injury cascades, and interventions based on these advances are demonstrably effective in animal models. Unfortunately to date, these successes have not generalized to human disorders. More success has been evident in the areas of enhancement of recovery and augmentation of residual skills. To date these efforts focus primarily on modulation of central cholinergic and catecholaminergic tone. Exciting progress in neurogenetics, neurogenesis, neural plasticity and cell transplantation strategies will likely play much bigger roles in the near future.

ACKNOWLEDGMENTS

Dr. McAllister's work was supported by NICHD grant # RO1 HD048176, NICHD grant # R01 HD047242-01, the Ira DeCamp Foundation, and New Hampshire Hospital.

Dr. Arnsten's work was supported by R37 AG06036 from NIA, P50 MH 068789 from NIMH, Shire Pharmaceuticals, and the Kavli Institute of Neuroscience at Yale University.

Dr. Arnsten and Yale University have license agreements with Shire Pharmaceuticals for the development of guanfacine for the treatment of attention deficit hyperactivity disorder, and with Marinus Pharmaceuticals for the development of chelerythrine for the treatment of bipolar disorder and schizophrenia.

REFERENCES

Andlin-Sobocki, P., Jonsson, B., Wittchen, H.-U., & Olesen, J. (2005). Cost of disorders of the brain in Europe. *European Journal of Neurology*, **12**, *Suppl. 1*, 1–27.

Aquilani, R., Iadarola, P., Boschi, F. *et al.* (2003). Reduced plasma levels of tyrosine, precursor of brain catecholamines, and of essential amino acids in patients with severe traumatic brain injury after rehabilitation. *Archives of Physical Medicine and Rehabilitation*, **84**, 1258–1265.

Aquilani, R., Verri, M., Iadarola, P. *et al.* (2004). Plasma precursors of brain catecholaminergic and serotonergic neurotransmitters in rehabilitation patients with ischemic stroke. *Archives of Physical Medicine and Rehabilitation*, **85**, 779–784.

Arciniegas, D. B. (2003). The cholinergic hypothesis of cognitive impairment caused by traumatic brain injury. *Current Psychiatry Reports*, **5**, 391–399.

Arciniegas, D. B., & Silver, J. M. (2006). Pharmacotherapy of posttraumatic cognitive impairments. *Behavioural Neurology*, **17**, 25–42.

Arciniegas, D., McAllister, T. W., & Kaufer, D. (2007). Cognitive impairment. In C. Coffey, T. W. McAllister, & J. Silver (Eds.), *Handbook of Neuropsychiatric Therapeutics* (pp. 24–78). Philadelphia: Williams & Wilkins.

Arnsten, A. F. T. (1998). Catecholamine modulation of prefrontal cortical cognitive function. *Trends in Cognitive Sciences*, **2**, 436–447.

Arnsten, A. F., & Goldman-Rakic, P. S. (1985). Alpha 2-adrenergic mechanisms in prefrontal cortex associated with cognitive decline in aged nonhuman primates. *Science*, **230**, 1273–1276.

Arnsten, A. F. T., & Li, B.-M. (2005). Neurobiology of executive functions: catecholamine influences on prefrontal cortical functions. *Biological Psychiatry*, **57**, 1377–1384.

Arnsten, A. F., Cai, J. X., & Goldman-Rakic, P. S. (1988). The alpha-2 adrenergic agonist guanfacine improves memory in aged monkeys without sedative or hypotensive side effects: evidence for alpha-2 receptor subtypes. *Journal of Neuroscience*, **8**, 4287–4298.

Arnsten, A. F. T., Cai, J. X., Murphy, B. L., & Goldman-Rakic, P. S. (1994). Dopamine D1 receptor mechanisms in the cognitive performance of young adult and aged monkeys. *Psychopharmacology*, **116**, 143–151.

Artal-Sanz, M., & Tavernarakis, N. (2005). Proteolytic mechanisms in necrotic cell death and neurodegeneration. *FEBS Letters*, **579**, 3287–3296.

Barch, D. M. (2004). Pharmacological manipulation of human working memory. *Psychopharmacology*, **174**, 126–135.

Barch, D. M., & Carter, C. S. (2005). Amphetamine improves cognitive function in medicated individuals with schizophrenia and in healthy volunteers. *Schizophrenia Research*, **77**, 43–58.

Ben-Yishay, Y., & Diller, L. (1993). Cognitive remediation in traumatic brain injury: update and issues. *Archives of Physical Medicine and Rehabilitation*, **74**, 204–213.

Berridge, C. W., Devilbiss, D. M., Andrzejewski, M. E. *et al.* (2006). Methylphenidate preferentially increases catecholamine neurotransmission within the prefrontal cortex at low doses that enhance cognitive function. *Biological Psychiatry*, **60**, 1111–1120.

Biederman, J., Monuteaux, M. C., Doyle, A. E. *et al.* (2004). Impact of executive function deficits and attention-deficit/hyperactivity disorder (ADHD) on academic outcomes in children. *Journal of Consulting and Clinical Psychology*, **72**, 757–766.

Birnbaum, S., Gobeske, K. T., Auerbach, J., Taylor, J. R., & Arnsten, A. F. (1999). A role for norepinephrine in stress-induced cognitive deficits: alpha-1-adrenoceptor mediation in the prefrontal cortex. *Biological Psychiatry*, **46**, 1266–1274.

Birnbaum, S., Yuan, P. X., Wang, M. *et al.* (2004). Protein kinase C overactivity impairs prefrontal cortical regulation of working memory. *Science*, **306**, 882–884.

Boyeson, M. G., & Feeney, D. M. (1984). The role of norepinephrine in recovery from brain injury. *Society of Neuroscience Abstracts*, **10**, 68.

Budson, A. E., & Price, B. H. (2005). Memory dysfunction. *New England Journal of Medicine*, **352**, 692–699.

Cai, J. X., & Arnsten, A. F. (1997). Dose-dependent effects of the dopamine D1 receptor agonists A77636 or SKF81297 on spatial working memory in aged monkeys. *Journal of Pharmacology and Experimental Therapeutics*, **283**, 183–189.

Carlson, S., Tanila, H., Rama, P., Mecke, E., & Pertovaara, A. (1992). Effects of medetomidine, an alpha-2 adrenoceptor agonist, and atipamezole, an alpha-2 antagonist, on spatial memory performance in adult and aged rats. *Behavioral and Neural Biology*, **58**, 113–119.

Chao, M. V. (2003). Neurotrophins and their receptors: a convergence point for many signalling pathways. *Nature Reviews Neuroscience*, **4**, 299–309.

Cicerone, K. D. (2002). Remediation of "working attention" in mild traumatic brain injury. *Brain Injury*, **16**, 185–195.

Clark, W., Raps, E. C., Tong, D. C., & Kelly, R. E. (2000). Cervene (Nalmefene) in acute ischemic stroke: final results of a phase III efficacy study. *Stroke*, **31**, 1234–1239.

DeKosky, S., Goss, J., Miller, P. *et al.* (1994). Upregulation of nerve growth factor following cortical trauma. *Experimental Neurology*, **130**, 173–177.

DeKosky, S. T., Kochanek, P. M., Clark, R. S. B., Ciallella, J. R., & Dixon, C. E. (1998). Secondary injury after head trauma: subacute and long-term mechanisms. *Seminars in Clinical Neuropsychiatry*, **3**, 176–185.

Devi, G., & Silver, J. (2000). Approaches to memory loss in neuropsychiatric disorders. *Seminars in Clinical Neuropsychiatry*, **5**, 259–265.

Dewar, D., & Graham, D. I. (1996). Depletion of choline acetyltransferase but preservation of M1 and M2 muscarinic receptor binding sites temporal cortex following head injury: a preliminary human postmorten study. *Journal of Neurotrauma*, **13**, 181–187.

Dixon, C. E., Liu, S. J., Jenkins, L. W. *et al.* (1995). Time course of increased vulnerability of cholinergic neurotransmission following traumatic brain injury in the rat. *Behavioural Brain Research*, **70**, 125–131.

Dixon, C. E., Flinn, P., Bao, J., Venya, R., & Hayes, R. L. (1997). Nerve growth factor attenuates cholinergic deficits following traumatic brain injury in rats. *Experimental Neurology*, **146**, 479–490.

Elkind, M. S. V. (2005). Implications of stroke prevention trials: treatment of global risk. *Neurology India*, **65**, 17–21.

Elliot, R., Sahakian, B. J., Matthews, K. *et al.* (1997). Effects of methylphenidate on spatial working memory and planning in healthy young adults. *Psychopharmacology*, **131**, 196–206.

Elovic, E., & Zafonte, R. (2005). Prevention. In J. Silver, T. W. McAllister, & S. Yudofsky (Eds.), *Textbook of Traumatic Brain Injury* (pp. 727–748). Washington, DC: American Psychiatric Publishing, Inc.

Faden, A. I., Jacobs, T., & Holaday, J. (1981). Opiate antagonist improves neurologic recovery after spinal injury. *Science*, **211**, 493–494.

Fan, J. B., Zhang, C. S., Gu, N. F. *et al.* (2005). Catechol-O-methyltransferase gene Val/Met functional polymorphism and risk of schizophrenia: a large-scale association study plus meta-analysis. *Biological Psychiatry*, **57**, 139–144.

Feeney, D. M., & Hovda, D. A. (1983). Amphetamine and apomorphine restore tactile placing after motor cortex injury in the cat. *Psychopharmacology*, **79**, 67–71.

Feeney, D. M., & Sutton, R. L. (1987). Pharmacotherapy for recovery of function after brain injury. *Critical Review of Neurobiology*, **1987**, 135–197.

Feeney, D. M., Boyeson, M. G., Linn, R. T., Murray, H. M., & Dail, W. G. (1981). Responses to cortical injury. 1. Methodology and local effects of contusions in the rat. *Brain Research*, **211**, 67–77.

Flamm, E. S., Young, W., Demopoulos, H., Descrescito, V., & Tamasula, J. (1982). Experimental spinal cord injury: treatment with naloxone. *Neurosurgery*, **10**, 227–231.

Franowicz, J. S., & Arnsten, A. F. (1998). The alpha-2a noradrenergic agonist, guanfacine, improves delayed response performance in young adult rhesus monkeys. *Psychopharmacology*, **136**, 8–14.

Friedlander, R. M. (2003). Apoptosis and caspases in neurodegenerative diseases. *New England Journal of Medicine*, **348**, 1365–1375.

Gennarelli, T., & Graham, D. (2005). Neuropathology. In J. Silver, T. W. McAllister, & S. Yudofsky (Eds.), *Textbook of Traumatic Brain Injury* (pp. 27–50). Washington, DC: American Psychiatric Press, Inc.

Gentile, N., Smith, D., Burhans, C., & McIntosh, T. (1993). Cognitive and neurologic functions and hippocampal neuronal loss after nimodipine in fluid percussion brain injury. *Journal of Neurotrauma*, **10**, S193.

Gilby, K. L., Sydserff, S. G., & Robertson, H. A. (2005). Differential neuroprotective effects for three GABA-potentiating compounds in a model of hypoxia-ischemia. *Brain Research*, **1035**, 196–205.

Gladstone, D., Black, S., & Hakim, A. (2002). Toward wisdom from failure: lessons from neuroprotective stroke trials and new therapeutic directions. *Stroke*, **33**, 2123–2136.

Gladstone, D. J., Danells, C. J., Armesto, A. *et al.* (2006). Physiotherapy coupled with dextroamphetamine for rehabilitation after hemiparetic stroke: a randomized, double-blind, placebo-controlled trial. *Stroke*, **37**, 179–185.

Goldstein, L. B. (2003). Neuropharmacology of TBI-induced plasticity. *Brain Injury*, **17**, 685–694.

Goldstein, L., & Hanley, G. (2006). Advances in primary stroke prevention. *Stroke*, **37**, 317–319.

Granholm, A. C., Reyland, M., Albeck, D. *et al.* (2000). Glial cell line-derived neurotrophic factor is essential for postnatal survival of midbrain dopamine neurons. *Journal of Neuroscience*, **20**, 3182–3190.

Greene, Y. M., Tariot, P. N., Wishart, H. *et al.* (2000). 12 week open trial of donepezil HCL in multiple sclerosis patients with associated cognitive impairment. *Journal of Clinical Psychopharmacology*, **20**, 350–356.

Gutteridge, J., & Halliwell, B. (1990). The measurement and mechanism of lipid peroxidation in biological systems. *Trends in Biochemical Sciences*, **15**, 129–135.

Hall, E., Yonkers, P., McCall, J., & Braughler, J. (1988). Effects of the 21-aminosteroid U74006F on experimental head injury in mice. *Journal of Neurosurgery*, **68**, 456–461.

Hall, E., Yonkers, P., Horan, K., & Braughler, J. (1989). Correlation between attenuation of post-traumatic spinal cord ischemia and preservation of tissue vitamin E by the 21-aminosteroid U74006F. Evidence for an in vivo antioxidant mechanism. *Journal of Neurotrauma*, **6**, 169–176.

Hayes, R., Galinet, B., Kulkarne, P., & Becker, D. (1983). Effects of naloxone on systemic and cerebral responses to experimental concussive brain injury in cats. *Journal of Neurosurgery*, **58**, 720–728.

Hermann, D., Kilic, E., Kugler, S., Isenmann, S., & Bahr, M. (2001). Adenovirus-mediated glial cell line-derived neurotrophic factor (GDNF) expression protects against subsequent cortical cold injury in rats. *Neurobiology of Disease*, **8**, 964–973.

Hicks, R. R., Numan, S., Dhillon, H. S., Prasad, M. R., & Seroogy, K. B. (1997). Alterations in BDNF and NT-3 mRNAs in rat hippocampus after experimental brain trauma. *Molecular Brain Research*, **48**, 401–406.

Hicks, R. R., Zhang, L., Dhillon, H. S., Prasad, M. R., & Seroogy, K. B. (1998). Expression of trkB mRNA is altered in rat hippocampus after experimental brain trauma. *Molecular Brain Research*, **59**, 264–268.

Horn, J., & Limburg, M. (2000). Calcium antagonists for acute ischaemic stroke. *Cochrane Database of Systematic Reviews*, **2**, CD001928.

Hovda, D., Sutton, R., & Feeney, D. (1984). Amphetamine with experience promotes recovery of locomotor function after unilateral frontal cortex injury in the cat. *Brain Research*, **298**, 358–361.

Hovda, D., Sutton, R., & Feeney, D. (1989). Amphetamine-induced recovery of visual cliff performance after bilateral visual cortex ablation in cats: measurements of depth perception thresholds. *Behavioural Neuroscience*, **103**, 574–584.

Hovda, D. A., Yoshino, A., Kawamata, T., Katayama, Y., & Becker, D. P. (1991). Diffuse prolonged depression of cerebral oxidative metabolism following concussive brain injury in the rat: A cytochrome oxidase histochemistry study. *Brain Research*, **567**, 1–10.

Jadad, A. R., Boyle, M., Cunningham, C., Kim, M., & Schachar, R. (1999). Treatment of attention-deficit/hyperactivity disorder. *Evidence Report: Technology Assessment*, **11**, i–viii.

Kempermann, G., Gast, D., & Gage, F. H. (2002). Neuroplasticity in old age: sustained fivefold induction of hippocampal neurogenesis by long-term environmental enrichment. *Annals of Neurology*, **52**, 135–143.

Kim, B. T., Rao, V. L., Sailor, K. A., Bowen, K. K., & Dempsey, R. J. (2001). Protective effects of glial cell line-derived neurotrophic factor on hippocampal neurons after traumatic brain injury in rats. *Journal of Neurosurgery*, **95**, 674–679.

Kline, A. E., Yu, J., Massucci, J. L., Zafonte, R. D., & Dixon, C. E. (2002). Protective effects of the 5-HT1A receptor agonist 8-hydroxy-2-(di-n-propylamino)tetralin against traumatic brain injury-induced cognitive deficits and neuropathology in adult male rats. *Neuroscience Letters*, **333**, 179–182.

Kobori, N., & Dash, P. K. (2006). Reversal of brain injury-induced prefrontal glutamic acid decarboxylase expression and working memory deficits by D1 receptor antagonism. *Journal of Neuroscience*, **26**, 4236–4246.

Ladurner, G., Kalvach, P., & Moessler, H. (2005). Neuroprotective treatment with cerebrolysin in patients with acute stroke: a randomised controlled trial. *Journal of Neural Transmission*, **112**, 415–428.

Lang, U. E., Jockers-Scherubl, M. C., & Hellweg, R. (2004). State of the art of the neurotrophin hypothesis in psychiatric disorders: implications and limitations. *Journal of Neural Transmission*, **111**, 387–411.

Langlois, J., Rutland-Brown, W., & Thomas, K. (2004). *Traumatic Brain Injury in the United States: Emergency Department Visits, Hospitalizations, and Deaths.* Atlanta, GA: Centers for Disease Control and Prevention, National Center for Injury Prevention and Control.

Li, B. M., & Mei, Z. T. (1994). Delayed-response deficit induced by local injection of the alpha 2-adrenergic antagonist yohimbine into the dorsolateral prefrontal cortex in young adult monkeys. *Behavioral and Neural Biology*, **62**, 134–139.

Lim, K. C., Lim, S. T., & Federoff, H. J. (2003). Neurotrophin secretory pathways and synaptic plasticity. *Neurobiology of Aging*, **24**, 1135–1145.

Lodder, J., van Raak, L., Hilton, A., Hardy, E., & Kessels, A. (2006). Diazepam to improve acute stroke outcome: results of the early GABA-Ergic activation study in stroke trial. a randomized double-blind placebo-controlled trial. *Cerebrovascular Diseases*, **21**, 120–127.

Luciana, M., & Collins, P. F. (1997). Dopaminergic modulation of working memory for spatial but not object cues in normal humans. *Journal of Cognitive Neuroscience*, **9**, 330–347.

Luciana, M., Depue, R. A., Arbisi, P., & Leon, A. (1992). Facilitation of working memory in humans by a D2

dopamine receptor agonist. *Journal of Cognitive Neuroscience*, **4**, 58–68.

Lyden, P., Jacoby, M., Schim, J. *et al.* (2001). The Clomethiazole Acute Stroke Study in tissue-type plasminogen activator-treated stroke (CLASS-T): final results. *Neurology*, **57**, 1199–1205.

Lyden, P., Shuaib, A., Ng, K. *et al.* (2002). Clomethiazole Acute Stroke Study in Ischemic Stroke (CLASS-I): final Results. *Stroke*, **33**, 122–129.

Martinsson, L., & Eksborg, S. (2004). Drugs for stroke recovery: the example of amphetamines. *Drugs and Aging*, **21**, 67–79.

Martinsson, L., & Wahlgren, N. G. (2003). Safety of dexamphetamine in acute ischemic stroke: a randomized, double-blind, controlled dose-escalation trial. *Stroke*, **34**, 475–481.

Mauler, F., & Horvath, E. (2005). Neuroprotective efficacy of repinotan HCl, a 5-HT1A receptor agonist, in animal models of stroke and traumatic brain injury. *Journal of Cerebral Blood Flow and Metabolism*, **25**, 451–459.

Mauler, F., Fahrig, T., Horvath, E., & Jork, R. (2001). Inhibition of evoked glutamate release by the neuroprotective 5-HT(1A) receptor agonist BAY x 3702 in vitro and in vivo. *Brain Research*, **888**, 150–157.

McAllister, T. W., Flashman, L. A., Sparling, M. B., & Saykin, A. J. (2004). Working memory deficits after mild traumatic brain injury: catecholaminergic mechanisms and prospects for catecholaminergic treatment – a review. *Brain Injury*, **18**, 331–350.

McDermott, K., Raghupathi, R., Fernandez, S. *et al.* (1997). Delayed administration of basic fibroblast growth. *Journal of Neurotrauma*, **14**, 191–200.

McDowell, S., Whyte, J., & D'Esposito, M. (1998). Differential effect of a dopaminergic agonist on prefrontal function in traumatic brain injury patients. *Brain*, **121**, 1155–1164.

McIntosh, T. K. (1994). Neurochemical sequelae of traumatic brain injury: therapeutic implications. *Cerebrovascular and Brain Metabolism Reviews*, **6**, 109–162.

McIntosh, T., Hayes, R., DeWitt, D. S., Agura, V., & Faden, A. I. (1987). Endogenous opioids may mediate secondary damage after experimental brain injury. *American Journal of Physiology*, **253**, E565–E574.

McIntosh, T., Fernyah, S., & Faden, A. I. (1991). The effects of naloxone hydrochloride treatment after experimental traumatic brain injury in the rat. *Journal of Cerebral Blood Flow and Metabolism, Suppl. 2*, S734.

McIntosh, T., Thomas, M., Smith, D., & Banbury, M. K. (1992). The novel 21-aminosteroid U74006F attenuates cerebral edema and improves survival after brain injury in the rat. *Journal of Neurotrauma*, **9**, 33–40.

McIntosh, T. K., Juhler, M., & Wieloch, T. (1998). Novel pharmacologic strategies in the treatment of experimental traumatic brain injury: 1998. *Journal of Neurotrauma*, **15**, 731–769.

Miller, L., Lyeth, B., Jenkins, L. *et al.* (1990). Excitatory amino acid receptor subtype binding following traumatic brain injury. *Brain Research*, **526**, 103–107.

Miller, N., & Adams, J. (2005). Alcohol and drug disorders. In J. Silver, T. W. McAllister, & S. Yudofsky (Eds.), *Textbook of Traumatic Brain Injury* (pp. 509–532). Washington, DC: American Psychiatric Publishing, Inc.

Miner, L., Jedema, H., Moore, F. *et al.* (2006). Chronic stress increases the plasmalemmal distribution of the norepinephrine transporter and the coexpression of tyrosine hydroxylase in norepinephrine axons in the prefrontal cortex. *Neuroscience and Behavioral Physiology*, **26**, 1571–1578.

Monaghan, D., & Cotman, C. (1986). Identification and properties of N-methyl-D-aspartate receptors in rat brain plasma membranes. *Proceedings of the National Academy of Sciences of the United States of America*, **83**, 7532–7536.

Murdoch, I., Perry, E. K., Court, J. A., Graham, D. I., & Dewar, D. (1998). Cortical cholinergic dysfunction after human head injury. *Journal of Neurotrauma*, **15**, 295–305.

Murdoch, I., Nicoll, J. A., Graham, D. I., & Dewar, D. (2002). Nucleus basalis of Meynert pathology in the human brain after fatal head injury. *Journal of Neurotrauma*, **19**, 279–284.

Nakanishi, S. (1992). Molecular characterization of the family of metabotropic glutamate receptors. In R. Simon (Eds.), *Excitatory Amino Acids* (pp. 21–22). New York, NY: Time Medical Publishers.

Narayan, R., Michel, M., Ansell, B. *et al.* (2002). Clinical trials in head injury. *Journal of Neurotrauma*, **19**, 503–557.

Ohman, J., Braakman, R., & Legout, V. (2001). Repinotan (BAY x 3702): a 5HT1A agonist in traumatically brain injured patients. *Journal of Neurotrauma*, **18**, 1313–1321.

Okiyama, K., Smith, D., Thomas, M., & McIntosh, T. (1992). Evaluation of a novel calcium channel blocker, (s)-emopamil, on regional cerebral edema and neurobehavioral function after experimental brain injury. *Journal of Neurosurgery*, **77**, 607–615.

Oyesiku, N., Evans, C., Houston, S. *et al.* (1999). Regional changes in the expression of neurotrophic factors and their receptors following acute traumatic brain injury in the adult rat brain. *Brain Research*, **833**, 161–172.

Philips, M. F., Mattiasson, G., Wieloch, T. *et al.* (2001). Neuroprotective and behavioral efficacy of nerve growth factor-transfected hippocampal progenitor cell transplants after experimental traumatic brain injury. *Journal of Neurosurgery*, **94**, 765–774.

Povlishock, J., & Katz, D. (2005). Update of neuropathology and neurological recovery after traumatic brain injury. *Journal of Head Trauma Rehabilitation*, **20**, 76–94.

Prasad, M. R., Tzigaret, C., Smith, D. H., Soares, H., & McIntosh, T. K. (1993). Decreased alpha-adrenergic receptors after experimental brain injury. *Journal of Neurotrauma*, **9**, 269–279.

Rama, P., Linnankoski, I., Tanila, H., Pertovaara, A., & Carlson, S. (1996). Medetomidine, atipamezole, and guanfacine in delayed response performance of aged monkeys. *Pharmacology, Biochemistry and Behavior*, **55**, 415–422.

Ramos, B., Colgan, L., Nou, E. *et al.* (2005). The beta-1 adrenergic antagonist, betaxolol, improves working memory performance in rats and monkeys. *Biological Psychiatry*, **58**, 894–900.

Ramos, B. P., Stark, D., Verduzco, L., van Dyck, C. H., & Arnsten, A. F. T. (2006). α2A-adrenoceptor stimulation improves prefrontal cortical regulation of behavior through inhibition of cAMP signaling in aging animals. *Learning and Memory*, **13**, 770–776.

Ray, S., Dixon, C., & Banik, N. (2002). Molecular mechanisms in the pathogenesis of traumatic brain injury. *Histology and Histopathology*, **17**, 1137–1152.

Raz, A. (2004). Anatomy of attentional networks. *Anatomical Record New Anatomist*, **281**, 21–36.

Raz, A., & Buhle, J. (2006). Typologies of attentional networks. *Nature Reviews Neuroscience*, **7**, 367–379.

Robinson, S., Lyeth, B. G., Jenkins, L. *et al.* (1987). The effect of naloxone pretreatment on behavioral responses to concussive brain injury in the rat. *Neuroscience Abstracts*, **2**, 1254.

Romhanyi, R., Tandian, D., Hovda, D. A. *et al.* (1990). Catecholaminergic stimulation enhances recovery of function following concussive brain injury. *Journal of Neurotrauma*, **9**, 164.

Royo, N., Schouten, J., Fulp, C. *et al.* (2003). From cell death to neuronal regeneration: building a new brain after traumatic brain injury. *Journal of Neuropathology and Experimental Neurology*, **62**, 801–811.

Saatman, K. E., Murai, H., Bartus, R. *et al.* (1996). Calpain inhibitor AK295 attenuates motor and cognitive deficits following experimental brain injury in the rat. *Proceedings of the National Academy of Sciences of the United States of America*, **93**, 3428–3433.

Samochocki, M., & Strosznaider, J. (1993). Modulatory action of arachidonic acid on GABAA/chloride channel receptor function in adult and aged brain cortex membranes. *Neurochemistry International*, **23**, 261–267.

Sanada, T., Nakamura, T., Nishimura, M., Isayama, K., & Pitts, L. S. (1993). Effect of U74006F on neurologic function and brain edema after fluid percussion injury in rats. *Journal of Neurotrauma*, **10**, 65–71.

Sanossian, N., & Oybiagele, B. (2006). Multimodality stroke prevention. *The Neurologist*, **12**, 14–31.

Sariola, H., & Saarma, M. (2003). Novel functions and signalling pathways for GDNF. *Journal of Cell Science*, **116**, 3855–3862.

Sawaguchi, T., & Goldman-Rakic, P. S. (1991). D1 dopamine receptors in prefrontal cortex: involvement in working memory. *Science*, **251**, 947–950.

Schaffer, D. V., & Gage, F. H. (2004). Neurogenesis and neuroadaptation. *NeuroMolecular Medicine*, **5**, 1–9.

Schaper, C., Zhu, Y., Kouklei, M., Culmsee, C., & Krieglstein, J. (2000). Stimulation of 5-HT(1A) receptors reduces apoptosis after transient forebrain ischemia in the rat. *Brain Research*, **883**, 41–50.

Schwartz-Bloom, R. D., & Sah, R. (2001). Gamma-aminobutyric acid(A) neurotransmission and cerebral ischemia. *Journal of Neurochemistry*, **77**, 353–371.

Schwartz-Bloom, R., Cook, T., & Yu, X. (1996). GABA-gated chloride channels in brain by the arachidonic acid metabolite, thromboxane A2. *Neuropharmacology*, **35**, 1347–1353.

Shimizu, S., Royo, N., & Saatman, K. (2002). Evaluation of the temporal and regional alterations in endogenous GDNF expression after experimental traumatic brain injury. *Journal of Neurotrauma*, **19**, 1344.

Shimizu, S., Fulp, C., Royo, N., & McIntosh, T. (2005). Pharmacotherapy of prevention. In J. Silver, T. W. McAllister, & S. Yudofsky (Eds.), *Textbook of Traumatic Brain Injury* (pp. 699–726). Washington, DC: American Psychiatric Publishing, Inc.

Smith, W. (2004). Pathophysiology of focal cerebral ischemia: a therapeutic perspective. *Journal of Vascular and Interventional Radiology*, **15**, S3–S12.

Steere, J. C., & Arnsten, A. F. (1997). The alpha-2A noradrenergic receptor agonist guanfacine improves visual object discrimination reversal performance in aged rhesus monkeys. *Behavioral Neuroscience*, **111**, 883–891.

Stroemer, R. P., Kent, T. A., & Hulsebosch, C. E. (1998). Enhanced neocortical neural sprouting, synaptogenesis, and behavioral recovery with D-amphetamine therapy after neocortical infarction in rats. *Stroke*, **29**, 2381–2393.

Sutton, R. L., & Feeney, D. M. (1992). Alpha-noradrenergic agonists and antagonists affect recovery and maintenance of beam-walking ability after sensorimotor cortex ablation in the rat. *Restorative Neurology and Neuroscience*, **4**, 1–11.

Sutton, R., Hovda, D., & Feeney, D. (1989). Amphetamine accelerates recovery of locomotor function following bilateral frontal cortex ablation in cats. *Behavioural Neuroscience*, **103**, 837–841.

Tandian, D., Romhanyi, R., Hovda, D. A. *et al.* (1990). Amphetamine enhances both behavior and metabolic recovery following fluid percussion brain injury. *Journal of Neurotrauma*, **9**, 174.

Tanila, H., Rama, P., & Carlson, S. (1996). The effects of prefrontal intracortical microinjections of an alpha-2 agonist, alpha-2 antagonist and lidocaine on the delayed alternation performance of aged rats. *Brain Research Bulletin*, **40**, 117–119.

Teal, P., Silver, F. L., & Simard, D. (2005). The BRAINS study: safety, tolerability, and dose-finding of repinotan in acute stroke. *Canadian Journal of Neurological Sciences*, **32**, 61–67.

Teasdale, G. (1991). A randomized trial of nimodipine in severe head injury: HIT 1. *Journal of Neurotrauma*, **37**, S545–S550.

Tekin, S., & Cummings, J. L. (2002). Frontal-subcortical neuronal circuits and clinical neuropsychiatry: an update. *Journal of Psychosomatic Research*, **53**, 647–654.

Tobias, C., & Bullock, M. (2004). Critical appraisal of neuroprotection trials in head injury: what have we learned. *NeuroRx*, **1**, 71–79.

Vijayraghavan, S., Wang, M., Birnbaum, S. *et al.* (2007). Inverted-U dopamine D1 receptor actions on prefrontal neurons engaged in working memory. *Nature Neuroscience*, **10**, 376–384.

Vink, R., McIntosh, T., Romhanyi, R., & Faden, A. I. (1990). Opiate antagonist nalmefene improves intracellular free Mg^{2+}, bioenergetic state and neurological outcome following traumatic brain injury in rats. *Journal of Neuroscience*, **10**, 3524–3530.

Wade, D. T. (1996). Epidemiology of disabling neurological disease: how and why does disability occur? *Journal of Neurology, Neurosurgery and Psychiatry*, **61**, 242–249.

Wahlgren, N. G., & Ahmed, N. (2004). Neuroprotection in cerebral ischaemia: facts and fancies: the need for new approaches. *Cerebrovascular Diseases*, **17**, *Suppl. 1*, 153–166.

Wahlgren, N. G., Ranasinha, K. W., Rosolacci, T. *et al.* (1999). Clomethiazole acute stroke study (CLASS): results of a randomized, controlled trial of clomethiazole versus placebo in 1360 acute stroke patients. *Stroke*, **30**, 21–28.

Walker-Batson, D., Curtis, S., Nataraian, R. *et al.* (2001). A double-blind, placebo-controlled study of the use of amphetamine in the treatment of aphasia. *Stroke*, **32**, 2093–2098.

Wang, M., Ramos, B., Paspalas, C. *et al.* (2007). A-2A-adrenoceptors strengthen working memory networks by inhibiting cAMP-HCN channel signaling in prefrontal cortex. *Cell*, **129**, 397–410.

Whyte, J., Polansky, M., Cavallucci, C. *et al.* (1996). Inattentive behavior after traumatic brain injury. *Journal of the International Neuropsychological Society*, **2**, 274–281.

Whyte, J., Vaccaro, M., Grieg-Neff, P., & Hart, T. (2002). Psychostimulant use in the rehabilitation of individuals with traumatic brain injury. *Journal of Head Trauma Rehabilitation*, **17**, 284–299.

Williams, G. V., & Goldman-Rakic, P. S. (1995). Modulation of memory fields by dopamine D1 receptors in prefrontal cortex. *Nature*, **376**, 572–575.

Young, W. F., Flamm, E. S., Demopoulos, H., Tomasula, J., & Decrescito, V. (1981). Naloxone ameliorates post-traumatic ischemia in experimental spinal contusion. *Journal of Neurosurgery*, **55**, 209–219.

Zhu, J., Hamm, R. J., Reeves, T. M., Povlishock, J. T., & Phillips, L. L. (2000). Postinjury administration of L-deprenyl improves cognitive function and enhances neuroplasticity after traumatic brain injury. *Experimental Neurology*, **166**, 136–152.

18

Pharmacologic treatment of cognitive impairment after traumatic brain injury

John Whyte

Neuropathology of traumatic brain injury

- Diffuse axonal injury (DAI) and focal cortical contusions are the leading forms of neuropathology in traumatic brain injury (TBI); both forms of injury can disrupt normal neurotransmitter levels and directly and indirectly interfere particularly with prefrontal function.
- The hippocampus, important for development of new episodic memories, may be damaged by the "excitotoxic cascade."

Traumatic brain injury can produce a wide range of cognitive impairments, owing to the diffuse and multifocal nature of the injury. Diffuse axonal injury and focal cortical contusions are the hallmark lesions of TBI and, although their distribution is somewhat predictable, individual differences in injury mechanism and resulting neuropathology may occur. Diffuse axonal injury predominantly affects the dense white matter tracts of the corpus callosum, as well as the midbrain and the reticular system that courses through it (Blumbergs *et al.*, 1995). Because of this, DAI may cause disruption of any or all of the modulating neurotransmitter systems that contribute to the reticular system. At a minimum, delivery of dopamine, norepinephrine, serotonin and acetylcholine may be disturbed. Transmission is thought to be particularly seriously affected by the disruption of richly dopaminergic fiber tracts coursing toward the prefrontal cortex.

Focal contusions predominantly affect the anterior temporal lobes and orbitofrontal cortex, potentially providing a second mechanism for impairment of frontal cortex function (Clifton *et al.*, 1980). In addition, many individuals with significant TBIs experience secondary cytotoxic damage from the outpouring of excitatory neurotransmitters such as glutamate, to which the hippocampus is particularly susceptible (Clausen & Bullock, 2001). Collectively, then, the typical patterns of TBI-related neuropathology tend to produce impairments in executive function, attention and anterograde memory.

Traumatic brain injury varies greatly in its severity, with objective evidence of cognitive deficits in "mild" TBI generally clearing within months of injury, although subjective cognitive complaints may continue for much longer (Dikmen *et al.*, 1986; Levin *et al.*, 1987). At the most severe end of the spectrum, TBI may result in a permanent state of unconsciousness, the vegetative state, which typically involves profound bilateral thalamic damage (Kinney *et al.*, 1994). Given the variation in location and severity of TBI-associated neuropathology, it is unlikely that specific pharmacologic treatments will prove useful to all individuals with TBI. In individuals who have suffered nearly total damage to specific processing networks, it seems unlikely that pharmacologic intervention could restore their operation. However, for individuals in whom network function has been degraded by partial damage, pharmacologic augmentation may be able to restore efficiency to a partially preserved system. Similarly, pharmacologic agents that enhance mechanisms of neural regeneration or sprouting may have important but still unknown roles in the recovery process.

Cognitive Neurorehabilitation, Second Edition: Evidence and Application, ed. Donald T. Stuss, Gordon Winocur and Ian H. Robertson. Published by Cambridge University Press. © Cambridge University Press 2008.

Cognitive sequelae of traumatic brain injury

- Deficits in attention, memory and executive function are common after TBI, and can be related to the prevalent forms of neuropathology individually or in combination.

Across the severity spectrum of TBI, the above domains of attention, memory and executive function appear to be the most commonly affected (Whyte *et al.*, 2004). In mild TBI, the primary cognitive complaints are typically difficulties with distractibility and concentration, as well as poor recall of recent information (McAllister, 1994). More severe injuries regularly result in a prolonged interval of post-traumatic amnesia followed by varying degrees of ongoing anterograde memory impairment, reports by clinicians and caregivers of inattentiveness, and difficulties with problem solving, abstract reasoning, social interaction and goal maintenance typical of executive dysfunction (Whyte *et al.*, 2004a).

Recent research also suggests inter-relationships among the cognitive systems commonly affected by TBI. Those aspects of attention that are most seriously deranged by TBI are not the basic attention mechanisms of orienting or switching, but rather the linkage of efficient attention mechanisms to higher-level behavioral goals, i.e., the interaction between attention and executive function. Similarly, although severe memory disorders are thought to be due to excitotoxic damage to the hippocampus, failure of executive mechanisms that support strategic searches for memorial material probably contribute, particularly in milder memory impairments.

Rationale for pharmacologic treatment in traumatic brain injury

- Neurotransmitters contained in the reticular system (dopamine, norepinephrine, acetylcholine and serotonin) have widespread modulatory effects throughout the brain and may be disrupted by TBI.

The nature of TBI-associated neuropathology, coupled with knowledge of the resulting cognitive sequelae, suggests a plausible role for therapeutic manipulation of several neurotransmitters. As mentioned, the reticular system is rich in neurotransmitters that are distributed to higher cortical areas, including dopamine, norepinephrine, acetylcholine and serotonin (Robbins & Everitt, 1995). Moreover, preliminary research in TBI, as well as research in other clinical populations, suggests that these same neurotransmitters are relevant to attention, memory and executive function. For example, Posner and colleagues have described a model of attentional function that involves three interacting neural networks largely controlled by norepinephrine, acetylcholine and dopamine (Fernandez-Duque & Posner, 2001) and a number of dopaminergic and noradrenergic medications have proved useful in attention deficit disorder (Mehta *et al.*, 2000; Michelson *et al.*, 2003; Spencer *et al.*, 2001). Augmenting cholinergic tone has therapeutic benefit in improving memory and independence in Alzheimer's disease (Tales *et al.*, 2002) and psychostimulants are also often found to enhance memory performance, though perhaps secondarily through attention or retrieval efficiency mechanisms (Siddall, 2005). There is also some evidence that dopaminergic drugs may enhance certain aspects of executive function (Kimberg *et al.*, 2001; Luciana *et al.*, 1992; McDowell *et al.*, 1998).

Current state of the science of drug treatment of TBI

- There are currently no drugs for which the evidence supports a treatment standard in improving cognitive function or enhancing recovery after TBI, though many drugs have been suggested to have such effects.
- A number of recurring methodologic difficulties have limited the value of psychopharmacologic research on TBI done to date.

Despite the logical prediction that manipulation of several important neurotransmitter systems might have therapeutic value in TBI, there is still no efficacy data of sufficient rigor to arrive at practice standards based on Class I evidence (Warden *et al.*, 2006). On a logical basis, there are four main questions to focus on when considering psychopharmacologic intervention:

1. Are there drugs that sedate or otherwise undermine cognitive recovery or performance, such that discontinuing these drugs or replacing them with more benign agents can enhance cognitive performance?
2. Are there drugs which provide a lasting benefit (lasting beyond the treatment interval) with respect to the pace of cognitive recovery and/or its final outcome?
3. Are there drugs which provide this type of lasting benefit specifically when coupled with appropriate treatment or training?
4. Are there drugs which can improve cognitive performance and real world functioning during the treatment interval ("symptomatic treatment")?

A number of recurrent methodologic challenges have prevented the studies conducted to date from addressing these goals (Warden *et al.*, 2006; Whyte, 2002). These methodologic limitations are summarized in Table 18.1.

Many of these limitations stem from the small sample sizes that are typical in published studies, as well as the fact that they are often conducted during periods of rapid spontaneous recovery. It appears that many authors attempt to conduct treatment trials with their local clinical populations and little or no outside resources – leading to small trials that are excessively constrained by clinically prevailing time frames and patient characteristics. Moreover, since much cognitive rehabilitation treatment is conducted during periods of relatively rapid clinical recovery, cross-over designs are rarely interpretable since cognitive function is unlikely to return to baseline when an active drug is discontinued. Cross-over designs are also logically inappropriate when considering goal #2 above, since they assume the reversibility of treatment effects. Even parallel group studies must enroll larger samples to cope with the pace and variability of spontaneous recovery.

Although psychopharmacologic practice standards for TBI do not yet exist, there has been progress in preliminary research in several cognitive areas and with respect to several specific medications, resulting in recommendations at the "guideline" level. This suggests that larger randomized trials are now called for, at least for these drugs.

Some of the largest and most rigorous studies to date have focused on the effects of several anticonvulsants, given to prevent post-traumatic epilepsy, on cognitive recovery. With respect to these medications, there is now reasonably strong evidence that phenytoin (Dilantin) may depress cognitive function in the acute post-injury period. Thus, anticonvulsant treatment with phenytoin should be of limited duration and those who need chronic

Table 18.1. Recurring methodologic limitations in psychopharmacologic research in traumatic brain injury.

Inclusion criteria that do not include valid measures of the target cognitive problem
Outcome measures that are not validated and/or that bear a tenuous relationship to the known actions of the study drug
Small samples with inadequate statistical power
Failure to achieve group comparability through simple randomization (particularly in small studies)
Use of cross-over designs during neurologic recovery
Inadequate control of bias (lack of placebo condition, blinded treatment and outcome assessment)
Incomplete or biased collection of outcome data (including failure to use intention-to-treat analysis)
Inappropriate statistical analysis (including failure to control for baseline performance differences)
Failure to follow promising but inconclusive pilot studies with definitive trials

treatment should be transitioned to carbamazepine (Tegretol) or valproate (Depakene/Depakote), two anticonvulsants that appear to have fewer cognitive side effects, at least at moderate doses. Other drugs, such as neuroleptics, have been suggested, based on animal research (Feeney et al., 1982), to slow neurologic recovery, but no rigorous research on this topic in TBI exists. Moreover, whether atypical antipsychotics or benzodiazepines, often used as substitutes for neuroleptics in patients with neurobehavioral disturbances, are any safer from this perspective is unknown.

Similarly, little research has been done to identify drugs that may positively influence the pace or level of cognitive recovery. A few studies purport to show a speeding of recovery during drug treatment which is maintained after drug discontinuation, (e.g., Kaelin et al., 1996). Unfortunately, this pattern of maintained benefit after treatment is consistent *either* with a lasting treatment effect *or* with imbalance between experimental groups in the pace of spontaneous recovery. Only larger, better controlled studies will be able to distinguish between these vastly different possibilities. Indeed, a large multicenter parallel group study of a drug intervention to enhance the pace of recovery from the vegetative and minimally conscious states (J. Giacino, J. Whyte, Principal Investigators) has intentionally included a post-treatment washout period in both groups to determine whether any treatment-related gains are lost when the active drug is stopped. Although many of the reported drug studies involved patients also receiving other forms of rehabilitation therapy, very little research on TBI has assessed the impact of linking drug administration with specific treatment or learning experiences, despite accumulating evidence, in animal and human studies, that drugs such as amphetamine, may specifically enhance the response to experience-based treatments (Walker-Batson et al., 1995, 2001).

The bulk of the suggestive evidence supporting psychopharmacologic intervention concerns symptomatic treatment (i.e., goal #4 above). There is evidence that methylphenidate, a psychostimulant that augments dopaminergic and noradrenergic function, can help to counteract the slowing in thought and action that is so common in TBI (Whyte et al., 1997, 2004b). It may also decrease the amount of off-task behavior seen during independent work tasks, and enhance caregiver ratings of attentiveness (Whyte et al., 1997, 2004b) as well as improve anterograde memory (Siddall, 2005), working memory (Kim et al., 2006), and mood (Lee et al., 2005). Although this drug is quite safe in short-term use, recent reports of an increased incidence of sudden death with stimulants has led to greater concern about long-term use (Nissen, 2006). Similarly, donepezil, which augments cholinergic function, appears to have some beneficial effects on both attention and memory (Zhang et al., 2004). To date, however, its effects on immediate memory and information processing speed/mental control (i.e., the PASAT) are more clear cut than its impact on anterograde memory (Zhang et al., 2004). Bromocriptine, a dopamine agonist acting primarily at the D2 receptor, has enhanced certain aspects of executive function, including dual-task performance, in individuals with TBI (McDowell et al., 1998) as well as elderly individuals with reduced working memory span (Kimberg et al., 2001). The initial studies reporting this finding used a single low-dose protocol. Recent research from our laboratory using chronic administration of a larger dose failed to replicate these findings, suggesting that more research is needed to understand the generality of these benefits and whether there is a narrow efficacy window for achieving them. In addition, controversy remains about which of the dopamine receptor subtypes are most closely linked to specific domains of cognitive function. Bromocriptine is primarily a D2 receptor subtype agonist. Thus, studies of drugs with greater activity at other receptor sites are also warranted.

All three of these drugs appear to be promising clinical agents, but each has only been studied to date in small and selected samples. Larger trials are now needed to establish optimal dosing, to measure the magnitude of drug impact on measures of real-world functioning, to identify predictors of a positive drug response, and to allow rational drug selection among pharmacologically similar agents.

Applying current knowledge to clinical practice

- Evaluating the impact of psychoactive medications in clinical practice is made more difficult by the simultaneous occurrence of spontaneous recovery and/or learning; the considerable day-to-day performance variability typical in TBI; and the complex correspondence between the cellular targets of psychoactive drugs vs. the behavioral targets of treatment.

In the absence of clear evidence-based practice standards, clinicians are left to rely on other sources of support for any psychopharmacologic interventions they may undertake. Practice in this context of uncertainty, then, should consider several key conceptual issues, as discussed below.

Spontaneous recovery

The presence of brisk spontaneous recovery in the cognitive domain under consideration makes it extremely challenging to determine whether any psychoactive drug contributes to that recovery. Thus, a clinician intervening in this context will rarely be any more sure of the value of treatment after the intervention than before. Certainly it is possible that formal research will determine that a particular agent makes brisk recovery even brisker. But that cannot be ascertained by watching the outcome of individual patients undergoing treatment. Thus, until such research is available, it would appear unwise for clinicians to intervene when recovery is proceeding well.

Variability in performance

Cognitive and behavioral variability are hallmarks of TBI and other neurologic conditions. Variability may be particularly pronounced in the context of frontal executive deficits (Stuss *et al.*, 1989, 2003) and the minimally conscious state (Giacino *et al.*, 2002; Whyte *et al.*, 1999) but exists throughout the severity spectrum. Determining whether an individual patient benefits from a psychopharmacologic intervention and whether they are on the optimal dose, requires comparing their cognitive and/or behavioral performance on and off the drug or on multiple doses of the drug. But, just as in formal research, the more variable performance is within a single drug condition, the more measurements in each drug condition will be required to make a legitimate comparison. If the measures being used to assess medication response are subject to practice effects, this further complicates sequential comparison within patients.

The goal of treatment

There is no drug that is specific to "attention," "memory" or any other cognitive domain. Indeed, most of the drugs in use clinically in TBI alter the activity of diffuse modulatory neurotransmitter systems, such as those in the reticular system, which project to numerous brain regions involved in many different cognitive and behavioral processes. Thus, for any particular drug intervention, one must engage in reasoning that attempts to link the fundamental actions of the psychopharmacologic agent to specific cognitive processes, to behaviors and tasks that are meaningful in the real world. At the same time, one must be open to the possibility of inadvertent effects of the treatment on other neurocognitive systems and resulting behaviors.

With these comments in mind, it would seem that individualized off-label assessment of psychoactive medications is most feasible in certain specific circumstances, which are summarized in Table 18.2. When these conditions cannot be realistically met, there is little alternative but to seek to enroll patients in traditional parallel group studies.

Table 18.2. Assessing the appropriateness of single subject experimental assessments. Adapted with permission from Sackett *et al.* (1991).

Is a single subject experimental assessment indicated for this patient and problem?

Is the effectiveness of the treatment in doubt?

Will the treatment, if effective, be continued long term?

Is the patient eager to collaborate in designing and carrying out a single-subject assessment?

Is a single subject experimental assessment feasible in this patient?

Does the treatment have a rapid onset?

Does the treatment cease to act soon after it is discontinued?

Is an optimal duration of treatment feasible?

Can clinically relevant treatment targets be measured (ideally at multiple conceptual levels)?

Can sensible criteria for stopping the trial be established?

Should an unblinded run-in period be conducted (particularly to assess performance variability and trend)?

Is a single subject experimental assessment feasible in this clinical setting?

Is there a pharmacist who will collaborate on preparation of the treatment phases?

Are strategies in place for collecting and analysing the data?

Is a single subject experimental assessment ethical?

Applying single subject experimental methods

- Single subject experimental methods can be valuable in assessing the impact of unproven drug treatments in individual patients, and if rigorously conducted they can also be combined into group analyses with greater generalizability.
- These methods can only be realistically applied in more chronic treatment settings, with certain specific drugs, and in relation to certain specific treatment goals. Questions not amenable to this type of design continue to require traditional parallel group study protocols.

Single subject experimental methods can be used to assess the impact of an unproven treatment, or to determine an individual's response to a proven treatment, since that "proof" nearly always represents an average treatment benefit with considerable individual variability in treatment response. These methods have the added benefit of examining whether treatment improves real-world outcomes of importance to the patient, since even proven treatments have typically been tested against one or two primary outcome measures. Single subject methods have been applied to a wide range of individualized clinical questions, including responses to theophylline in chronic airway disease (Mahon *et al.*, 1996), quinine in leg cramps (Woodfield *et al.*, 2005), various drugs for osteoarthritis (Nikles *et al.*, 2005), cannabis for chronic pain (Notcutt *et al.*, 2004), and generic vs. brand name warfarin (Pereira *et al.*, 2005). In addition, although the effectiveness of methylphenidate to treat ADHD is well established, concerns about overprescribing and the presence of treatment nonresponders remain. Single subject experimental designs have met with high family satisfaction as a way to ensure appropriate use of this drug (Kent *et al.*, 1999).

Guyatt *et al.* (1990) have written extensively about applications of these methods to many different treatments in internal medicine. In a review of the results from their "n of 1" consultation service, they note an unknown number of cases that were not deemed amenable to single subject assessment methods after a preliminary discussion. Of 70 trials begun, 13 were not completed (mostly because of patient noncompliance or concurrent illness). Of the 57 trials completed 48 produced "clinically definite" results, of which 19 were "statistically definite," while nine were inconclusive (Guyatt *et al.*, 1990).

Applications of these methods to clinical management is an evolving field, with considerable controversy remaining about precisely when they are most useful (Larson, 1990), how to weigh the evidence from group studies vs. individual assessments (Schluter & Ware, 2005; Zucker *et al.*, 1997), as well as how to optimally design and analyse the single subject experiments themselves (Bagne & Lewis, 1992; Guyatt & Jaeschke, 1990; Hersen & Barlow, 1976; Jacobs *et al.*, 1996; Ottenbacher & Hinderer,

2001). However, if the clinician is determined to intervene pharmacologically, it seems likely that a systematic quantitative approach to the intervention will be superior to subjective clinical judgment regardless of the precise details of assessment design and data analysis.

In our experience, pharmacologic intervention begins with a formulation of the treatment goal at several levels, corresponding to the levels of the *International Classification of Functioning, Disability and Health*. First one needs to characterize the clinical problem from the patient's perspective with reference to real-world behaviors or tasks where performance is suboptimal and where the patient wishes improvement (i.e., at the activity level). Through discussion with the patient and caregivers, one hopes to arrive at a measurable index of the problem, individually tailored to the patient's circumstances. Questions such as, "How does this problem show itself in everyday life?" or "How would you recognize it if this problem improved?" can be helpful in designing individually tailored measures that are sensitive to treatment effects and relevant to the patient's concerns.

To the extent possible, these measures should be operationalized into observable outcomes. Ideally, one also selects a standardized measure of the problem, if such exists. For example, if the complaint in everyday life is of slowness of thought and action, affecting the ability to complete household chores in a reasonable amount of time, one might include a measure of impairment in mental and motor speed (i.e., a body structure/function level measure) such as the Digit Symbol subtest, along with an individualised activity measure, such as the time required to prepare dinner. For drugs that also have easily detectable physiologic effects (e.g., heart rate or alertness for psychostimulants), it is helpful to measure this level as well, since it can help ensure that adequate drug is being taken and absorbed, particularly if behavioral effects are not seen at the dose tested.

Implicit in this process is the formulation of hypotheses linking specific impairments to difficulties in specific activities (Whyte, 1997). In the above example, one hypothesizes that the length of time required to make dinner is *particularly* related to the speed of information processing, and less so to inattention, forgetting the steps of the cooking task, motor inco-ordination in chopping the food, etc. If there are no important life tasks for which this is true, then it is unclear that the patient will benefit clinically from an improvement in processing speed, should it occur. It is, of course, possible that performance of certain activities is dependent on several capacities *including* processing speed. If so, it may be useful to pursue treatment of this impairment as long as treatments are also available for the other contributing impairments.

An attempt at baseline measurement of these various indices before the intervention is undertaken is ideal. This allows one to clarify any confusion about how the effects should be measured, and to address pre-treatment variability and trend in the measures, since this will be relevant to how the drug effect will be analysed. In some instances, one may discover that the act of discussing and concretely measuring the treatment goal, itself, may result in considerable resolution, obviating the need for treatment. Or one may discover that the problem, while still present, is not well measured by the indices chosen. One should arrive at one or more feasible and interpretable measures before undertaking the actual trial. Finally, one may observe brisk improvement during the baseline assessment, indicating that the problem may be resolved before a trial can be completed.

When it is time for the intervention to begin, one must decide on the optimal assessment design. The three simplest designs, in order of rigor are A-B, A-B-A, and multiple cross-over. In the A-B design, one collects a sequential set of pre-treatment scores during the A phase, then introduces the drug and continues to collect the same measures during the treatment (B) phase. Some variation of the celeration line approach is used to assess whether performance in the B phase differs from that in the A phase. In the celeration line approach, the data from the A phase are used to construct a trend line which is continued through the B phase. The proportion of data points in the B phase that lie above and below this line serves as an index of the degree to which post-treatment performance differs from the expected trend (Ottenbacher, 1986).

The A-B design is the simplest and most feasible because it conforms to typical clinical practice. But it also has serious limitations. Any residual spontaneous recovery or practice effects will tend to favor the B phase. Although the trend line seeks to control for such non-treatment effects, the nature of the trend line always involves mathematical assumptions (i.e., linear, exponential, etc.) which are difficult to support without extensive baseline data. In addition, when there is considerable pre-treatment performance variability, the confidence interval around the trend line may be quite wide, leaving almost any deviation from expectation during treatment as a plausible chance effect.

The A-B-A design is similar to the A-B design except that one withdraws the treatment again after an interval of measurement on treatment, with the expectation that performance will decline (or decelerate its improvement). This controls more completely for spontaneous recovery and practice than the A-B design and, by providing a second phase of nontreatment data, can narrow the confidence interval around the trend line constructed through the nontreatment data. Although this approach has important advantages over the A-B design, the patient, caregiver, or clinician may be reluctant to withdraw a medication that is perceived to have led to improvement when it was introduced. One may be more likely to implement this method when treatment effects are modest, leading to a biased use of the method.

Still more rigorous is the repeated crossover design where multiple A and B phases of random length are constructed with continuous measurement throughout. This results in equal allocation of treatment and nontreatment data points throughout the data sequence, so that overall trend, however complex, is not confounded with drug condition. One can construct a trend line through all of the nontreatment data and examine the proportion of treatment data on either side of that line. One can also compute a linear regression with a drug variable and a session

variable, although the P value calculated from such an analysis may be distorted by autocorrelation (lack of independence) in the performance data. The most serious limitation of this method is that it can be applied only to short-acting drugs that can be quickly delivered and withdrawn (such that each phase in the crossover design can be one or a few days long), or else it will require a very long period to conduct.

Practical aspects to conducting quantitative single subject drug assessments

- Conducting single subject assessments requires an infrastructure including drug preparation, data collection oversight and data analysis skills.
- Controversies remain about the optimal assessment design, method of randomisation and data analysis, but it is likely that any carefully conducted quantitative trial has advantages over informal assessment.

The methods of single subject experimental design, while relatively simple in conceptual terms, present numerous operational challenges. Before undertaking such an evaluation, it is helpful to ensure that the patient will value the outcome of the assessment in terms of treatment decisions (Woodfield *et al.*, 2005). That is, if the patient strongly favors a particular treatment and is not truly collaborating on the assessment, the outcome may not be implemented. Assuming one wishes to go forward, the ethical standing of these trials should be checked at the local institutional level. In our institution, the Institutional Review Board has concluded that these trials do not require individual IRB approval, nor do they need to be presented to families as experiments requiring informed consent, as long as the treatment being studied is already in routine clinical use, the outcome measures being obtained are typical of clinical assessment approaches, and the goal of the trial is to answer an individual clinical question. The IRB's reasoning is that it would be ironic to require informed consent and IRB oversight when a doctor meticulously assesses a treatment, but not when that assessment is done more casually. Nevertheless, because the word "placebo" carries research connotations, and because almost all of the drugs we routinely evaluate are being used "off label," we always meet with the patient and/or caregiver to explain both the off label status of the drug and the rationale for the "experimental" assessment method. In cases where there is a plan to assemble a set of single subject assessments into a group analysis, we recommend IRB approval. In this context, the investigator has a conflict of interest between running the trial in the way most likely to provide a clear answer for the individual patient and running it in a way that will be cleanly analysed with other patients' data.

When undertaking such a trial, one must address how the performance data will be obtained. Patients who are continuously involved in some kind of therapy program (e.g., community re-entry, vocational rehabilitation program, etc.) are the most straightforward. Staff members in such programs can be involved in the treatment planning and measure development process, and treatment-related measures that are observable within that milieu can be chosen. Treatment staff can also communicate regularly with the patient and caregivers to supervise their data collection, where applicable. Patients not involved in ongoing services are more challenging to evaluate. Caregivers or the patients themselves can participate in the design of measures and the data collection. However, considerable effort and training are often required to achieve satisfactory reliability and, for patients in particular, memory and executive impairments may lead to failures to record the necessary data.

Blinded multiple crossover trials are superior to open label trials, particularly if the outcome measures are somewhat subjective in nature or easily influenced by expectation. Even A-B and A-B-A trials are somewhat strengthened if the precise timing of treatment initiation and withdrawal are not known by those involved in the evaluation. When conducting blinded trials, one must have the cooperation of a pharmacist to prepare the drug and placebo in identical form. The simplest method is to obtain opaque gelatin capsules in several sizes. The pill containing the active drug can be inserted whole into a capsule of appropriate size and filled out with an inactive substance (e.g., sugar), whereas the placebo capsules are filled with the inactive substance alone. Patients and caregivers obviously must be trained to take the correct medication on the correct day.

In the multiple cross-over method, the treatment periods should be randomly allocated to active drug and placebo (or one vs. another dose). The length of each treatment epoch depends both on the pharmacokinetics of the drug (i.e., anticipated speed of onset and dissipation of effects), and also on the amount of data to be collected in each epoch. Suppose a short-acting drug is being studied, that can be delivered in 2-day epochs, and one plans 5 epochs in each treatment condition (resulting in 10 epochs and 20 days for the trial). One will have the greatest statistical power if the 10 epochs are randomized collectively, since this allows for any ordering of the 10 different conditions. However, this method also runs the risk that several treatment epochs or several placebo epochs may occur sequentially, increasing the risk that irrelevant concurrent events might masquerade as treatment effects. Randomizing the treatment conditions in pairs (i.e., each 4-day block contains one treatment and one placebo epoch) lowers overall statistical power, but increases control of concurrent events (Guyatt & Jaeschke, 1990).

Data storage and analysis also present challenges. If single subject drug evaluations are conducted routinely, it may be cost effective to use personal digital assistants with cuing alarms to assist in data recording and allow direct downloading of the entries for analysis. In many instances, data will be recorded on paper and will need to be entered into a spreadsheet for analysis. Care should be taken that those completing the data collection do so at the time of the treatment rather than after the fact from memory. The odds of this can be increased by collecting the data frequently and checking it for quality.

Analysis, itself, will likely require several iterations. The initial baseline data must be analysed for problems that suggest confusion about the measures, and to determine when sufficient data have been obtained and whether a trend is present. At least one further analysis is then required to examine drug effects in relation to this baseline. Simple graphic presentation of the data may be sufficient if the effects are dramatic, but studies have shown poor agreement among different individuals interpreting the same graphs (Gottman & Glass, 1978). More quantitative approaches have also been described (Bagne & Lewis, 1992; Ottenbacher & Hinderer, 2001; Schluter & Ware, 2005; Zucker *et al.*, 1997). However, as noted by Guyatt and colleagues (1990), the results of such trials may be deemed sufficient to guide clinical practice even in the absence of traditional statistical significance and in almost all cases, the effort at least contributes to greater clarity in defining the goals of treatment and the patient's current status.

Prescribing outside of single subject assessments

A clinician seeking to help individuals with TBI with difficult cognitive and social problems is in a difficult predicament. As we have noted above, no drug can currently be chosen based on rigorous research, and the clinical circumstances and/or drug pharmacokinetics may make rigorous single subject assessments difficult. How, then, should a clinician respond to the many clinical situations where little reliable evidence exists to guide treatment, and a rigorous n-of-1 assessment does not appear feasible? It is possible, of course, to prescribe based on logical parallels to other disease states where evidence is more advanced. For example, one might choose to administer a drug such as donepezil for an individual with memory impairment, based on the parallel to Alzheimer's disease. One may also prescribe based on logical inferences from basic psychopharmacology research and animal models. For example, one might prescribe a dopamine agonist

to an individual with TBI who appears apathetic and lacking in initiative, because of dopamine's association with arousal and action systems in the anterior part of the brain.

Choosing drugs in this fashion, while very common in clinical practice, is not without difficulties. If the pace of spontaneous recovery or the degree of variability truly preclude arriving at any judgment about the drug's effects on behavior, then what has really been achieved? And how would one ever decide to stop the drug in the future? Every drug carries a financial cost and most have at least minor physical risks, so prescribing with no hope of assessing the outcome is of unclear value.

In addition, it is clear that logical parallels from animals to humans or basic research to clinical trials are often flawed. The brain is a complex and highly interactive network. Thus, patients whose surface behavior appears similar may not have similar underlying neurochemical profiles and, in turn, may not respond similarly to a medication. Even within the TBI population, it is likely that future drug prescribing will have to be done not simply in response to behavioral profiles, but in relation to finer-grained analysis of the neural network imbalances responsible for the individual's performance difficulties.

The final risk of prescribing in the absence of a rigorous evaluation system is a "cultural" risk rather than a patient risk. In our experience, institutions and programs that are active in prescribing off-label medications develop a culture that supports such interventions as the standard of care. When such attitudes prevail, it becomes exceedingly challenging to conduct more rigorous studies, particularly ones that involve placebo, because such studies involve "denying" patients this standard of care. In our recent recruiting for a study of the effects of amantadine HCl (vs. placebo) on recovery from severe disorders of consciousness, for example, one exclusion criterion is previous treatment with amantadine. We have encountered an acute care institution that routinely starts all their seriously injured patients on amantadine (and hence makes them all ineligible for this study). When questioned about their logic in doing so, since there is no compelling evidence to support this choice, and since it actually undermines the attempt to assemble such evidence, their explanation was that many of these patients lack generous insurance coverage for rehabilitation services and therefore, it is important for them to "do all they can" as quickly as possible to stimulate recovery.

While we do not claim never to have treated a patient outside of a formal study or a single subject assessment, we recommend minimizing such practice wherever possible because the logic that guides such treatment is tenuous, the ability to evaluate its impact is limited, and it undermines a culture of equipoise.

Conclusions

Traumatic brain injury results in significant disruption of neurotransmitter function, providing a rational basis for psychoactive drug treatment. Psychoactive medications may have a role in permanently enhancing the learning and recovery process, and/or in improving cognitive function symptomatically during their use. Unfortunately, the evidence that they can do this is only suggestive at present. Structured single subject assessments may assist clinical practice until more rigorous evidence is available, and, if properly conducted, may contribute to the generation of that evidence. However, this method is most applicable to the chronic phase of injury and to short-acting medications and reversible clinical problems. Drug treatment during rapid spontaneous recovery, treatment of problems that may not recur after treatment, and treatment with longer-acting drugs will require group research with parallel group designs.

ACKNOWLEDGMENTS

The author would like to thank Mary Czerniak for assistance in preparing the manuscript.

REFERENCES

Bagne, C. A., & Lewis, R. F. (1992). Evaluating the effects of drugs on behavior and quality of life: an alternative strategy for clinical trials. *Journal of Consulting and Clinical Psychology*, **60**, 225–239.

Blumbergs, P. C., Scott, G., Manavis, J., Wainwright, H., & Simpson, D. A. (1995). Topography of axonal injury as defined by amyloid precursor protein and the sector scoring method in mild and severe closed head injury. *Journal of Neurotrauma*, **12**, 565–572.

Clausen, T., & Bullock, R. (2001). Medical treatment and neuroprotection in traumatic brain injury. *Current Pharmacology Research*, **7**, 1517–1532.

Clifton, G. L., Grossman, R. G., Makela, M. E. *et al.* (1980). Neurological course and correlated computerized tomography findings after severe closed head injury. *Journal of Neurosurgery*, **52**, 611–624.

Dikmen, S., McLean, A., & Temkin, N. (1986). Neuropsychological and psychosocial consequences of minor head injury. *Journal of Neurology, Neurosurgery and Psychiatry*, **49**, 1227–1232.

Feeney, D. M., Gonzalez, A., & Law, W. A. (1982). Amphetamine, haloperidol, and experience interact to affect the rate of recovery after motor cortex injury. *Science*, **217**, 855–857.

Fernandez-Duque, D., & Posner, M. I. (2001). Brain imaging of attentional networks in normal and pathological states. *Journal of Clinical and Experimental Neuropsychology*, **23**, 74–93.

Giacino, J. T., Ashwal, S., Childs, N. *et al.* (2002). The minimally conscious state: definition and diagnostic criteria. *Neurology*, **58**, 349–353.

Gottman, J. M., & Glass, G. V. (1978). Analysis of interrupted time-series experiments. In T. R. Kratochwill (Eds.), *Single-subject Research Strategies for Evaluating Change* (pp. 241–262). New York, NY: Academic Press.

Guyatt, G. H., & Jaeschke, R. (1990). N-of-1 randomized trials – where do we stand? *Western Journal of Medicine*, **152**, 67–68.

Guyatt, G. H., Keller, J. L., Jaeschke, R. *et al.* (1990). The n-of-1 randomized controlled trial: clinical usefulness. Our three-year experience. *Annals of Internal Medicine*, **112**, 293–299.

Hersen, M., & Barlow, D. H. (1976). *Single-case experimental designs: Strategies for studying behavior change*. New York, NY: Pergamon Press.

Jacobs, A., Put, E., Ingels, M., Put, T., & Bossuyt, A. (1996). One-year follow-up of technetium-99m-HMPAO SPECT in mild head injury. *Journal of Nuclear Medicine*, **37**, 1605–1609.

Kaelin, D. L., Cifu, D. X., & Matthies, B. (1996). Methylphenidate effect on attention deficit in the acutely brain-injured adult. *Archives of Physical Medicine and Rehabilitation*, **77**, 6–9.

Kent, M. A., Camfield, C. S., & Camfield, P. R. (1999). Double-blind methylphenidate trials: Practical, useful, and highly endorsed by families. *Archives of Pediatric and Adolescent Medicine*, **153**, 1292–1296.

Kim, Y. H., Ko, M. H., Na, S. Y., Park, S. H., & Kim, K. W. (2006). Effects of single-dose methylphenidate on cognitive performance in patients with traumatic brain injury: a double-blind placebo-controlled study. *Clinical Rehabilitation*, **20**, 24–30.

Kimberg, D. Y., Aguirre, G. K., Lease, J., & D'Esposito, M. (2001). Cortical effects of bromocriptine, a D-2 dopamine receptor agonist, in human subjects, revealed by fMRI. *Human Brain Mapping*, **12**, 246–257.

Kinney, H. C., Korein, J., Panigrahy, A., Dikkes, P., & Goode, R. (1994). Neuropathological findings in the brain of Karen Ann Quinlan – the role of the thalamus in the persistent vegetative state. *New England Journal of Medicine*, **330**, 1469–1475.

Larson, E. B. (1990). N-of-1 clinical trials. A technique for improving medical therapeutics. *Western Journal of Medicine*, **152**, 52–56.

Lee, H., Kim, S. W., Kim, J. M. *et al.* (2005). Comparing effects of methylphenidate, sertraline and placebo on neuropsychiatric sequelae in patients with traumatic brain injury. *Human Psychopharmacology*, **20**, 97–104.

Levin, H. S., Mattis, S., Ruff, R. M. *et al.* (1987). Neurobehavioral outcome following minor head injury: a three-center study. *Journal of Neurosurgery*, **66**, 234–243.

Luciana, M., Depue, R. A., Arbisi, P., & Leon, A. (1992). Facilitation of working memory in humans by a D2 dopamine receptor agonist. *Journal of Cognitive Neuroscience*, **4**, 58–68.

Mahon, J., Laupacis, A., Donner, A., & Wood, T. (1996). Randomised study of n of 1 trials versus standard practice. *British Medical Journal*, **312**, 1069–1074.

McAllister, T. W. (1994). Mild traumatic brain injury and the postconcussive syndrome. In J. M. Silver, S. C. Yudofsky, & R. E. Hales (Eds.), *Neuropsychiatry of Traumatic Brain Injury* (pp. 357–392). Washington, DC: American Psychiatric Press, Inc.

McDowell, S., Whyte, J., & D'Esposito, M. (1998). Differential effect of a dopaminergic agonist on prefrontal function in traumatic brain injury patients. *Brain*, **121**, 1155–1164.

Mehta, M. A., Owen, A. M., Sahakian, B. J. *et al.* (2000). Methylphenidate enhances working memory by modulating discrete frontal and parietal lobe regions in the human brain. *Journal of Neuroscience*, **20**, RC65:1–6.

Michelson, D., Adler, L., Spencer, T. *et al.* (2003). Atomoxetine in adults with ADHD: two randomized placebo-controlled studies. *Biological Psychiatry*, **53**, 112–120.

Nikles, C. J., Clavarino, A. M., & Del Mar, C. B. (2005). Using n-of-1 trials as a clinical tool to improve prescribing. *British Journal of General Practice*, **55**, 175–180.

Nissen, S. E. (2006). ADHD drugs and cardiovascular risk. *New England Journal of Medicine*, **354**, 2296.

Notcutt, W., Price, M., Miller, R. *et al.* (2004). Initial experiences with medicinal extracts of cannabis for chronic pain: results from 34 "N of 1" studies. *Anaesthesia*, **59**, 440–452.

Ottenbacher, K. J. (1986). *Evaluating Clinical Change*. Baltimore, MD: Williams & Wilkins.

Ottenbacher, K. J., & Hinderer, S. R. (2001). Evidence-based practice: methods to evaluate individual patient improvement. *American Journal of Physical Medicine and Rehabilitation*, **80**, 786–796.

Pereira, J. A., Holbrook, A. M., Dolovich, L. *et al.* (2005). Are brand-name and generic warfarin interchangeable? Multiple n-of-1 randomized, crossover trials. *Annals of Pharmacotherapy*, **39**, 1188–1193.

Robbins, T. W., & Everitt, B. J. (1995). Arousal systems and attention. In M. S. Gazzaniga (Eds.), *The Cognitive Neurosciences* (pp. 703–720). Cambridge, MA: MIT Press.

Sackett, D. L., Haynes, R. B., Guyatt, G. H., & Tugell, P. (1991). *Clinical Epidemiology: A Basic Science for Clinical Medicine (2nd Edition)*. Boston, MA: Little Brown & Co.

Schluter, P. J., & Ware, R. S. (2005). Single patient (n-of-1) trials with binary treatment preference. *Statistics in Medicine*, **24**, 2625–2636.

Siddall, O. M. (2005). Use of methylphenidate in traumatic brain injury. *Annals of Pharmacotherapy*, **39**, 1309–1313.

Spencer, T., Biederman, J., Heiligenstein, J. *et al.* (2001). An open-label, dose-ranging study of atomexetine in children with attention deficit hyperactivity disorder. *Journal of Child and Adolescent Psychopharmacology*, **11**, 251–265.

Stuss, D. T., Stethem, L. L., Hugenholtz, H. *et al.* (1989). Reaction time after head injury: fatigue, divided and focused attention, and consistency of performance.

Journal of Neurology, Neurosurgery, and Psychiatry, **52**, 742–748.

Stuss, D. T., Murphy, K. J., Binns, M. A., & Alexander, M. P. (2003). Staying on the job: the frontal lobes control individual performance variability. *Brain*, **126**, 2363–2380.

Tales, A., Muir, J. L., Bayer, A., & Snowden, R. J. (2002). Spatial shifts in visual attention in normal ageing and dementia of the Alzheimer type. *Neuropsychologia*, **40**, 2000–2012.

Walker-Batson, D., Smith, P., Curtis, S., Unwin, H., & Greenlee, R. (1995). Amphetamine paired with physical therapy accelerates motor recovery after stroke: Further evidence. *Stroke*, **26**, 2254–2259.

Walker-Batson, D., Curtis, S., Natarajan, R. *et al.* (2001). A double-blind, placebo-controlled study of the use of amphetamine in the treatment of aphasia. *Stroke*, **32**, 2093–2098.

Warden, D. L., Gordon, B., McAllister, T. W. (2006). Guidelines for the pharmacologic treatment of neurobehavioral sequelae of traumatic brain injury. *Journal of Neurotrauma*, **10**, 1468–1501.

Whyte, J. (1997). Assessing medical rehabilitation practices: distinctive methodologic challenges. In M. J. Fuhrer (Ed.), *The Promise of Outcomes Research, Vol.2* (pp. 43–59) Baltimore, MD: Brookes.

Whyte, J. (2002). Pharmacologic treatment of cognitive impairments: conceptual and methodological considerations. In P. Eslinger (Ed.), *Neuropsychological Interventions* (pp. 59–79). New York, NY: Guilford Publications.

Whyte, J., Hart, T., Schuster, K., *et al.* (1997). The effects of methylphenidate on attentional function after traumatic brain injury: a randomized, placebo-controlled trial.

American Journal of Physical Medicine and Rehabilitation, **76**, 440–450.

Whyte, J., DiPasquale, M., & Vaccaro, M. (1999). Assessment of command-following in minimally conscious brain injured patients. *Archives of Physical Medicine and Rehabilitation*, **80**, 1–8.

Whyte, J., Hart, T., Laborde, A., & Rosenthal, M. (2004a). Rehabilitation issues in traumatic brain injury. In J. A. DeLisa, B. M. Gans, & W. L. Bockenek (Eds.), *Rehabilitation Medicine: Principles and Practice* (pp. 1677–1713). Philadelphia, PA: Lippincott.

Whyte, J., Hart, T., Vaccaro, M., *et al.* (2004b). The effects of methylphenidate on attention deficits after traumatic brain injury: a multi-dimensional randomized controlled trial. *Journal of Physical Medicine and Rehabilitation*, **83**, 401–420.

Woodfield, R., Goodyear-Smith, F., & Arroll, B. (2005). N-of-1 trials of quinine efficacy in skeletal muscle cramps of the leg. *British Journal of General Practice*, **55**, 181–185.

World Health Organization *International Classification of Functioning, Disability and Health*. (www3.who.int/icf/icftemplate.cfm).

Zhang, L., Plotkin, R. C., Wang, G., Sandel, M. E., & Lee, S. (2004). Cholinergic augmentation with donepezil enhances recovery in short-term memory and sustained attention after traumatic brain injury. *Archives of Physical Medicine and Rehabilitation*, **85**, 1050–1055.

Zucker, D. R., Schmid, C. H., McIntosh, M. W. *et al.* (1997). Combining single patient (N-of-1) trials to estimate population treatment effects and to evaluate individual patient responses to treatment. *Journal of Clinical Epidemiology*, **50**, 401–410.

19

Pharmacologic interventions for cognition in dementia

John M. Ringman and Jeffrey L. Cummings

Introduction

With the aging of the population, the prevalence of dementia is increasing dramatically. Interventions that can prevent, slow, or even reverse the underlying pathology of these progressive neurodegenerative illnesses are desperately needed. There is scant evidence that existing Food and Drug Administration (FDA)-approved treatments for Alzheimer's disease (AD) achieve these goals. However, progress has been made towards effectively treating the cognitive and behavioral symptoms of the dementias. In this chapter we will briefly review the relevant pathology of these illnesses, discuss approaches to evaluating the efficacy of medications for cognition, and summarize the evidence for cognitive benefits of pharmacologic treatments for these disorders.

Brief review of pathology with an emphasis on neurotransmitter systems

- Alzheimer's disease and mild cognitive impairment (MCI).
- Frontotemporal lobar degenerations.
- Parkinson's disease and dementia with Lewy bodies.
- Vascular dementia.

Alzheimer's disease

Alzheimer's disease is the most common cause of dementia, accounting for about 60% of cases (Mendez *et al.*, 1992). Insidious onset of deficits in recent episodic memory is the classic presentation, though atypical initial cognitive manifestations can occur (Galton *et al.*, 2000). As the illness progresses, executive function, language, and global cognitive decline results. Attention was initially drawn to the pathological hallmarks that currently define the illness by Alois Alzheimer in 1906 (Alzheimer *et al.*, 1995). Intraneuronal neurofibrillary tangles (NFTs) in the medial temporal lobe characterize the earliest stages of the disorder with these changes spreading to the neocortex as the illness progresses. These consist of abnormal cytoskeletal elements that indicate dead or dying neurons whose severity and distribution are closely associated with the clinical manifestations of the illness (Gómez-Isla *et al.*, 1997). Also required for the pathological diagnosis of AD are abundant senile and neuritic plaques (SP and NPs) that are extracellular aggregates of various forms of beta-amyloid (Aβ) protein in addition to other proteins and dystrophic cell processes. Neuritic plaques contain hyperphosphorylated tau protein as is found in NFTs. Senile plaques and NPs are present in the hippocampus in the medial temporal lobe and in association cortex. Data from genetic studies that suggest over-production of the 42 amino acid-length version of Aβ is a key factor in the etiology of AD have contributed to the focus of disease-modifying treatment efforts on preventing or eliminating Aβ deposition (Selkoe, 2005). Other neuropathological changes present to varying degrees in persons dying with AD include Hirano bodies, granulovacuolar degeneration and congophilic angiopathy.

Cognitive Neurorehabilitation, Second Edition: Evidence and Application, ed. Donald T. Stuss, Gordon Winocur and Ian H. Robertson. Published by Cambridge University Press. © Cambridge University Press 2008.

It is well recognized that persons who ultimately develop AD go through a stage in which they have a milder degree of cognitive impairment and do not yet meet criteria for dementia. In order to identify this early stage, various criteria for "mild cognitive impairment," or "MCI," have been proposed. A commonly used set of criteria was proposed by Petersen (Petersen et al., 1999) in which a relatively isolated memory deficit is present. Studies have suggested that persons meeting criteria for this amnestic subtype of MCI progress to dementia, usually AD, at a rate of 10–15% per year (Petersen et al., 2001). Postmortem studies of persons dying while fitting criteria for amnestic MCI have indeed confirmed that in most cases the neuropathological changes found are consistent with a transitional state between normal aging and AD (Petersen et al., 2006).

As AD progresses, synaptic elements are lost and neurons die, resulting in an overall decrease in brain size ("atrophy"). Since the 1980s a relatively selective and severe loss of neurons in the basal forebrain that employ acetylcholine (Ach) as a neurotransmitter was recognized in the disorder (Whitehouse et al., 1982). Loss of these cells that project to limbic as well as temporal, frontal and other areas of cortex is thought to be responsible for the diminished immunostaining for acetylcholinesterase (AChE), the enzyme that hydrolyzes ACh, seen in these areas. Reduced numbers of nicotinic ACh receptors in temporal cortex is a consistent finding in AD whereas significant muscarinic receptor loss is more equivocal (Nordberg, 1992). Neurofibrillary degeneration of brainstem cholinergic nuclei that project to the thalamus has also been observed (Jellinger, 1988) and decreased AChE staining has been found in the thalamus as well as the striatum (Perry et al., 1998). Dysfunction of these limbic, cortical and subcortical cholinergic systems might be expected to result in the deficits of memory, arousal and behavior that are seen in AD. Correlations between cognitive and behavioral status and cholinergic indices in autopsied brain have been explicitly sought. Dournaud et al. (1995) found a correlation between performance on the Blessed Dementia Scale and staining for choline acetyltransferase (ChAT), an enzyme involved in the synthesis of ACh, that was greatest for the parietal lobe. The cholinergic deficit in AD likely contributes to the visual hallucinations seen in the illness (Perry et al., 1990) as well as to other psychiatric manifestations of the disease such as delusions, apathy and agitation (Cummings & Kaufer, 1996).

These findings provided a target for drug development in AD. That is, enhancement of cholinergic neurotransmission by providing precursors for acetycholine, reducing the breakdown of acetycholine through drugs that inhibit AChE, or stimulation of acetycholine receptors by exogenous agents might serve to ameliorate the cognitive or behavioral symptoms of the disease. Of the five FDA-approved medications for the treatment of AD, four are thought to mediate their effects through AChE inhibition.

Glutamate is the major excitatory neurotransmitter in input pathways to the hippocampus from the entorhinal cortex and in cortico-cortical pathways and as such plays an important role in memory. These pathways have been demonstrated to be dramatically affected in AD (Hyman et al., 1987). An association between loss of brainstem serotonergic and noradrenergic neurons and depression in AD has been reported but is controversial (Syed et al., 2005; Thomas et al., 2006). Studies of losses in other neurotransmitter systems in early AD have been less consistent though most pathways studied are ultimately affected late in the disease.

In addition to helping reveal the causes of AD, knowledge gained about the genetics of this disorder also holds promise in refining the ability to treat it. One allele of the apolipoprotein E gene (the ApoE ε4 allele) has been repeatedly shown to be a risk factor for the illness (Corder et al., 1993) and a recent study of a PPAR-γ agonist yielded results suggesting that persons with AD not carrying this allele were more likely to benefit from the medication (Risner et al., 2006). Though speculative at present, this finding brings to light the possibility that certain genetic subpopulations with greater or lesser responses to a given intervention might be defined.

Frontotemporal lobar degenerations

The frontotemporal lobar degenerations (FTLDs) are a diverse group of neuropathological entities linked to similar clinical syndromes. Subtle changes in mood or personality are frequently the initial symptoms that typically worsen such that decreased initiative and deficits in judgment and social behavior ultimately result. Executive dysfunction and language deficits are typically the earliest cognitive difficulties with sparing of visual perception and memory compared to AD. Motor deficits such as ideomotor apraxia, Parkinsonism and motor neuron disease are variably present, depending in part on the nature and location of the underlying pathology. Persons may be classified according to the predominant clinical syndrome: the behavioral variant (FTD-bv) in which social behavior and personality changes are most evident, primary progressive aphasia (PPA) in which a nonfluent aphasia predominates, and semantic dementia (SD) in which there is a prevalent loss of concepts and comprehension (Neary *et al.*, 1998).

These clinical presentations were initially associated with relatively selective atrophy of the frontal and temporal lobes and later designated Pick's disease (Pick, 1892). The neuropathology has since been characterized in more detail with multiple different entities being described. Two broad pathological categories are generally accepted; those with and without neuronal inclusions that stain with antibodies to tau protein. The tau-positive group is composed of Pick's disease (PiD), corticobasal degeneration (CBD) and progressive supranuclear palsy (PSP) with the tau-negative group consisting of cases with ubiquitin-positive inclusions (frontotemporal lobar degeneration with ubiquitin-positive inclusions – FTLD-U) and those lacking distinctive pathology (dementia lacking distinctive histopathology – DLDH). All subtypes are characterized microscopically, at least to some extent, by loss of large pyramidal neurons in the frontal and temporal lobes with spongiosis, astrogliosis and ballooned neurons. Round argyrophilic neuronal inclusions, or Pick bodies, are found in the upper layers of the cingulate, parietal and temporal cortices as well as in the hippocampus and subcortical nuclei such as the putamen and the locus ceruleus in the brainstem in PiD. Though there is a statistical tendency for tau-positive pathology to be associated with PPA and Parkinsonian presentations and for tau-negative pathology to be associated with FTD-bv and SD, it is difficult to predict the underlying pathology from the clinical presentation (Forman *et al.*, 2006; Kertesz *et al.*, 2005).

Generalized synaptic loss occurs in the FTLDs as in AD (Weiler *et al.*, 1990), but otherwise the neurochemical changes appear to be distinctive. Loss of postsynaptic serotonin receptors have been demonstrated in the orbital- and medial-frontal cortex using in vivo neuroimaging techniques (Franceschi *et al.*, 2005) as well as postmortem histochemical staining. Presynaptic serotonin markers are spared (Sparks & Markesbery, 1991) though loss of neurons in the raphe nucleus has also been observed. In vivo imaging of patients with FTLD has demonstrated decreased binding of markers of presynaptic dopaminergic nerve terminals in the basal ganglia (Rinne *et al.*, 2002), possibly indicating a substrate for the Parkinsonism sometimes seen in these disorders. Loss of dopaminergic neurotransmission in the striatum has been reported using histochemical methods as have decreases in gamma amino butyric acid levels (Kanazawa *et al.*, 1988). The basal nucleus of Meynert is relatively spared in PiD (Mizukami & Kosaka, 1989).

Parkinson's disease and dementia with Lewy Bodies

Parkinsonian motor symptoms (bradykinesia, rest tremor, rigidity) may be accompanied by cognitive impairment in a number of neurodegenerative conditions and as a consequence of cerebrovascular ischemia (vascular dementia or VaD). Dementia occurs in association with dementia with Lewy bodies (DLB), is seen with increasing frequency in advancing stages of idiopathic Parkinson's disease (PD), and occurs in other neurodegenerative diseases associated with parkinsonism (e.g., multi-system atrophy and some of the FTLDs described above). Vascular dementia will be discussed below. We will focus here on DLB and the dementia associated with PD.

Dementia with Lewy bodies is thought to be the second most common cause of degenerative dementia (McKeith *et al.*, 1996). Lewy bodies are intracellular eosinophilic inclusion bodies that stain positive for ubiquitin and alpha-synuclein and are found in the cerebral cortex in at least 25% of dementia patients (Barker *et al.*, 2002). When present, they are typically associated with the motor features of Parkinsonism, visual hallucinations, and fluctuating mental status in addition to depression, apathy and REM sleep behavior disorder (Boeve *et al.*, 1998; McKeith *et al.*, 1996). Neuropathological studies of persons with DLB have demonstrated a more severe loss of cortical cholinergic input indexed by decreased levels of choline acetyltransferase (ChAT) with relatively preserved postsynaptic muscarinic receptors (Perry *et al.*, 1994). This pathology may underlie the more dramatic behavioral disturbances occurring in DLB and suggests the possibility of an enhanced response to cholinergic treatments.

Lewy bodies occurring in the substantia nigra are characteristic of idiopathic PD. Approximately 40% of patients with PD have cognitive impairment severe enough to meet criteria for dementia (Cummings, 1988). The incidence of dementia increases with the duration of PD. The classic pathology of PD that is thought to be most closely related to the motor symptoms is decreased dopaminergic innervation of the striatum due to loss of pigmented neurons in the pars compacta of the substantia nigra in the midbrain. Apathy (Ringman *et al.*, 2002) and deficits in aspects of executive function (Zgaljardic *et al.*, 2003) are consistently described in PD and it is thought that associated loss of dopaminergic neurons projecting from the midbrain to portions of the limbic or neocortical areas might also contribute to these abnormalities (Taylor *et al.*, 1986). Decreases in norepinephrine, serotonin (Mayeux *et al.*, 1984) and acetylcholine (Perry *et al.*, 1985) neurotransmission have been described

in PD as well. There is uncertainty regarding the pathological changes most closely correlated with cognitive decline in PD but a role for the cholinergic system is supported by the positive influence of AChE inhibitors in PD (Emre *et al.*, 2004).

Vascular dementia

Approximately one quarter of persons with stroke meet criteria for dementia 3 months to 3 years later (Henon *et al.*, 2001; Tatemichi *et al.*, 1993). Such cognitive impairment is likely due at least in part to ischemic brain damage. Brain damage from cerebral ischemia itself may take many forms including that due to cortical strokes, multiple subcortical lacunar strokes and diffuse white matter ischemia not always associated with clinical events. It is also difficult to rule out the simultaneous presence of AD pathology in most patients with or at-risk for cerebral ischemia. Attempts to study treatments in VaD are therefore complicated by the underlying pathologic heterogeneity of this population.

The neuropathology of vascular dementia is discussed in depth by Vinters and Carmichael in Chapter 21, this volume. For the current chapter, we should note that deficits in acetylcholinergic neurotransmission have been sought and found in VaD. The hippocampus, in which cholinergic neurotransmission is important and which plays a critical role in memory formation, is sensitive to ischemia and is atrophied in VaD (Vinters *et al.*, 2000). Furthermore, the cholinergic projections to cortex from the basal nucleus of Meynert pass through white matter areas known to be affected by subcortical ischemia (Selden *et al.*, 1998). These observations have inspired attempts to treat VaD with cholinomimetic drugs.

How do we study the effects of interventions in dementia?

- Cognitive outcome measures.
- Global outcome measures.
- General clinical trial design issues.

The development of medications for the symptoms of dementia is a relatively new field. As dementia is a multidimensional illness not only affecting cognition but also having tremendous impact on patients' psychiatric state, behavior, activities of daily living (ADLs) and overall quality of life, the specific target symptoms of an intended intervention must be defined. In addition, it is hoped that treatments might be developed that slow the progression of the disease. Such disease-modifying treatments may or may not have any detectable impact on symptoms. In this chapter we will focus on symptomatic treatment of cognition.

Regulatory agencies have stated that for an intervention to be approved for the treatment of dementia, it must have a measurable and clinically relevant impact on a specific symptom (e.g., cognition). This has been operationalized as a statistically significant difference on a test of cognition and on an assessment of overall clinical or functional status.

Many scales have been used to measure cognition in clinical trials in dementia. The Mini-Mental Status Examination (MMSE) (Folstein *et al.*, 1975) is easy to administer but lacks sensitivity and therefore is principally used currently as a screening tool for dementia severity. The cognitive subportion of the Alzheimer's Disease Assessment Scale (ADAS-Cog) is the most widely employed cognitive outcome measure in AD clinical trials (Mohs & Cohen, 1988). This is a 70-point scale that assesses orientation, memory, language, construction and praxis in which a higher score indicates poorer performance. Variability in scores tends to be limited in both very early dementia and advanced disease (i.e., ceiling and floor effects) and therefore it is of maximal utility in moderate stages of AD. As it was developed for use in AD and does not test perceptual or executive function, it is less relevant in non-AD dementias in which these areas of cognition are more likely to be affected (e.g., DLB, FTLD). Because of the floor effects seen on the ADAS-Cog, the Severe Impairment Battery (SIB) was developed and shows validity and reliability as a measure of cognitive function in more advanced AD (Panisset *et al.*, 1994). In order to study the effects of drugs on cognition in early phases of dementia such as MCI, instruments more sensitive to change in such persons are needed. A modification to the ADAS-Cog that includes a maze test, delayed recall of a word list, and a letter cancellation test has been employed in this context (Mohs *et al.*, 1997). Other batteries that include more challenging memory tests (e.g., the Buschke–Fuld Selective Reminding Test (Buschke & Fuld, 1974), more extensive screening tests (the Modified Mini-Mental Status Exam; Loewenstein *et al.*, 2000), or combinations of commonly employed neuropsychological tests (the "Neuropsychological Test Battery") are also being studied (Gilman *et al.*, 2005).

In addition to a benefit in cognition, an overall global benefit must be demonstrated in order for an anti-dementia agent to be approved by the US Food and Drug Administration (FDA). Various such scales exist but all have the common theme of a clinician surveying the patient's cognition, behavior, social function, and activities of daily living and producing a single composite measure. The Clinician's Global Impression of Change (CGIC) (Schneider *et al.*, 1997) and the Clinician's Interview Based Impression of Change with caregiver input (CIBIC-plus) (Reisberg *et al.*, 1997) are two of the most commonly used such scales. The Clinical Dementia Rating scale (CDR) (Reisberg, 1997 – see discussion by Morris therein) is a structured interview of both the patient and caregiver from which a single summary score or individual scores in different aspects of function may be derived. These global scales measure diverse aspects of patients' status and provide a measure of a clinically observable and therefore presumably relevant impact of a drug on the illness.

The most commonly employed study design for phase III studies in dementia compares scores (or change in scores) on a given test or tests between the treatment group and a control group after some period of time (typically 6 months). The control group generally consists of placebo-treated subjects though due to ethical considerations, approved and indicated treatments (e.g., acetycholinesterase inhibitors – AChEIs) are now generally permitted in all treatment arms. Another approach employed more often when testing putative disease-modifying agents is survival time to a particular endpoint (e.g., loss of ADLs, nursing home placement). The length of a study varies depending on the goal of the study. Medications expected to have an impact on symptoms may have a duration of 6–24 weeks whereas it takes longer (e.g., 24–96 weeks) to demonstrate a disease-modifying effect. The use of surrogate outcome measures of disease status (e.g., neuroimaging or biochemical markers) hold promise in reducing both the length of and number of patients required in trials of potentially disease-modifying agents (Dickerson & Sperling, 2005; Frank et al., 2003).

Review of clinical trial results

- Alzheimer's disease and MCI.
    Acetylcholinesterase inhibitors
    Memantine
- Frontotemporal lobar degenerations.
- Parkinson's disease and dementia with Lewy bodies.
- Vascular dementia.

Alzheimer's disease and MCI

Acetylcholinesterase inhibitors

Tacrine, an AChEI, was demonstrated to be effective in improving cognition and global status compared with placebo in persons with mild-to-moderate AD in a 12-week randomized double-blind, placebo-controlled trial (Farlow et al., 1992). It is now rarely used because of a high incidence of hepatoxicity and a difficult dosing regimen. Nonetheless, tacrine was the first medication to be approved by the US FDA for the treatment of AD and its development helped to establish the current paradigm by which potential drugs for AD are evaluated.

Donepezil is a reversible cholinesterase inhibitor that was shown in two randomized studies to be superior to placebo after 12 and 24 weeks at 5 and 10 mg per day in change scores on the ADAS-Cog in

persons with mild-to-moderate AD (Rogers et al., 1998a, 1998b). The difference in mean change scores between donepezil- and placebo-treated patients was approximately three points on this 70-point scale. Donepezil was also statistically superior to placebo on the CIBIC-plus, a scale of overall clinical status that is based on a structured interview with both the patient and a caregiver. In these studies discontinuation of donepezil resulted in a decline on the ADAS-Cog to a level comparable to placebo-treated subjects.

A one-year, placebo-controlled study of donepezil in AD was performed in Europe. This study provided evidence that treatment with donepezil had benefits on cognition and activities of daily living (ADLs) over this longer time interval (Winblad et al., 2001) as well. Another one-year placebo-controlled study in the USA demonstrated that treatment with donepezil significantly decreased the likelihood of progression of functional decline during this interval (Mohs et al., 2001). Longer placebo-controlled studies of AChEIs are now ethically difficult to do secondary to their demonstrated, albeit small, degree of efficacy.

Some argue that the consistent yet small benefits of donepezil on cognitive and global assessments are not clinically significant and therefore long-term treatment with donepezil is not cost-effective. Investigators in the UK set out to ascertain the long-term effects of donepezil vs. placebo on nursing home placement and progression of disability in a population of persons with dementia not as strictly defined as AD as in most prior drug studies (Courtney et al., 2004). These authors also collected cognitive and neuropsychiatric measures as secondary outcomes in addition to performing an economic evaluation. They confirmed a small benefit of donepezil on MMSE scores and on a scale measuring activities of daily living after 2 years but failed to find a significant effect on institutionalization, progression of disability, or behavioral symptoms. They concluded that treatment with donepezil was associated with higher overall costs than placebo and was therefore not cost-effective.

In order to ascertain if treatment with donepezil or an antioxidant have effects on the rate at which persons with MCI progress to dementia, a 3-year study of donepezil vs. vitamin E vs. placebo in persons with MCI was performed in which a survival to diagnosis of dementia analysis was the primary outcome (Petersen *et al.*, 2004). Donepezil increased the mean time of progression to AD for about 12 months but after 3 years' time there were no differences in the likelihood of being diagnosed with dementia between any of the three groups. Vitamin E at 2000 i.u. per day had no measurable effect on progression of disease in this study. The effects of medications on cognition and disease progression in persons with MCI is currently a growing area of research.

The efficacy of donepezil has been studied in persons in a more advanced stage of AD. In a 6-month study of persons with MMSE scores between 1 and 10 who were living in assisted care homes in Sweden, differences in SIB scores and scores on a scale of ADLs favored treatment with donepezil (Winblad *et al.*, 2006). Though statistically significant, the magnitude of the differences was smaller than the authors felt a priori to be clinically relevant. Furthermore, there was a large number of drop-outs (26%) due to adverse effects in the donepezil group.

Donepezil is approved by the FDA for both mild-to-moderate and severe AD. It is administered orally once per day. Treatment is initiated at 5 mg/day which can be increased to 10 mg/day with a decreased likelihood of side effects with slower titration. It is generally tolerated well in persons with mild to moderate disease with transient adverse effects occurring approximately 10% of the time. All AChEIs have similar side-effect profiles that consist of nausea, diarrhea, vomiting, muscle cramps, anorexia and dizziness.

Rivastigmine is a carbamate-based AChEI that binds to the esteratic site of the enzyme but dissociates slowly. Its effect is therefore described as "pseudoirreversible." It has few drug–drug interactions due to its degradation by butyryl- and acetylcholinesterase (Spencer & Noble, 1998). Rivastigmine was demonstrated to have an effect superior to placebo on changes in the ADAS-Cog, CIBIC-plus, MMSE and two scales of overall disease progression after 26 weeks in persons with mild-to-moderate AD (Corey-Bloom *et al.*, 1998). High dose (6–12 mg/day) had a greater effect than low dose (1–4 mg/day) rivastigmine on all measures with the difference between placebo and high-dose rivastigmine-treated groups on the ADAS-Cog being 5 points. The drop-out rates due to adverse effects were greater on the higher dose (29% vs. 8%) of rivastigmine. A parallel study in Europe showed similar efficacy and tolerability (Rosler *et al.*, 1999).

A study attempted to ascertain the effects of delayed treatment with rivastigmine by comparing patients that received the drug throughout the trial to those that were not treated for the initial 6 months. In an open-label extension of the 26-week pivotal trial described above, patients initially on placebo were subsequently put on rivastigmine with the dose increased as tolerated up to a maximum of 6 mg BID (Farlow *et al.*, 2000). An initial improvement in the mean ADAS-Cog score was seen in this group (mean daily dose 8.5 mg) that after 52 weeks was statistically lower than the group treated with high-dose rivastigmine (mean dose 9.4 mg) throughout. Weight loss has been associated with rivastigmine treatment and should be monitored in treated patients. Rivastigmine is administered in doses from 1.5 mg/day to 6 mg BID. The dose is advanced at 1 month intervals from 1.5 mg BID, to 3 mg BID, 4.5 mg BID and 6 mg BID. The agent should be administered with food.

Galantamine is a tertiary alkaloid that is a competitive and reversible inhibitor of AchE (Harvey, 1995). In addition to inhibiting AchE, it is thought to enhance cholinergic neurotransmission by allosterically sensitizing nicotinic receptors to the effects of acetylcholine (Maelicke *et al.*, 2001). In a study of 978 patients randomized to placebo, 8, 16, or 24 mg of galantamine per day in two divided doses, the difference in mean change in ADAS-Cog scores between the placebo and 24 mg treatment groups was 3.6 in the observed case analysis after 21 weeks of treatment ($P < 0.001$) (Tariot *et al.*, 2000). Change in CIBIC-plus ($P < 0.001$) was significantly better than placebo in the 24 mg galantamine group in this study and this group did not differ from the 18 mg/day group on these measures. In another study, patients received either placebo, 24 mg/day or 32 mg/day of galantamine (Raskind *et al.*, 2000). After 6 months the 24 mg/day and 32 mg/day galantamine groups had better mean changes in ADAS-Cog score and on the CIBIC-plus. At 6 months' time, patients on placebo were switched to 24 mg/day whereas those on 32 mg/day were switched to 24 mg/day for another 6 months. The ADAS-Cog scores initially improved in subjects formerly given placebo though at 6 months' time they scored significantly worse on this scale than subjects treated with 24 mg of galantamine throughout the study. Though initially available as a twice-a-day formulation, an extended release form of the medication that is given only once a day has been more recently released.

Despite the superiority of the AChEIs to placebo on measures of cognition in AD outlined above, clinical experience with these medications is at times disappointing. This in part reflects the small absolute effect of these medications. For instance, in a pivotal 24-week trial of donepezil, the mean difference in change in ADAS-Cog scores of approximately 150 subjects per group was approximately 3 points on this 70 point scale (Rogers *et al.*, 1998b). Other authors have pointed out methodological limitations to studies of AChEIs that might also contribute to an apparent discrepancy between trial results and clinical experience (Kaduszkiewicz *et al.*, 2005). For example, they note that in the statistical analyses of most such clinical trials, no corrections for multiple comparisons are made, intention to treat analyses are often not performed, and that the Last Observation Carried Forward (LOCF) analysis that is frequently used is inappropriate for a progressive illness. In the LOCF technique, the last data point prior to a subject's dropping out of the study is used in the final analysis. As drop-outs tend to be more common in the drug-treated group and it can be assumed that some degree of worsening will occur over time in all

subjects, carrying this data point forwards biases results in favor of the intervention being tested.

A common misinterpretation of study results is that AChEIs necessarily improve memory. However, the cognitive outcome measures typically used in AD clinical trials measure general cognitive function rather than memory alone. Of the 70 points in the ADAS-Cog for example, 27 are related to memory with the rest of the points being distributed among other cognitive realms. Improvements in cognition seen in response to treatment AChEIs may reflect enhanced levels of arousal rather than improved memory per se.

Memantine

Memantine is a moderate-affinity uncompetitive N-methyl-D-aspartate (NMDA) receptor blocker that has been used in Germany since 1982 for symptomatic treatment of Parkinson's disease and other neurological conditions. It was subsequently studied in AD and was approved by the US FDA for use in moderate-to-severe AD in late 2003.

The efficacy of memantine in a nursing home population of persons with severe dementia (MMSE scores <10) was studied (Winblad & Poritis, 1999). In this 12-week study, in which 49% of patients were diagnosed with AD and 51% with vascular dementia, memantine was found to improve CGIC scores significantly more often than placebo (73% vs. 45%). In a subsequent placebo-controlled 28 week study of memantine performed in moderate-to-severe AD patients (mean MMSE score = 8), the SIB was used as the cognitive outcome measure. The CIBIC-plus, Alzheimer's Disease Cooperative Study – Activities of Daily Living scale (ADCS-ADLsev) scale and the Functional Assessment STaging scale (FAST) were also employed. Memantine was superior to placebo on the SIB in both the observed case analysis and the LOCF analysis. In a randomized, placebo-controlled 24-week add-on study of memantine in patients with moderate-to-severe AD already on stable doses of donepezil, those treated with memantine did better on the SIB and the

ADCS-ADLsev (primary outcome measures) as well as on the CIBIC-Plus, and other secondary outcome measures in the LOCF analysis (Tariot *et al.*, 2004).

Memantine, both alone and in combination with donepezil, therefore has demonstrated efficacy on cognition and other outcome measures in moderate-to-severe AD. Though it would be expected that "neuroprotectant" NMDA receptor antagonists should exert their effect on disease progression over the long run, experience has been that there can be an immediate, if modest, improvement in treated patients' status, bringing into question the relevant mechanism of action of the drug. Memantine is very well tolerated with adverse events occurring with essentially equal frequency in the placebo group in controlled trials. Clinical experience with the drug, however, has shown that reversible worsening of agitation and somnolence may occur. Treatment with memantine is begun at 5 mg/day and titrated upward to 10 mg/BID.

Frontemporal lobar degenerations

There have been few randomized, placebo-controlled studies of pharmacological interventions in the FTLDs in part due to the relative rarity of the condition. There are, however, multiple small open-label studies that have been published in which the effects of various interventions on the behavioral symptoms of the disorder have been described. In light of their tolerability and the serotonergic deficit described in FTLD, the selective serotonin reuptake inhibitors (SSRIs) are the most commonly studied. Anecdotal experience and open-label studies suggest improvement in behavior with paroxetine (Moretti *et al.*, 2003) and fluvoxamine (Ikeda *et al.*, 2004). However, a randomized, placebo-controlled, double-blind study of paroxetine in ten patients suggested worsening in behavior as measured with the Neuropsychiatric Inventory (NPI) as well as in cognition (Deakin *et al.*, 2004). Trazodone, a weak SSRI, has been studied in a randomized, double-blind, placebo-controlled, cross-over study in 26 FTLD patients (Lebert *et al.*, 2004). Favorable improvements in NPI scores were observed though

no change in MMSE score was seen and adverse effects were common.

Despite the lack of a significant cholinergic deficit in FTLD, treatment of the condition with the cholinesterase inhibitors has been attempted. In the face of anecdotal evidence to the contrary, a benefit of rivastigmine on the behavioral symptoms in 20 patients with FTLD was observed in an open-label trial (Moretti *et al.*, 2004). No improvement in cognition was seen in this study. In fact, there is minimal evidence for any medication having beneficial effects on cognition in FTLD. This may be due in part to the conventional use of cognitive outcome measures such as the ADAS-Cog and MMSE instruments which are less sensitive to the deficits in executive function most characteristic of FTLD.

Parkinson's disease and dementia with Lewy bodies

In light of the cholinergic deficit seen in DLB described above, AChEIs have been studied as a therapeutic intervention. The efficacy of rivastigmine in patients with clinically defined DLB was investigated in a multinational, randomized, double-blind, placebo-controlled study in which cognition measured with a computerized battery and behavioral abnormalities as measured with the NPI were the primary outcome measures (McKeith *et al.*, 2000). After 20 weeks, patients treated with rivastigmine at a maximum mean dose of 9.4 mg performed better on the cognitive assessments. Rivastigmine also was superior to placebo with regard to reduced severity of apathy, anxiety, delusions, hallucinations, and aberrant motor behavior but the CGIC was not significantly different between groups.

A 24-week randomized, placebo-controlled study of rivastigmine in patients with idiopathic PD was performed using the ADAS-Cog and CIBIC-plus as primary outcome measures (Emre *et al.*, 2004); 541 subjects were randomized of which 410 completed the study. Mean dose of rivastigmine was 8.3 mg in the 263 active treatment patients that completed the study. In the LOCF analysis, persons treated with rivastigmine had significantly superior scores on the

ADAS-Cog and CIBIC-plus as well as on the secondary outcome measures of the ADCS-ADL, NPI, and the cognitive tests (MMSE, computerized battery, verbal fluency and clock drawing). Adverse effects paralleled those seen in other studies of rivastigmine though a higher rate of worsened tremor occurred in treated patients (10.2% vs. 3.9%). The results of this study suggest that rivastigmine and perhaps other cholinesterase inhibitors have benefits in cognition in idiopathic PD though may in some cases worsen tremor. Rivastigmine is approved by the FDA for use in dementia in the context of idiopathic PD.

Vascular dementia

In a 24-week study of donepezil 5 mg/day or 10 mg/day vs. placebo involving 616 subjects with probable (76%) or possible (24%) VaD, treatment with either dose of donepezil was associated with better scores on the ADAS-Cog and the CIBIC-plus (Wilkinson et al., 2003). The placebo-treated group did not decline on these measures, and therefore the difference was accounted for by an improvement of about 2 points on the ADAS-Cog in the donepezil 10 mg/day group. Statistically significant improvement was seen on the MMSE (approximately 1 point) and the CDR. There were no major differences in efficacy between the donepezil 5 mg and 10 mg group with more adverse effects in the 10 mg group suggesting that the lower dose of donepezil should be considered in patients with VaD. A large study of galantamine in VaD and mixed AD-VaD yielded similar results (Erkinjuntti et al., 2002). These studies provide evidence for efficacy of cholinesterase inhibitors in VaD though perhaps of a smaller degree than is seen in AD. Whether the response to cholinesterase inhibitors is due to a deficit from ischemic damage or to concurrent AD pathology is currently an unresolved issue.

Ginkgo biloba is a plant extract used in Chinese herbal medicine for a variety of ailments. It is approved in Germany for the treatment of dementia. Its mechanism of action is unknown though it has antioxidant and platelet-inhibiting properties.

In a one-year study of 309 persons with mild-to-moderate dementia (76% with AD, 24% characterized as having multi-infarct dementia), small but statistically significant differences favoring ginkgo biloba were seen on the ADAS-Cog (1.5 points) and the Geriatric Evaluation by Relative's Rating Instrument (GERRI) but not on the CGIC (Le Bars et al., 1997). The effect of ginkgo biloba is small and its use in AD is not widely recommended, in part due to its action on platelet aggregation. Its utility preventing VaD and AD is currently being evaluated in a large study (DeKosky et al., 2006).

Conclusions

Because of the aging of the population, tremendous effort is going into developing pharmacologic interventions to improve cognition in persons with dementia. Alzheimer's disease is the most common form of dementia and has received the most attention. Drugs from two classes (AChEIs and NMDA antagonists) have been approved in the USA for treatment of AD. Statistical superiority of these medications over placebo in cognitive and global outcome measures has been shown consistently in AD and preliminarily in VaD and dementia associated with Parkinsonism. To date, an intervention that improves cognition in persons with FTLD has not been identified. The effects of AChEIs and memantine, though consistent, are small in magnitude and better treatments are needed.

Declaration of interest

Dr. Ringman has received honoraria for speaking on behalf of Pfizer, Eisai, Astra-Zenaca, and Novartis Pharmaceuticals as well as Forest Laboratories. He has also received compensation for serving on an advisory board for Avanir Pharmaceuticals. Total compensation from each of these companies totals less than $10000.

Dr. Cummings has provided consulation to Eisai, Janssen, Forest, Lundbeck, Novartis, Merz, and Pfizer pharmaceutical companies relevant to this chapter. Total annual compensation from each of these companies totals less than $10000.

REFERENCES

Alzheimer, A., Stelzmann, H., Schnitzlein, N., & Murtagh, F. R. (1995). An English translation of Alzheimer's 1907 paper, "über eine eigenartige erkankung der hirnrinde". *Clinical Anatomy*, **8**, 429–431.

Barker, W. W., Luis, C. A., Kashuba, A. *et al.* (2002). Relative frequencies of Alzheimer disease, Lewy body, vascular and frontotemporal dememtia, and hippocampal sclerosis in the State of Florida Brain Bank. *Alzheimer Disease and Associated Disorders*, **16**, 203–212.

Boeve, B. F., Silber, M. H., Ferman, T. J. *et al.* (1998). REM sleep behaviour disorder and degenerative dementia: an association likely reflecting Lewy body disease. *Neurology*, **51**, 363–370.

Buschke, H., & Fuld, P. A. (1974). Evaluating storage, retention, and retrieval in disordered memory and learning. *Neurology*, **24**, 1019–1025.

Corder, E. H., Saunders, A. M., Strittmatter, W. J. *et al.* (1993). Gene dose of apolipoprotein E type 4 allele and the risk of Alzheimer's disease in late onset families. *Science*, **261**, 921–923.

Corey-Bloom, J., Anand, R., & Veach, J. (1998). A randomized trial evaluating the efficacy and safety of ENA 713 (rivastigmine tartrate), a new acetylcholinesterase inhibitor, in patients with mild to moderately severe Alzheimer's disease. *International Journal of Geriatric Psychiatry*, **1**, 55–65.

Courtney, C., Farrell, D., Gray, R. *et al.* (2004). Long-term donepezil treatment in 565 patients with Alzheimer's disease (AD2000): randomized double-blind trial. *Lancet*, **363**, 2105–2115.

Cummings, J. L. (1988). The dementias of Parkinson's disease: prevalence, characteristics, neurobiology, and comparison with dementia of the Alzheimer type. *European Neurology*, **28**, *Suppl. 1*, 15–23.

Cummings, J. L., & Kaufer, D. (1996). Neuropsychiatric aspects of Alzheimer's disease: the cholinergic hypothesis revisited. *Neurology*, **47**, 876–883.

Deakin, J. B., Rahman, S., Nestor, P. J., Hodges, J. R., & Sahakian, B. J. (2004). Paroxetine does not improve symptoms and impairs cognition in frontotemporal dementia: a double-blind randomized controlled trial. *Psychopharmacology*, **172**, 400–408.

DeKosky, S. T., Fitzpatrick, A., Ives, D. G. *et al.* (2006). The Ginkgo Evaluation of Memory (GEM) study: design and baseline data of a randomized trial of Ginkgo biloba extract in prevention of dementia. *Contemporary Clinical Trials*, **27**, 238–253.

Dickerson, B. C., & Sperling, R. A. (2005). Neuroimaging biomarkers for clinical trials of disease-modifying therapies in Alzheimer's disease. *NeuroRx*, **2**, 348–360.

Dournaud, P., Delaere, P., Hauw, J. J., & Epelbaum, J. (1995). Differential correlation between neurochemical deficits, neuropathology, and cognitive status in Alzheimer's disease. *Neurobiology of Aging*, **16**, 817–823.

Emre, M., Aarsland, D., Albanese, A. *et al.* (2004). Rivastigmine for dementia associated with Parkinson's disease. *New England Journal of Medicine*, **351**, 2509–2518.

Erkinjuntti, T., Kurz, A., Gauthier, S. *et al.* (2002). Efficacy of galantamine in probable vascular dementia and Alzheimer's disease combined with cerebrovascular disease: a randomized trial. *Lancet*, **359**, 1283–1290.

Farlow, M., Gracon, S. I., Hershey, L. A. *et al.* (1992). A controlled trial of tacrine in Alzheimer's disease. *Journal of the American Medical Association*, **268**, 2523–2529.

Farlow, M., Anand, R., Messina, J., Hartman, R., & Veach, J. (2000). A 52-week study of the efficacy of rivastigmine in patients with mild to moderately severe Alzheimer's disease. *European Neurology*, **44**, 236–241.

Folstein, M. F., Folstein, S. E., & McHugh, P. R. (1975). "Mini-Mental State": a practical method for grading the cognitive state of patients for the clinician. *Journal of Psychiatric Research*, **12**, 189–198.

Forman, M. S., Farmer, J., Johnson, J. K. *et al.* (2006). Frontotemporal dementia: clinicopathological correlations. *Annals of Neurology*, **59**, 952–962.

Franceschi, M., Anchisi, D., Pelati, O. *et al.* (2005). Glucose metabolism and serotonin receptors in the frontotemporal lobe degeneration. *Annals of Neurology*, **57**, 216–225.

Frank, R. A., Galasko, D., Hampel, H. *et al.* (2003). Biological markers for therapeutic trials in Alzheimer's disease. Proceedings of the biological markers working group; NIA initiative on neuroimaging in Alzheimer's disease. *Neurobiology of Aging*, **24**, 521–536.

Galton, C. J., Patterson, K., Xuereb, J. H., & Hodges, J. R. (2000). Atypical and typical presentations of Alzheimer's disease: a clinical, neuropsychological, neuroimaging and pathological study of 13 cases. *Brain*, **123**, 484–498.

Gilman, S., Koller, M., Black, R. S. *et al.* (2005). Clinical effects of A[beta] immunization (AN1792) in patients with AD in an interrupted trial. *Neurology*, **64**, 1553–1562.

Gómez-Isla, T., Hollister, R., West, H. *et al.* (1997). Neuronal loss correlates with but exceeds neurofibrillary tangles in Alzheimer's disease. *Annals of Neurology*, **41**, 17–24.

Harvey, A. L. (1995). The pharmacology of galanthamine and its analogues. *Pharmacology and Therapeutics*, **68**, 113–128.

Henon, H., Durieu, I., Guerouaou, D. *et al.* (2001). Poststroke dementia: incidence and relationship to pre-stroke cognitive decline. *Neurology*, **57**, 1216–1222.

Hyman, B. T., Van Hoesen, G. W., & Damasio, A. R. (1987). Alzheimer's disease: glutamate depletion in the hippo-campal perforant pathway zone. *Annals of Neurology*, **22**, 37–40.

Ikeda, M., Shigenobu, K., Fukuhara, R. *et al.* (2004). Efficacy of fluoxamine as a treatment for behavioural symptoms in frontotemporal lobar degeneration patients. *Dementia and Geriatric Cognitive Disorders*, **17**, 117–121.

Jellinger, K. (1988). The pedunculopontine nucleus in Parkinson's disease, progressive supranuclear palsy and Alzheimer's disease. *Journal of Neurology, Neurosurgery, and Psychiatry*, **51**, 540–543.

Kaduszkiewicz, H., Zimmerman, T., Beck-Bornholdt, H.-P., & van den Bussche, H. (2005). Cholinesterase inhibitors for patients with Alzheimer's disease: systematic review of randomised clinical trials. *British Medical Journal*, **331**, 321–323.

Kanazawa, I., Kwak, S., Sasaki, H. *et al.* (1988). Studies on neurotransmitter markers of the basal ganglia in Pick's disease, with special reference to dopamine reduction. *Journal of the Neurological Sciences*, **83**, 63–74.

Kertesz, A., McMonagle, P., Blair, M., Davidson, W., & Munoz, D. G. (2005). The evolution and pathology of frontotemporal dementia. *Brain*, **128**, 1996–2005.

Le Bars, P. L., Katz, M. M., Berman, N. *et al.* (1997). A placebo-controlled, double-blind, randomized trial of an extract of Ginkgo biloba for dementia. *Journal of the American Medical Association*, **278**, 1327–1332.

Lebert, F., Stekke, W., Hasenbroekx, C., & Pasquier, F. (2004). Frontotemporal dementia: a randomized, con-trolled trial with trazodone. *Dementia and Geriatric Cognitive Disorders*, **17**, 355–359.

Loewenstein, D. A., Barker, W. W., Harwood, D. G. *et al.* (2000). Utility of a modified Mini-Mental State Examination with extended delayed recall in screening for mild cognitive impairment and dementia among community dwelling elders. *International Journal of Geriatric Psychiatry*, **15**, 434–440.

Maelicke, A., Samochocki, M., Jostock, R. *et al.* (2001). Allosteric sensitization of nicotinic receptors by galant-amine, a new treatment strategy for Alzheimer's disease. *Biological Psychiatry*, **49**, 279–288.

Mayeux, R., Stern, Y., Cote, L., & Williams, J. B. W. (1984). Altered serotonin metabolism in depressed patients with Parkinson's disease. *Neurology*, **34**, 642–646.

McKeith, I. G., Galasko, D., Kosaka, K. *et al.* (1996). Consensus guidelines for the clinical and pathologic diagnosis of dementia with Lewy bodies (DLB): report of the consortium on DLB international workshop. *Neurology*, **47**, 1113–1124.

McKeith, I., Del Ser, T., Spano, P. *et al.* (2000). Efficacy of rivastigmine in dementia with Lewy bodies: a random-ized, double-blind, placebo-controlled international study. *Lancet*, **356**, 2031–2036.

Mendez, M. F., Mastri, A. R., Sung, J. H., & Frey, W. H. I. (1992). Clinically diagnosed Alzheimer disease: neuro-pathologic findings in 650 cases. *Alzheimer Disease and Associated Disorders*, **6**, 35–43.

Mizukami, K., & Kosaka, K. (1989). Neuropathological study on the nucleus basalis of Meynert in Pick's disease. *Acta Neuropathologica*, **78**, 52–56.

Mohs, R. C., & Cohen, L. (1988). Alzheimer's Disease Assessment Scale (ADAS). *Psychopharmacology Bulletin*, **24**, 627–628.

Mohs, R. C., Knopman, D., Petersen, R. C. *et al.* (1997). Development of cognitive instruments for use in clinical trials of antidementia drugs: additions to the Alzheimer's disease assessment scale that broaden its scope. *Alzheimer Disease and Associated Disorders*, **11**, *Suppl. 2*, S13–S21.

Mohs, R. C., Doody, R. S., Morris, J. C. *et al.* (2001). A 1-year, placebo-controlled preservation of function survival study of donepezil in AD patients. *Neurology*, **57**, 481–488.

Moretti, R., Torre, P., Antonello, R. M., Cazzato, G., & Bava, A. (2003). Frontotemporal dementia: paroxetine as a possible treatment of behaviour symptoms: a random-ized, controlled, open 14-month study. *European Neurology*, **49**, 13–19.

Moretti, R., Torre, P., Antonello, R. M. *et al.* (2004). Rivastigmine in frontotemporal dementia: an open-label study. *Drugs and Aging*, **21**, 931–937.

Neary, D., Snowden, J. S., Gustafson, L. *et al.* (1998). Frontotemporal lobar degeneration. A consensus on clinical diagnostic criteria. *Neurology*, **51**, 1546–1554.

Nordberg, A. (1992). Neuroreceptor changes in Alzheimer disease. *Cerebrovascular and Brain Metabolism Reviews*, **4**, 303–328.

Panisset, M., Roudier, M., Saxton, J., & Boller, F. (1994). Severe impairment battery: a neuropsychological test for severely demented patients. *Archives of Neurology*, **51**, 41–45.

Perry, E. K., Curtis, M., Dick, D. J. *et al.* (1985). Cholinergic correlates of cognitive impairment in Parkinson's disease: comparisons with Alzheimer's disease. *Journal of Neurology, Neurosurgery, and Psychiatry*, **48**, 413–421.

Perry, E. K., Kerwin, J., Perry, R. H., Blessed, G., & Fairbairn, A. F. (1990). Visual hallucinations and the cholinergic system in dementia. *Journal of Neurology, Neurosurgery, and Psychiatry*, **53**, 88.

Perry, E. K., Haroutunian, V., Davis, K. L. *et al.* (1994). Neocortical cholinergic activities differentiate Lewy body dementia from classical Alzheimer's disease. *NeuroReport*, **5**, 747–749.

Perry, E., Court, J., Goodchild, R. *et al.* (1998). Clinical neurochemistry: developments in dementia research based on brain bank material. *Journal of Neural Transmission*, **105**, 915–933.

Petersen, R. C., Smith, G. E., Waring, S. C. *et al.* (1999). Mild cognitive impairment: clinical characterization and outcome. *Archives of Neurology*, **56**, 303–308.

Petersen, R. C., Stevens, J. C., Ganguli, M. *et al.* (2001). Practice parameter: Early detection of dementia: Mild cognitive impairment (an evidence-based review): report of the Quality Standards Subcommittee of the American Academy of Neurology. *Neurology*, **56**, 1133–1142.

Petersen, R., Grundman, M., Thomas, R., & Thal, L. J. (2004). Donepezil and vitamin E as treatments for mild cognitive impairment. *Program and Abstracts of the 9th International Conference on Alzheimer's Disease and Related Disorders, July 17–22*, Philadelphia, Pennsylvania.

Petersen, R. C., Parisi, J. E., Dickson, D. W. *et al.* (2006). Neuropathologic features of amnestic mild cognitive impairment. *Archives of Neurology*, **63**, 665–672.

Pick, A. (1892). Über die beziehungen der senilen hirnatrophie zur aphasie. *Prager Medicinische Wochenschrift*, **17**, 165–167.

Raskind, M. A., Peskind, E. R., Wessel, T., & Yuan, W. (2000). Galantamine in AD: a 6-month randomized, placebo-controlled trial with a 6-month extension. *Neurology*, **54**, 2261–2268.

Reisberg, B. (1997). Functional and global evaluations: Discussion. *International Psychogeriatrics*, **9**, *Suppl. 1*, 177–178.

Reisberg, B., Schneider, L., Doody, R. *et al.* (1997). Clinical global measures of dementia: position paper from the International Working Group on Harmonization of Dementia Drug Guidelines. *Alzheimer Disease and Associated Disorders*, **11**, *Suppl. 3*, 8–18.

Ringman, J. M., Diaz-Olavarrieta, C., Rodriguez, Y., Fairbanks, L., & Cummings, J. L. (2002). The prevalence and correlates of neuropsychiatric symptoms in a population with Parkinson's disease in Mexico. *Neuropsychiatry, Neuropsychology and Behavioural Neurology*, **15**, 99–105.

Rinne, J. O., Laine, M., Kaasinen, V. *et al.* (2002). Striatal dopamine transporter and extrapyramidal symptoms in frontotemporal dementia. *Neurology*, **58**, 1489–1493.

Risner, M. E., Saunders, A. M., Altman, J. F. B. *et al.* (2006). Efficacy of rosiglitazone in a genetically defined population with mild-to-moderate Alzheimer's disease. *Pharmacogenomics Journal*, **6**, 246–254.

Rogers, S. L., Doody, R. S., Mohs, R. C., & Friedhoff, L. T. (1998a). Donepezil improves cognition and global function in Alzheimer disease. *Archives of Internal Medicine*, **158**, 1021–1031.

Rogers, S. L., Farlow, M. R., Doody, R. S., Mohs, R., & Friedhoff, L. T. (1998b). A 24-week, double-blind, placebo-controlled trial of donepezil in patients with Alzheimer's disease. *Neurology*, **50**, 136–145.

Rosler, M., Anand, R., Cicin-Sain, A. *et al.* (1999). Efficacy and safety of revastigmine in patients with Alzheimer's disease: international randomised controlled trial. *British Medical Journal*, **318**, 633–638.

Schneider, L. S., Olin, J. T., Doody, R. S. *et al.* (1997). Validity and reliability of the Alzheimer's Disease cooperative study: clinical global impression of change. *Alzheimer Disease and Associated Disorders*, **11**, *Suppl. 2*, S22–S32.

Selden, N. R., Gitelman, D. R., Salamon-Murayama, N., Parrish, T. B., & Mesulam, M.-M. (1998). Trajectories of cholinergic pathways within the cerebral hemispheres of the human brain. *Brain*, **121**, 2249–2257.

Selkoe, D. J. (2005). Defining molecular targets to prevent Alzheimer disease. *Archives of Neurology*, **62**, 192–195.

Sparks, D. L., & Markesbery, W. R. (1991). Altered serotonergic and cholinergic synaptic markers in Pick's disease. *Archives of Neurology*, **48**, 796–799.

Spencer, C. M., & Noble, S. (1998). Rivastigmine: a review of its use in Alzheimer's disease. *Drugs and Aging*, **13**, 391–411.

Syed, A., Chatfield, M., Matthews, F. *et al.* (2005). Depression in the elderly: pathological study of raphe and locus ceruleus. *Neuropathology and Applied Neurobiology*, **31**, 405–413.

Tariot, P. N., Solomon, P. R., Morris, J. C. *et al.* (2000). A 5-month, randomized, placebo-controlled trial of galantamine. *Neurology*, **54**, 2269–2276.

Tariot, P. N., Farlow, M. R., Grossberg, G. T. *et al.* (2004). Memantine treatment in patients with moderate to severe Alzheimer disease already receiving donepezil: a randomized controlled trial. *Journal of the American Medical Association*, **291**, 317–324.

Tatemichi, T. K., Desmond, D. W., Paik, M. *et al.* (1993). Clinical determinants of dementia related to stroke. *Annals of Neurology*, **33**, 568–575.

Taylor, A. E., Saint-Cyr, J. A., & Lang, A. E. (1986). Frontal lobe dysfunction in Parkinson's disease: the cortical focus of neostriatal outflow. *Brain*, **109**, 845–883.

Thomas, A. J., Hendriksen, M., Piggott, M. *et al.* (2006). A study of the serotonin transporter in the prefrontal cortex in late-life depression and Alzheimer's disease with and without depression. *Neuropathology and Applied Neurobiology*, **32**, 296–303.

Vinters, H. V., Ellis, W. G., Zarow, C. *et al.* (2000). Neuropathologic substrates of ischemic vascular dementia. *Journal of Neuropathology and Experimental Neurology*, **59**, 931–945.

Weiler, R., Lassmann, H., Fischer, P., Jellinger, K., & Winkler, H. (1990). A high ratio of chromogranin A to synaptin/synaptophysin is a common feature of brains in Alzheimer and Pick disease. *FEBS Letters*, **263**, 337–339.

Whitehouse, P. J., Price, D. L., Struble, R. G. *et al.* (1982). Alzheimer's disease and senile dementia: loss of neurons in the basal forebrain. *Science*, **215**, 1237–1239.

Wilkinson, D., Doody, R., Helme, R. *et al.* (2003). Donepezil in vascular dementia: a randomized, placebo-controlled study. *Neurology*, **61**, 479–486.

Winblad, B., & Poritis, N. (1999). Memantine in severe dementia: results of the M-BEST Study (benefit and efficacy in severely demented patients during treatment with memantine). *International Journal of Geriatric Psychiatry*, **14**, 135–146.

Winblad, B., Engedal, K., Soininen, H. *et al.* (2001). A 1-year, randomized, placebo-controlled study of donepezil in patients with mild to moderate AD. *Neurology*, **57**, 489–495.

Winblad, B., Kilander, L., Eriksson, S. *et al.* (2006). Donepezil in patients with severe Alzheimer's disease: double-blind, parallel-group, placebo-controlled study. *Lancet*, **367**, 1057–1065.

Zgaljardic, D. J., Borod, J. C., Foldi, N. S., & Mattis, P. (2003). A review of the cognitive and behavioural sequelae of Parkinson's disease: relationship to frontostriatal circuitry. *Cognitive and Behavioural Neurology*, **16**, 193–210.

20

Neurogenesis-based regeneration and cognitive therapy in the adult brain. Is it feasible?

J. Martin Wojtowicz

Adult neurogenesis

- Adult brain can generate new neurons (neurogenesis). The process is well defined in terms of specific phases of cell growth but still not completely understood as far as its regulation and functional significance are concerned.
- "Use it or lose it" rule applies to neurogenesis.
- Neurogenesis is commonly observed in hippocampus but is also being found in other brain regions.

A dogma that neurons in adult mammalian brain cannot regenerate is no longer true. Persistent reports dating back as far as 1962 suggested that some cells in adult brain can divide through mitosis and grow as neurons. Joseph Altman and colleagues reported that incorporation of a DNA-synthesis marker [3]H Thymidine did in fact occur in the adult rodent hippocampus and were first to propose that adult neurogenesis is a bona fide phenomenon (Altman, 1962; Altman & Das, 1965, 1967). Although suggestive, these studies were hampered by lack of convincing demonstration that new-born cells were properly matured and functionally relevant neurons. It was not even clear if they were neurons at all. This was in contrast to the common acceptance of proliferation of glial cells within the adult brain, especially after injury. The renaissance in the field became possible with the availability of the novel DNA-synthesis marker bromodeoxyuridine (BrdU) (Gratzner, 1982). Bromodeoxyuridine appears to be more sensitive and selective than [3]H Thymidine and allows for colabeling with specific antibodies raised against proteins that are expressed in neurons at specific developmental stages. By now a catalogue of markers is available that can be used to chart the neuronal development as cells divide, differentiate, migrate and mature (Figure 20.1).

The progression from stem cell proliferation to maturation and functional integration has been documented with increasing accuracy by numerous studies. Perhaps the most informative are those that used pulse-labeling with BrdU and tracked cell maturation by measuring morphological parameters and marker expression at different stages. Figure 20.2 illustrates progression from the undifferentiated precursor cells to mature phenotype (Espósito et al., 2005; Kempermann et al., 2004; McDonald & Wojtowicz, 2005).

A remarkable feature of this process is that it follows the same pattern in both young and mature animals with the main difference being the number of cells that are produced. It is not yet clear if this is due to the depletion of the precursor cells with age or to a change in the microenvironment that grows more hostile to cell division and neuronal differentiation. In either case, extrapolation of these results to other ages predicts that the number of new neurons present at any given age declines exponentially during the animal's lifespan. This model fits well with experimental observations of the total number of immature neurons per dentate gyrus.

The model and the data illustrate a dramatic decline in neurogenic capacity of the hippocampus

Cognitive Neurorehabilitation, Second Edition: Evidence and Application, ed. Donald T. Stuss, Gordon Winocur and Ian H. Robertson. Published by Cambridge University Press. © Cambridge University Press 2008.

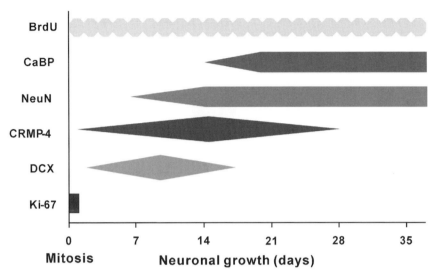

Figure 20.1. Markers of neurogenesis. The age and extent of growth of a newly born neuron can be measured by double-labeling with bromodeoxyuridine (BrdU), a substance that is incorporated into the DNA during cell division, and with specific antibodies for one of the proteins expressed during cell development. Bromodeoxyuridine stays in the cell from day one until staining is done. The other markers are expressed transiently according to the time scale shown in the graph. Doublecortin (DCX) and CRMP-4 are immature neuronal markers. Neuron specific nuclear protein (NeuN) and CaBP are mature neuronal markers. CRMP-4 – collapsin response mediator protein; Ki-67 – a nuclear protein expressed during cell division; CaBP – calcium binding protein.

by middle age in laboratory animals. However, a much slower decline can be seen in those species of rodents that live in their natural habitat in the wild (Barker *et al.*, 2005). For example, a comparison of the decline in the number of young neurons produced in lab rats vs. wild squirrels suggests that living conditions may dictate the rate of decline of neurogenesis with age. Indeed, numerous studies on laboratory rodents, such as mice and rats, have demonstrated that improved living conditions, so-called enriched environment, can enhance neurogenesis (Olson *et al.*, 2006). Even more significantly, the enhanced neurogenesis occurs in parallel with enhanced ability to perform various behavioral tasks involving learning and memory (van Praag *et al.*, 1999). It is still uncertain whether there is a causal relationship between enhanced memory and neurogenesis, since so many other physiological

functions are changed by improved living conditions (Meshi *et al.*, 2006). Some hippocampus-dependent learning tasks, such as contextual learning, are very sensitive to changes in neurogenesis while others, e.g., spatial navigation, are not (Leuner *et al.*, 2006). Nevertheless, the maintenance of the normal young cell population within the dentate gyrus would appear to be a requirement for normal functioning of the hippocampal formation as a whole. A particularly important issue may be restoration of neurogenesis after brain injury or disease. The presence of an innate homeostatic mechanism maintaining the appropriate rate of neurogenesis is suggested by spontaneous enhancement of neuronal production after brain ischemia such as during stroke (Macas *et al.*, 2006; Wang *et al.*, 2005).

As more laboratories begin to study adult neurogenesis and the methodology evolves, the

Time line of neurogenesis

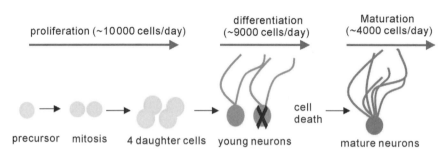

proliferation (~10000 cells/day)   differentiation (~9000 cells/day)   Maturation (~4000 cells/day)

precursor   mitosis   4 daughter cells   young neurons   cell death   mature neurons

1 day   2 weeks   4 weeks

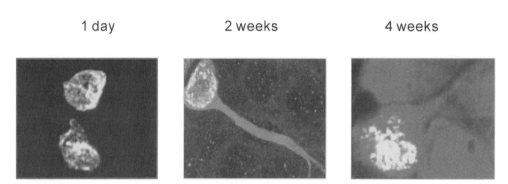

Figure 20.2. (This figure is reproduced in the color plate section at the front of this volume.) Stages of neurogenesis. Neurogenesis progresses from proliferation (division of precursors into several daughter cells) to differentiation (growth of neurites), cell attrition (presumably only the synaptically active and functional neurons survive), and maturation when neurons form a complete dendritic tree and are incorporated into the hippocampal circuitry. In a juvenile rat approximately 9000 cells are produced at the proliferation stage every 24 hours per dentate gyrus. However, only 4000 survive to the maturation stage. The complete process takes four weeks. Typical labeled cells seen at each stage of development are illustrated. The yellow stain represents bromodeoxyuridine (BrdU) within the nuclei of two cells that had just divided one day before. The yellow nuclear stain combined with the green cytoplasmic marker shows co-presence of BrdU and doublecortin in 1–2-week-old neurons. The red marker, calbindin, together with BrdU indicates the state of neuronal maturation at 4 weeks after the cell birth.

phenomenon is being detected in more and more brain regions. It is now established that cells born in anterior brain regions adjacent to the lateral ventricles migrate to the olfactory bulb and become neurons (Lledo *et al.* 2006; Macas *et al.*, 2006). In the hypothalamus, progenitor cells derived from the wall of the third ventricle differentiate into glia and neurons (Kokoeva *et al.*, 2005). The striatum can also acquire new neurons from the subventricular zone although in this case additional trophic support is needed (Chmielnicki *et al.*, 2004). Some regions of the cortex and the striatum can give rise to differentiated, apparently GABA-ergic neurons (Dayer *et al.*, 2005). Aside from the proven ongoing neurogenesis in the adult hippocampus, the emerging picture is that central nervous system (CNS) tissue has the potential for regeneration even though under normal conditions this regeneration is only marginally effective in terms of functional recovery. The problem appears to be in providing the appropriate tissue environment that would nurture the existing neuronal precursors to grow up as neurons. The only brain regions that provide such favorable environments are the hippocampus and the olfactory bulb. Tissue samples from the subventricular zone of the forebrain ventricles are a rich source of multipotent neural stem cells. The brain white matter gives rise to astroglia and oligodendrocytes, but retains multilineage competence and can produce neurons in culture (Goldman, 2005).

Thus, contrary to the previously held view that brain tissue does not regenerate, recent studies show that the CNS, including the brain, is a potently neurogenic tissue, albeit neurogenesis is usually limited by the local cellular microenvironment. These studies set the stage for investigation of the regenerative potential of the adult brain. Several such lines of investigation are being pursued, all involving some type of insult or injury to the brain.

Neurogenesis and cognition

- Neurogenesis is essential for some types of learning.
- Neurogenesis is stimulated by hippocampal activity.
- Neurogenesis is use-dependent.

Ever since hippocampal neurogenesis was discovered in the 1960s and re-discovered in the 1990s, its involvement in memory has been postulated in theory and probed experimentally. The idea that new-born neurons pass through a critical period during the second week of their development and can be rescued by a hippocampus-dependent learning task was originally proposed by Gould and colleagues (Gould *et al.*, 1999a). Although not universally accepted, this concept is still under investigation and remains a working hypothesis for ongoing experimental work.

Following the original work of Gould and colleagues there is substantial, albeit indirect, experimental evidence to support the notion that neuronal recruitment can improve memory. Young

neurons exhibit enhanced synaptic plasticity in comparison to the mature ones (Piatti *et al.*, 2006). In principle, this plasticity could be utilized to form new memory traces. There are, in fact, several aspects to the relationship between the young neurons and learning. On the one hand, learning is dependent on the presence of the young neurons as shown by the ablation studies using irradiation (Wojtowicz, 2006). On the other hand, perhaps more relevant from the perspective of cognitive therapy, is the evidence that learning (or just plain afferent activity in the hippocampus) can stimulate proliferation and survival of new neurons. For example, survival of new neurons can be enhanced by the experimentally induced afferent activity in the dentate gyrus (Bruel-Jungerman *et al.*, 2006). Enriched environment or running can substantially enhance neurogenesis, synaptic plasticity and subsequent learning (van Praag *et al.*, 1999). Such evidence indicates that any procedure or treatment that enhances the availability of the new neurons could be beneficial. Although the direct contribution of neurogenesis to these enhancements is not clear, the evidence is consistent with the idea that new neurons play a significant role in memory. Aging laboratory rodents show drastically reduced neurogenesis by middle age. Some evidence suggests that the age-dependent reduction relates to impaired performance (Drapeau *et al.*, 2003). However, this has not been a consistent finding and more studies have to be done taking into account different hippocampal tasks.

Reduced neurogenesis has been linked to depression. The evidence is largely correlative and still awaits verification in human subjects (Becker & Wojtowicz, 2007). Nevertheless, the animal experimentation shows that antidepressants, such as selective serotonin reuptake inhibitors (SSRIs), enhance neurogenesis at a specific developmental stage (Encinas *et al.*, 2006). Furthermore, this enhancement is a requirement for SSRI action in an animal model of depression (Santarelli *et al.*, 2003). Thus, abnormal emotional responses in addition to memory deficits could be dependent on hippocampal neurogenesis.

How can neurogenesis be harnessed for regeneration and treatment of cognitive deficits?

- The question is not if, but how, the inherent regenerative capacity of brain tissue can be harnessed for brain repair.
- Non-neurogenic brain regions could be stimulated to induce neuronal production.
- Neurogenic brain regions can be specifically stimulated to raise neurogenesis from abnormally low levels.

Epilepsy, ischemia, chemotoxic or mechanical injuries are all known to induce compensatory neurogenesis but it is still not known whether the new cells that are produced after these injuries are significantly beneficial for functional recovery (Lichtenwalner & Parent, 2006). Nevertheless, since at least some new cells are produced, and progressively more information is available about their properties and regulation, there is a realistic hope that physiological recovery can be achieved if the natural process of neurogenesis can be harnessed and substantially enhanced. Until now, most cases of reactive neurogenesis after injury have been quantitatively insignificant and therefore functionally questionable. In the hippocampal dentate gyrus, where constitutive neurogenesis is robust, its acceleration after ischemia is transient and contributes relatively small numbers of new neurons to the overall pre-existing neuronal population. Paradoxically, the neuronal loss in dentate gyrus is usually less severe than in the adjacent hippocampal regions, thus there is less need for regeneration. Neuronal recruitment after ischemia has been reported in CA1, but it is still an open question if this "recovery" process is reproducible and quantitatively and functionally significant (Kokaia & Lindvall, 2003; Nakatomi et al., 2002; Schmidt & Reymann, 2002; Wang et al., 2005).

Analysis of post-injury neurogenesis is made difficult by the fact that numerous other cellular processes apart from neuronal recruitment can contribute to the recovery. These include general reduction in GABA-ergic inhibition and enhancement of glutamate-ergic synaptic plasticity in peri-infarct regions of the injured brain (Nudo et al., 2001). These symptoms of "adaptive plasticity" have been observed in the non-neurogenic brain regions such as the motor cortex and therefore could be independent of neurogenesis. Such generalized responses could occur in parallel with neurogenesis, making it difficult to dissect the responses attributed directly to the neurogenesis alone. All studies of recovery should take into consideration the rules of engagement that are being derived from ongoing studies of the physiologically occurring neurogenesis and from its age-dependence. Unlike the simplistic ideas of implanting stem cells into the injured tissue and expecting a miraculous recovery, neurogenesis-based strategies would involve stimulation of a nearby source of adult stem cells within the brain, guiding the migration of the progeny of these cells towards the site of injury, and nursing their development through the essential stages outlined in Figure 20.2. This would have to include formation of appropriate synaptic connections on afferent and efferent sides of the injured region. Furthermore, the new cells would have to be "trained" to respond to incoming stimuli, as the normal cells presumably are during their normal ontogenic development. We are far from understanding such regenerative processes.

Somewhat more feasible are the approaches for rehabilitation of cognitive functions that rely on neurogenesis in the neurogenic niche of the hippocampus, the dentate gyrus. Here a logical approach would be simply to "exercise" the neuronal circuit to produce more neurons. The idea of the critical window discussed above would suggests that in order to rescue the neurons from cell death one would exercise the subjects at 1–2 weeks after a cohort of cells had been produced. In cases when cell production is at abnormally low levels, e.g., during aging, one would first increase cell proliferation with physiological (e.g., running) or pharmacological (e.g., antidepressant SSRI) stimuli, wait for 1–2 weeks and stimulate the cells by appropriate brain activity (e.g., learning).

Gonadal hormones such as testosterone and estrogens have complex but generally stimulatory effects on neurogenesis (Galea *et al.*, 2006). Considering a sharp decline of neurogenesis and the circulating levels of these hormones with age, there exists an obvious possibility for linking the hormonal effects, neurogenesis and cognitive decline in old age. However, this field still awaits animal experimentation.

Therapeutic potential of neurogenesis

- A specific protocol for tissue regeneration is described by taking the rules derived from basic studies of adult neurogenesis into account.
- Proliferation of neuronal precursors, creation of a neurogenic niche with trophic support and synaptogenesis are the first necessary steps in neurogenesis.
- Exercising the new circuit with physiological activity may be a second necessary phase in therapy.

The central question is to what extent can a CNS lesion be repaired? For example, can we repair the damage caused by a stroke that leaves a gaping hole in the hippocampus, cortex or the striatum? Can spinal cord damage resulting from a mechanical insult be filled-in by appropriate neuronal circuitry? Conceptually, several steps need to be followed to enable such recovery. (1) One needs to orchestrate a controlled proliferation and migration of neuroimmune microglia, that have a natural tendency to invade the spaces previously occupied by injured neurons. Although this inflammatory reaction is probably useful in removing the debris of the injured cells, it may also produce excessive release of cytotoxic substances (cytokines) that will exacerbate cell damage (Simard & Rivest, 2006). The activated astrocytes, if uncontrolled, will rapidly surround a space created by the lesion and prevent neuronal regeneration. Thus, careful control of these potentially harmful processes may be essential to permit regeneration. In theory, this may be accomplished by transient application of anti-inflammatory drugs and specific growth factors that inhibit glia cell formation (Chmielnicki *et al.*,

2004). (2) One needs to promote and orchestrate growth of neurons in the injured area. This is a delicate process of "guiding" the precursors through a series of steps involving at first the expression and later downregulation of specific genes responsible for functions such as growth of dendrites and axons, formation of synapses, insertion of appropriate receptors, etc. This is a tall order with our imperfect knowledge of the controlling factors in neurogenesis, but it should be attempted. The task may be easier for brain regions that are located near normally neurogenic areas such as the walls of the cerebral ventricles. More remote locations within the brain tissue will require guided migration of progenitors to the site of injury. This may be facilitated by judicial application of chemotaxic substances that are known to function within the brain; conveniently, chemotaxy is often triggered by cell death. However, cellular migration is not easy within the tightly packed CNS tissue, so a path may have to be created to make sufficient cell movement feasible. Interestingly, there is an organized pathway of this type, the rostral migratory stream, that leads neurons over a considerable distance from the lateral ventricles to the olfactory bulb (Lledo *et al.*, 2006). This may become a useful model for the migratory paths required to propel progenitors towards the lesion after injury. (3) One should permit the endothelial and glial cells, including myelin-forming oligodendrocytes, to generate the normal infrastructure where glia, neurons and capillaries can interact with each other (Palmer *et al.*, 2000). (4) One may have to "train" the circuit to act in an appropriate electrophysiological manner, i.e., respond to incoming neural impulses with appropriately balanced excitation and inhibition that, in turn, will produce an appropriate efferent output to the target brain region. Otherwise, it can be envisaged that an unsuitable circuit will disrupt rather than improve normal brain recovery. An example of unsuitable neurogenesis is the uncontrolled proliferation of the dentate gyrus granule neurons following the epileptic seizures. The excess of neurons created by reactive neurogenesis may cause abnormal excitability of the hippocampal circuit (Lichtenwalner & Parent, 2006). (5) The final outcome of this regenerative process would provide the functional circuitry and infrastructure that ultimately would restore proper behavior in an individual organism.

It is encouraging to see that steps 1–5 are being increasingly well understood through investigation of normal, physiological neurogenesis in dentate gyrus and elsewhere. Ultimately, the developmental steps outlined in Figure 20.2 can be related to the putative steps required for regeneration shown in Figure 20.3.

All previous experimental attempts to accomplish brain tissue recovery have been limited to one or two of these essential steps. The main line of experimentation has been to induce tissue damage by artificial means or use a genetic mouse model of a disease that resulted in a significant behavioral deficit. After a delay, the recovery process is initiated with application of a neurotrophic factor to promote stem cell mitotic activity and differentiation into neurons. There are now many neurotrophins to choose from and some of them have been shown to act on well-defined stages of neuronal development. Most experiments used mechanical infusions or growth factor delivery with viral vectors (Nakatomi et al., 2002). Others used "physiologic" stimuli such as physical activity, analogues to what may be expected from physiotherapy approaches, to promote recovery (Komitova et al., 2005). Various degrees of functional recovery have been claimed, but the simplistic design of all these efforts, in comparison to what should be considered only a "bare bones" approach, underlines the shortcomings of such studies. The main problem, conceptually, would appear to be the lack of attention for proper timing of the applications of regulatory factors. Also, the concentrations and the methods of delivery of the regulatory substances will need to be worked out.

What are the prospects? Increasingly rational experimental approaches to tissue regeneration and functional recovery are becoming possible. Technically, one can now apply a series of neurotrophins that would inhibit the excessive growth of

astrocytes and microglia and, at the same time, encourage migration, proliferation and growth of neurons. The obvious experimental approach is to infuse the appropriate growth factors into the ventricles or into the injured area in appropriate sequence. In addition, the recent results also suggest that small-molecule transmitters (GABA and glutamate agonists) or their blockers could help in the appropriate formation of synaptic connections since they have trophic effects of their own (Espósito et al., 2005). This concept is particularly encouraging since the logistics of introducing small molecules, e.g., transmitters, into the brain may be much easier to overcome than applications of large neurotrophic peptides. Finally, physiotherapy-like physiological stimulation may be required at the appropriate stages of circuit formation to ensure functional integration and training of new neurons. The timing of all these steps is crucial, considering typical needs of neurons for so-called "critical periods." Wrong timing of these steps could defeat the desired outcomes.

What are the specific physiological stimuli that could be used to promote the neurogenesis-based regeneration? It appears that the stimuli that engage the brain regions where neurogenesis takes place could provide a significant stimulus to enhance cell survival. A fascinating example of this effect is the enhanced survival of new-born neurons resulting from hippocampus-dependent learning. As described above, the subgranular, proliferative zone of the dentate gyrus produces an oversupply of potential young neurons, of which less than half survive to maturity. Learning tasks that specifically involve the hippocampus and consequently the dentate gyrus, such as spatial learning in the water maze or the trace eye blink conditioning, appear to promote neuronal survival during the 1–2 week period following the cell's birth (Leuner et al., 2006). Although the mechanism of this phenomenon is not yet known, its astonishing specificity for hippocampal learning and its strict time-dependence suggest a great promise for future efforts to stimulate regional brain regeneration. In the case of the dentate gyrus, the microinfrastructure is

Five steps in tissue regeneration

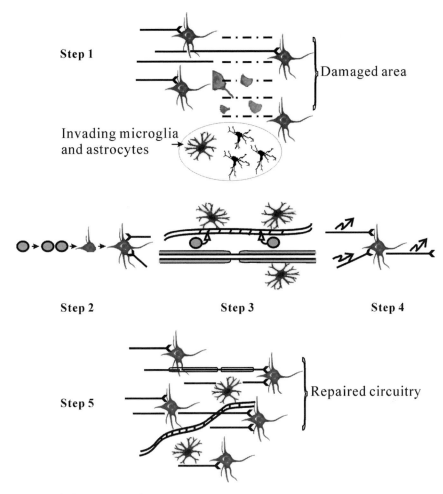

Figure 20.3. Five steps in tissue regeneration.

Step 1 requires controlled inhibition of activated neuroimmune cells to prevent excessive release of cytokines having possible harmful effects on the surviving neurons and inhibition of astrocytes forming a scar that would prevent neuronal regeneration.

Step 2 involves stimulation of neurogenesis with appropriate growth factors. This would presumably follow the sequence outlined in Figure 20.2 but may have to be preceded by guidance of neural precursors from a nearby source such as the subventricular zone.

Step 3 involves stimulation of glial precursors required for production of oligodendrocytes that in turn would form the myelin sheath around the axons of regenerating neurons. Also, angiogenesis needs to be promoted through proliferation of endothelial cells.

Step 4 would involve activation of the new circuit to assure its integration into the existing brain structure. This may take the form of physiotherapy or training that would partly simulate sequence of events during ontogenic development.

Step 5 represents a complete regenerated circuit with glial support, axonal projections, synaptic connections and blood supply.

already there in terms of glia and blood supply, as well as afferent and efferent synaptic projections. Nevertheless, the phenomenon of activity-induced cell survival should be applicable to any potential site of regeneration. The second physiological stimulus is voluntary running behavior that robustly enhances cell proliferation and survival (Olson *et al.*, 2006). Although it may be too much to expect of any injured animal to exercise by running after injury, specific types of exercise that would involve limited neuronal circuits should prove useful in recruiting the endogenous regenerative mechanisms. It must be emphasized that all evidence in favor of such specific physiological regulatory factors is still controversial and not readily reproducible in all laboratories (Leuner *et al.*, 2006; Snyder *et al.*, 2005). Nevertheless, the promise of at least some of the studies remains under active investigation and should be clarified in the near future.

How much of this is applicable to humans?

- Translational opportunities exist for protecting and promoting a healthy progenitor cell population in the adult brain.
- Physiologic and pharmacologic factors can be employed to enhance regeneration.

Adult neurogenesis in primates and humans is not well understood. With the exception of a pioneering study on patients that were given BrdU and showed surviving cells with neuronal phenotype in the dentate gyrus for several years afterwards (Eriksson *et al.*, 1998), other evidence in humans for physiological neurogenesis is still missing. Nevertheless, studies on monkeys showed that BrdU labeling of identifiable neurons is present in the dentate gyrus (Gould *et al.*, 1999b). According to some views, primates have little use for adult neurogenesis but there is no doubt that neuronal progenitor/stem cells can be obtained from adult brain tissue and expanded into neuronal phenotype in culture. There is also accumulating evidence from several reports using postmortem human tissue that the cells expressing proliferation marker Ki-67 and

specific neuronal progenitor markers are present in the hippocampus and in the subventricular/olfactory system (Macas *et al.*, 2006; Reif *et al.*, 2006). Thus, the potential for regeneration exists providing that the proper environment can be recreated within the normally non-neurogenic adult tissue. Some therapeutic procedures such as radiotherapy and chemotherapy, will make this environment even more inhospitable due to depletion of the endogenous progenitors and inhibition of ongoing endothelial renewal (Monje & Palmer, 2003). On the other hand many of the neurogenesis-promoting treatments and drugs would seem to be easy to apply to patients on experimental basis. These include running, learning exercises, hormones, antidepressants and many others.

Recovery from stroke, anoxia or ischemia could involve some of the required regenerative mechanisms described earlier, but their success will clearly be dependent on the size of the lesions and the age of the individual. It is well known that patients suffering from brain injury can continue to recover for months or even years. Physiotherapy is believed to improve such recovery (Nudo *et al.*, 2001), and the results from animal work can be translated into clinical practice to involve neurogenesis in this process. This may be particularly relevant to the "training" phase of the regeneration process and cognitive therapy (see Figure 20.3), when the circuitry is present but its function not fully established or underperforming. The earlier phases of regeneration, steps 1–4 in Figure 20.3, are not easily accessible to manipulation in humans, although better understanding of the physiologic and pharmacologic factors affecting neurogenesis, particularly actions of small molecules such as transmitter agonists, should create future translational opportunities. One dominant factor that will affect the effectiveness of tissue regeneration via neurogenesis is the age of an individual. In laboratory animals, the rate of neurogenesis declines drastically by middle-age. We also know that an animal's physical and mental activity can slow down this decline. In fact, animals living in their natural environment show persistent neurogenesis even at the end of their life span (Figure 20.4).

Decreased density of young neurons with age

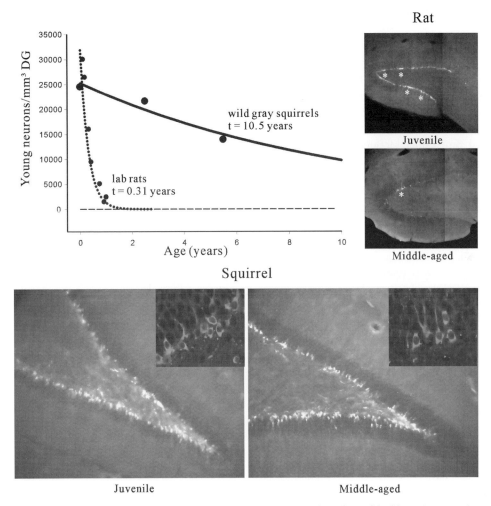

Figure 20.4. Exponential decay of neurogenesis with animal's age. Normalized numbers of doublecortin-expressing cells in laboratory rats and wild gray squirrels. Exponential decay curve was fitted to the experimental data obtained in rats of different ages. Time constant of 0.3 years is only about 10% of the rat's life span in a standard housing cage. The time constant for the squirrels is approximately equal to their average life span of 10–12 years. This comparison suggests a regulated production of new neurons that may depend on need for hippocampal plasticity. Histological sections show dentate gyrus in two species for comparison. The narrow but dense band of young neurons present in a young rat (asterisks) disappears by middle-age. In squirrels robust neurogenesis persists for their whole life.

However, we still do not know how these findings relate to humans: where does the average sedentary person in our society fall on this scale between laboratory and wild animals? It would appear that maintenance of a healthy precursor cell population should be a prerequisite for brain tissue regeneration, but more work on aging laboratory rodents and ultimately on primates and humans is needed before the feasibility of clinically relevant regeneration in the human brain can be assessed.

ACKNOWLEDGMENTS

This work was supported by the CIHR and NSERC research grants. The expert technical support of Ms. Y. F. Tan is greatly appreciated.

Figures 20.2 and 20.4 have been adapted from data collected by Heather McDonald and Jenn Barker during their graduate work in JMWs laboratory.

REFERENCES

Altman, J. (1962). Are new neurons formed in the brains of adult animals. *Science*, **135**, 1127–1128.

Altman, J., & Das, G. D. (1965). Autoradiographic and histological evidence of postnatal hippocampal neurogenesis in rats. *Journal of Comparative Neurology*, **124**, 319–336.

Altman, J., & Das, G. D. (1967). Postnatal neurogenesis in the guinea pig. *Nature*, **214**, 1089–1101.

Barker, J., Wojtowicz, J. M., & Boonstra, R. (2005). Where is my dinner? Adult neurogenesis in free-living food-storing rodents. *Genes, Brain and Behavior*, **4**, 89–98.

Becker, S., & Wojtowicz, J. M. (2007). A model of hippocampal neurogenesis in memory and mood disorders. *Trends in Cognitive Sciences*, **11**, 70–76.

Bruel-Jungerman, E., Davis, S., Rampon, C., & Laroche, S. (2006). Long-term potentiation enhances neurogenesis in the adult dentate gyrus. *Journal of Neuroscience*, **26**, 5888–5893.

Chmielnicki, E., Benraiss, A., Economides, A. N., & Goldman, S. A. (2004). Adenovirally expressed noggin and brain derived neurotrophic factor cooperate to induce new medium spiny neurons from resident progenitor cells in the adult striatal ventricular zone. *Journal of Neuroscience*, **24**, 2133–2142.

Dayer, A. G., Cleaverm, K. M., Abouantoun, T., & Cameron, H. A. (2005). New GABAergic interneurons in the adult neocortex and striatum are generated from different precursors. *Journal of Cell Biology*, **168**, 415–427.

Drapeau, E., Mayo, W., Aurousseau, C. *et al.* (2003). Spatial memory performances of aged rats in the water maze predict levels of hippocampal neurogenesis. *Proceedings of the National Academy of Sciences of the United States of America*, **100**, 14385–14390.

Encinas, J. M., Vaahtokari, A., & Enikolopov, G. (2006). Fluoxetine targets early progenitor cells in the adult brain. *Proceedings of the National Academy of Sciences of the United States of America*, **103**, 8233–8238.

Eriksson, P. S., Perfilieva, E., Bjork-Eriksson, T. *et al.* (1998). Neurogenesis in the adult human hippocampus. *Nature Medicine*, **4**, 1313–1317.

Espósito, M. S., Piatti, V. C., Laplange, D. A. *et al.* (2005). Neuronal differentiation in the adult hippocampus recapitulates embryonic development. *Journal of Neuroscience*, **25**, 10074–10086.

Galea, L. A. M., Spritzer, M. D., Barker, J. M., & Pawluski, J. L. (2006). Gonadal hormone modulation of hippocampal neurogenesis in the adult. *Hippocampus*, **16**, 225–232.

Goldman, S. (2005). Stem and progenitor cell-based therapy of the human central nervous system. *Nature Biotechnology*, **23**, 862–871.

Gould, E., Reeves, A. J., Graziano, M. S., & Gross, C. G. (1999a). Neurogenesis in the neocortex of adult primates. *Science*, **286**, 548–552.

Gould, E., Reeves, A. J., Graziano, M. S., & Gross, C. G. (1999b). Neurogenesis in the neocortex of adult primates. *Science*, **286**, 548–552.

Gratzner, H. G. (1982). Monoclonal antibody to 5-Bromo- and 5-iododeoxyuridine: A new reagent for detection of DNA replication. *Science*, **218**, 474–475.

Kempermann, G., Jessberger, S., Steiner, B., & Kronenberg, G. (2004). Milestones of neuronal development in the adult hippocampus. *Trends in Neurosciences*, **27**, 446–452.

Kokaia, Z., & Lindvall, O. (2003). Neurogenesis after ischaemic brain insults. *Current Opinion in Neurobiology*, **13**, 127–132.

Kokoeva, M. V., Yin, H., & Flier, J. S. (2005). Neurogenesis in the hypothalamus of adult mice: potential role in energy balance. *Science*, **310**, 679–683.

Komitova, M., Zhao, L. R., Gido, G., Johansson, B. B., & Eriksson, P. S. (2005). Postischemic exercise attenuates whereas enriched environment has certain enhancing effects on lesion-induced subventricular zone activation in the adult rat. *Journal of Neuroscience*, **21**, 2397–2405.

Leuner, B., Gould, E., & Shors, T. J. (2006). Is there a link between adult neurogenesis and learning? *Hippocampus*, **16**, 216–224.

Lichtenwalner, R. J., & Parent, J. M. (2006). Adult neurogenesis and the ischemic forebrain. *Journal of Cerebral Blood Flow and Metabolism*, **26**, 1–20.

Lledo, P.-M., Alonso, M., & Grubb, M. S. (2006). Adult neurogenesis and functional plasticity in neuronal circuits. *Nature Neuroscience*, 7, 179–193.

Macas, J., Nern, C., Plate, K. H., & Momma, S. (2006). Increased generation of neuronal progenitors after ischemic injury in the aged adult human forebrain. *Journal of Neuroscience*, 26, 13114–13119.

McDonald, H. Y., & Wojtowicz, J. M. (2005). Dynamics of neurogenesis in the dentate gyrus of adult rats. *Neuroscience Letters*, 385, 70–75.

Meshi, D., Drew, M. R., Saxe, M. *et al.* (2006). Hippocampal neurogenesis is not required for behavioral effects of environmental enrichment. *Nature Neuroscience*, 9, 729–731.

Monje, M. L., & Palmer, T. D. (2003). Radiation injury and neurogenesis. *Current Opinion in Neurology*, 16, 129–134.

Nakatomi, H., Kuriu, T., Okabe, S. *et al.* (2002). Regeneration of hippocampal pyramidal neurons after ischemic brain injury by recruitment of endogenous neural progenitors. *Cell*, 110, 429–441.

Nudo, R. J., Plautz, E. J., & Frost, S. B. (2001). Role of adaptive plasticity in recovery of function after damage to motor cortex. *Muscle and Nerve*, 24, 1000–1019.

Olson, A. K., Eadie, B. D., Ernst, C., & Christie, B. R. (2006). Environmental enrichment and voluntary exercise massively increase neurogenesis in the adult hippocampus via dissociable pathways. *Hippocampus*, 16, 261–266.

Palmer, T. D., Willhoite, A. R., & Gage, F. G. (2000). Vascular niche for adult hippocampal neurogenesis. *Journal of Comparative Neurology*, 425, 479–494.

Piatti, V. C., Espósito, M. S., & Schinder, A. F. (2006). The timing of neuronal development in adult hippocampal neurogenesis. *The Neuroscientist*, 12, 463–468.

Reif, A., Fritzen, S., Finger, M. *et al.* (2006). Neural stem cell proliferation is decreased in schizophrenia, but not in depression. *Molecular Psychiatry*, 11, 514–522.

Santarelli, L., Saxe, M., Gross, C. *et al.* (2003). Requirement of hippocampal neurogenesis for the behavioral effects of antidepressants. *Science*, 301, 805–809.

Schmidt, W., & Reymann, K. G. (2002). Proliferating cells differentiate into neurons in the hippocampal CA1 region of gerbils after global cerebral ischemia. *Neuroscience Letters*, 334, 153–156.

Simard, A. R., & Rivest, S. (2006). Neuroprotective properties of the innate immune system and bone marrow stem cells in Alzheimer's disease. *Molecular Psychiatry*, 11, 327–335.

Snyder, J. S., Hong, N., McDonald, R. J., & Wojtowicz, J. M. (2005). A role for adult hippocampal neurogenesis in spatial long-term memory. *Neuroscience*, 130, 843–852.

van Praag, H., Christie, B. R., Sejnowski, T. J., & Gage, F. H. (1999). Running enhances neurogenesis, learning, and long-term potentiation in mice. *Proceedings of the National Academy of Sciences of the United States of America*, 96, 13427–13431.

Wang, S., Kee, N., Preston, E., & Wojtowicz, J. M. (2005). Electrophysiological correlates of neural plasticity compensating for ischemia-induced damage in the hippocampus. *Experimental Brain Research*, 165, 250–260.

Wojtowicz, J. M. (2006). Irradiation as an experimental tool in studies of adult neurogenesis. *Hippocampus*, 16, 261–266.

21

The impact of cerebral small vessel disease on cognitive impairment and rehabilitation

Harry V. Vinters and S. Thomas Carmichael

Introduction

- Cerebral microangiopathies in relation to ischemic vascular disease (IVD).
- Systemic factors that may contribute to IVD – the issue of ischemic necrosis vs. "subinfarctive" ischemia.
- Ischemic vascular disease in comparison to Alzheimer disease and "mixed" dementias.

It is impossible to consider the impact of various forms of cerebral small vessel disease ("*microangiopathies*") on the brain separately from that of ischemic vascular dementia (IVD). Several excellent reviews of IVD have appeared in recent years (Chui, 2005; del Ser *et al.*, 1990; Hulette *et al.*, 1997; Ince & Fernando, 2003; Jellinger, 2002; Kalaria *et al.*, 2004; Munoz, 1991; Pantoni *et al.*, 1996; Vinters *et al.*, 2000); a recent one has analysed IVD from neurobehavioral and morphologic points of view (Selnes & Vinters, 2006). From a neuropathologic perspective, the study of IVD can be reduced – accepting immediately that this is an oversimplification – to examining three major inter-related, yet functionally separable, pathophysiologic components: *cerebrovascular disease* (CVD) that affects both large and small arteries, *systemic* mediators of ischemic brain necrosis or anoxic-ischemic injury (which of course often interact with CVD), and the central nervous system (CNS) *parenchymal* lesions we recognize as being the *result* of combined CVD and systemic factors. Once irreversible brain injury has occurred, there are downstream and retrograde effects in the CNS that result from that insult – as a

function of Wallerian, trans-synaptic and other types of degeneration – which almost certainly impact upon subsequent neurobehavioral morbidity in ways that we do not yet fully understand (O'Brien *et al.*, 2003; Vinters *et al.*, 1998a). Subcortical axonal injury and loss, together with astrocytic gliosis, may be key elements in IVD pathogenesis and progression (Medana & Esiri, 2003). The neuropathologic substrates of *leukoaraiosis*, also affecting the subcortical white matter, are controversial but are now thought to include apoptosis of oligodendroglia, the key myelinating cell in the brain and spinal cord (Brown *et al.*, 2000).

Almost all autopsy studies of IVD have been on patients who (a) have been ill for many years, often decades, with various combinations of CVD that have caused complex ischemic brain lesions and associated neuropsychologic symptoms, and (b) are elderly and thus very likely to manifest significant "Alzheimerization" of the brain (Chui *et al.*, 2006). Deducing pathophysiologic mechanisms (from such studies) that may have been of major importance years or decades earlier, is an exercise fraught with peril. Careful neuropathologic investigations of cognitively normal elderly individuals have shown that small, old cerebral infarcts are common in such patients, though relatively few in number (Knopman *et al.*, 2003). Community-based investigations (e.g., the Religious Orders Study) have shown that almost 25% of brains from cognitively normal older patients show cerebral infarcts, though often neuropathologic details of the lesions are scanty (Bennett *et al.*, 2006). Sorting out

Cognitive Neurorehabilitation, Second Edition: Evidence and Application, ed. Donald T. Stuss, Gordon Winocur and Ian H. Robertson. Published by Cambridge University Press. © Cambridge University Press 2008.

Table 21.1. Neuropathologic substrates of ischemic vascular dementia

Multifocal or diffuse lesions

Sporadic

(1) Multiple atherosclerotic, atheroembolic and/or watershed (border-zone) cystic infarcts

(2) Cortical laminar necrosis (post-cardiac arrest, hypotensive episode[s])

(3) Multifocal cortical/white matter microinfarcts (*"Granular atrophy"* of the cortex)

(4) Lacunar infarcts in deep gray, subcortical white matter (caused by arteriosclerotic microangiopathy/lipohyalinosis, microatheroma, other factors to be defined)

(5) Binswanger subcortical (arteriosclerotic) leukoencephalopathy (BSLE)

(6) Cerebral amyloid angiopathy (CAA) – in elderly individuals including those with AD/SDAT

(7) Angiitis/vasculitis (e.g., primary angiitis of the CNS, granulomatous angiitis)

(8) Miscellaneous angiopathies affecting large arteries (fibromuscular dysplasia, Moyamoya disease)

Familial/Genetic

(1) *"Anti-phospholipid"* – related ischemia

(2) Cerebral Autosomal Dominant Arteriopathy with Subcortical Infarcts and Leukoencephalopathy (CADASIL)

(3) Cerebral amyloid angiopathy (e.g., *APP* codon 692,693,694,705 mutations) (Some show significant *"Alzheimerization"* of the brain in addition to CAA)

(4) Hereditary endotheliopathy with retinopathy, nephropathy and stroke (HERNS)

Focal lesions/ strategically placed infarcts

(1) Mesial temporal (hippocampal) sclerosis/ischemia/infarcts

(2) Caudate and thalamic infarcts (especially dorsomedial nucleus, bilateral damage)

(3) Anterior cerebral territory infarcts (e.g., fronto-cingulate)

(4) Angular gyrus infarcts in dominant cerebral hemisphere

Adapted from Vinters *et al.*, 2000.

neurobehavioral and neuroimaging correlates of ischemic brain lesions when these occur in the context of significant Alzheimer's disease (AD) alterations can be daunting. A more critical question is: what are the implications for brain structure and function of hypoxia-ischemia that *fails* to produce a visible area of cystic necrosis or encephalomalacia – but still may result in more subtle neurologic injury that is best characterized clinically as *vascular cognitive impairment* (VCI) (Ince & Fernando, 2003; O'Brien *et al.*, 2003)? A recent NINDS-Canadian Stroke Network workshop has proposed *"standards"* by which patients with suspected VCI are best studied – whether this be from clinical, neuroimaging, neuropsychologic or neuropathologic perspectives (Hachinski *et al.*, 2006). Table 21.1 summarizes the major neuropathologic substrates of IVD, including ones that result from cerebral microvascular disease (microangiopathies), the

emphasis of this chapter; several of these are described in greater detail below.

There is much debate as to the precise frequency and incidence of IVD. Clinicopathologic studies of various selected or unselected patient populations have shown a remarkable heterogeneity of vascular and brain parenchymal lesions in IVD patients (Chui, 2005; del Ser *et al.*, 1990; Erkinjuntti *et al.*, 1988; Fernando *et al.*, 2004; Munoz, 1991; Pantoni *et al.*, 1996; Wallin & Blennow, 1991). Many individuals with AD, especially those beyond 85 years of age, show significant vascular comorbidity – whether or not they have experienced clinical transient ischemic attacks or infarcts while alive – to the extent that they are more accurately characterized as having mixed vascular-AD dementia (Hansen & Crain, 1995). In longitudinal studies and large clinicopathologic case series with autopsy confirmation of neuropathologic findings, the observed anatomic substrates are largely determined by criteria used to recruit or enter patients into a given study. Necropsy investigations on individuals who develop dementia after large hemispheric cystic infarcts (usually involving both cortex and subcortical white matter) will show different vascular and parenchymal lesions than studies in which patients are selected for a high likelihood of having deep lacunar infarcts or subcortical white matter alterations, including leukoaraiosis (LA) (Kalimo, 2005; Vinters *et al.*, 2000). Such distinctive populations of patients are also likely to differ in terms of their clinical progression; those with small deep lacunar infarcts (especially within the white matter) or multiple neocortical micro-infarcts are *less* likely to show a stepwise progression of cognitive impairment than those with regions of substantial cystic encephalomalacia that have replaced significant functioning brain volume. In large autopsy series of demented patients, e.g., from Vienna, Austria, "*pure*" IVD was seen in 9.4% (out of 900 demented individuals) but in only 2.9% of patients with the *clinical* diagnosis of probable/possible AD (Jellinger, 2002). Some investigators suggest that IVD may account for only 2–3% of dementias (Hansen & Crain, 1995). An extreme view is that "*pure*" IVD is almost nonexistent in large dementia clinics, even when careful necropsies are performed on afflicted individuals (Nolan *et al.*, 1998). Cerebrovascular disease as a cause of dementia is considered to be much more common in Asia, accounting for an estimated 22–35% of such cases there; however, autopsy confirmation of the *cause* of dementia is much less common in Asia than in Europe or North America.

Neuropathologic substrates and correlates of IVD

- Neuropathologic findings in patients with suspected IVD (multi-infarct dementia).
- Spectrum of parenchymal lesions – cystic infarcts, lacunes, microinfarcts – etiology?
- Atherosclerosis and arteriolosclerosis/lipohyalinosis in relation to hypertension.

- Cerebral amyloid angiopathy (CAA) – sporadic (age-related), familial forms.
- Familial non-CAA cerebral microangiopathies – CADASIL, HERNS, etc.

Ischemic parenchymal lesions in IVD patients are extremely variable in size, distribution and total number, and therefore variable in the volume of brain parenchyma that has been lost. In a longitudinal California-wide study of patients preselected for a high likelihood of subcortical ischemic lesions, especially lacunar infarcts (based upon clinical assessment and antemortem neuroimaging studies), we have arbitrarily subcategorized infarcts seen at autopsy as cystic infarcts (larger than 1.0 cm in greatest dimension), lacunar infarcts or lacunes (grossly visible on cut sections of the brain but smaller than 1.0 cm in maximal size, Figure 21.1) and microinfarcts (not seen on gross inspection of the cut brain, but identified at microscopy) (Vinters *et al.*, 2000). Immunohistochemical stains that are especially helpful for demonstrating microinfarcts include those using primary antibodies against CD68 or any other reliable macrophage/microglial marker, and the astrocyte marker glial fibrillary acidic protein (GFAP). Both of these stains highlight areas of localized proliferation of cells that react to *irreversible* ischemic injury; put differently, they show tiny microscopic areas of brain "scarring," which are sometimes the result of occlusion of small brain vessels or atheroemboli from larger arteries (see below). The role of astrocytes and microglia, and factors they secrete, in the progression of *subinfarctive* or incomplete ischemia is not yet known. Abundant old cortical microinfarcts render the cortical surface irregular and pitted; an affected brain is sometimes described as showing "*granular atrophy*," even though the causal lesions are infarctive rather than atrophic or degenerative. It is somewhat curious that tissue reactions to ischemic infarcts, both large and small, within *human* brain have been the subject of relatively little systematic or quantitative study using modern immunohistochemical approaches. Recent preliminary work along these lines has emphasized the possibility of "*stroke-induced neurogenesis*"

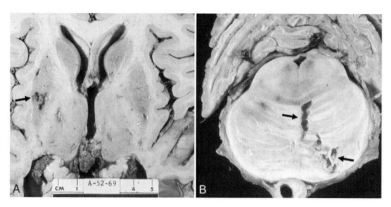

Figure 21.1. (This figure is reproduced in the color plate section at the front of this volume.) Lacunes/lacunar infarcts. (A) Axial cut of the fixed brain, at level of the 'V' configuration of the internal capsule. Note multiple lacunar infarcts in the left lentiform nucleus (arrow) and adjacent thalamus. (B) Fairly large lacunar infarcts (arrows) in the basis pontis of a known hypertensive. (Note also the severely atherosclerotic basilar artery seen at bottom of the specimen.) Lacunar infarcts are thought to be one consequence of longstanding hypertension, though that association has recently been questioned.

adjacent to brain infarcts (Jin *et al.*, 2006), but little attention has been paid to reparative events (adjacent to a region of necrosis) characterized by microglial/ macrophage, astrocyte and microvascular prolifera-tion, phenomena easily recognized by most neuro-pathologists (Vinters, 2001a).

Cystic infarcts are often the consequence of occlusion of large meningeal or basal arteries affected by atheroslcerosis, sometimes as a result of atheroemboli that lodge within them – such ath-eroemboli may also originate in complicated athero-sclerotic plaques within cervical carotid or vertebral arteries, especially when such unstable plaques undergo rupture or ulceration (Hulette *et al.*, 1997; Vinters, 2001a). They may also be seen as wedge-shaped regions of encephalomalacia in the water-shed or border-zone between two large territories of cerebral arteries (e.g., middle and anterior cerebral, middle and posterior cerebral). The view that a cer-tain threshold volume of brain tissue loss due to infarct(s) (e.g., 50–100 ml) predictably causes dementia is no longer widely accepted; strategically placed much smaller infarcts, e.g., in the deep central gray matter, may play an equally important (or greater) role in causing dementia (Chui, 2005; del Ser *et al.*, 1990). Lacunar infarcts have historically

been attributed to *arteriosclerotic* microangiopathy affecting cerebral parenchymal or meningeal arteries, a process sometimes described as *lipohya-linosis* and linked etiologically to longstanding hypertension. The strength of that association has recently been called into question (Kalimo, 2005; Lammie, 2002); the term "*hypertensive microvascular disease*" as a synonym for lipohyalinosis is thus best avoided. Lacunar infarcts have further been classi-fied into various subtypes based upon their neuro-pathologic elements, including types Ia (small cystic cavity containing small blood vessels and a few mac-rophages), Ib (*incomplete* necrosis with perivascular rarefaction and patchy astrocytic gliosis), and II (an old *microhemorrhage* with abundant hemosiderin-laden macrophages) (Lammie, 2002). Lipohyalinosis (cerebral arteriosclerosis) may also cause cerebral hemorrhage; when this occurs, small aneurysms (described as Charcot–Bouchard aneurysms) are sometimes seen at the edge of the hematoma, sug-gesting that their rupture produced the hemorrhage (Figure 21.2). (Once thought to be fairly specific for arteriosclerotic/hypertensive cerebral microvascular disease, Charcot–Bouchard aneurysms are now well described in numerous other brain microangi-opathies, especially CAA – see below.) A very small

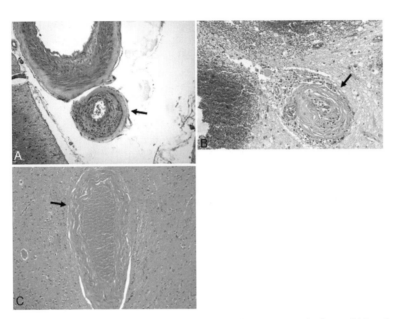

Figure 21.2. (This figure is reproduced in the color plate section at the front of this volume.) Various manifestations of cerebral microvascular disease in the CNS. (A) Severe "*onion skin*" type thickening of a meningeal artery (arrow). (B) Charcot–Bouchard type microaneurysm (arrow) adjacent to a typical "hypertensive" intracerebral hemorrhage. (C) Section of basal ganglia showing a small artery with microatheroma (arrow), noted as circumferential intimal thickening (superficial to the elastica) of a modest degree. Surrounding brain parenchyma appears largely "unaffected." (All micrographs are from H&E-stained sections.)

subset of hypertensive individuals develop extensive leukomalacia related to arteriosclerotic microangiopathy – a condition sometimes described as Binswanger's subcortical leukoencephalopathy, or BSLE (Figure 21.3) (Lim *et al.*, 2002). Binswanger's subcortical leukoencephalopathy is a term also now used to describe patients who have widespread white matter lacunar infarcts, an infrequent cause of dementia in affected individuals. Hippocampal injury, often resembling hippocampal sclerosis (HS) identified in the medial temporal lobes of patients with intractable temporal lobe epilepsy (with severe segmental neuron loss in the CA1 segment of the pyramidal cell layer and frequent preservation of CA2) is now recognized as a common neuropathologic finding in the CNS of very elderly demented patients, and is probably best considered as part of the spectrum of IVD (Dickson *et al.*, 1994; Vinters

et al., 2000). The precise etiology of this type of hippocampal injury is unknown, though it is unlikely to be strongly linked to cerebral microangiopathies.

Cerebral amyloid angiopathy

Cerebral amyloid angiopathy (CAA) describes an enigmatic microangiopathy that involves meningeal and cortical arterioles, venules and capillaries, whereby the normal vessel wall becomes replaced by fibrillar amyloid (Rensink *et al.*, 2003; Revesz *et al.*, 2002; Verbeek *et al.*, 2000). The most common form of CAA is an age-related vasculopathy, appears to be confined to the brain, and results from ABeta protein deposition within arteriolar media and the walls of capillaries and venules (ABeta is also the major protein component of senile plaques found in AD brain) (Vinters *et al.*, 1996). Microvascular

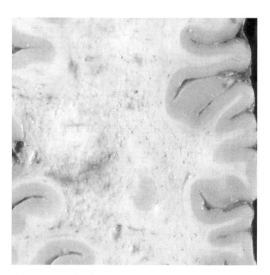

Figure 21.3. (This figure is reproduced in the color plate section at the front of this volume.) Binswanger's subcortical leukoencephalopathy (BSLE). Cut section of fixed brain. The cerebral cortex appears relatively normal, but note "motheaten" appearance of the subcortical white matter, with poorly defined regions of variably severe encephalomalacia.

amyloid may be widely distributed within the cerebral cortex and overlying meninges (Vinters & Gilbert, 1983), but is almost never found in the subcortical white matter, brainstem, deep central gray matter or cerebellum (except in the meninges overlying the latter structure). Cerebral amyloid angiopathy is strongly associated with AD, such that almost all AD patients have some degree of CAA when this is diligently sought by multiple brain sections in autopsy brains, especially using ABeta immunohistochemistry (Greenberg et al., 1993; Vinters, 1987; Vinters et al., 1996). The most severe cases of ABeta CAA are usually noted in patients with AD. Rare individuals with prominent CAA lack other neuropathologic stigmata of advanced AD (with abundant neocortical SPs, NFTs) and may not even be demented while alive (Vinters, 1992). Severe CAA, in which the medial layer of many or most cortical arterioles is completely replaced by amyloid, is comparatively rare (Figure 21.4). Replacement of

the smooth muscle cell layer of arteriolar media by fibrillar amyloid renders the involved vessel susceptible to rupture spontaneously, with mild increases in intravascular pressure or when thrombolytic agents are administered (Rensink et al., 2003; Vinters et al., 1994); nontraumatic lobar intracerebral (intraparenchymal) hemorrhage is a consequence of this, though it occurs infrequently when one considers the vast numbers of individuals who have *some degree* of CAA (Gilbert & Vinters, 1983; Vinters, 1987; Verbeek et al., 2000). Although the cerebral accumulation of many AD microscopic lesions appears to be, at least in part, mediated by the Apolipoprotein E *epsilon 4* allele, CAA-related brain hemorrhage is associated with the *epsilon 2* allele (Nicoll et al., 1997). The peripheral location (within brain) of CAA-related bleeds makes them quite easily distinguishable from centrencephalic hypertensive hemorrhages. In biopsy or autopsy brain specimens, antibodies to ABeta protein (especially ABeta 1–40 rather than 1–42) effectively immunolabel arteriolar and capillary walls, confirming that vascular amyloid in CAA is similar, though probably not identical, to SP amyloid (Revesz et al., 2002; Vinters et al., 1996; Verbeek et al., 2000).

A small subset of patients with sporadic or age-related CAA develop superimposed vasculitis/angiitis. This granulomatous vasculitis, often with a significant giant cell component, appears to *result from* amyloid deposition in arteriolar walls, rather than *causing* amyloid deposition (Anders et al., 1997; Gray et al., 1990) (Figure 21.5). The inflammatory reaction in this CAA variant, which can be quite destructive to cerebral arteries, appears to represent a puzzling and idiosyncratic reaction to the presence of large amounts of ABeta within the arterial walls. Recent studies have suggested that angiitis with CAA may present with a clinically distinctive syndrome of rapid cognitive decline and seizures, rather than cerebral hemorrhage (Eng et al., 2004). There is also growing interest in the likelihood that patients with severe CAA may represent an underappreciated *variant* of IVD (Haglund et al., 2004). In our California-wide longitudinal study of

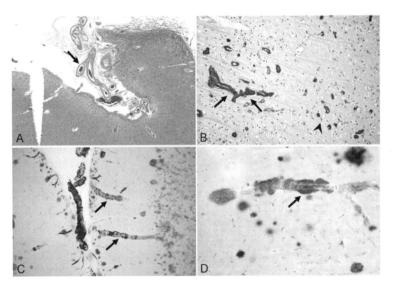

Figure 21.4. (This figure is reproduced in the color plate section at the front of this volume.) Cerebral amyloid (congophilic) angiopathy. (A) H&E-stained section shows many markedly thickened meningeal arteries, some of which have a "double barrel" lumen appearance, typical of severe CAA. (B) Section stained with primary antibodies to ABeta. Note that virtually all ABeta immunoreactivity is confined to the walls of cerebral vessels, including small arteries/arterioles (arrows) and capillaries (arrowhead). (C,D). Images are from 100 μm thick sections stained with the Campbell-Switzer technique (preparations courtesy of Professor Heiko Braak, Frankfurt-am-Main, Germany). At low magnification (panel C), penetration of amyloid-containing arteries (arrows) through the cortex is appreciated. At higher magnification (D), the focally accentuated deposition (e.g., indicated by arrow) of amyloid at various points along the arteriolar wall is highlighted.

individuals at high risk for IVD, as many as 8–10% of those examined at necropsy (admittedly a highly selected group) show severe CAA, often with associated cortical microinfarcts and/or severe subcortical leukoencephalopathy. Whereas the prediction would be that all of these individuals also have advanced (Braak stage V–VI) AD, in fact a subset of them show Alzheimerization of the CNS that does *not* extend to the isocortical stage. Further characterization of this interesting patient group is in progress. Many of these patients with severe ABeta CAA show extensive neocortical microinfarcts, which are best appreciated using CD68 immunohistochemistry (Figure 21.6). One suspects that this extensive multifocal ischemic necrosis affecting large areas of cortex might well be one substrate for slowly progressive dementia in such individuals. In large case control studies, ABeta CAA has now clearly been

established as a risk factor for cerebral ischemic infarcts (Cadavid *et al.*, 2000).

Familial cerebral amyloid angiopathy (fCAA)

An autosomal dominant syndrome of dementia and stroke (both cerebral hemorrhage and infarcts) characterized by extensive, often overwhelming and widely distributed meningocortical CAA, results from an *APP* codon 693 point mutation. The resulting disease, observed in circumscribed North Sea coastal regions in the Netherlands (especially Katwijk and Scheveningen), is described as hereditary cerebral hemorrhage with amyloidosis, Dutch type (HCHWA-D) (Verbeek *et al.*, 2000; Vinters *et al.*, 1998b; Zhang-Nunes *et al.*, 2006). Of interest, dementia in these patients clearly appears linked to the severity or burden of CAA rather than SP

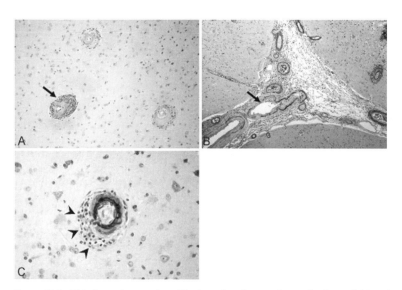

Figure 21.5. (This figure is reproduced in the color plate section at the front of this volume.) ABeta cerebral amyloid angiopathy with associated (granulomatous) angiitis. (A) Three amyloid-laden arteries, all markedly thickened, one of which (arrow) shows prominent adventitial lymphocytes. (B,C) Micrographs are from sections immunostained with primary antibodies against ABeta protein. Panel B shows extensive ABeta-immunoreactive arterial walls in both meningeal and parenchymal vessels. Note marked surrounding inflammation. Arrow indicates a large meningeal artery that appears to be in the early stages of microaneurysm formation. Panel C shows ABeta-immunoreactive parenchymal artery with surrounding mononuclear inflammatory cells (arrowheads). A single multinucleated giant cell is seen inferiorly immediately adjacent to the ABeta-immunoreactive vessel wall material.

and NFT density (Natte *et al.*, 2001). This suggests that sporadic, age- or AD-associated CAA, especially when severe, may be a significant – perhaps defining – factor in the cognitive decline in *this* disorder as well, though the effects of CAA in this context are difficult to parse out from the effects of AD parenchymal lesions, even when the latter are not necessarily overwhelming. Other familial syndromes in which a dominant neuropathologic finding is that of ABeta-immunoreactive CAA result from mutations at *APP* codon 692–694, including one described in an Iowa kindred (Grabowski *et al.*, 2001; Rensink *et al.*, 2003; Verbeek *et al.*, 2000). Very recently, a neuropathologically "*pure*" form of CAA has been identified in association with an autosomal dominant *APP* L705V mutation within the ABeta sequence (Obici *et al.*, 2005). Similar disorders are likely to emerge to pique the curiosity of

neurologists, pathologists, geneticists and basic neuroscientists in coming years. The molecular pathogenesis of CAA, often studied using transgenic animal models that carry familial AD *APP* mutations, is the subject of intense research. The details of this work are beyond the scope of the current review, but are amply summarized in several excellent recent reviews and monographs (Herzig *et al.*, 2006; Verbeek *et al.*, 2000; Zhang-Nunes *et al.*, 2006). As one might expect, ABeta deposition in arteriolar walls is believed to represent a derangement of the balance between excessive production and/or cleavage of APP protein within or near arterioles, together with impaired clearance mechanisms of Abeta protein from the vessel wall or its adventitia.

Nor are all forms of fCAA associated with abnormalities of ABeta protein deposition, or mutations in the *APP* gene. An Icelandic form of autosomal

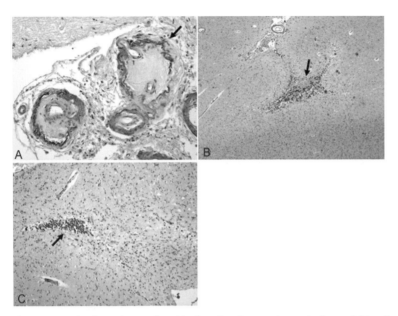

Figure 21.6. (This figure is reproduced in the color plate section at the front of this volume.) Severe cerebral amyloid angiopathy with extensive neocortical microinfarcts. (A) ABeta-immunostained section shows meningeal arteries/arterioles with prominent immunoreactive protein in their vessel walls (e.g., arrow). Notice that lumen of affected artery (arrow) is severely compromised by non-ABeta-immunoreactive material. (B,C) Micrographs are from sections immunostained with CD68, a microglial/macrophage marker. Both sections show small linear infarcts (arrows) in the cortex, highlighted by the presence of macrophages and vaguely defined cystic microcavitation.

dominant CAA (HCCAA, previously hereditary cerebral hemorrhage with amyloidosis, Icelandic type, abbreviated as HCHWA-I) results from mutations in the cystatin C (gamma trace) gene – cystatin C is an inhibitor of several cysteine proteases, including cathepsins. The resulting deposition of cystatin C in the media of cerebral arterioles leads to degeneration of affected vessel walls, with resultant predisposition for these arterioles/arteries to rupture, producing debilitating or fatal cerebral hemorrhage in young adults, usually in the third or fourth decade of life (Palsdottir *et al.*, 2006; Verbeek *et al.*, 2000; Wang *et al.*, 1997). Familial British and Danish dementias are very rare disorders that result from mutations in the *BRI2* gene on chromosome 13. This appears to cause extensive amyloid and pre-amyloid deposition throughout the CNS. The CNS amyloid deposits are largely (though not exclusively) composed of proteins ABri and ADan, and are seen to be widely distributed within both brain parenchyma and cerebral blood vessel walls in affected patients (Ghiso *et al.*, 2006). The molecular pathogenesis of these dementias is intriguing, insofar as the responsible *BRI2* mutations cause longer-than-normal protein products, and lead to the release of the ABri and ADan proteins. Stroke or stroke-like episodes, however, do not appear to be major features of the clinical spectrum in patients with familial British or Danish dementia.

Familial (non-CAA) syndromes of cerebral microangiopathy

Cerebral autosomal dominant arteriopathy with subcortical infarcts and leukoencephalopathy (CADASIL) is an entity characterized by cognitive

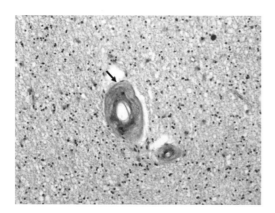

Figure 21.7. (This figure is reproduced in the color plate section at the front of this volume.) Cerebral autosomal dominant arteriopathy with subcortical infarcts and leukoencephalopathy (CADASIL). PAS-stained section of white matter shows a thickened vessel (arrow) containing PAS positive granular material, and thickening of its media and adventitia; this material corresponds to the "GOMs" noted by electron microscopy . Surrounding white matter shows "rarefaction" and astrocytic gliosis.

decline resulting from widespread deep white matter infarcts. It results from either a gain or loss of 1 or 3 cysteine residues in the extracellular N-terminal region of the *Notch3* gene (chromosome 19p13) (Gray *et al.*, 1994; Kalimo *et al.*, 2002; Miao *et al.*, 2004). Affected deep cerebral arteries show destruction of the smooth muscle cell layer in their media, accompanied by progressive wall thickening, and luminal narrowing caused by this and fibrosis (Figure 21.7). Characteristic ultrastructural features include the presence of "GOMs" (granular osmiophilic material) adjacent to smooth muscle cells of involved arterioles, a change that can be detected in cutaneous microvessels as well. Other familial stroke syndromes resulting from cerebral microangiopathies (e.g., HERNS) are less well characterized and/or identified in much smaller numbers of patients (Auerbach *et al.*, 2003; Jen *et al.*, 1997; Ringelstein & Nabavi, 2005). A common theme links many of these disorders of the cerebral microvasculature, including lipohyalinosis, CAA, and the less common disorders

described: degeneration of the (smooth muscle rich) media of cerebral arteries and arterioles, sometimes associated with abnormal smooth muscle cell proliferation, and often with deposition of insoluble proteins (beta-pleated sheet or otherwise) in the abnormal arteriolar media. The observation of smooth muscle cell degeneration as a common feature in these disorders has led to the suggestion that they are best described by the term cerebral "*angiomyopathies*" (Auerbach *et al.*, 2003; Vinters, 2001b).

Cerebral microangiopathy and cognitive reserve – implications for neurorehabilitation

- Cerebral small vessel disease – neuroimaging correlates.
- "White matter hyperintensities" on MRI and their meaning.
- Deep white matter "ischemia" and its relationship to brain aging.
- Cerebral small vessel disease – a substrate that partly determines outcome/rehabilitation potential after stroke.
- The brain's potential "regenerative" capacity.

Cerebral small vessel disease is most commonly clinically defined from MRI imaging results. Hyperintensities on T2 or FLAIR (fluid attenuated inversion recovery) sequences in the white matter identify presumed cerebral small vessel ischemia (Barkhof & Scheltens, 2002). These hyperintensities are found most commonly in periventricular locations, in which they cap the lateral ventricles or extend from the anterior and posterior regions of the lateral ventricles; or within deep subcortical white matter, such as the corona radiata (Figure 21.8). However, ischemia caused by small vessel disease may present with other pathologic manifestations, such as with cortical and subcortical microinfarcts (Kovari *et al.*, 2004). The incidence of cerebral small vessel disease sharply increases with age. In "non-diseased" community populations, 30% of people younger than 75 and 63% of those older than 75 have evidence of cerebral small vessel disease (Ylikoski *et al.*, 1995). With quantitative MRI measurements, there is a ten-fold increase in white

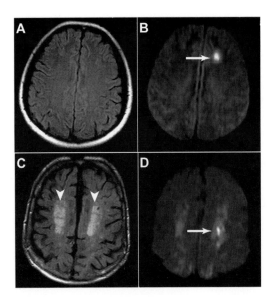

Figure 21.8. Cerebral small vessel disease (microangiopathy) and subcortical stroke. All panels show MRI sequences taken 8–12 hours after an acute stroke. Panels A and C are FLAIR sequences, panels B and D are diffusion-weighted images (DWI). (A,B) 49-year-old patient with no subcortical white matter hyperintensities on FLAIR (panel A), and a small acute subcortical infarct near the "leg" area of the motor strip (arrow in B). This patient recovered full use of her right leg with two weeks of neurorehabilitation. (C,D) 84-year-old patient with substantial cerebral small vessel disease in the corona radiata (arrowheads in C), and a small acute subcortical infarct near the face and arm area of the motor homunculus (arrow in D). This patient recovered incompletely over 4 weeks of inpatient rehabilitation.

matter hyperintensities after age 55 (Hopkins *et al.*, 2006). Cerebral small vessel disease is also associated with vascular risk factors for small vessel disease in other organs, including hypertension and diabetes (Roman *et al.*, 2002).

The pathologic damage from cerebral small vessel disease has an effect on cognitive function in the normal aging population. The amount of subcortical white matter hyperintensities correlates with tests of processing speed and executive function, both in aged populations (Prins *et al.*, 2005; Soderlund *et al.*, 2006) and in middle-aged groups

(Sachdev *et al.*, 2005). Cerebral small vessel disease also increases the rate of cognitive decline with age (de Groot *et al.*, 2002). Cerebral small vessel disease impacts physical independence and motor control. Patients with white matter lesions have difficulties with tests of fine motor coordination and report poorer physical health (Sachdev *et al.*, 2005). As with cognitive function, serial testing of physical function, such as walking speed or ability to carry out activities of daily living, indicates a greater rate of physical decline in normal elderly adults with white matter lesions (Rosano *et al.*, 2005).

Two important methodologic issues influence this analysis of the effect of cerebral small vessel disease on behavioral function in normal aging. First, it is clear that cerebral small vessel disease produces behavioral deficits that are unlike the early stages of cortical dementias, such as Alzheimer's or frontotemporal dementias. The deficits from cerebral small vessel disease are in cognitive processing speed, planning and attentional tests (Ferro & Madureira, 2002) and may not reveal themselves in the battery of tests usually applied to bedside cognitive testing, such as the Mini-Mental State Examination (MMSE). Thus early studies that utilized behavioral tests with a strong component of declarative memory testing may have missed important cognitive effects of cerebral small vessel disease. However, these behavioral deficits from cerebral small vessel disease, often characterized as frontal or executive dysfunction (Roman *et al.*, 2002), have major impacts on community function and overall assessments of well-being (Rosano *et al.*, 2005, 2006; Sachdev *et al.*, 2005).

A second methodologic issue in the clinical analysis of cerebral small vessel disease relates to the actual definition of this entity. Cerebral small vessel disease has been defined with MRI or neuropathologic findings of white matter hyperintensities in periventricular and focal and diffuse deep subcortical locations, as well as cortical and subcortical microinfarcts and lacunar infarcts (Barkhof & Scheltens, 2006; Giannakopoulos *et al.*, 2007). As noted above, the clinical convention most commonly classifies cerebral small vessel disease as ischemic change within subcortical white matter. There may be a differential contribution of lesion location and subtype to cognitive dysfunction, with periventricular white matter lesions most significantly associated with cognitive decline (de Groot et al., 2002; Soderlund et al., 2006; van den Heuvel et al., 2006). However, the clinical history of cerebral small vessel disease is that it is progressive (Schmidt et al., 2004). With progression there is often not a clear radiologic distinction between these periventricular and isolated deep white matter lesions. The majority of white matter hyperintensities are often described as "*periventricular*," as they can be physically traced as a continuous white matter hyperintensity to the lateral ventricular surface (Barkhof & Scheltens, 2006). Thus overall it can be said that white matter hyperintensities on MRI which are contiguous with the lateral ventricles affect cognitive speed, fine motor skills, activities of daily living and self-reports of well-being in normal aged individuals.

Many neurologic diseases show an increased incidence with age. The most numerically important neurological diseases of aging are stroke and Alzheimer's disease. For example, with an aging population in the USA, the incidence of stroke is expected to almost double in the coming quarter century despite aggressive control of the treatable risk factors (Broderick, 2004). If the incidence of cerebral small vessel disease increases with age, and this entity produces deficits in cognitive function and fine motor skill in normal adults, it might be expected that the presence of cerebral small vessel disease would exacerbate the behavioral effect of a superimposed stroke or Alzheimer's disease. Indeed, there is an overall increased effect of cerebral small vessel disease in terms of cognitive decline with advancing age in general (Garde et al., 2000).

The processes that lead to cerebral small vessel disease overlap with both stroke and Alzheimer's disease; indeed one type of small vessel disease, CAA, is strongly associated with AD (see above). Thus, only recently have studies with large numbers of patients pathologically segregated cases with

small vessel disease, larger strokes and Alzheimer's disease pathologic changes (Giannakopoulos et al., 2007). Patients with early Alzheimer's disease and superimposed cerebral small vessel disease perform less well on cognitive tests than those *without* small vessel disease. This includes poorer performance on measures of information processing speed, visual memory and executive function (Burns et al., 2005). Thus, cerebral small vessel disease may compound the behavioral effects of emerging Alzheimer pathologic change. Such a relationship between cerebral small vessel disease and recovery of function after stroke has not been demonstrated. However, aged individuals, who are highly likely to have an increased burden of cerebral small vessel disease (see previous), recover less well from stroke (Dobkin, 2003).

Neurologic recovery after stroke occurs in large part through reorganization and repair in adjacent brain areas, such as peri-infarct cortex (Carmichael, 2006). Brain areas adjacent to the stroke assume cognitive functions of the infarct site, sprout new connections and participate in the regeneration of new neurons (Carmichael, 2006; Ohab et al., 2006). If these brain areas, or their connections, have microinfarcts, demyelination and chronic inflammation related to ischemia, it might be expected that they will exhibit less neuronal plasticity and recovery. It has long been recognized by neurorehabilitation specialists that patients with moderate to severe cerebral small vessel disease exhibit a greater neurologic deficit and reduced neurologic recovery following ischemic strokes (Figure 21.8). However, there have been no systematic studies of the effect of quantified levels of cerebral small vessel disease on neurologic *recovery* after stroke. This is clearly an area of study that will provide important insights into the process of neurologic recovery in the aged brain after injury.

In summary, cerebral small vessel disease manifests as an age-related disease that physically and cognitively "*slows patients down*." Normal, community-dwelling people with cerebral small vessel disease have reduced cognitive processing speed, planning and attention; reduced fine motor skill and performance in activities of daily living and a greater rate of cognitive and physical decline with age. Cerebral small vessel disease also compounds the effects of other neurologic diseases of aging, by worsening the behavioral effects of Alzheimer pathology and likely by impacting the neuroplasticity that underlies recovery after stroke. The basic neurobiological mechanisms through which white matter lesions impair cognitive function or recovery after neurologic injury has not been well defined. Small vessel disease in white matter tracts may impact the remapping of cognitive operations that is seen in these diseases, as well as the cellular processes of axonal sprouting, neurogenesis and adaptive plasticity in cortical areas that connect *through* damaged white matter.

ACKNOWLEDGMENTS

Work in H. Vinters' laboratory supported by PHS grants P50 AG 16570, NS 44378 and P01 AG 12435. Technical assistance and help with preparation of the manuscript, including illustrations, was provided by Justine Pomakian, Matthew Lynch and Carol Appleton. HVV supported in part by the Daljit S. & Elaine Sarkaria Chair in Diagnostic Medicine. Some of the illustrations are from the archival collection of the late Dr. Uwamie Tomiyasu, formerly neuropathologist at the West Los Angeles VAMC.

REFERENCES

Anders, K. H., Wang, Z. Z., Kornfeld, M. *et al.* (1997). Giant cell arteritis in association with cerebral amyloid angiopathy: immunohistochemical and molecular studies. *Human Pathology*, **28**, 1237–1246.

Auerbach, I. D., Sung, S. H., Wang, Z., & Vinters, H. V. (2003). Smooth muscle cells and the pathogenesis of cerebral microvascular disease ("angiomyopathies"). *Experimental and Molecular Pathology*, **74**, 148–159.

Barkhof, F., & Scheltens, P. (2002). Imaging of white matter lesions. *Cerebrovascular Disease*, **13**, *Suppl. 2*, 21–30.

Barkhof, F., & Scheltens, P. (2006). Is the whole brain periventricular? *Journal of Neurology, Neurosurgery and Psychiatry*, **77**, 143–144.

Bennett, D. A., Schneider, J. A., Arvanitakis, Z. *et al.* (2006). Neuropathology of older persons without cognitive impairment from two community based studies. *Neurology*, **66**, 1837–1844.

Broderick, J. P. (2004). William M. Feinberg Lecture. Stroke therapy in the year 2025: burden, breakthroughs, and barriers to progress. *Stroke*, **35**, 205–211.

Brown, W. R., Moody, D. M., Thore, C. R., & Challa, V. R. (2000). Apoptosis in leukoaraiosis. *American Journal of Neuroradiology*, **21**, 79–82.

Burns, J. M., Church, J. A., Johnson, D. K. *et al.* (2005). White matter lesions are prevalent but differentially related with cognition in aging and early Alzheimer disease. *Archives of Neurology*, **62**, 1870–1876.

Cadavid, D., Mena, H., Koeller, K., & Frommelt, R. R. (2000). Cerebral beta amyloid angiopathy is a risk factor for cerebral ischemic infarction. A case control study in human brain biopsies. *Journal of Neuropathology and Experimental Neurology*, **59**, 768–773.

Carmichael, S. T. (2006). Cellular and molecular mechanisms of neural repair after stroke: making waves. *Annals of Neurology*, **59**, 735–742.

Chui, H. (2005). Neuropathology lessons in vascular dementia. *Alzheimer Disease and Associated Disorders*, **19**, 45–52.

Chui, H. C., Zarow, C., Mack, W. J. *et al.* (2006). Cognitive impact of subcortical vascular and Alzheimer's disease pathology. *Annals of Neurology*, **60**, 677–687.

de Groot, J. C., de Leeuw, F. E., Oudkerk, M. *et al.* (2002). Periventricular cerebral white matter lesions predict rate of cognitive decline. *Annals of Neurology*, **52**, 335–341.

del Ser, T., Bermejo, F., Portera, A. *et al.* (1990). Vascular dementia. A clinicopathological study. *Journal of the Neurological Sciences*, **96**, 1–17.

Dickson, D. W., Davies, P., Bevona, C. *et al.* (1994). Hippocampal sclerosis: a common pathological feature of dementia in very old (greater than 80 year of age) humans. *Acta Neuropathologica*, **88**, 212–221.

Dobkin, B. (2003). *The Clinical Science of Neurologic Rehabilitation*. Oxford, UK: Oxford University Press.

Eng, J. A., Frosch, M. P., Choi, K., Rebeck, W. G., & Greenberg, S. M. (2004). Clinical manifestations of cerebral amyloid angiopathy-related inflammation. *Annals of Neurology*, **55**, 250–256.

Erkinjuntti, T., Haltia, M., Palo, J., Sulkava, R., & Paetau, A. (1988). Accuracy of the clinical diagnosis of vascular dementia: a prospective clinical and post-mortem neuropathological study. *Journal of Neurology, Neurosurgery and Psychiatry*, **51**, 1037–1044.

Fernando, M. S., Ince, P. G., & Group, on behalf of the MRC Cognitive Function and Ageing Neuropathology Study Group (2004). Vascular pathologies and cognition in a population-based cohort of elderly people. *Journal of the Neurological Sciences*, **226**, 13–17.

Ferro, J. M., & Madureira, S. (2002). Age-related white matter changes and cognitive impairment. *Journal of the Neurological Sciences*, **203–204**, 221–225.

Garde, E., Mortensen, E. L., Krabbe, K., Rostrup, E., & Larsson, H. B. (2000). Relation between age-related decline in intelligence and cerebral white-matter hyperintensities in healthy octogenarians: a longitudinal study. *Lancet*, **356**, 628–634.

Ghiso, J., Rostagno, A., Tomidokoro, Y. *et al.* (2006). Genetic alterations of the BRI2 gene: familial British and Danish dementias. *Brain Pathology*, **16**, 71–79.

Giannakopoulos, P., Gold, G., Kovari, E. *et al.* (2007). Assessing the cognitive impact of Alzheimer disease pathology and vascular burden in the aging brain: the Geneva experience. *Acta Neuropathologica*, **113**, 1–12.

Gilbert, J. J., & Vinters, H. V. (1983). Cerebral amyloid angiopathy: Incidence and complications in the aging brain. I. Cerebral hemorrhage. *Stroke*, **14**, 915–923.

Grabowski, T. J., Cho, H. S., Vonsattel, J. P. G., Rebeck, G. W., & Greenberg, S. M. (2001). Novel amyloid precursor protein mutation in an Iowa family with dementia and severe cerebral amyloid angiopathy. *Annals of Neurology*, **49**, 697–705.

Gray, F., Vinters, H. V., Le Noan, H. *et al.* (1990). Cerebral amyloid angiopathy and granulomatous angiitis: immunohistochemical study using antibodies to the Alzheimer A4 peptide. *Human Pathology*, **21**, 1290–1293.

Gray, F., Robert, F., Labrecque, R. *et al.* (1994). Autosomal dominant arteriopathic leuko-encephalopathy and Alzheimer's disease. *Neuropathology and Applied Neurobiology*, **20**, 22–30.

Greenberg, S. M., Vonsattel, J. P. G., Stakes, J. W., Gruber, M., & Finklestein, S. P. (1993). The clinical spectrum of cerebral amyloid angiopathy: presentations without lobar hemorrhage. *Neurology*, **43**, 2073–2079.

Hachinski, V., C., I., Petersen, R. C. *et al.* (2006). National Institute of Neurological Disorders and Stroke – Canadian Stroke Network Vascular Cognitive Impairment Harmonization Standards. *Stroke*, **37**, 2220–2241.

Haglund, M., Sjobeck, M., & Englund, E. (2004). Severe cerebral amyloid angiopathy characterizes an underestimated variant of vascular dementia. *Dementia and Geriatric Cognitive Disorders*, **18**, 132–137.

Hansen, L. A., & Crain, B. J. (1995). Making the diagnosis of mixed and non-Alzheimer dementias. *Archives of Pathology and Laboratory Medicine*, **119**, 1023–1031.

Herzig, M. C., Van Nostrand, W. E., & Jucker, M. (2006). Mechanism of cerebral beta-amyloid angiopathy: murine and cellular models. *Brain Pathology*, **16**, 40–54.

Hopkins, R. O., Beck, C. J., Burnett, D. L. *et al.* (2006). Prevalence of white matter hyperintensities in a young healthy population. *Journal of Neuroimaging*, **16**, 243–251.

Hulette, C., Nochlin, D., McKeel, D. *et al.* (1997). Clinical-neuropathologic findings in multi-infarct dementia: a report of six autopsied cases. *Neurology*, **48**, 668–672.

Ince, P. G., & Fernando, M. S. (2003). Neuropathology of vascular cognitive impairment and vascular dementia. *International Psychogeriatrics*, **15**, Suppl. 1, 71–75.

Jellinger, K. A. (2002). The pathology of ischemic-vascular dementia: an update. *Journal of the Neurological Sciences*, **203–204**, 153–157.

Jen, J., Cohen, A. H., Yue, Q. *et al.* (1997). Hereditary endotheliopathy with retinopathy, nephropathy, and stroke (HERNS). *Neurology*, **49**, 1322–1330.

Jin, K., Wang, X., Xie, L. *et al.* (2006). Evidence for stroke-induced neurogenesis in the human brain. *Proceedings of the National Academy of Sciences of the United States of America*, **103**, 13198–13202.

Kalaria, R. N., Kenny, R. A., Ballard, C. G. *et al.* (2004). Towards defining the neuropathological substrates of vascular dementia. *Journal of the Neurological Sciences*, **226**, 75–80.

Kalimo, H. (2005). *Pathology and Genetics. Cerebrovascular Disease.* Basel, Switzerland: ISN Neuropath Press.

Kalimo, H., Ruchoux, M.-M., Viitanen, M., & Kalaria, R. N. (2002). CADASIL: a common form of hereditary arteriopathy causing brain infarcts and dementia. *Brain Pathology*, **12**, 371–384.

Knopman, D. S., Parisi, J. E., Salviati, A. *et al.* (2003). Neuropathology of cognitively normal elderly. *Journal of Neuropathology and Experimental Neurology*, **62**, 1087–1095.

Kovari, E., Gold, G., Herrmann, F. R. *et al.* (2004). Cortical microinfarcts and demyelination significantly affect cognition in brain aging. *Stroke*, **35**, 410–414.

Lammie, G. A. (2002). Hypertensive cerebral small vessel disease and stroke. *Brain Pathology*, **12**, 358–370.

Lim, G. T., Mendez, M. F., Bronstein, Y. L., Jouben-Steele, L., & Vinters, H. V. (2002). Clinicopathologic case report: akinetic mutism with findings of white matter hyperintensity.

Journal of Neuropsychiatry and Clinical Neuroscience, **14**, 214–221.

Medana, I. M., & Esiri, M. M. (2003). Axonal damage: a key predictor of outcome in human CNS diseases. *Brain*, **126**, 515–530.

Miao, Q., Paloneva, T., Tuominen, S. *et al.* (2004). Fibrosis and stenosis of the long penetrating cerebral arteries: the cause of the white matter pathology in cerebral autosomal dominant arteriopathy with subcortical infarcts and leukoencephalopathy. *Brain Pathology*, **14**, 358–364.

Munoz, D. G. (1991). The pathological basis of multi-infarct dementia. *Alzheimer Disease and Associated Disorders*, **5**, 77–90.

Natte, R., Maat-Schieman, M. L. C., Haan, J. *et al.* (2001). Dementia in hereditary cerebral hemorrhage with amyloidosis – Dutch type is associated with cerebral amyloid angiopathy but is independent of plaques and neurofibrillary tangles. *Annals of Neurology*, **50**, 765–772.

Nicoll, J. A. R., Burnett, C., Love, S. *et al.* (1997). High frequency of apolipoprotein E epsilon 2 allele in hemorrhage due to cerebral amyloid angiopathy. *Annals of Neurology*, **41**, 716–721.

Nolan, K. A., Lino, M. M., Seligmann, A. W., & Blass, J. P. (1998). Absence of vascular dementia in an autopsy series from a dementia clinic. *Journal of the American Geriatrics Society*, **46**, 597–604.

Obici, L., Demarchi, A., de Rosa, G. *et al.* (2005). A novel AbetaPP mutation exclusively associated with cerebral amyloid angiopathy. *Annals of Neurology*, **58**, 639–644.

O'Brien, J. T., Erkinjuntti, T., Reisberg, B. *et al.* (2003). Vascular cognitive impairment. *Lancet Neurology*, **2**, 89–98.

Ohab, J. J., Fleming, S., Blesch, A., & Carmichael, S. T. (2006). A neurovascular niche for neurogenesis after stroke. *Journal of Neuroscience*, **26**, 13007–13016.

Palsdottir, A., Snorradottir, A. O., & Thorsteinsson, L. (2006). Hereditary cystatin C amyloid angiopathy: genetic, clinical, and pathological aspects. *Brain Pathology*, **16**, 55–59.

Pantoni, L., Garcia, J. H., & Brown, G. G. (1996). Vascular pathology in three cases of progressive cognitive deterioration. *Journal of the Neurological Sciences*, **135**, 131–139.

Prins, N. D., van Dijk, E. J., den Heijer, T. *et al.* (2005). Cerebral small-vessel disease and decline in information processing speed, executive function and memory. *Brain*, **128**, 2034–2041.

Rensink, A. A. M., de Waal, R. M. W., Kremer, B., & Verbeek, M. M. (2003). Pathogenesis of cerebral amyloid angiopathy. *Brain Research Reviews*, **43**, 207–223.

Revesz, T., Holton, J. L., Lashley, T. *et al.* (2002). Sporadic and familial cerebral amyloid angiopathies. *Brain Pathology*, **12**, 343–357.

Ringelstein, E. B., & Nabavi, D. G. (2005). Cerebral small vessel diseases: cerebral microangiopathies. *Current Opinion in Neurology*, **18**, 179–188.

Roman, G. C., Erkinjuntti, T., Wallin, A., Pantoni, L., & Chui, H. C. (2002). Subcortical ischaemic vascular dementia. *Lancet Neurology*, **1**, 426–436.

Rosano, C., Kuller, L. H., Chung, H. *et al.* (2005). Subclinical brain magnetic resonance imaging abnormalities predict physical functional decline in high-functioning older adults. *Journal of the American Geriatrics Society*, **53**, 649–654.

Rosano, C., Brach, J., Longstreth, W. T. J., & Newman, A. B. (2006). Quantitative measures of gait characteristics indicate prevalence of underlying subclinical structural brain abnormalities in high-functioning older adults. *Neuroepidemiology*, **26**, 52–60.

Sachdev, P. S., Wen, W., Christensen, H., & Jorm, A. F. (2005). White matter hyperintensities are related to physical disability and poor motor function. *Journal of Neurology, Neurosurgery and Psychiatry*, **76**, 362–367.

Schmidt, R., Scheltens, P., Erkinjuntti, T. *et al.* (2004). White matter lesion progression: a surrogate endpoint for trials in cerebral small-vessel disease. *Neurology*, **63**, 139–144.

Selnes, O. A., & Vinters, H. V. (2006). Vascular cognitive impairment. *Nature Clinical Practice Neurology*, **2**, 538–547.

Soderlund, H., Nilsson, L. G., Berger, K. *et al.* (2006). Cerebral changes on MRI and cognitive function: the CASCADE study. *Neurobiology of Aging*, **27**, 16–23.

van den Heuvel, D. M., ten Dam, V. H., de Craen, A. J. *et al.* (2006). Increase in periventricular white matter hyperintensities parallels decline in mental processing speed in a non-demented elderly population. *Journal of Neurology, Neurosurgery and Psychiatry*, **77**, 149–153.

Verbeek, M. M., de Waal, R. M. W., & Vinters, H. V. (2000). *Cerebral Amyloid Angiopathy in Alzheimer's Disease and Related Disorders*. Dordrecht, the Netherlands: Kluwer Academic Publishers.

Vinters, H. V. (1987). Cerebral amyloid angiopathy: a critical review. *Stroke*, **18**, 311–324.

Vinters, H. V. (1992). Cerebral amyloid angiopathy and Alzheimer's disease: two entities or one? *Journal of the Neurological Sciences*, **112**, 1–3.

Vinters, H. V. (2001a). Cerebrovascular disease – practical issues in surgical and autopsy pathology. *Current Topics in Pathology*, **95**, 51–99.

Vinters, H. V. (2001b). Cerebral amyloid angiopathy: a microvascular link between parenchymal and vascular dementia? *Annals of Neurology*, **49**, 691–693.

Vinters, H. V., & Gilbert, J. J. (1983). Cerebral amyloid angiopathy: incidence and complications in the aging brain. II. The distribution of amyloid vascular changes. *Stroke*, **14**, 924–928.

Vinters, H. V., Secor, D. L., Read, S. L. *et al.* (1994). The microvasculature in brain biopsy specimens from patients with Alzheimer's disease: an immunohistochemical and ultrastructural study. *Ultrastructural Pathology*, **18**, 333–348.

Vinters, H. V., Wang, Z. Z., & Secor, D. L. (1996). Brain parenchymal and microvascular amyloid in Alzheimer's disease. *Brain Pathology*, **6**, 179–195.

Vinters, H. V., Farrell, M. A., Mischel, P. S., & Anders, K. H. (1998a). Basic neurobiology and cellular responses in nervous system diseases. In H. V. Vinters (Ed.), *Diagnostic Neuropathology* (pp. 1–49). New York, NY: Marcel Dekker Inc.

Vinters, H. V., Natte, R., Maat-Schieman, M. L. C. *et al.* (1998b). Secondary microvascular degeneration in amyloid angiopathy of patients with hereditary cerebral hemorrhage with amyloidosis, Dutch type (HCHWA-D). *Acta Neuropathologica*, **95**, 235–244.

Vinters, H. V., Ellis, W. G., Zarow, C. *et al.* (2000). Neuropathologic substrates of ischemic vascular dementia. *Journal of Neuropathology and Experimental Neurology*, **59**, 931–945.

Wallin, A., & Blennow, K. (1991). Pathogenetic basis of vascular dementia. *Alzheimer Disease and Associated Disorders*, **5**, 91–102.

Wang, Z. Z., Jensson, O., Thorsteinsson, L., & Vinters, H. V. (1997). Microvascular degeneration in hereditary cystatin C amyloid angiopathy. *Acta Pathologica, Microbiologica et Immunologica Scandinavica*, **105**, 41–47.

Ylikoski, A., Erkinjuntti, T., Raininko, R., Sarna, S., Sulkava, R., & Tilvis, R. (1995). White matter hyperintensities on MRI in the neurologically nondiseased elderly. Analysis of cohorts of consecutive subjects aged 55 to 85 years living at home. *Stroke*, **26**, 1171–1177.

Zhang-Nunes, S. X., Maat-Schieman, M. L. C., van Duinen, S. G. *et al.* (2006). The cerebral beta-amyloid angiopathies: hereditary and sporadic. *Brain Pathology*, **16**, 30–39.

22

Intrinsic and extrinsic neural stem cell treatment of central nervous system injury and disease

Trudi Stickland, Samuel Weiss and Bryan Kolb

Introduction

Neural stem cells (NSC) display three main characteristics; they are derived from the central nervous system and can generate neural tissue, they are able to self-renew, and they are multipotent (Gage, 2000). The adult mammalian brain has retained the capacity for neurogenesis, presenting a promising avenue for disease treatment (Lledo *et al.*, 2006). Stem cell treatment can take the form of either intrinsic repair through the mobilization of endogenous precursors, or through stem cell transplantation. Both have their strengths and weaknesses, however mobilization of endogenous stem cells to aid in recovery may represent the most practical and ethical means of stem cell treatment.

Harnessing endogenous NSCs for therapeutic purposes has been investigated within a number of disease models including stroke (Arvidsson *et al.*, 2002; Jin *et al.*, 2003; Nakatomi *et al.*, 2002;), multiple sclerosis (Calza *et al.*, 2002; Danilov *et al.*, 2006; Picard-Riera *et al.*, 2002), Parkinson's disease (Cooper & Isacson, 2004; Fallon *et al.*, 2000), and Huntington's disease (Curtis *et al.*, 2003; Lazic *et al.*, 2006). Different diseases require replacement of different cell phenotypes, different migratory routes, and different treatment regimes in order to be successful (Lindvall *et al.*, 2004). For example, in order for stem cell treatment to be successful in treating stroke, cells must not only replace those that have been lost, but must be incorporated into the existing circuitry in order to reestablish connections necessary for functional recovery to pre-stroke levels. Furthermore, not only do neurons need to be replaced, but also the glia, including astrocytes and oligodendrocytes, require replacement. Although there has been much progress in understanding various diseases and how stem cells may be of use in supporting recovery, to date, no treatment has proven to be 100% effective. Most likely, stem cell therapy will have to be supplemented with other types of rehabilitation in order to promote a more complete recovery.

Basic research, using animal models of disease, provides an avenue for investigating stem cell treatments. Furthermore, basic research allows for a greater understanding of the disease process, and how recovery may manifest. The focus of the following chapter is on the role of stem cells in recovery following injury or disease of the central nervous system, with special emphasis on intrinsic mobilisation of stem cells for the treatment of stroke.

Clinical stroke

- Stroke is a devastating disease with few treatment options.
- Animal models of stroke provide an opportunity to understand the pathology and recovery process following stroke.

Stroke can be classified into two types: hemorrhagic or ischemic. Hemorrhagic stroke, accounting for roughly 20% of strokes, involves a rupture of blood vessels in the brain resulting in death of the tissue in contact with the blood. The remaining 80% of

Cognitive Neurorehabilitation, Second Edition: Evidence and Application, ed. Donald T. Stuss, Gordon Winocur and Ian H. Robertson. Published by Cambridge University Press. © Cambridge University Press 2008.

strokes are ischemic, which result from a disruption in blood flow, typically caused by a clot, with death to the tissue of the areas normally fed by the blocked blood vessel. Stroke is the fourth leading cause of death in Canada, and approximately 300000 Canadians are living with the resulting disabilities. Deficits following a stroke can include disruptions to gross and fine movements as well as coordination of movements, disruptions to the sensory system, and problems with communication – including speaking, understanding language, reading, writing and the ability to do arithmetic, as well as changes in personality (Santos *et al.*, 2006). Very few survivors show recovery to levels of pre-stroke functioning. Most stroke sufferers must rely on family and care-givers to help them through day-to-day life, and adjust to a significantly reduced quality of life with an increased risk of depression (Nys *et al.*, 2006).

With stroke being such a prevalent, and disabling, disease, finding new treatments that can aid in recovery are of paramount importance. To date, the most effective treatment for ischemic stroke involves the administration of recombinant tissue plasminogen activator (rtPA), a thrombolytic agent that can break up clots and restore blood flow, resulting in a rescue of much of the ischemic penumbra. Unfortunately, the administration of rtPA must occur during the first 3–4 hours of stroke onset, making the window of administration very narrow (Kindler *et al.*, 2000). Less than 4% of stroke patients receive rtPA, and of those who do receive it, reperfusion and complete recovery occurs only 50% of the time (Davalos, 2005). In the event that rtPA cannot be administered, or the patient presents with hemorrhagic stroke, surgery may be required to break up the clot, remove excess blood or repair vasculature.

Following the acute period of stroke, rehabilitation therapy can be used in order to help the patient regain strength and dexterity of the paretic limb. One such therapy involves constraining the good limb thereby forcing the patient to use the paretic limb, a method termed constraint-induced movement therapy (CIMT). This form of treatment arose from the observation that forelimb deafferentation

in the monkey resulted in non-use of the forelimb, even though they were physically capable of using it, a condition referred to as "learned non-use" (Taub *et al.*, 1994). It was found that the monkey could be forced to use the paretic limb if the good limb was restrained, and furthermore that if the monkey was left in the restraining device for a pro-longed period of time, use of the deafferented limb substantially increased after the device was removed, which was retained for at least 4 years (Taub, 1977, 1980). In 1980, Taub transferred this technique to human patients who had suffered a stroke and had reached a plateau in their recovery. The results were exceptionally encouraging, dem-onstrating that CIMT could help to restore quality of movement, functional ability and strength well beyond initial recovery. Since then, this method of rehabilitation has received much attention as an intervention following stroke (Dromerick *et al.*, 2000; Liepert *et al.*, 2000; Lincoln *et al.*, 1999; Pierce *et al.*, 2003; Schaechter *et al.*, 2002; Taub *et al.*, 2006), and other forms of brain injury (Charles *et al.*, 2006; Shaw *et al.*, 2005). Furthermore, advances in imaging techniques have revealed that CIMT induces reor-ganisation of cortical areas responsible for motor output (Hamzei *et al.*, 2006; Ro *et al.*, 2006), a finding that parallels what has been found in animal studies (Frost *et al.*, 2003; Nudo & Milliken, 1996). (See Chapter 23 by Morris and Taub in this volume.)

While motor deficits are most prevalent following stroke, the incidence of cognitive deficits can range from 10–82% (Rasquin *et al.*, 2004). Studies inves-tigating cognitive recovery following stroke have indicated that the most affected cognitive domains involve calculation, executive functioning and vis-ual perception (Nys *et al.*, 2005). Recovery of these deficits is as high as 80% within the first year follow-ing stroke and has been attributed to neural reor-ganisation (del Ser *et al.*, 2005).

Although no current treatment can lead to com-plete recovery, combining known treatments involving drug therapy and methods of rehabilita-tion will likely be needed. Gaining an understanding of how the brain responds to stroke and the natural progression of spontaneous recovery can give important insight into creating better treatments. A plethora of animal models have been used to mimic clinical stroke, allowing for a greater understanding of the neuropathology of stroke and the mechanisms underlying the recovery process.

Animal models allow for a deeper understanding of stroke

Many human neurological disorders are modeled in animals (Schallert *et al.*, 2000), with the rat being the most common. Animal disease models allow for in-depth examination of the disease time course, molecular underpinnings, behavioral manifestations and recovery. There is apprehension regarding the use of animal models for clinical disease, due to the notion that the animal models cannot possibly replicate the human disease exactly. However, so long as the manifestations of the disease are based primarily on functional similarities this need not be a concern (Cenci *et al.*, 2002). As such, it is important to recognize how the animal would manifest a given symptom, instead of supposing that it would manifest as it would in the human. For example, when conducting behavioral analysis of motor deficits following primary motor cortex stroke, the scale used to assess the impairment will be different for rat and human, however the interpretation of the extent of deficit, and the underlying circuitry, may not. Once this is understood and implemented animal models of human disease become essential for furthering our understanding of disease.

In diseases such as stroke, the rat provides an excellent model for gaining insights into deficits and recovery (Aspey *et al.*, 1998). Not only are motor deficits one of the most common disabilities following human stroke, but also some motor behaviors in the rat (such as reaching) parallel those seen in humans (Iwaniuk & Whishaw, 2000; Metz & Whishaw, 2000). Likewise, a number of tasks measuring such cognitive abilities as learning and memory can be employed. Furthermore, a rat model can allow for use of a wide array of behavioral testing paradigms, and also lends well to histochemical and molecular techniques.

Neural stem cells

- Neural stem cells are multipotent, self-renewing, proliferative cells that can be found within the adult mammalian CNS.
- Injury and disease can alter adult neurogenesis.

Since the discovery of multipotential stem cells in the adult forebrain (Altman, 1969; Altman & Das, 1965), there has been much interest in harnessing these endogenous precursors for prospective therapeutic use. The ability to tap into endogenous stem cells to aid in recovery following injury or disease would negate issues surrounding the use of embryonic stem cells for transplantation as well as the need for immunosuppression. The following section reviews adult neural stem cells, their role following injury and disease, and the relationship between stem cells and functional recovery.

Neural stem cells: what are they?

In a general sense, neural stem cells (NSC) can be thought of as multipotent, self-renewing cells that can proliferate in order to produce the different cell types required for the development and maintenance of neural tissue (Gage, 2000). A true stem cell has the ability to self-renew for the entire lifetime of the organism, an important attribute given the existence of many types of progenitor cells that have a limited self-renewal life span (van der Kooy & Weiss, 2000). There are three types of stem cells, distinguished according to their origin. Embryonic stem cells arise from the inner cell mass of the blastocyst of the embryo, are totipotent and differentiate to form the germ layers. Fetal stem cells are a more restricted progenitor, which can be harvested from tissue. However, there are many ethical and legal concerns over embryonic and fetal stem cells that restrict their therapeutic use. Adult neural stem cells are multipotent, allowing them the ability to differentiate into the three main cell types of the central nervous system: astrocytes, oligodendrocytes and neurons (Figure 22.1). In the adult mammalian brain there are two main regions of neurogenesis; the subventricular zone (SVZ) (Altman, 1969;

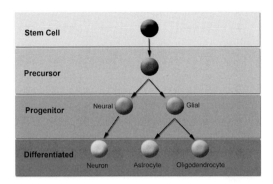

Figure 22.1. Lineage of adult neural stem cells. Adult neural stem cells are self-renewing, with the capacity to differentiate into the three major cell types of the central nervous system: neurons, astrocytes and oligodendrocytes.

Morshead & van der Kooy, 1992) and the subgranular zone of the dentate gyrus (Altman & Das, 1965).

In rodents, stem cells resident in the adult SVZ (Craig *et al.*, 1996; Morshead *et al.*, 1994; Reynolds & Weiss, 1992), will migrate through the rostral migratory stream (RMS) to the olfactory bulb where they differentiate into a neuronal phenotype (Lois & Alvarez-Buylla, 1994). While some of these cells incorporate into the existing circuitry, others will die almost immediately (Morshead & van der Kooy, 1992), suggesting equilibrium of cell death and replacement within the tissue.

Neural stem cells resident in the adult mammalian subgranular zone of the dentate gyrus produce progenitor cells that migrate to the nearby dentate granule cell layer, where they differentiate into granule neurons (Kuhn *et al.*, 1996), and functionally integrate into the existing circuitry (Carlen *et al.*, 2002; Markakis & Gage, 1999).

Intrinsic vs. extrinsic stem cell treatment

- Environmental manipulations can increase growth factor levels and increase neurogenesis, both of which may work to ameliorate functional deficits following injury or disease.

- Administration of various agents can increase neurogenesis and support neural stem cell differentiation.
- Transplantation of stem cells allows for a specific cell phenotype to be introduced to a specific area of injury or disease.
- Genetic manipulations allow for the manufacturing of stem cells secreting specific agents to be transplanted into the adult CNS.

The ultimate goal of stem cell therapy in injury and disease is to replace lost or damaged cells and re-establish functional circuitry, which may lead to significant improvement of behavioral deficits. Stem cells can be utilised therapeutically via two primary methods: endogenous recruitment, or transplantation. Both have their strengths and weaknesses, which will be discussed.

Environmental manipulations and neurogenesis

Intrinsically, adult hippocampal neurogenesis can be modulated by a variety of external factors including exercise (van Praag *et al.*, 1999a, 1999b, 2005), environmental enrichment (Kempermann *et al.*, 1997; Komitova *et al.*, 2005a), and learning (Gould *et al.*, 1999). It has been shown that hippocampal expression of vascular endothelial growth factor (VEGF) is increased by spatial learning (Cao *et al.*, 2004), exercise (Fabel *et al.*, 2003) and enriched housing (Matthew & Cao, 2006). Vascular endothelial growth factor has also been known to act as a neurotrophic factor (Jin *et al.* 2000; Oosthuyse *et al.*, 2001) and to have neurogenic effects on neural progenitors (Jin *et al.*, 2002). Studies have demonstrated that mice with increased VEGF expression will show enhanced neurogenesis and improvements in hippocampal-dependent learning (Cao *et al.*, 2004; Matthew & Cao, 2006). Furthermore, decreased VEGF expression can abolish enrichment-induced neurogenesis (Cao *et al.*, 2004). Thus, VEGF may be necessary for mediating the beneficial effects of environmentally induced neurogenesis, learning and memory.

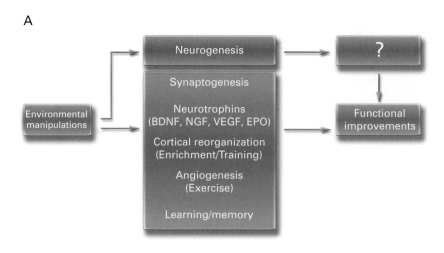

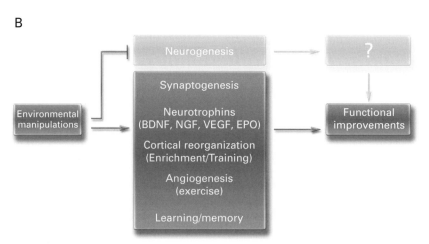

Figure 22.2. Environmental manipulations and functional recovery. (A) Environmental manipulations are known to increase neurogenesis as well as influence plasticity and neurotrophin release, resulting in functional improvements. Although plasticity and neurotrophin release can directly influence recovery, neurogenesis most likely influences recovery indirectly, acting through an as of yet unknown mechanism. (B) Recent research has suggested that blocking environmentally mediated neurogenesis does not ablate the functional benefits of this manipulation. This suggests that large-scale alterations in plasticity and increases in neurotrophins may have greater impact on functional restitution following injury and disease.

Until recently, it had been hypothesized that following environmental manipulations, the resulting increase in neurogenesis was responsible for improved hippocampal dependent learning and memory (Snyder *et al.*, 2005; Winocur *et al.*, 2006) and reduced anxiety (Roy *et al.*, 2001) (Figure 22.2A). This concept was challenged by Meshi and colleagues (Meshi *et al.*, 2006), who used focal X-irradiation to halt neurogenesis within the hippocampus of rats before providing them with either an enriched environment, or standard laboratory housing. If neurogenesis is necessary for behavioral changes associated with enriched housing then those rats that received the X-irradiation should demonstrate behavior akin to their littermates that were housed in standard conditions. These behaviors would include maintenance of baseline memory functioning and a moderate level of anxiety behaviors. Surprisingly, what they found was that although the X-irradiation did in fact abolish hippocampal neurogenesis, there was no reduction in the behavioral phenotype seen with enriched housing. Thus, hippocampal neurogenesis does not appear to be required for the behavioral effects of environmental enrichment (Figure 22.2B). Environmental enrichment is known to have other effects, including the ability to induce widespread changes in synaptic organization, which likely underlie the behavioral effects of this manipulation (Kolb & Whishaw, 1998).

Although it is known that neurogenesis correlates negatively with aging, such that as age increases there is a reduction in neurogenesis (Enwere *et al.*, 2004; Jin *et al.*, 2004; Luo *et al.*, 2006), there may be methods to ameliorate this. For instance, it has been shown that voluntary running will significantly increase hippocampal neurogenesis in aged rats, concomitant with improvement in a spatial memory task (van Praag *et al.*, 2005). Furthermore, long-term housing in an enriched environment has been demonstrated to increase neurogenesis in the aging rodent brain, concomitant with increases in cognitive functioning (Kempermann *et al.*, 2002). These findings, that exercise and environmental enrichment can impact neurogenesis and aid in functional improvement in the aged animal, has important implications as many diseases strike at later ages when neurogenesis is reduced. It is important to keep in mind that the relationship between neurogenesis and behavioral improvements resulting from environmental interventions is not necessarily causally linked, emphasizing the need for combining treatments. Although the exact mechanism

underlying the positive impact that neurogenesis has on disease recovery is still unknown, finding methods to increase neurogenesis in the aging brain may be important for replacing lost cells or indirectly aiding in functional recovery.

If an enriched environment or exercise can increase neurogenesis in the intact brain, can it also have positive effects in the damaged or diseased brain? Recent results suggest that this is true following fluid percussion injury (Gaulke *et al.*, 2005), epilepsy (Auvergne *et al.*, 2002) and stroke (Komitova *et al.*, 2002). For example, Komitova and colleagues (Komitova *et al.*, 2005a, 2005b) demonstrate that rats housed in an enriched environment following MCAo will have significantly increased neurogenesis in the subventricular zone compared with those rats housed in standard laboratory cages. It should be noted, however, that these new cells did not differentiate into mature neurons. Interestingly, there was significant motor improvement observed in the enriched rats despite the lack of neuronal replacement, further supporting the hypothesis that wide-scale alterations in synaptic organization following enrichment may be responsible for the observed beneficial response.

The effective duration of the complex housing has not been studied systematically but we have shown that 2 hours/day for 5 months is not sufficient to produce significant functional benefit after motor cortex stroke whereas 8 hours/day for only a month does provide significant benefit (Kolb, unpublished). This observation is likely important as we think about the design of human rehabilitation treatments.

Another question that remains unanswered is whether enriched housing can provide benefits to brain-injured animals on cognitive functions. Kolb & Gibb (1991) showed that although there was some general benefit from complex housing after large bilateral frontal injuries, there was no benefit to cognitive behaviors. It is unclear if this is because the injuries were bilateral or because the functional measures were cognitive rather than motor. However, there are benefits of complex housing on cognitive behavior in perinatally bilaterally brain-injured animals (e.g., Kolb & Elliott, 1987), although such effects may depend on the specific circumstances, such as the specific age at which injury is incurred.

One of the effects of enriched housing is to increase the production of a variety of neurotrophic factors including brain-derived neurotrophic factor (BDNF), nerve growth factor (NGF) and basic fibroblast growth factor (bFGF) (e.g., Dahlqvist *et al.*, 1999; Johansson, 2000). Although direct administration of these factors has been used as a treatment for brain injury (e.g., Kawamata *et al.*, 1997; Kolb *et al.*, 1997; Schäbitz *et al.*, 2004), the functional recovery is generally far from complete. However, the interplay between behavioral therapies and neurotrophic factors has not been well examined to date. Treatments incorporating various modes of rehabilitation following stem cell transplantation or administration of agents aimed at increasing neural stem cell proliferation may allow for the greatest degree of recovery following injury or disease. Recently, Witt-Lajeunesse *et al.* (submitted) investigated this possibility. Following injury to the motor cortex, a variety of treatments including basic FGF alone, reach training, complex housing, reach training with basic FGF or complex housing with basic FGF were employed. Interestingly, it was found that although different treatments could induce improvement in different facets of forepaw motor function, only when complex housing was used in conjunction with basic FGF treatment was functional improvement noted in all motor tasks assessed. Basic FGF is known to have a number of effects including the ability to increase neurogenesis (Kuhn *et al.*, 1997) and synaptic plasticity (Johansson, 2000), which, along with the aforementioned benefits of enrichment, may further enhance recovery. Although the mechanism underlying this recovery is unknown, immediate administration of basic FGF followed by complex housing beginning 3 days post lesion may result in the greatest benefit. Others have shown that early initiation of rehabilitation following cortical injury results in greater functional improvement than rehabilitation initiated at later time points (Biernaskie *et al.*, 2004). Understanding these critical periods will enhance

our ability to initiate effective treatments that allow for greater recovery, and can be applied to the clinical setting in order to improve functional outcomes following injury and disease.

The specific roles of newly generated cells as well as the mechanism underlying the functional improvement observed following exercise or enrichment remain unclear. Nevertheless, the effects of enrichment or exercise on neurogenesis and functional restitution following disease and injury in the adult cannot be overlooked as vital components of rehabilitation treatments.

Exogenous stimulation of adult neural stem cells

Unfortunately, many diseases and illnesses leave the patient unable to engage in the type of activity required to promote neurogenesis. As such, an understanding of the various agents that can be exogenously administered in order to enhance neurogenesis in the adult brain is necessary. By no means exhaustive, some of these agents include epidermal growth factor (EGF) (Craig *et al.*, 1996; Kuhn *et al.*, 1997), prolactin (PRL) (Shingo *et al.*, 2003), fibroblast growth factor-2 (FGF-2) (Palmer *et al.*, 1995; Kuhn *et al.*, 1997), insulin-like growth factor-1 (IGF-1) (Aberg *et al.*, 2000), VEGF and erythropoietin (EPO) (Shingo *et al.*, 2001; Wang *et al.*, 2006) (Table 22.1).

Perhaps the most commonly used neural stem cell mitogens are FGF-2 and EGF. In the developing mammalian brain, two populations of neural stem cells can be dissociated based on their responsiveness to these two mitogens (Tropepe *et al.*, 1999). In the adult, cells dissociated from the subventricular zone require FGF-2 or EGF in order to proliferate (Gritti *et al.*, 1999; Palmer *et al.*, 1995; Reynolds & Weiss, 1992; Richards *et al.*, 1992). In vivo, Craig *et al.* (1996) show that an infusion of EGF into the ventricle will increase proliferation of SVZ neural stem cells, yet does not promote cells to differentiate into neurons. Thus, an additional agent must be used in order to induce differentiation into a neuronal phenotype if these cells are to be of use

Table 22.1. Agents influencing adult stem cell proliferation, differentiation, and recovery of function

Agent	Impact on neurogenesis	Impact on recovery	References
Brain-derived neurotrophic factor (BDNF)	Increases number of newly generated neurons	Increases synaptic plasticity, neurite growth	Pencea *et al.* (2001)
Epidermal growth factor (EGF)	Administered intracerebroventricularly (icv) to increase subventricular zone (SVZ) neurogenesis	Limited ability to promote neurite outgrowth, may increase neurotrophic factors to have an indirect effect on recovery	Craig *et al.* (1996); Shetty & Turner (1999)
Prolactin (PRL)	Administered either peripherally, or icv to increase neurogenesis	None to date	Shingo *et al.* (2003)
Fibroblast growth factor-2 (FGF-2)	Peripheral administration to increase SVZ and hippocampal neurogenesis, and enhance neuronal survival	Promotes neurotrophic factors, aids in recovery following neonatal injury, improves sensorimotor deficits following ischemia	Li & Stephenson (2002); Monfils *et al.* (2005); Palmer *et al.* (1995)
Erythropoietin (EPO)	Peripheral administration has been shown to increase neurogenesis, and support neuronal differentiation	Promotes restoration of spatial memory following tramatic brain injury	Shingo *et al.* (2001); Lu *et al.* (2005)
Insulin-like growth factor-1 (IGF-1)	Peripheral administration can increase hippocampal neurogenesis, enhances survival of new neurons in the SVZ	Mimics effects of exercise or BDNF – increases synaptogenesis and brain plasticity	Aberg *et al.* (2000); Perez-Martin *et al.* (2003); Koopmans *et al.* (2006)
Vascular endothelial growth factor (VEGF)	Exogenous administration has been shown to increase hippocampal neurogenesis	Increases hippocampal dependent learning, works as a neurotrophin	Widenfalk *et al.* (2003); Cao *et al.* (2004)

therapeutically. In 2001, Shingo *et al.* demonstrated that erythropoietin (EPO) could be administered both in vitro and in vivo in order to induce differentiation of these SVZ precursors to a neuronal phenotype. Furthermore, EPO has been shown to have an effect on angiogenesis (Wang *et al.*, 2004) and neuronal survival (Siren *et al.*, 2001), both of which are important factors when considering recovery following stroke. Investigation into the administration of exogenous agents has shown that FGF-2 administration to mice expressing Huntington's disease-like symptoms show increased proliferation of neural stem cells, migration of these cells to the striatum where they replace the medium spiny neurons that had been lost with the disease, and a reduction in behavioral deficits associated with the disease (Jin *et al.*, 2005). These results demonstrate that exogenous administration of various neurogenic agents

can have beneficial effects following brain injury and disease in the absence of environmental manipulation. This is an important consideration when injury or disease leaves the victim unable to engage in strenuous activity.

Stem cell transplantation and disease

Although stem cell transplantation can be more invasive than intrinsic mobilization, it allows for the introduction of cells that have the specific phenotype required for a particular injury or disease. Furthermore with transplantation, stem cells can be introduced to optimal locations for recovery. For instance, it has been shown that following spinal cord injury in the rodent, stem cells can be transplanted into the injured area, which, when combined with infusions of growth factors, can enhance cell survival and differentiation of these cells into oligodendrocytes, which will help to remyelinate the damaged axons of the spinal cord and support functional recovery (Karimi-Abdolrezaee *et al.*, 2006). Unfortunately, it has also been demonstrated that although transplantation of adult neural stem cells into the injured spinal cord of adult mice can help improve sensory and motor deficits, it will also cause neuropathic pain (allodynia). When left on their own, transplanted stem cells will differentiate predominantly into a glial phenotype (Ogawa *et al.*, 2002; Vroemen *et al.*, 2003), which may secrete trophic factors that work to improve recovery indirectly (Lu *et al.*, 2003). Several studies show that administration of trophic factors will improve behavioral recovery in rodents, yet also result in allodynia (Hao *et al.*, 2000; Jubran & Widenfalk, 2003). In order to dissociate the effect of transplanted stem cells differentiating into astrocytes versus neurons and their effect on allodynia, Hofstetter and colleagues (Hofstetter *et al.*, 2005) performed stem cell transplants of either naive or stem cells transduced to express neurogenin-2, a transcription factor involved in determination and differentiation of neuronal lineages, into spinal-cord injured mice. They found that naive neural stem cell transplants became predominantly astrocytes and improved function following the spinal-cord injury, but also caused allodynia. Interestingly, those stem cells transduced to express neurogenin-2 did in fact differentiate predominantly into oligodendrocytes, allowed for further sensory and motor recovery, and did not cause allodynia. Thus, ensuring that transplanted neural stem cells differentiate into a phenotype that can support recovery without unfavorable side effects is an important consideration.

Recently, it has been shown that primate embryonic stem cells transplanted into the ischemic mouse brain will survive for at least 28 days, differentiate into the various types of neurons and glia required for recovery following MCAo, and appear to integrate into the existing circuitry (Hayashi *et al.*, 2006). Although this study is compelling, there is no evidence that the new cells are directly supporting

functional recovery. Without the inclusion of behavioral analysis it is very difficult to determine the extent to which these transplanted stem cells are supporting recovery in a manner that is clinically relevant. In a rodent Huntington's disease model, Vazey and colleagues transplanted adult neural progenitor cells into the lesioned striatum, and found that a portion of these transplanted cells were able to survive and differentiate into striatal medium spiny projection neurons and interneurons, with concomitant motor recovery (Vazey *et al.*, 2006). Although there is evidence of functional restitution, this study does not address whether these new cells integrate into the existing circuitry to influence recovery directly or whether the effects of the transplanted cells on recovery are indirect.

Advances in genetics may allow cells, manufactured to secrete necessary proteins or trophic factors, to be delivered to specific locations in order to assist disease recovery. This method of delivery may be a practical solution to the invasiveness required for intracerebroventricular administration, which has been used in clinical trials. For example, in Parkinson's disease there is a need to replace cells responsible for producing dopamine. In animal models of Parkinson's disease, delivery of glial cell line-derived neurotrophic factor (GDNF) has been shown to be important in the development and maintenance of dopaminergic neurons (Lin *et al.*, 1993), and also to increase sprouting of dopaminergic fibers with concomitant improvement of motor deficits (Beck *et al.*, 1995; Tomac *et al.*, 1995). So compelling was the outcome, that similar infusions were performed in clinical trials, and were met with success (Gill *et al.*, 2003; Love *et al.*, 2005). Unfortunately, in these studies GDNF was infused directly into the striatum via a catheter and pump. In order to improve upon the method of administration, human neural stem cells genetically modified to release GDNF have been produced (Behrstock *et al.*, 2006). These studies, using both rodents and primates, show that, once transplanted, the cells migrate within the damaged striatum and release physiologically relevant levels of GDNF, sufficient to increase dopamine neuron survival and increase fiber outgrowth concomitant with functional improvements. Similarly, human neural stem cells, manipulated to express L-Dopa, a precursor of dopamine, can be transplanted into a rodent model of Parkinson's disease, resulting in significantly increased dopamine, which works to ameliorate behavioral deficits associated with the disease (Kim *et al.*, 2006).

Endogenous neural stem cells and stroke

- Following stroke, stem cells redirect their migration toward the ischemic boundary.
- Various agents can be administered following stroke in order to increase neurogenesis and stem cell differentiation, and to assist functional recovery.

When assessing repair through endogenous neural stem cells, several questions are of interest (Lichtenwalner & Parent, 2006). First, is there a baseline level of spontaneous repair following injury? Second, if we can increase neurogenesis following injury will that be sufficient to induce functional recovery? Finally, is it necessary for the new cells to become integrated into the existing circuitry in order to allow for functional recovery?

Brain injury has been shown to alter the proliferation of neural stem cells in the adult brain (Liu *et al.*, 1998; Parent *et al.*, 1997). As previously mentioned, FGF-2 has an integral role in stem cell proliferation during development and in the adult brain. Yoshimura and colleagues (Yoshimura *et al.*, 2001) showed that mice genetically deficient in FGF-2 do not display the increase in neurogenesis following either kainic acid injection or MCAo compared to their wild-type littermates. Furthermore, the increased neurogenesis following injury could be rescued in the FGF-2 deficient mice through injection of a vector carrying the FGF-2 gene. These results indicate that FGF-2 is both necessary and sufficient to stimulate the proliferation and differentiation of neural progenitor cells in the adult brain following brain injury. In experimental models of stroke, it has been shown that both global

and focal ischemia will induce proliferation of stem cells resident in the SVZ (Arvidsson *et al.*, 2002; Jin *et al.*, 2001; Parent *et al.*, 2002) and/or dentate gyrus (Ernst & Christie, 2006; Kluska *et al.*, 2005; Yagita *et al.*, 2001). Not only is there an increase in neural stem cell proliferation in the SVZ following MCAo, but also neuronal migration is rerouted from the RMS to the damaged cortex and striatum (Jin *et al.*, 2003; Zhang *et al.*, 2004). Likewise, cells resident in the dentate gyrus will migrate to the lesion site within the hippocampus (Jin *et al.*, 2001). Once at the lesion site, these new cells incorporate into the ischemic penumbra. Although most of these cells die within the first few weeks (Arvidsson *et al.*, 2002), those cells that do survive appear to differentiate into the predominant neuronal or glial phenotype and integrate into the existing circuitry (Arvidsson *et al.*, 2002; Gu *et al.*, 2000; Parent *et al.*, 2002). Unfortunately, this small number of surviving cells is not enough to support full functional recovery. As such, methods aimed at further increasing proliferation, differentiation and survival is required to make optimal use of intrinsic stem cells.

In order to support intrinsic repair it may be necessary to administer various agents aimed at increasing neurogenesis and differentiation. One convincing example of how administration of mitogens may be of benefit following stroke was provided by Nakatomi and colleagues (Nakatomi *et al.*, 2002). They showed that activation of endogenous neural progenitors through infusions of EGF and FGF-2 led to significant regeneration of hippocampal pyramidal neurons following ischemic insult. Furthermore, they showed that these new neurons were able to integrate into the existing brain circuitry and improve functional deficits. Unfortunately, this study was not able to show that, once the new neurons are removed, the behavioral deficit returns. As such, it cannot be determined that the new neurons were directly responsible for the recovery.

As previously mentioned, EPO not only has the ability to influence the phenotype of stem cells, but can affect angiogenesis (Jelkmann & Wagner, 2004; Wang *et al.*, 2004) and neuronal survival (Liu *et al.*, 2006), both of which are important in enhancing repair following ischemia. The ability to ameliorate damage following stroke by combining EGF, to increase proliferation of stem cells (Craig *et al.*, 1996), with EPO, to induce a neuronal phenotype was elegantly demonstrated by Kolb *et al.* (2007). In this study, rats were given an ischemic lesion to the primary motor cortex and three days later received EGF followed by EPO. This treatment resulted in tissue regeneration concomitant with motor recovery. Importantly, when this new tissue was removed following behavioral recovery the deficit re-emerged, demonstrating the importance of the new tissue to recovery (Kolb *et al.*, 2007). Albeit, the exact role the new tissue plays in supporting recovery is not known. For instance, it may be re-establishing lost connections, or playing an indirect role through enhancing cortical plasticity.

Stem cells and mechanisms of recovery

• Stem cells may support functional improvements following injury or disease via two routes: indirectly through the secretion of trophic factors, or directly through re-establishing lost circuitry.

The biggest challenge in studies seeking to demonstrate that regeneration is responsible for behavioral outcomes is elucidating the core mechanism(s) responsible. For instance, the new cells may be replacing lost neurons and incorporating into the existing circuitry, or they may be secreting factors that aid in the plasticity of surrounding intact tissue. In the case of brain injury, the idea that new neurons will not only repopulate a lesion site, but also re-establish connections in the same manner as pre-lesion is unlikely given the innumerable associations that would have to be made within a harsh environment that is already reorganizing to deflect the damage. More likely is the idea that new neurons, or astrocytes, will work to restore function indirectly, possibly by secreting agents that allow for greater plasticity (Lu *et al.*, 2003). Although this has not been proven in the case of stroke, there is evidence that alludes to its likelihood. For instance, Kolb *et al.* (2007) studied rats with cortical ischemia

and showed that infusions of EGF followed by EPO will lead to a regrowth of cortical tissue with concomitant behavioral recovery. If these new neurons and glia within the regenerated tissue are directly responsible for functional recovery, once the new tissue is removed the deficit will return to the level originally associated with the initial lesion. When Kolb and colleagues removed the tissue re-growth they observed a reinstatement of the original deficit, but not immediately following tissue removal. Instead, the deficit returned slowly over the following week, pointing to an indirect role of the new tissue for functional restitution. One possibility is that the new tissue secreted growth factors that increase plasticity of the adjacent tissue, having the effect of promoting functional improvement.

Neonatal injury provides an exciting avenue for exploring cortical regeneration in a model where new cells do in fact functionally integrate into surrounding tissue. Studies demonstrate that treatment with FGF-2 following motor cortex injury at postnatal day 10 will result in tissue regeneration and improvements in motor function (Monfils *et al.*, 2005, 2006). Using intracortical microstimulation they were able to demonstrate that this new cortical tissue will generate motor responses, indicating that these cells are incorporating into the existing circuitry (Monfils *et al.*, 2005). This is remarkable given that the new tissue generated in the adult using EGF and EPO does not integrate into existing circuitry. None the less, these studies are extremely encouraging as they suggest that it is possible for newly generated tissue to functionally integrate following cortical injury. Future studies will seek to understand how to prompt an aged brain to respond in a way similar to what is observed in the young brain.

If the ultimate goal for stem cell therapy is to restore functional circuitry to pre-lesion or pre-disease status, allowing for total functional recovery, then it may be necessary to engage concomitant strategies of treatment aimed at integrating the new cells into existing circuitry. For instance, following ischemic insult to the primary motor cortex rats display a fair amount of spontaneous recovery of forelimb functioning. This is due to cortical reorganization, where regions adjacent to (or in the homologous contralateral hemisphere) take on the function of the lesioned area in rats (Biernaskie *et al.*, 2005; Gharbawie *et al.*, 2005), primates (Frost *et al.*, 2003; Nudo & Milliken, 1996) and humans (Lotze *et al.*, 2006). During development, integration of cells into networks is established through experience. For instance, monocular deprivation during a critical period will result in significant reduction of neuronal response to visual input from the deprived eye (Hubel & Wiesel, 1970). Similarly, experience has been shown to be imperative for proper organisation of sensory systems (Shatz, 1990) and for corticospinal terminations (Martin, 2005). For example, Chakrabarty & Martin (2005) have shown that if activity within the primary motor cortex is blocked for the duration of the critical period during development it will never display full organization, however, if it is disrupted following the critical period during adulthood the effects are transient. In the adult brain, new cells also require activity in order to survive (Kempermann *et al.*, 1997; van Praag *et al.*, 1999a) and become functionally integrated (Ge *et al.*, 2006; Tashiro *et al.*, 2006).

The "use it or lose it" notion may be helpful in understanding the integration of new cells (either endogenous or transplanted) into existing circuitry following brain injury in adulthood. At the same time, it is likely that compensation and reorganization have already begun by the time the new cells are in place to be used. Thus, the new cells may not be needed in the same capacity as pre-lesion, and may not have the opportunity to become fully integrated in a functional sense. As we learn more about plasticity, reorganization, and the behavior of new cells following stroke, we will be better equipped to develop treatments aimed at achieving complete recovery.

Summary

Stroke is the fourth leading cause of death in Canada, and approximately 300000 people are living with resulting disabilities. To date, the most effective therapy involves the administration of rtPA, which has a very narrow window of therapeutic use. Rehabilitative therapies, such as constraint-induced movement therapy, provide an excellent avenue for recovery.

Animal models of injury and disease are important for allowing a greater understanding of mechanisms underlying deficits and recovery. These models have been employed in order to investigate various treatments, such as those involving stem cells. Stem cell therapy can take the form of intrinsic mobilization or transplantation.

Environmental manipulations can induce neurogenesis and have great benefit for functional recovery. When strenuous physical activity cannot be achieved, exogenous administration of agents can increase neurogenesis concomitant with functional recovery. Stem cell transplantation can allow for the introduction of specialized cell types specific for the injury or disease. Furthermore, the ability to choose the location of transplantation might allow for greater viability of the cells.

The mechanism(s) underlying functional (both motor and cognitive) recovery observed following stem cell treatment remains unknown. The new cells may be allowing for recovery directly through re-establishing lost circuitry, or indirectly through increasing plasticity. A combination of stem cells treatment and rehabilitation may represent the most beneficial regime for functional recovery following injury and disease.

REFERENCES

Aberg, M. A., Aberg, N. D., Hedbacker, H., Oscarsson, J., & Eriksson, P. S. (2000). Peripheral infusion of IGF-1 selectively induces neurogenesis in the adult rat hippocampus. *Journal of Neuroscience*, **20**, 2896–2903.

Altman, J. (1969). Autoradiographic and histological studies of postnatal neurogenesis. IV. Cell proliferation and migration in the anterior forebrain, with special reference to persisting neurogenesis in the olfactory bulb. *Journal of Comparative Neurology*, **137**, 433–458.

Altman, J., & Das, G. D. (1965). Autoradiographic and histological evidence of postnatal hippocampal neurogenesis in rats. *Journal of Comparative Neurology*, **124**, 319–336.

Arvidsson, A., Collin, T., Kirik, D., Kokaia, Z., & Lindvall, O. (2002). Neuronal replacement from endogenous precursors in the adult brain after stroke. *Nature Medicine*, **8**, 963–970.

Aspey, B. S., Cohen, S., Patel, Y., Terruli, M., & Harrison, M. J. G. (1998). Middle cerebral artery occlusion in the rat: consistent protocol for a model of stroke. *Neuropathology and Applied Neurobiology*, **24**, 487–497.

Auvergne, R., Lere, C., ElBehh, B. *et al.* (2002). Delayed kindling epileptogenesis and increased neurogenesis in adult rats housed in an enriched environment. *Brain Research*, **954**, 277–285.

Beck, K. D., Valverde, J., Alexi, T. *et al.* (1995). Mesencephalic dopaminergic neurons protected by GDNF from axotomy-induced degeneration in the adult brain. *Nature*, **373**, 339–341.

Behrstock, S., Ebert, A., McHugh, J. *et al.* (2006). Human neural progenitors deliver glial cell line-derived neurotrophic factor to parkinsonian rodents and aged primates. *Gene Therapy*, **13**, 379–388.

Biernaskie, J., Chernenko, G., & Corbett, D. (2004). Efficacy of rehabilitative experience declines with time after focal ischemic brain injury. *Journal of Neuroscience*, **24**, 1245–1254.

Biernaskie, J., Szymanska, A., Windle, V., & Corbett, D. (2005). Bi-hemispheric contribution to functional motor recovery of the affected forelimb following ischemic brain injury in rats. *European Journal of Neuroscience*, **21**, 989–999.

Calza, L., Fernandez, M., Giuliani, A., Aloe, L., & Giardino, L. (2002). Thyroid hormone activates oligodendrocyte precursors and increases a myelin-forming protein and NGF content in the spinal cord during experimental allergic encephalomyelitis. *Proceedings of the National Academy of Sciences of the United States of America*, **99**, 3258–3263.

Cao, L., Jiao, X., Zuzga, D. S. *et al.* (2004). VEGF links hippocampal activity with neurogenesis, learning and memory. *Nature Genetics*, **36**, 827–835.

Carlen, M., Cassidy, R. M., Brismar, H. *et al.* (2002). Functional integration of adult-born neurons. *Current Biology*, **12**, 606–608.

Cenci, M. A., Whishaw, I. Q., & Schallert, T. (2002). Animals models of neurological deficits: how relevant is the rat? *Nature Reviews Neuroscience*, **3**, 574–579.

Chakrabarty, S., & Martin, J. H. (2005). Motor but not sensory representation in motor cortex depends on

postsynaptic activity during development and in maturity. *Journal of Neurophysiology*, **94**, 3192–3198.

Charles, J. R., Wolf, S. L., Schneider, J. A., & Gordon, A. M. (2006). Efficacy of a child-friendly form of constraint-induced movement therapy in hemiplegic cerebral palsy: a randomized control trial. *Developmental Medicine and Child Neurology*, **48**, 635–642.

Cooper, O., & Isacson, O. (2004). Intrastiatal transforming growth factor alpha delivery to a model of Parkinson's disease induces proliferation and migration of endogenous adult neural progenitor cells without differentiation into dopaminergic neurons. *Journal of Neuroscience*, **41**, 8924–8931.

Craig, C. G., Tropepe, V., Morshead, C. M. *et al.* (1996). In vivo growth factor expansion of endogenous subependymal neural precursor cell populations in the adult mouse brain. *Journal of Neuroscience*, **16**, 2649–2658.

Curtis, M. A., Peney, E. B., Pearson, A. G. *et al.* (2003). Increased cell proliferation and neurogenesis in the adult human Huntington's disease brain. *Proceedings of the National Academy of Sciences of the United States of America*, **100**, 9023–9027.

Dahlqvist, P., Zhao, L., Johansson, I. M. *et al.* (1999). Environmental enrichment alters nerve growth factor-induced gene A and glucocorticoid receptor messenger RNA expression after middle cerebral artery occlusion in rats. *Neuroscience*, **93**, 527–535.

Danilov, A. I., Covacu, R., Moe, M. C. *et al.* (2006). Neurogenesis in the adult rat spinal cord in an experimental model of multiple sclerosis. *European Journal of Neuroscience*, **23**, 394–400.

Davalos, A. (2005). Thrombolysis in acute ischemic stroke: successes, failures, and new hopes. *Cerebrovascular Disease*, **2**, 135–139.

del Ser, T., Barba, R., & Morin, M. M. (2005). Evolution of cognitive impairment after stroke and risk factors for delayed progression. *Stroke*, **36**, 2670–2675.

Dromerick, A. W., Edwards, D. F., & Hahn, M. (2000). Does the application of constraint-induced movement therapy during acute rehabilitation reduce arm impairment after ischemic stroke? *Stroke*, **31**, 2984–2988.

Enwere, E., Shingo, T., Gregg, C. *et al.* (2004). Aging results in reduced epidermal growth factor receptor signaling, diminished olfactory neurogenesis, and deficits in fine olfactory discrimination. *Journal of Neuroscience*, **24**, 8354–8365.

Ernst, C., & Christie, B. R. (2006). Temporally specific proliferation events are indeed in the hippocampus following acute focal injury. *Journal of Neuroscience Research*, **15**, 349–361.

Fabel, K., Fabel, K., Tam, B. *et al.* (2003). VEGF is necessary for exercise-induced adult hippocampal neurogenesis. *European Journal of Neuroscience*, **18**, 2803–2812.

Fallon, J., Reid, S., Kinyamu, R. *et al.* (2000). In vivo induction of massive proliferation, directed migration, and differentiation of neural cells in the adult mammalian brain. *Proceedings of the National Academy of Sciences of the United States of America*, **26**, 14686–14691.

Frost, S. B., Barbay, S., Friel, K. M., Plautz, E. J., & Nudo, R. J. (2003). Reorganization of remote cortical regions after ischemic brain injury: a potential substrate for stroke recovery. *Journal of Neurophysiology*, **89**, 3205–3214.

Gage, F. H. (2000). Mammalian neural stem cells. *Science*, **287**, 1433–1438.

Gaulke, L. J., Horner, P. J., Fink, A. J., McNamara, C. L., & Hicks, R. R. (2005). Environmental enrichment increases progenitor cell survival in the dentate gyrus following lateral fluid percussion injury. *Molecular Brain Research*, **141**, 138–150.

Ge, S., Goh, E. L. K., Sailor, K. A., Kitabatake, J., Ming, G., & Song, H. (2006). GABA regulates synaptic integration of newly generated neurons in the adult brain. *Nature*, **439**, 589–593.

Gharbawie, O. A., Gonzalez, C. L. R., Williams, P. T., Kleim, J. A., & Whishaw, I. Q. (2005). Middle cerebral artery (MCA) stroke produces dysfunction in adjacent motor cortex as detected by intracortical microstimulation in rats. *Neuroscience*, **130**, 601–610.

Gill, S. S., Patel, N. K., Hotton, G. R. *et al.* (2003). Direct brain infusion of glial cell line-derived neurotrophic factor in Parkinson disease. *Nature Medicine*, **9**, 589–595.

Gould, E., Beylin, A., Tanapat, P., Reeves, A., & Shors, T. J. (1999). Learning enhances adult neurogenesis in the hippocampal formation. *Nature Neuroscience*, **2**, 260–265.

Gritti, A., Frolichsthal-Schoeller, P., Galli, R. *et al.* (1999). Epidermal and fibroblast growth factors behave as mitogenic regulators for a single multipotent stem cell-like population from the subventricular region of the adult mouse forebrain. *Journal of Neuroscience*, **19**, 3287–3297.

Gu, W., Brannstrom, T., & Wester, P. (2000). Cortical neurogenesis in adult rats after reversible photothrombotic stroke. *Journal of Cerebral Blood Flow and Metabolism*, **20**, 1166–1173.

Hamzei, F., Liepert, J., Dettmers, C. W., & Rijntjes, M. (2006). Two different reorganization patterns after rehabilitative therapy: an exploratory study with fMRI and TMS. *NeuroImage*, **31**, 710–720.

Hao, J., Ebendal, T., Xu, X., Wiesenfeld-Hallin, Z., & Eriksdotter, M. J. (2000). Intracerebroventricular infusion of nerve growth factor induces pain-like response in rats. *Neuroscience Letters*, **286**, 208–212.

Hayashi, J., Takagi, Y., Fukuda, H. *et al.* (2006). Primate embryonic stem cell-derived neuronal progenitors transplanted into ischemic brain. *Journal of Cerebral Blood Flow and Metabolism*, **26**, 906–914.

Hofstetter, C. P., Holmstrom, N. A. V., Lilja, J. A. *et al.* (2005). Allodynia limits the usefulness of intraspinal neural stem cell grafts; directed differentiation improves outcome. *Nature Neuroscience*, **8**, 347–353.

Hubel, D. H., & Wiesel, T. N. (1970). The period of susceptibility to the physiological effects of unilateral eye closure in kittens. *Journal of Physiology*, **206**, 419–436.

Iwaniuk, A. N., & Whishaw, I. Q. (2000). On the origin of skilled forelimb movements. *Trends in Neurosciences*, **23**, 372–376.

Jelkmann, W., & Wagner, K. (2004). Beneficial and ominous aspects of the pleiotropic action of erythropoietin. *Annuals of Hematology*, **83**, 673–686.

Jin, K. L., Mao, X. O., & Greenberg, D. A. (2000). Vascular endothelial growth factor: direct neuroprotective effect in in vitro ischemia. *Proceedings of the National Academy of Science*, **97**, 10242–10247.

Jin, K., Minami, M., Lan, J. Q. *et al.* (2001). Neurogenesis in dentate subgranular zone and rostral subventricular zone after focal cerebral ischemia in the rat. *Proceedings of the National Academy of Sciences of the United States of America*, **98**, 4710–4715.

Jin, K., Zhu, Y., Sun, Y. *et al.* (2002). Vascular endothelial growth factor (VEGF) stimulates neurogenesis in vivo. *Proceedings of the National Academy of Sciences of the United States of America*, **99**, 11950–11964.

Jin, K., Sun, Y., Xie, L. *et al.* (2003). Directed migration of neuronal precursors into the ischemic cerebral cortex and striatum. *Molecular Cellular Neuroscience*, **24**, 171–189.

Jin, K., Minami, M., Xie, L. *et al.* (2004). Ischemia-induced neurogenesis is preserved but reduced in the aged rodent brain. *Aging Cell*, **3**, 373–377.

Jin, K., LaFevre-Bernt, M., Sun, Y. *et al.* (2005). FGF-2 promotes neurogenesis and neuroprotection and prolongs survival in a transgenic mouse model of Huntington's disease. *Proceedings of the National Academy of Sciences of the United States of America*, **102**, 18189–18194.

Johansson, B. B. (2000). Brain plasticity and stroke rehabilitation: the Willis Lecture. *Stroke*, **31**, 223–230.

Jubran, M., & Widenfalk, J. (2003). Repair of peripheral nerve transections with fibrin sealant containing neurotrophic factors. *Experimental Neurology*, **181**, 204–212.

Karimi-Abdolrezaee, S., Eftekarpour, E., Wang, J., Morshead, C. M., & Fehlings, M. G. (2006). Delayed transplantation of adult neural precursor cells promotes remyelination and functional neurological recovery after spinal cord injury. *Journal of Neuroscience*, **26**, 3377–3389.

Kawamata, T., Dietrich, W. D., Schallert, T. *et al.* (1997). Intracisternal basic fibroblast growth factor enhances functional recovery and up-regulates the expression of a molecular marker of neuronal sprouting following focal cerebral infarction. *Proceedings of the National Academy of Sciences of the United States of America*, **94**, 8179–8184.

Kempermann, G., Kuhn, H. G., & Gage, G. H. (1997). More hippocampal neurons in adult mice living in an enriched environment. *Nature*, **386**, 493–495.

Kempermann, G., Gast, D., & Gage, F. H. (2002). Neuroplasticity in old age: sustained fivefold induction of hippocampal neurogenesis by long-term environmental enrichment. *Annals of Neurology*, **52**, 135–143.

Kim, S. U., Park, I. H., Kim, T. H. *et al.* (2006). Brain transplantation of human neural stem cells transduced with tyrosine hydroxylase and GTP cyclohydrolase 1 provides functional improvement in animal models of Parkinson disease. *Neuropathology*, **26**, 129–140.

Kindler, D. D., Lopez, G. A., Worrall, B. B., & Johnston, K. C. (2000). Update on therapies for acute ischemic stroke. *Neurosurgical Focus*, **8**, 1–5.

Kluska, M. M., Witte, O. W., Bolz, J., & Redecker, C. (2005). Neurogenesis in the adult dentate gyrus after crtical infarcts: effects of infarct location, N-methyl-D-aspartate receptor blockade and anti-inflammatory treatment. *Neuroscience*, **135**, 723–735.

Kolb, B., & Elliot, W. (1987). Recovery from early cortical damage in rats. II. Effects of experience on anatomy and behavior following frontal lesions at 1 or 5 days of age. *Behavioral Brain Research*, **26**, 47–56.

Kolb, B., & Gibb, R. (1991). Sparing of function after neonatal frontal lesions correlates with increased cortical dendritic branching: a possible mechanism for the Kennard effect. *Behavioral Brain Research*, **43**, 51–56.

Kolb, B., & Whishaw, I. Q. (1998). Brain plasticity and behavior. *Annual Reviews in Psychology*, **49**, 43–64.

Kolb, B., Gorny, G., Côte, S., Ribeiro-da-Silva, A., & Cuella, A. C. (1997). Nerve growth factor stimulates growth of cortical pyramidal neurons in young adult rats. *Brain Research*, **751**, 289–294.

Kolb, B., Morshead, C., Gonzalez, C. *et al.* (2007). Growth factor-stimulated generation of new cortical tissue and functional recovery after stroke damage to the motor cortex of rats. *Journal of Cerebral Blood Flow and Metabolism*, **27**, 983–997.

Komitova, M., Perfilieva, E., Mattsson, B., Eriksson, P. S., & Johansson, B. B. (2002). Effects of cortical ischemia and postischemic environmental enrichment on hippocampal cell genesis and differentiation in the adult rat. *Journal of Cerebral Blood Flow and Metabolism*, **22**, 852–860.

Komitova, M., Mattsson, B., Johansson, B. B., & Eriksson, P. S. (2005a). Enriched environment increases neural stem/progenitor cell proliferation and neurogenesis in the subventricular zone of stroke-lesioned adult rats. *Stroke*, **36**, 1278–1282.

Komitova, M., Zhao, L. R., Gido, G., Johansson, B. B., & Eriksson, P. S. (2005b). Postischemic exercise attenuates whereas enriched environment has certain enhancing effects on lesion-induced subventricular zone activation in the adult rat. *Journal of Neuroscience*, **21**, 2397–2405.

Koopmans, G. C., Brans, M., Gómez-Pinilla, F. *et al.* (2006). Circulating insulin-like growth factor 1 and functional recovery from spinal cord injury under enriched housing conditions. *European Journal of Neuroscience*, **23**, 1035–1046.

Kuhn, H. G., Dickinson-Anson, H., & Gage, F. H. (1996). Neurogenesis in the dentate gyrus of the adult rat: age-related decrease of neuronal progenitor proliferation. *Journal of Neuroscience*, **16**, 2027–2033.

Kuhn, G. H., Winkler, J., Kempermann, G., Thal, L. J., & Gage, F. H. (1997). Epidermal growth factor and fibroblast growth factor-2 have different effects on neural progenitors in the adult rat brain. *Journal of Neuroscience*, **17**, 5820–5829.

Lazic, S. E., Grote, H. E., Blakemore, C. *et al.* (2006). Neurogenesis in the R6/1 transgenic mouse model of Huntington's disease: effects of environmental enrichment. *European Journal of Neuroscience*, **23**, 1829–1838.

Li, Q., & Stephenson, D. (2002). Postischemic administration of basic fibroblast growth factor improves sensorimotor function and reduces infarct size following permanent focal cerebral ischemia in the rat. *Experimental Neurology*, **177**, 531–537.

Lichtenwalner, R. J., & Parent, J. M. (2006). Adult neurogenesis and the ischemic forebrain. *Journal of Cerebral Blood Flow and Metabolism*, **26**, 1–20.

Liepert, J., Bauder, H., Miltner, W. H. R., Taub, E., & Weiller, C. (2000). Treatment-induced cortical reorganization after stroke in humans. *Stroke*, **31**, 1210–1216.

Lin, L. F., Doherty, D. H., Lile, J. D., Dektesh, S., & Collins, F. (1993). GDNF: a glial cell line-derived neurotrophic factor for midbrain dopaminergic neurons. *Science*, **260**, 1130–1132.

Lincoln, N. B., Parry, R. H., & Vass, C. D. (1999). Randomized, controlled trial to evaluate increased intensity of physiotherapy treatment of arm function after stroke. *Stroke*, **30**, 573–579.

Lindvall, O., Kokaia, Z., & Martinez-Serrano, A. (2004). Stem cell therapy for human neurodegenerative disorders – how to make it work. *Nature Medicine*, **10**, S42–S50.

Liu, J., Solway, K., Messing, R. O., & Sharp, F. R. (1998). Increased neurogenesis in the dentate gyrus after transient global ischemia in gerbils. *Journal of Neuroscience*, **18**, 7768–7778.

Liu, R., Suzuki, A., Guo, Z., Mizuno, Y., & Urabe, T. (2006). Intrinsic and extrinsic erythropoietin enhances neuroprotection against ischemia and reperfusion injury in vitro. *Journal of Neurochemistry*, **96**, 1101–1110.

Lledo, P. M., Alonso, M., & Grubb, M. S. (2006). Adult neurogenesis and functional plasticity in neuronal circuits. *Nature Reviews Neuroscience*, **7**, 179–193.

Lois, C., & Alvarez-Buylla, A. (1994). Long-distance neuronal migration in the adult mammalian brain. *Science*, **264**, 1145–1148.

Lotze, M., Markert, J., Sauseng, P. *et al.* (2006). The role of multiple contralesional motor areas for complex hand movements after internal capsular lesion. *Journal of Neuroscience*, **26**, 6096–6102.

Love, S., Plaha, P., Patel, N. K. *et al.* (2005). Glial cell line-derived neurotrophic factor induces neuronal sprouting in human brain. *Nature Medicine*, **11**, 703–704.

Lu, D., Mahmood, A., Qu, C. *et al.* (2005). Erythropoietin enhances neurogenesis and restores spatial memory in rats after traumatic brain injury. *Journal of Neurotrauma*, **22**, 1011–1017.

Lu, P., Jones, L. L., Snyder, E. Y., & Tuszynski, M. H. (2003). Neural stem cells constitutively secrete neurotrophic factors and promote extensive host axonal growth after spinal cord injury. *Experimental Neurology*, **181**, 115–129.

Luo, J., Daniels, S. B., Lennington, J. B., Notti, R. Q., & Conover, J. C. (2006). The aging neurogenic subventricular zone. *Aging Cell*, **5**, 139–152.

Markakis, E. A., & Gage, F. H. (1999). Adult-generated neurons in the dentate gyrus send axonal projections to field CA3 and are surrounded by synaptic vesicles. *Journal of Comparative Neurology*, **406**, 449–460.

Martin, J. H. (2005). The corticospinal system: from development to motor control. *Neuroscientist*, **11**, 161–173.

Matthew, J., & Cao, L. (2006). VEGF, a mediator of the effect of experience on hippocampal neurogenesis. *Current Alzheimer Research*, **3**, 29–33.

Meshi, D., Drew, M. R., Saxe, M. *et al.* (2006). Hippocampal neurogenesis is not required for behavioral effects of environmental enrichment. *Nature Neuroscience*, **9**, 729–731.

Metz, G. A., & Whishaw, I. Q. (2000). Skilled reaching an action pattern: stability in rat (*Rattus norvegicus*) grasping movements as a function of changing food pellet size. *Behavioral Brain Research*, **116**, 111–122.

Monfils, M. H., Driscoll, I., Vandenberg, P. M. *et al.* (2005). Basic fibroblast growth factor stimulates functional recovery after neonatal lesions of motor cortex in rats. *Neuroscience*, **134**, 1–8.

Monfils, M.-H., Driscoll, I., Kamitakahara, H. *et al.* (2006). FGF-2-induced cell proliferation stimulates anatomical, neurophysiological and functional recovery from neonatal motor cortex injury. *European Journal of Neuroscience*, **24**, 739–749.

Morshead, C. M., & van der Kooy, D. (1992). Postmitotic death is the fate of constitutively proliferating cells in the subependymal layer of the adult mouse brain. *Journal of Neuroscience*, **12**, 249–256.

Morshead, C. M., Reynolds, B. A., Craig, C. G. *et al.* (1994). Neural stem cells in the adult mammalian forebrain: a relatively quiescent subpopulation of subependymal cells. *Neuron*, **13**, 1071–1082.

Nakatomi, H., Kuriu, T., Okabe, S. *et al.* (2002). Regeneration of hippocampal pyramidal neurons after ischemic brain injury by recruitment of endogenous neural progenitors. *Cell*, **110**, 429–441.

Nudo, R. J., & Milliken, G. W. (1996). Reorganization of movement representations in primary motor cortex following focal ischemic infarcts in adult squirrel monkeys. *Journal of Neurophysiology*, **75**, 2144–2149.

Nys, G. M. S., van Zandvoort, M. J. E., & de Kort, P. L. M. (2005). Domain-specific cognitive recovery after first-ever stroke: a follow-up study of 111 cases. *Journal of International Neuropsychological Society*, **11**, 795–806.

Nys, G. M. S, van Zandvoort, M. J. E., van der Worp, H. B. *et al.* (2006). Early cognitive impairment predicts long-term depressive symptoms and quality of life after stroke. *Journal of Neurological Sciences*, **247**, 149–156.

Ogawa, Y., Sawamoto, K., Miyata, T. *et al.* (2002). Transplantation of in vitro-expanded fetal neural progenitor cells results in neurogenesis and functional recovery after spinal cord contusion injury in adult rats. *Journal of Neuroscience Research*, **69**, 925–933.

Oosthuyse, B., Moons, L., Storkebaum, E. *et al.* (2001). Deletion of the hypoxia-response element in the vascular endothelial growth factor promoter causes motor neuron degeneration. *Nature Genetics*, **28**, 131–138.

Palmer, T. D., Ray, J., & Gage, F. H. (1995). FGF-2-responsive neuronal progenitors reside in proliferative and quiescent regions of the adult rodent brain. *Molecular and Cellular Neuroscience*, **6**, 474–486.

Parent, J. M., Yu, T. W., Leibowitz, R. T. *et al.* (1997). Dentate granule cell neurogenesis is increased by seizures and contributes to aberrant network reorganization in the adult rat hippocampus. *Journal of Neuroscience*, **17**, 3727–3738.

Parent, J. M., Vexler, Z. S., Gong, C., Derugin, N., & Ferriero, D. M. (2002). Rat forebrain neurogenesis and striatal neuron replacement after focal stroke. *Annals of Neurology*, **52**, 802–813.

Pencea, V., Bingaman, K. D., Wiegand, S. J., & Luskin, M. B. (2001). Infusion of brain-derived neurotrophic factor into the lateral ventricle of the adult rat leads to new neurons in the parenchyma of the striatum, septum, thalamus and hypothalamus. *Journal of Neuroscience*, **21**, 6706–6717.

Perez-Martin, M., Cifuentes, M., Grondona, J. M. *et al.* (2003). Neurogenesis in explants from the walls of the lateral ventricle of adult bovine brain: role of endogenous IGF-1 as a survival factor. *European Journal of Neuroscience*, **17**, 205–211.

Picard-Riera, N., Decker, L., Delarasse, C. *et al.* (2002). Experimental autoimmune encephalomyelitis mobilizes neural progenitors from the subventricular zone to undergo oligodendrogenesis in adult mice. *Proceedings of the National Academy of Sciences of the United States of America*, **99**, 13211–13216.

Pierce, S. R., Gallagher, K. G., Schaumburg, S. W. *et al.* (2003). Home forced use in an outpatient rehabilitation program for adults with hemiplegia: a pilot study. *Neurorehabilitation and Neural Repair*, **17**, 214–219.

Rasquin, S. M., Lodder, J., & Ponds, R. W. (2004). Cognitive functioning after stroke: a one-year follow-up study. *Dementia and Geriatric Cognitive Disorders*, **18**, 138–144.

Reynolds, B. A., & Weiss, S. (1992). Generation of neurons and astrocytes from isolated cells of the adult mammalian central nervous system. *Science*, **255**, 1613–1808.

Richards, L. J., Kilpatrick, T. J., & Bartlett, P. F. (1992). De novo generation of neuronal cells from the adult mouse

brain. *Proceedings of the National Academy of Sciences of the United States of America*, **89**, 8591–8595.

Ro, T., Noser, E., Boake, C. *et al.* (2006). Functional reorganization and recovery after constraint-induced movement therapy in subacute stroke: case reports. *Neurocase*, **12**, 50–60.

Roy, V., Belzung, C., Delarue, C., & Chapillon, P. (2001). Environmental enrichment in BALB/c mice: effects of classical tests of anxiety and exposure to a predatory odor. *Physiology and Behavior*, **74**, 313–320.

Santos, C. O., Caeiro, L., Ferro, J. M., Albuquerque, R., & Figueira, M. L. (2006). Anger, hostility and aggression in the first days of acute stroke. *European Journal of Neurology*, **13**, 351–358.

Schäbitz, W. R., Berger, C., Kollmar, R. *et al.* (2004). Effect of brain-derived neurotrophic factor treatment and forced arm use on functional motor recovery after small cortical ischemia. *Stroke*, **35**, 992–997.

Schaechter, J. D., Draft, E., Hilliard, T. S. *et al.* (2002). Motor recovery and cortical reorganization after constraint-induced movement therapy in stroke patients: a preliminary study. *The American Association of Neurorehabilitation*.

Schallert, T., Fleming, S. M., Leasure, J. L., Tillerson, J. L., & Bland, S. T. (2000). CNS plasticity and assessment of forelimb sensorimotor outcome in unilateral rat models of stroke, cortical ablation, parkinsonism and spinal cord injury. *Neuropharmacology*, **39**, 777–787.

Shatz, C. J. (1990). Impulse activity and the patterning of connections during CNS development. *Neuron*, **5**, 745–756.

Shaw, S. E., Morris, D. M., Uswatte, G. *et al.* (2005). Constraint-induced movement therapy for recovery of upper-limb function following traumatic brain injury. *Journal of Rehabilitation Research and Development*, **42**, 769–778.

Shetty, A. K., & Turner, D. A. (1999). Neurite outgrowth from progeny of epidermal growth factor-responsive hippocampal stem cells is significantly less robust than from fetal hippocampal cells following grafting onto organotypic hippocampal slice cultures: effect of brain-derived neurotrophic factor. *Journal of Neurobiology*, **38**, 391–413.

Shingo, T., Sorokan, S., Shimazaki, T., & Weiss, S. (2001). Erythropoietin regulates the in vitro and in vivo production of neuronal progenitors by mammalian forebrain neural stem cells. *Journal of Neuroscience*, **21**, 9733–9743.

Shingo, T., Gregg, C., Enwere, E. *et al.* (2003). Pregnancy-stimulated neurogenesis in the adult female forebrain mediated by prolactin. *Science*, **299**, 117–120.

Siren, A. L., Fratelli, M., Brines, M. *et al.* (2001). Erythropoietin prevents neuronal apoptosis after cerebral ischemia and metabolic stress. *Proceedings of the National Academy of Sciences of the United States of America*, **98**, 4044–4049.

Snyder, J. S., Hong, N. S., McDonald, R. J., & Wojtowicz, J. M. (2005). A role for adult neurogenesis in spatial long-term memory. *Neuroscience*, **130**, 843–852.

Tashiro, A., Sandler, V. M., Toni, N., Zhao, C., & Gage, F. H. (2006). NMDA-receptor-mediated, cell-specific integration of new neurons in adult dentate gyrus. *Nature, **2006***, 929–933.

Taub, E. (1977). Movement in nonhuman primates deprived of somatosensory feedback. *Exercise and Sports Sciences Reviews*, **4**, 335–374.

Taub, E. (1980). *Somatosensory Deafferentation Research with Monkeys: Implications for Rehabilitation Medicine.* New York, NY: Williams & Wilkins.

Taub, E., Crago, J. E., Burgio, L. D. *et al.* (1994). An operant approach to rehabilitation medicine: overcoming learned nonuse by shaping. *Journal of the Experimental Analysis of Behavior*, **61**, 281–293.

Taub, E., Uswatte, G., King, D. K. *et al.* (2006). A placebo-controlled trial of constraint-induced movement therapy for upper extremity after stroke. *Stroke*, **37**, 1045–1049.

Tomac, A., Lindqvist, E., Lin, L. F. *et al.* (1995). Protection and repair of the nigrostriatal dopaminergic system by GDNF in vivo. *Nature*, **373**, 335–339.

Tropepe, V., Sibilia, M., Ciruna, B. G. *et al.* (1999). Distinct neural stem cells proliferate in response to EGF and FGF in the developing mouse telencephalon. *Developmental Biology*, **208**, 166–188.

van der Kooy, D., & Weiss, S. (2000). Why stem cells? *Science*, **287**, 1439–1441.

van Praag, H., Christie, B. R., Sejnowski, T. J., & Gage, F. H. (1999a). Running enhances neurogenesis, learning, and long-term potentiation in mice. *Proceedings of the National Academy of Sciences of the United States of America*, **96**, 13427–13431.

van Praag, H., Kempermann, G., & Gage, F. H. (1999b). Running increases cell proliferation and neurogenesis in the adult mouse dentate gyrus. *Nature Neuroscience*, **2**, 266–270.

van Praag, H., Shubert, T., Zhao, C., & Gage, F. H. (2005). Exercise enhances learning and hippocampal neurogenesis in aged mice. *Journal of Neuroscience*, **25**, 8680–8685.

Vazey, E. M., Chen, K., Hughes, S. M., & Connor, B. (2006). Transplanted adult neural progenitor cells survive, differentiate and reduce motor function impairment in a rodent model of Huntington's disease. *Experimental Neurology*, **199**, 384–396.

Vroemen, M., Aigner, L., Winkler, J., & Weidner, N. (2003). Adult neural progenitor cell grafts survive after acute spinal cord injury and integrate along axonal pathways. *European Journal of Neuroscience*, **18**, 743–751.

Wang, L., Zhang, Z., Wang, Y., Zhang, R., & Chopp, M. (2004). Treatment of stroke with erythropoietin enhances neurogenesis and angiogenesis and improves neurological function in rats. *Stroke*, **35**, 1732–1737.

Wang, L., Zhang, Z. G., Zhang, R. L. *et al.* (2006). Matrix metalloproteinase 2 (MMP2) and MMP9 secreted by erythropoietin-activated endothelial cells promote neural progenitor cell migration. *Journal of Neuroscience*, **26**, 5996–6003.

Widenfalk, J., Lipson, A., Jubran, M. *et al.* (2003). Vascular endothelial growth factor improves functional outcome and decreases secondary degeneration in experimental spinal cord contusion injury. *Neuroscience*, **120**, 951–960.

Winocur, G., Wojtowicz, J. M., Sekeres, M., Snyder, J. S., & Wang, S. (2006). Inhibition of neurogenesis interferes with hippocampus-dependent memory function. *Hippocampus*, **16**, 296–304.

Witt-Lajeunesse, A., Cioe, J., & Kolb, B. (submitted). Rehabilitative experience interacts with bFGF to facilitate functional improvement after motor cortex injury.

Yagita, Y., Kitagawa, K., Ohtsuki, T. *et al.* (2001). Neurogenesis by progenitor cells in the ischemic adult rat hippocampus. *Stroke*, **32**, 1890–1896.

Yoshimura, S., Takagi, Y., Harada, J. *et al.* (2001). FGF-2 regulation of neurogenesis in adult hippocampus after brain injury. *Proceedings of the National Academy of Sciences of the United States of America*, **98**, 5874–5879.

Zhang, R., Zhang, Z., Wang, L. *et al.* (2004). Activated neural stem cells contribute to stroke-induced neurogenesis and neuroblast migration toward the infarct boundary in adult rats. *Journal of Cerebral Blood Flow and Metabolism*, **24**, 441–448.

Behavioral/ neuropsychological approaches

Introduction to Section 5

Ian H. Robertson and Donald T. Stuss

In this section of the book, we come to what is the core of what is generally meant by cognitive rehabilitation – the application of behavioral methods to alter brain function and behavior. The early textbooks of cognitive rehabilitation would have focused mainly on the areas covered by this section. Take *Neuropsychological Rehabilitation*, published in 1987 by Meier *et al.* (1987), a very influential early textbook. This had three sections: the first was on assessment and methodological issues – scanning nowhere on the rehabilitation horizon yet – while the second on application covered just a small number of pioneering rehabilitation methods by researchers such as Ben Yishay, Anna Basso and Harold Goodglass. The final section reviewed rehabilitation programs across a number of different countries. The developments in just 20 years in rehabilitation methods as outlined in this section of the book are dramatic.

Furthermore, it is a mark of the dramatic developments and growing sophistication in neuroscience in particular, and cognitive neuroscience in general, that the "core" of cognitive rehabilitation is only addressed in the fifth section of a large textbook. It is also absolutely correct: for cognitive rehabilitation to achieve its potential, it must be securely grounded in basic neuroscience, in the biology of the brain and in the relevant medical, psychological and social psychological contexts.

In Chapter 23, Morris and Taub outline one of the most important and influential developments in rehabilitation of the last 20 years, constraint-induced therapy (CIT). Its importance arises from

a number of reasons, including its grounding in a theoretical model of the underlying deficit and – more importantly – a theoretically based hypothesis as to the mechanism of rehabilitative recovery.

Taub's model proposed that injury to a limb results in neural shock and initial depression of function, leading to a learned non-use of that limb even when movements could potentially be made. This can be overcome – in cases where there is a minimum of residual function – through restricting movement of the intact limb in a way that can induce use of the deafferented limb. Practice, the use of conditioned responses, and shaping assists in maximising use of the impaired limb with several studies showing cortical reorganization corresponding to the behavioral improvements.

A second reason for according CIT such importance in the development of cognitive rehabilitation is that while being theoretically grounded, the therapy is also articulated into a coherent and replicable protocol which allows for the proper degree of assessment and replication that has been notably lacking in a landscape littered with one-off protocols of uncertain efficacy. The fact that CIT has been evaluated in over 400 patients worldwide, with a mean effect size of 3.3, is a mark of the maturity and critical importance of this milestone in rehabilitation.

Kramer, Erickson and McAuley (Chapter 24) have also introduced a ground-breaking approach to rehabilitation that could not have been conceived of in a 1980s textbook of rehabilitation – the role of aerobic exercise on brain structure and function. A particular strength of this approach is – as in the

Cognitive Neurorehabilitation, Second Edition: Evidence and Application, ed. Donald T. Stuss, Gordon Winocur and Ian H. Robertson. Published by Cambridge University Press. © Cambridge University Press 2008.

case of Taub's CIT – it allows for evaluation of a standard intervention protocol across studies, and indeed across species, allowing for molecular and cellular assays as well as cognitive and imaging ones. It is clear that – in some populations at least – the cognitive, functional imaging and structural imaging effects of aerobic exercise greatly exceed many pharmacotherapeutic effects, and hence must be evaluated with a range of different pathologies. This is particularly the case given that animal models of neurological disease have also reported behavioral benefits of exercise, including Parkinson's, Alzheimer's and Huntington's disease. Kramer and his colleagues also show that exercise effectively induces angiogenesis in several brain areas, suggesting this may be an important factor in recovery from stroke.

Leon, Nadeau, de Riesthal, Crosson, Rosenbek and Gonzalez Rothi (Chapter 25) do us a considerable service by systematically reviewing one of the oldest methods of cognitive rehabilitation – that aimed at the language system. Their review concludes that effective treatments exist for word retrieval, for aspects of sentence use and for verbal fluency, among others. They further conclude, however, that the evidence for generalization of these effective treatments is weak, and offer an insightful and important analysis as to how to improve generalisation, including training more complex rather then less complex structures, activating wider concept representations, activating intentional biases to use spoken language, and training cognitive resources that underlie effective language use. These important ideas have implications far beyond the area of language rehabilitation.

Singh-Curry and Husain (Chapter 26) comprehensively review another area which – as is the case for language – has a long track record as a target for cognitive rehabilitation – spatial neglect. What is notable about neglect rehabilitation research is a relatively strong basis in models of normal brain functioning and the resulting developments of non-intuitive rehabilitation methods such as vibro-tactile stimulation, prism adaptation therapy, limb activation training and sustained attention training.

Singh-Curry and Husain show evidence for a range of promising treatments, but none with the degree of support and replication as pertains to CIT. Given the multidimensional nature of spatial neglect, however, this is not surprising, and it may be that a single treatment akin to CIT will be unlikely to emerge, but rather different types of rehabilitation for different subtypes of neglect.

Levine, Turner and Stuss, in Chapter 27, offer a groundbreaking approach to rehabilitation of executive dysfunction through embedding their assessment of treatment effectiveness within an important new typology of frontal functions – energization, executive, self-regulation and metacognition respectively. They observe that executive functions should not be used synonymously with frontal lobe disorders, as executive dysfunction is only one of at least four different types of frontal lobe dysfunction. Their rigorous review found only nine randomized controlled trials out of a total of 55 studies of frontal dysfunction rehabilitation, mostly in groups with acquired brain injury. This scholarly chapter will become the starting off point for a new approach to the rehabilitation of this crucially important set of cognitive deficits – at the moment, again in marked contrast to the body of evidence accumulated for CIT – the field badly needs to carry out repeated evaluations of a small number of rehabilitation protocols aimed at distinct subtypes of frontal dysfunction. The authors also give a valuable mention of the importance of awareness in rehabilitation – a dimension of importance across the range of domains of cognitive rehabilitation, and not just for frontal lobe dysfunction.

Hanten and Levin (Chapter 28) clearly outline the important differences in considering frontal lobe dysfunction in the developing brain, particularly given that different types of dysfunction appear to have different developmental strategies. They highlight the important bidirectional relationships between two particular sources of frontal lobe dysfunction in children – traumatic brain injury and attention deficit hyperactivity disorder. They highlight the differences in treatment for these two otherwise quite similar disorders – largely pharmacological for ADHD and behavioral for TBI. It is clear that opportunities exist for these two hitherto largely separated domains of therapeutic endeavor to learn from each other.

Ponsford (Chapter 29) takes us further into the domain of frontal lobe dysfunction, in the context of one of the major causes of such dysfunction – traumatic brain injury and the attentional deficits that characterize it. As in the case of aphasia rehabilitation, this author argues that while effective training exists in terms of laboratory effects, the generalization of attentional rehabilitation to everyday life tasks in TBI remains elusive; where training focuses on these real life tasks then real life effects related to these tasks are more likely to be observed. Ponsford is careful to highlight the other potential sources of attentional disturbance, including pain, medication, post-traumatic stress, anxiety and depression, and, like Singh-Curry and Husain, emphasizes the importance of awareness in rehabilitation success.

Wilson and Kapur, in Chapter 30, continue on the theme of generalization and the need to focus on real life tasks in their consideration of memory problems in neurological disorders. Mnemonic strategies can work in laboratory settings, but, Wilson and Kapur argue, most brain-injured people do not use them spontaneously. They give important practical advice as to how to enhance cognitive strategies such as the use of imagery, and urge the individual preferences of individuals to be taken on board, with the recognition that different strategies may benefit some individuals but not others. They argue that the main benefit of mnemonics and strategies is to teach individuals new information, rather than for them to use themselves in everyday life. This raises issues of awareness, self-monitoring and attentional capacity that are raised in the aphasia chapter by Leon *et al.*

Glisky and Glisky (Chapter 31) review evidence suggesting that older people can be trained to use mnemonic and other strategies, but not if suffering from severe memory deficits as are seen in Alzheimer's disease: this may explain in part the difference between Wilson and Kapur on the one

hand, and Glisky and Glisky on the other – perhaps they have more and less severe amnesics in mind when considering the effectiveness of what Glisky and Glisky describe as methods for "optimization of existing or residual memory function." This first class of memory rehabilitation they distinguish from the substitution of intact function for lost or declining function on the one hand, and external compensation for lost or reduced function on the other; the latter, as Wilson and Kapur would agree, is the method of choice for those with severe memory dysfunction. Glisky and Glisky argue that improvement or maintenance of memory function may also be achieved through general non-mnemonic methods such as practice, aerobic exercise, stimulating lifestyles and nonprescription drugs.

A number of important lessons can be learned from the chapters in this section. First, there is a pressing need to develop some standardized methods in each domain of dysfunction, so that the degree of evaluation and replication that is evident in CIT can be reached in these other domains. Second, while very exciting results are achieved in laboratories, finding generalization across time and into everyday life is a much more elusive goal: as Levine and colleagues point out, there is a pressing need for better measures of everyday life functioning so that we can better assess the effectiveness of new methods against this criterion.

All this having been said, it is heartening to see the significant amount of progress that has been made in just 20 years of research, particularly when the level of research funding for rehabilitation research has been tiny in comparison to that available for other domains of neuroscience and medicine. The financial tide may be changing, and the future for neurorehabilitation research may be vastly different in the next 20 years. In the USA, the Veterans Administration Health System has developed Centers of Excellence in rehabilitation, and several of the chapters in the book derive from scientists working in these centers. In the Province of Ontario, Canada, the Heart and Stroke Foundation has made a major commitment to stroke recovery creating a virtual "Centre for Stroke Recovery" (see website listed below), consisting of three different institutions (Sunnybrook Health Sciences Centre, Baycrest Centre, Ottawa Health Research Institute) in two Ontario cities (Ottawa and Toronto), and neurorehabilitation research is a key component of this commitment. The Heart and Stroke Foundation has recognized correctly, as have several contributors to this volume, including Fitzpatrick and Robertson in their summary chapter, that the largest gains are most likely to occur when neurorehabilitation is practiced in a context where there are linkages from molecular to brain and behavior, through stages of recovery, and from behavior to brain mechanisms as demonstrated by imaging.

REFERENCES

http://www.heartandstroke-centrestrokerecovery.ca/.

Meier, M. J., Benton, A. L., & Diller, L. (1987). *Neuropsychological Rehabilitation*. Edinburgh and New York: Churchill Livingston.

23

The use of constraint-induced movement therapy (CI therapy) to promote motor recovery following stroke

David M. Morris and Edward Taub

Introduction

- Stroke is the third leading cause of death, with high economic costs.
- There are a limited number of experimentally verified therapeutic interventions to enhance motor performance; however, there is a growing body of evidence to support the benefit of constraint-induced (CI) therapy.
- This chapter details the individual components of CI therapy techniques.

Stroke is the third leading cause of death after heart disease and cancer and a leading cause of serious, long-term disability. Profoundly impaired motor dysfunction is a major consequence of stroke (American Heart Association, 2005). As a result, a large number of the more than 700 000 people in America sustaining a stroke each year have limitations in motor ability and compromised quality of life. From the early 1970s to the early 1990s, the estimated number of noninstitutionalized survivors of stroke increased from 1.5 million to 2.4 million (Centers for Disease Control and Prevention, 2004). Medicare spent $3.6 billion in 1998 on stroke survivors discharged from short-stay hospitals. The American Heart Association estimates that the current direct and indirect costs of stroke are $43.3 billion per year. The great prevalence of stroke and its high economic costs make the reduction of stroke-related disability a national healthcare priority.

Unfortunately, the number of therapeutic interventions shown in controlled experiments to enhance motor function and promote independent use of an impaired upper extremity (UE) following stroke is quite limited (Duncan, 1997). In our past work, derived from basic research with animals and human subjects, we have developed a set of techniques that reduce the incapacitating movement deficits of many persons in the chronic phase of stroke recovery and increase their independence. The techniques, termed Constraint-Induced Movement therapy or CI therapy, involve a variety of procedures that promote repetitive use of the more-impaired upper extremity (UE) for many hours a day, in the research laboratory, clinical and home settings, during the intervention period (Morris et al., 1997; Morris & Taub, 2001; Taub et al., 1993, 1999; Uswatte & Taub, 2005).

Over the last 20 years, a large body of evidence has accumulated to support the efficacy of CI therapy for hemiparesis following chronic stroke (i.e., >1-year post-injury) (Taub et al., 1999). Evidence for efficacy includes results from: the initial small, randomized controlled trial (RCT) of CI therapy in individuals with UE hemiparesis secondary to chronic stroke (Taub et al., 1993); a larger placebo-controlled trial in individuals of the same chronicity and level of impairment (Taub et al., 2006); and a large, multi-site RCT in individuals with UE hemiparesis in the subacute phase of recovery (i.e., 3–9 months post-stroke) (Wolf et al., 2006). Positive findings regarding CI therapy after chronic stroke are also published in several studies employing within-subjects control procedures and numerous

Cognitive Neurorehabilitation, Second Edition: Evidence and Application, ed. Donald T. Stuss, Gordon Winocur and Ian H. Robertson. Published by Cambridge University Press. © Cambridge University Press 2008.

case studies (Dettmers *et al.*, 2005; Kunkel *et al.*, 1999; Miltner *et al.*, 1999; Sterr *et al.*, 2002; Uswatte & Taub, 2005). Moreover, the most recent post-stroke clinical care guidelines describe CI therapy as an intervention that has evidence of benefit for survivors of stroke with mild-to-moderate UE hemiparesis (Duncan *et al.*, 2005). To date over 200 papers making use of CI therapy have been published. To our knowledge the results of all studies have been positive.

The primary purpose of this chapter is to describe the CI therapy protocol with emphasis placed on detailing the individual components constituting the package of CI therapy techniques.

Theoretical basis underlying CI therapy

- The efficacy of CI therapy is based on basic neuroscience research. Injury to a limb's afferent supply results in neural shock and initial depression of function, leading to a learned non-use of that limb even when movements could potentially be made.
- Restricting movement of the intact limb can induce use of the deafferented limb. Practice, use of conditioned responses and shaping assists in maximizing use of the impaired limb.

Overcoming learned non-use

CI therapy is derived from basic behavioral neuroscience research with primates by Edward Taub. When a single forelimb is deafferented in a monkey, the animal does not make use of it in the free situation (Knapp *et al.*, 1958; Mott & Sherrington, 1895; Twitchell, 1954). Several converging lines of evidence suggested that non-use of a single deafferented limb is a learning phenomenon involving a conditioned suppression of movement. (For a description of the experimental analysis leading to this conclusion, see Taub, 1980.)

The trauma induced by the deafferentation surgical procedure leads to a depression in all neural function (sensory and motor); a phenomenon commonly referred to as neural shock. The process responsible for the initial depression of function and the later gradual recovery of function, which occurs at the level of both the spinal cord and the brain, is at present incompletely understood. However, regardless of the mechanism, recovery processes come into operation following deafferentation so that after a period of time movements can once again, *at least potentially*, be expressed. In monkeys the initial period of depressed function lasts from 2–6 months following forelimb deafferentation (Taub, 1980).

Thus, immediately after operation, the monkeys cannot use a deafferented limb; recovery from the initial depression of function requires considerable time. An animal with one deafferented limb tries to use that extremity in the immediate postoperative situation but it cannot. The monkey functions effectively in the laboratory environment on three limbs and is therefore positively reinforced for this pattern of behavior, which, as a result, is strengthened. Moreover, continued attempts to use the deafferented limb often lead to painful and otherwise aversive consequences, such as incoordination and falling and loss of food objects. In general, the monkey fails with any attempts to use the deafferented limb functionally. These aversive consequences constitute punishment. Many learning experiments have demonstrated that punishment results in the suppression of behavior (Azrin & Holz, 1966; Catania, 1998; Estes, 1944; Lashley, 1924). This response tendency persists, and consequently the monkeys never learn that several months after operation (after neural shock subsides) the limb has become potentially useful. In addition, following stroke (Liepert *et al.*, 1998, 2000) and presumably after extremity deafferentation, there is marked contraction in the size of the cortical representation of the limb; this is probably correlative with the report of patients with stroke that movement of that extremity is effortful. These three processes (failure of attempts to use the deafferented limb, reward of use of just one forelimb, a degraded pattern of coordination, and contraction of the cortical representation zone leading to more effortful movement) interact to produce a vicious spiral downward

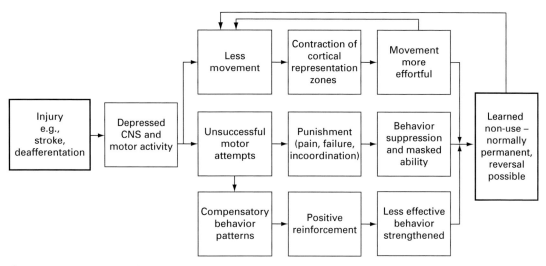

Figure 23.1. Schematic model for development of learned non-use.

that results in a learned non-use of the affected extremity that is normally permanent (illustrated in Figure 23.1).

However, the monkey can be induced to use the deafferented extremity by restricting movement of the intact limb (Taub, 1980). When the movements of the intact limb are restricted several months after unilateral deafferentation, the situation is changed dramatically. The animal either uses the deafferented limb or it cannot with any degree of efficiency feed itself, walk or carry out a large portion of its normal activities of daily life. This change in motivation overcomes the learned non-use of the deafferented limb, and consequently the animal uses it. However, if the movement-restricting device is removed a short while after the early display of purposive movement, the newly learned use of the deafferented limb acquires little strength and is, therefore, quickly overwhelmed by the well-learned tendency not to use the limb. If the movement restriction device is left on for several days or longer, however, use of the deafferented limb acquires strength and is then able to compete successfully with the well-learned habit of non-use of that limb in the free situation (see Figure 23.2). Conditioned response and shaping techniques are another

behavioral means of overcoming the inability to use a single deafferented limb (Taub, 1980) in primates. The conditioned response and shaping, just like the restriction of the intact limb, also involve major alterations in motivation. For a fuller account of these alterations, see Taub (1980).

A similar analysis could also be relevant to human patients after brain injury (e.g., stroke). The period of temporary, organically based inability to use a more-impaired UE would be due to cortical mechanisms rather than processes associated with deafferentation at the level of the spinal cord. With respect to humans, the models do not incorporate all modifiers, such as comorbidities, psychosocial support, motivation and some types of cognitive deficits that could potentially influence the mechanisms underlying learned non-use and those that overcome it. However, the fact that some patients with a given extent and locus of lesion recover more movement than other patients with stroke having similar lesions suggests that additional factors may be involved. One of these factors might be the operation of a learned non-use mechanism. Support for this view comes from the fact that a measure of learned non-use developed in this laboratory (i.e., a measure of ability to use a more-affected

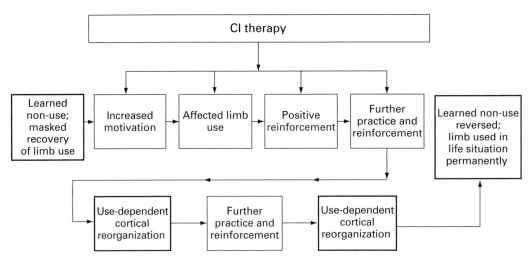

Figure 23.2. Schematic model of mechanism for overcoming learned non-use.

extremity when asked to do so in the laboratory minus a measure of actual amount of use of that extremity in the life situation) correlates $r = 0.47$ ($P < 0.0001$), with CI therapy treatment outcome, while the component measures of this index correlate either not at all (initial laboratory motor function) or significantly but weakly (initial life situation use) with treatment outcome (Mark & Taub, 2004). The strength of the correlation of treatment outcome with a presumed measure of learned non-use suggests that this measure is an index of a real entity.

Use-dependent cortical reorganization: a linked but independent mechanism

- Constraint-induced therapy leads to cortical reorganization, as indexed by various imaging techniques.
- The size of the cortical representation of a body part in adult humans after therapy depends on the amount of use of that part.

An intracortical microstimulation (ICMS) study with monkeys and multiple studies with humans making use of focal transcranial magnetic stimulation (TMS), neuroelectric source imaging, PET, analysis of the readiness potential, and fMRI carried out by five groups of investigators, suggest that cortical reorganization may be associated with the therapeutic effect of CI therapy. Following the seminal work of Jenkins, Recanzone, Merzenich and co-workers on use-dependent cortical reorganization in monkeys (Jenkins *et al.*, 1990; Recanzone *et al.*, 1992a, 1992b, 1992c), imaging studies showed that the same phenomenon occurs in humans. For example, Elbert and coworkers (Elbert *et al.*, 1995) found that the cortical somatosensory representation of the digits of the left hand was larger in string players, who use their left hand for the dexterity-demanding task of fingering the strings, than in nonmusician controls. Moreover, the representation of the fingers of blind Braille readers, who use several fingers simultaneously to read, was enlarged (Sterr *et al.*, 1998). These results, in conjunction with research on cortical reorganization in adult monkeys (Pons *et al.*, 1991) and persons with phantom limb pain (Flor *et al.*, 1995), suggest that the size of the cortical representation of a body part in adult humans depends on the amount of use of that part. The ICMS study by Nudo and co-workers, the first of a series of incisive experiments, demonstrated in adult squirrel monkeys that were surgically given an ischemic infarct in the cortical area controlling the movements of a hand, that training of the

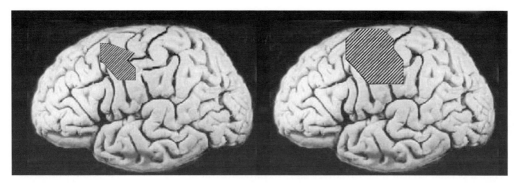

Figure 23.3. (right) Pretreatment cortical map of the contralateral abductor pollicus brevis in a single participant with stroke, determined by TMS, superimposed on an unlesioned postmortem brain to indicate approximate size and location. (left) Post-treatment TMS map in same patient. Modified from Liepert *et al.* (1998) with permission. (Diagram by V. Mark.)

more-affected limb resulted in a cortical reorganization. Specifically, the area surrounding the infarct not normally involved in control of the hand came to participate in that function (Nudo *et al.*, 1996). These findings suggested the possibility that the increase in more-affected arm use produced by CI therapy results in a use-dependent increase in the cortical representation of the more-impaired UE, which provides the neural basis for a permanent increase in the use of that extremity. This hypothesis has been confirmed in TMS studies which showed that the cortical region from which EMG responses of a hand muscle can be elicited by TMS were almost doubled after CI therapy in chronic stroke patients compared to the pretreatment period (Liepert *et al.*, 1998, 2000). Figure 23.3 illustrates the approximate location and size of cortical changes seen in the TMS studies conducted. This experimental evidence suggests that CI therapy is associated with a use-dependent increase in cortical reorganization and has been further confirmed by convergent data from three other laboratories with which Taub collaborated (Bauder *et al.*, 1999; Kopp *et al.*, 1999; Wittenberg *et al.*, 2003) and by two fMRI studies (Levy *et al.*, 2001; Miltner *et al.*, submitted). These studies represent a demonstration of an alteration in brain organization or function associated with a therapy-induced improvement in the rehabilitation of movement after neurological injury in humans.

Application of CI therapy to recovery of upper extremity function following stroke in humans

- Constraint-induced therapy has been used in over 400 patients in the chronic stage of recovery after stroke in this laboratory. The value of the procedure is indexed by a mean effect size of 3.3 for increase of use of the more affected extremity in the life situation.

Studies by Bach-y-Rita and Franz, not operating within a CI therapy context, demonstrated that improvements in UE use in patients with chronic stroke, whose greatly impaired motor function was presumably not amenable to further recovery, was possible (Bach-y-Rita, 1993; Bach-y-Rita & Bach-y-Rita, 1990; Franz *et al.*, 1915). The initial work with patients with stroke that made explicit use of part of the CI therapy approach was carried out by first Ince (1969) and then Halberstam and colleagues (Halberstam *et al.*, 1971) who used one of the simple conditioned response paradigms developed in the deafferentation research with monkeys (noted above) in successful attempts to improve motor capacity following stroke. For some time this work was not followed up.

In the 1980s, Wolf and co-workers employed one of the two suggested techniques, restriction of the less-affected extremity, to induce a significant remediation of motor impairment in chronic stroke patients (Ostendorf & Wolf, 1981; Wolf *et al.*, 1989). However, the effect size was quite small ($d' = 0.2$). Taub and co-workers expanded the protocol using two components: restriction and a variant of the shaping component (i.e., simple practice of use of the more-impaired UE) in a small-sample pilot experiment (Taub *et al.*, 1993). The participants were chronic patients with stroke experienced from 1 to 18 years earlier. Patients with this degree of chronicity had traditionally been presumed to have reached a plateau in their motor recovery and were not expected to exhibit any further improvement for the rest of their lives even if therapy (of whatever type) was administered. This, in fact, was the reason that patients with chronic stroke were chosen as subjects because if there were any improvement in the short span of 2 weeks, it would be unlikely to be due to spontaneous recovery. Nine persons who met the initial study's inclusion criteria, including ability to extend at least 20° at the more-impaired wrist and 10° at each of the more impaired finger joints, were assigned by a random process either to an experimental group ($n = 4$) or an attention-placebo control comparison group ($n = 5$). Patients in the experimental group signed a behavioral contract in which they agreed to wear a sling on their less-impaired UE for a target of 90% of waking hours for 14 days. On 10 of those days, the treatment subjects received six hours of supervised task practice using their more affected arm on a variety of tasks interspersed with one hour of rest. Additional behavioral techniques were used that emphasized transfer of therapeutic gains in the laboratory to the life situation. Treatment efficacy was evaluated using two laboratory motor function tests and the motor activity log or MAL (Taub *et al.*, 1993; Uswatte & Taub, 1999, 2005; Uswatte *et al.*, 2005, 2006). The MAL tracks arm use in a number of activities of daily living through a structured interview administered independently to patients and caregivers (Uswatte & Taub, 1999). The treatment group demonstrated a significant increase in motor ability, as measured by both laboratory motor tests e.g., Wolf Motor Function Test (WMFT) (Morris *et al.*, 2001; Taub *et al.*, 1993; Wolf *et al.*, 2001),

Arm Motor Ability Test (AMAT) (Kopp *et al.*, 1997; McCulloch *et al.*, 1988; Taub *et al.*, 1993) over the treatment period, whereas the control patients showed no change or a decline in arm motor ability. The improvement on the WMFT was approximately eight times as great as in the work of Wolf and colleagues (Wolf *et al.*, 1989). This presumably reflects the effect of expanding the protocol by adding practiced, repetitive movements to motor restriction of the unaffected limb. Indeed, subjects given intensive training only and no restraint exhibit 80% of the full treatment effect post-treatment (Taub *et al.*, 1998). On the MAL, the treatment group showed a very large increase in real-world arm use over the 2-week period and demonstrated a further small (but nonsignificant) increase in use when tested 2 years after treatment. Thus, the improvement was long term. The control patients exhibited no change or a decline in arm use over the same period.

These results have since been confirmed in an experiment from this laboratory using less-affected UE restraint and training (by shaping) of the more-impaired UE instead of task practice, with a larger sample (20 subjects) and a credible placebo control group of equal size (Taub *et al.*, 1993). As in other experiments, the treatment group demonstrated a significant increase in motor ability, as measured by a laboratory motor function test and a very large increase in real-world arm use over the intervention period. The control subjects did not show a significant improvement at the end of treatment. These studies from our laboratory have been replicated in published studies from four other laboratories (Dettmers *et al.*, 2005; Kunkel *et al.*, 1999; Miltner *et al.*, 1999; Sterr *et al.*, 2002).

To date over 400 patients with chronic stroke have been treated in this laboratory and its associated clinic. The mean effect size (ES) for increase of use of the more affected extremity in the life situation over all studies that have been conducted here has been 3.3. By convention, a large ES is considered to be 0.8; thus the ES for real-world use of the more affected arm is extremely large. The magnitude of the treatment effect is not correlated with the amount of time since stroke onset. The mean chronicity of deficits from stroke across all studies is 4.4 years; the patient whose time elapsed from stroke was longest (50 years) had a better than laboratory-average outcome. Treatment gain is also not correlated with age. Our oldest patient to date was 92 years at time of treatment, and his results were approximately as good as the laboratory average. We have had equivalent success with numerous patients in their 80s. This suggests that the plasticity of the nervous system remains throughout the life span and extends well into old age.

The use of CI therapy has begun to spread. As of June 2006, there were over 150 published studies using either the original technique used here or in many cases a variant. The magnitude of the treatment effect has varied, in large part it would seem because of alterations in the methodology, but all studies report a positive outcome (Uswatte & Taub, 2005).

The CI therapy protocol

- Constraint-induced therapy is a therapeutic package, consisting of a number of different techniques.
- Evolving improvement of the CI therapy protocol has led to inclusion of three major components: (1) repetitive, task-oriented training for an extended period; (2) above and beyond training, constraining the patient to use the more-impaired UE during waking hours; (3) use of adherence-enhancing behavioral methods to transfer gains to the real-world environment.

Constraint-induced therapy is a "therapeutic package" consisting of a number of different techniques. Some of these intervention elements have been employed in neurorehabilitation before; yet usually as individual procedures and in a reduced intensity compared with CI therapy. The main novel feature of CI therapy is the combination of these treatment components and their application in a prescribed, integrated and systematic manner to induce a patient to use a more-impaired UE for many hours a day for a period of 2 or 3 consecutive weeks

(depending on the severity of the initial deficit). Constraint-induced therapy has evolved and undergone modification over the two decades of its existence. However, many of the original treatment elements remain part of the standard protocol. The present CI therapy protocol, as applied in our research and clinical setting, consists of three components (Mark & Taub, 2004). These include: (1) repetitive, task-oriented training of the more-impaired UE for several hours a day for 10 or 15 consecutive weekdays; (2) constraining the patient to use the more-impaired UE during waking hours over the course of treatment, sometimes by restraining the less-impaired UE; and (3) applying a package of adherence-enhancing behavioral methods designed to transfer gains made in the research laboratory or clinical setting to the patient's real-world environment. Each component is described in the following sections.

Repetitive, task-oriented training

On each of the weekdays during the intervention period, participants receive training, under the supervision of an interventionist, for several hours each day. The original protocol called for 6 hours/day for this training. More recent studies suggest that a shorter daily training period (i.e., 3 hours/day) may be as effective for higher functioning patients. Two distinct training procedures are employed as patients practice functional task activities: shaping or task practice. Shaping is a training method based on the principles of behavioral training (Morgan, 1974; Panyan, 1980; Skinner, 1938, 1968; Taub et al., 1994). In this approach, a motor or behavioral objective is approached in small steps, by successive approximation or the task is made more difficult in accordance with a participant's motor capabilities, or the requirement for speed of performance is progressively increased. Each functional activity is practiced for a set of 10 trials and explicit feedback is provided regarding the participant's performance on each trial. Figure 23.4 shows a research participant performing a shaping task with supervision from a therapist. Task practice is less

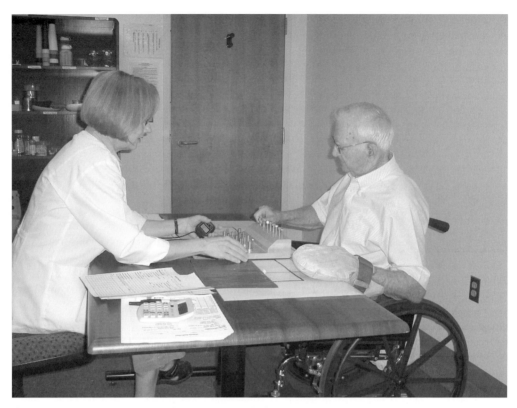

Figure 23.4. Patient participating in shaping activity with therapist supervision.

structured (for example, the tasks are not set up to be carried out as individual trials of discrete movements); it involves functionally based activities performed continuously for a period of 15–20 minutes (e.g., wrapping a present, writing). In successive periods of task practice, the spatial requirements of the activity, or other parameters (such as duration), can be changed to require more demanding control of limb segments for task completion. Global feedback about overall performance is provided at the end of the 15–20 minute period. A large bank of tasks has been created for each type of training procedure. Tables 23.1 and 23.2 provide a more detailed example of a shaping and a task practice activity, respectively. Training tasks are selected for each participant considering: (1) specific joint movements that exhibit the most pronounced deficits, (2) the joint movements that

trainers believe have the greatest potential for improvement, and (3) participant preference among tasks that have similar potential for producing specific improvement. Frequent rest intervals are provided through the training day and intensity of training (i.e., the number of trials/hour (shaping) or the amount of time spent on each training procedure (e.g., task practice)) is recorded.

In an attempt to reduce the intensive therapist supervision required during training, automation has been successfully incorporated into CI therapy training (Lum *et al.*, 2004, 2006; Taub *et al.*, 2005). A device called AutoCITE (Automated Constraint-Induced Therapy Extension) was developed in collaboration between the UAB team and Peter Lum and others at the VA Rehabilitation Research and Development Center in Palo Alto, CA. The AutoCITE

Table 23.1. Example of a shaping task: placing blocks onto box

Activity description	A box and several blocks are used for this task. The subject moves small wooden blocks from the table to the top of a box. The placement and height of the box depend on the movements desired. For example, the box can be placed directly in front of the subject to challenge shoulder flexion and elbow extension or placed to the side to challenge shoulder abduction and elbow extension.
Potential shaping progressions parameters	• Distance: The box can be moved farther away to challenge elbow extension. • Height: A higher box can be used to challenge shoulder flexion. • Size of object: Larger or smaller blocks can be used to challenge wrist and hand control.
Potential feedback parameters	• Number of repetitions: Number of blocks placed on the box in a given period of time • Time: Time required to place a set number of blocks on the box
Movements emphasized	• Pincer grasp • Wrist extension • Elbow extension • Shoulder flexion

Table 23.2. Example of a task practice activity: folding/sorting clothes

Activity description	Subjects sit/stand at a table with a laundry basket in front of them. The basket is filled with wash cloths/towels/clothes of different colors. The subjects remove the items and sort them into piles of different colors. After sorting, the subject proceeds to fold the items. Sorting items can be combined with the hanging clothes.
Adjusting difficulty/complexity	Folding items can be graded from wash cloths, to towels, to clothes.
Suggested feedback	• Number of items sorted/folded in a set period of time (e.g., 20 minutes). • Time required sorting and folding entire basket of laundry. • Quality of folding (e.g., wash cloths folded symmetrically). • Improvement in hand function in performing these tasks (e.g., thumb extension/opposition).

consists of a computer, eight task devices arrayed in a cabinet on four work surfaces, and an attached chair. The eight activities are: Reaching, Tracing, Peg board, Supination/Pronation, Threading, Arc-and-rings, Finger-tapping and Object-flipping. The computer provides simple one-step instructions on a monitor that guides the participant through the entire treatment session. Completion of each instruction is verified by sensors, which are built into the device. Task completion is recorded and displayed to participants before the next instruction is given. The participant is able to select tasks from a menu displayed on the monitor using two pushbuttons. Once a task has been chosen, the device automatically adjusts so that the appropriate work surface is at the correct height for task performance. The computer program guides the participant through a set of ten 30-s trials in which the objective is to repeat a task as many times as possible. After 10 trials, the task menu is displayed and the subject can select the next task. Several types of performance feedback and encouragement are provided on the computer monitor, simulating the type of verbal behavior engaged in by a therapist. The time remaining on each trial is shown on the computer monitor. The number of successful repetitions is displayed after each trial in the form of a bar added to a bar graph for each set of 10 trials. The activities are based upon tasks currently used in CI therapy. Studies using the AutoCITE during the CI therapy intervention indicate that gains achieved are substantial and comparable to those observed using CI therapy without automation (Lum *et al.*, 2004, 2006; Taub *et al.*, 2005).

Constraining use of the more-impaired UE

The most commonly applied CI therapy treatment protocol has incorporated use of a restraint (either sling or protective safety mitt) on the less-impaired UE to prevent participants from succumbing to the strong urge to use that UE during most or all functional activities, both with and without interventionist supervision. Over the last decade, the protective safety mitt has been preferred for restraint as it prevents functional use of the less-impaired UE for most purposes while still allowing protective extension of that UE in case of a loss of balance. When employed, participants are taught to put on and take off the mitt independently, and decisions are made with the interventionist as to when its use is feasible and safe. The goal for mitt use is 90% of waking hours. This so-called "forced use" is arguably the most visible element of the intervention to the rehabilitation community and is frequently and mistakenly described as synonymous with "CI therapy." However, Taub has stated "there is ... nothing talismanic about use of a sling, protective safety mitt or other constraining device on the less-affected UE" as long as the more-impaired UE is exclusively engaged in repeated practice (Taub *et al.*, 1999). "Constraint" was not intended to refer only to the application of a physical restraint, such as a mitt, but also to indicate a constraint of opportunity for the less-impaired UE to be used for functional activities (Taub *et al.*, 1999). As such, any strategy that encourages exclusive use of the more-impaired UE is viewed as a "constraining" component of the treatment package. For example, shaping was meant to be considered as constituting a very important constraint on behavior; either the participant succeeds at the task or he is not rewarded (e.g., by praise or knowledge of improvement).

Preliminary findings by Sterr *et al.* (2002) indicate a significant treatment effect using CI therapy without the physical restraint component. Likewise, our laboratory has obtained similar findings with a small group of participants ($n = 9$) when a CI therapy protocol, without physical restraint was employed (Taub *et al.*, 1998, 1999). However, our study suggested that this group experienced a larger decrement at the 2-year follow-up testing than groups where physical restraint was employed. If other treatment package elements, developed in our laboratory, are not used, our clinical experience suggests that routine reminders to not use the less-affected UE alone, without physical restraint, would not be as effective as using the mitt. Consequently, we use the mitt to minimize the need for the interventionist to remind or the participant to remember to limit use of the less-impaired UE during the intervention period.

Adherence-enhancing behavioral methods

One of the over-riding goals for CI therapy is to transfer gains made in the research or clinical setting into the participant's real-world environment (e.g., home and community settings). To achieve this goal, we employ a set of techniques that we term a "transfer package" which has the effect of making the patient accountable for adherence to the requirements of the therapy. The participant must be actively engaged in and adherent to the intervention without constant supervision from an interventionist. Attention to adherence must be directed towards wearing the mitt as much as possible (when it is safe to do so), using the more-impaired UE during functional tasks, and assuring appropriate assistance from caregivers if present (i.e., assistance to prevent the participant from struggling excessively but allowing them to try as many tasks as is feasible). Behavioral techniques currently employed include the daily administration of the MAL (monitoring), maintenance of a home diary (monitoring), a behavioral contract with the patient and the caregiver independently (behavioral contract + monitoring = patient accountability), problem solving to help overcome what the patient sees as barriers to use of the more affected arm, daily schedule, home skill assignment and home practice.

Behavioral contract (BC)

The behavioral contract (BC) is a formal, written agreement between the interventionist and participant that the participant will use the more-affected extremity for specific activities outside of the laboratory. In addition to increasing mitt use outside of the laboratory, the BC is helpful in assuring safety while wearing the mitt, engaging the participant in active problem-solving to increase adherence, and assuring participant accountability for adherence. The BC is completed after the first day of treatment when the interventionist has assessed the participant's functional motor capacity and the participant has experienced using the mitt.

Participants first list all activities of daily living (ADLs) performed on a typical day. These ADLs are then categorised on the contract into those to be done with (a) the more-affected UE and mitt on; (b) both UEs with the mitt off; and (c) less-affected UE only with the mitt off. The time agreed upon for "mitt off" activities is specified (i.e., when it is to be removed and put back on), and have mainly to do with safety and the use of water. Activities may be added to increase UE use during down times (e.g., periodically turning pages of a magazine during time spent watching television). Activities of daily living may be modified to allow more-affected UE use (e.g., using a spill-proof cup while drinking liquids, using a build-up orthotic device on a fork). The BC is signed by the interventionist, participant and a witness; this formality emphasizes the importance of the BC. The BC is often modified during treatment as the participant gains new movement skills.

The home diary (HD)

The home diary (HD) is a daily process wherein participants list their activities outside the laboratory and report whether they have used their more-affected extremity or not while performing different tasks. Daily administration of the MAL has the same effect. The HD and daily review of the MAL heightens participants' awareness of their use of the more-affected UE and emphasizes adherence to the BC and the patients' accountability for their own improvement. Discussion of the HD and MAL also provides a structured opportunity for discussing why the weaker extremity was not used for specific activities and for problem-solving on how to use it more. The HD and daily administration of the MAL directly support the BC.

Home skill assignment (HSA)

Wearing the mitt while away from the clinic/laboratory does not assure that participants will use the more-impaired UE to carry out ADLs that have been accomplished exclusively with the less-impaired UE, or not at all, since the stroke. The HSA process encourages the participant to try ADLs that they may not normally try with the more-impaired UE. To work up a HSA, the interventionist first reviews a list of common ADL tasks carried out in the home. The tasks are categorized according to the rooms in which they are usually performed (e.g., kitchen, bathroom, bedroom, office). Starting on the second day of the intervention period, participants are asked to select 10 ADL tasks from the list that they agree to try after they leave the laboratory/clinic and before they return for the next day of in-lab/clinic treatment. Tasks not on the list may be selected if desired by the participant. These tasks are to be carried out while wearing the mitt when possible and safe. Interventionists guide the participant to select five tasks that the participant believes will be relatively easy to accomplish and five they believe will be more challenging. The ten items selected are recorded on an assignment sheet and sent with the participant when they leave the laboratory or clinic for the day. The goal is for approximately 30 minutes to be devoted to trying the specified ADLs at home each day. The HSA sheet is reviewed during the first part of the next in-lab/clinic treatment day and 10 additional ADL tasks are selected for HSA for that evening. This process is repeated throughout the intervention period with efforts made to encourage use of the more-impaired UE during as many "different" ADL tasks in as many "different" rooms of the participant's home as possible.

Caregiver contract (CC)

The caregiver contract (CC) is a formal, written agreement between the interventionist and the participant's caregiver that the caregiver will be present and available while the participant is wearing the mitt and will aid in the at-home program and more generally in helping to increase more-affected UE use. The CC is completed after the terms of BC are shared with the caregiver. The CC (a) improves caregivers' understanding of the treatment program; (b) guides caregivers to assist appropriately; and (c) increases the safety of the participant. The CC is signed by the interventionist, participant and caregiver and thereby formally emphasizes the importance of the CC.

Daily schedule (DS)

Project staff record a detailed schedule of all clinical activities carried out on each day of the intervention. This DS includes time devoted to each activity listed. The schedule specifically notes the times when the restraint device is put on and taken off. The time and length of rest periods are also included. Specific shaping and task practice activities are listed on the DS. Wearing the mitt, and using only the more-affected UE during lunch, is included on the DS whenever it is feasible for the patient to come close to doing so. For this activity, the DS not only includes the length of time devoted to eating lunch, but also what foods were eaten and how this was accomplished. Information recorded on the DS is particularly helpful for demonstrating improvements in daily activities to the participant, which often has the effect of motivating them to try harder.

Home practice (HP)

During treatment, participants are asked to spend 15 to 30 minutes at home on a daily basis performing specific upper-extremity tasks repetitively with their more-affected arm; referred to as HP-during. The tasks typically employ materials that are commonly available (e.g., stacking styrofoam cups). This strategy is particularly helpful for individuals who are typically relatively inactive while in their home setting (e.g., spend long periods watching TV) and provides more structured opportunities to use the more-impaired UE. Care must be taken, however, to not overload the participant with too many assignments while away from the lab/clinic as this could prove de-motivating to the patient. As such, interventionists usually select HSA or HP-during to encourage more UE, rarely are both used. Towards the end of treatment, an individualized post-treatment home practice program is drawn up consisting of similar tasks; referred to as HP-after. For each participant, approximately 8–10 task practice-type activities are selected based on the participant's remaining movement deficits. These activities are detailed on a HP-after assignment sheet and participants are asked to demonstrate understanding and proficiency with all tasks before discharge. As with HP-during, these tasks usually employ commonly available equipment to increase the likelihood that they will be implemented. Participants are encouraged to select 1 or 2 tasks/day and to perform these tasks for 30 minutes daily. On the next day, 1 or 2 different tasks will be selected on the participants' HP-after assignment sheet. The HP-after activities are intended to be used indefinitely by participants.

Therapeutic factors: massing of practice and limb restraint

A characterization of conventional physical rehabilitation procedures is difficult to formulate because the treatments are so diverse and are not connected by a single conceptual framework. Though individual elements of CI therapy have been used before, the integrated treatment package represents a substantial change. The common goal of all the treatment components is to promote repeated practice of use of the more-impaired UE for many hours over the CI therapy intervention period. As such, any technique, such as a training method that induces a patient to use a more-affected extremity many hours a day for a period of consecutive days, should be therapeutically efficacious. Mauritz and co-workers have also shown that repetitive practice is an important factor in stroke rehabilitation (Butefisch *et al.*, 1995; Hesse *et al.*, 1994). This factor is likely to produce the activity-dependent cortical reorganization found to result from CI therapy (described above) and is presumed to be the basis for the long-term persistence of the increase in the amount of use of the more affected extremity. As stated earlier, it is not the restraint in CI therapy that is important. Multiple components of the CI therapy protocol encourage participants to use the more-impaired UE, thus promoting overcoming learned non-use and facilitating the development of use-dependent plastic brain reorganization. They operate by imposing a constraint (and not a restraint) on movement. Restraint of the less affected limb is employed, but it is also a kind of constraint – a physical constraint – though in any case it does not make a major contribution to treatment effect. Hence the formulation of the name of the intervention: constraint (not restraint)-induced movement therapy.

Conclusions: an impending paradigm shift in neurorehabilitation

Recent discoveries about how the central nervous system responds to injury and how to retrain or remediate behaviors have given rise to effective new therapies in other laboratories for the rehabilitation of function after neurological injury (Dobkin, 1989). Until now, neurorehabilitation has been largely static; few, if any, older treatments have received evidence-based demonstrations of efficacy. However, a current melding of basic behavioral

science with neuroscience gives promise of entirely new approaches to improving the behavioral, perceptual and possibly cognitive capabilities of individuals who have sustained neurological damage. The discoveries in a number of laboratories have been with respect to such phenomena as plastic brain reorganization, spinal cord regeneration, neurogenesis from endogenous stem cells, pharmacological intervention, and the substantial enhancement of dyslexia and extremity use by behavioral means (Kolb, 2003; see also Chapter 1 by Kolb and Gibb, Chapter 17 by McAllister and Arnsten, and Chapter 22 by Stickland, Weiss and Kolb in this volume for a review). Each of these new or promising treatments in the fields of rehabilitation and remediation either (a) emerge from behavioral research or research in behavior and neuroscience, (b) involve rehabilitation/behavioral techniques in conjunction with other types of interventions, or (c) make use of rehabilitation/behavioral methods to produce an advantageous effect on the nervous system (Taub *et al.*, 2002). These types of approaches are not entirely new, but their explicit formulation and the effectiveness with which they are currently being applied to the enhancement of impaired human abilities is. The current state of change in rehabilitation amounts to an impending paradigm shift (Taub *et al.*, 2002). The studies from this laboratory stemming from basic behavioral neuroscience research involving somatosensory deafferentation in monkeys that gave rise to CI therapy constitute one example of this new approach.

REFERENCES

American Heart Association (2005). Heart and Stroke Statistical Update. http://www.Americanheart.org/statistics/stroke.htm.

Azrin, N. H., & Holz, W. C. (1996). Punishment. In W. K. Honig (Ed.), *Operant Behavior: Areas of Research and Application* (pp. 380–447). New York, NY: Appleton-Century-Crofts.

Bach-y-Rita, P. (1993). Recovery from brain damage. *Journal of Neurological Rehabilitation*, **6**, 191–199.

Bach-y-Rita, P., & Bach-y-Rita, E. W. (1990). Biological and psychosocial factors in recovery from brain damage in humans. *Canadian Journal of Psychology*, **44**, 148–165.

Bauder, H., Sommer, M., Taub, E., & Miltner, W. H. R. (1999). Effect of CI therapy on movement-related brain potentials. *Psychophysiology*, **36**, S31.

Butefisch, C., Hummelsheim, H., Densler, P., & Mauritz, K.-H. (1995). Mauritz, K-H. Repetitive training of isolated movements improves the outcome of motor rehabilitation of the centrally paretic hand. *Journal of Neurological Science*, **130**, 59–68.

Catania, A. C. (1998). *Learning (4th Edition)*. Upper Saddle River, NJ: Prentice Hall.

Center for Disease Control and Prevention. (2004). Health, United States. http.//www.cdc.gov/nchs/hus.htm.

Dettmers, C., Teske, U., Hamzei, F. *et al.* (2005). Distributed form of constraint-induced movement therapy improves functional outcome and quality of life after stroke. *Archives of Physical Medicine and Rehabilitation*, **86**, 204–209.

Dobkin, B. H. (1989). Focused stroke rehabilitation programs do not improve outcome. *Archives of Neurology and Psychiatry*, **46**, 701–703.

Duncan, P. W. (1997). Synthesis of intervention trials to improve motor recovery following stroke. *Topics in Stroke Rehabilitation*, **3**, 1–20.

Duncan, P. W., Zorowitz, R., Bates, B. *et al.* (2005). Management of adult rehabilitation care: a clinical practice guideline. *Stroke*, **36**, e100–e143.

Elbert, T., Pantev, C., Wienbruch, C., Rockstroh, B., & Taub, E. (1995). Increased use of the left hand in string players associated with increased cortical representation of the fingers. *Science*, **220**, 21–23.

Estes, W. K. (1944). An experimental study of punishment. *Psychological Monographs*, **57**, (Serial No. 263).

Flor, H., Elbert, T., Knecht, S. *et al.* (1995). Phantom limb pain as a perceptual correlate of massive reorganization in upper limb amputees. *Nature*, **375**, 482–484.

Franz, S. I., Scheetz, M. E., & Wilson, A. A. (1915). The possibility of recovery of motor functioning in long-standing hemiplegia. *Journal of the American Medical Association*, **65**, 2150–2154.

Halberstam, J. L., Zaretsky, H. H., Brucker, B. S., & Guttman, A. (1971). Avoidance conditioning of motor responses in elderly brain-damaged patients. *Archives of Physical Medicine and Rehabilitation*, **52**, 318–328.

Hesse, S., Bertelt, C., Schaffrin, A., Malezic, M. S., & Mauritz, K.-H. (1994). Restoration of gait in nonambulatory hemiparetic patients by treadmill training with partial body-weight support. *Archives of Physical Medicine and Rehabilitation*, **75**, 1087–1093.

Ince, L. P. (1969). Escape and avoidance conditioning of response in the plegic arm of stroke patients: a preliminary study. *Psychonomic Science*, **16**, 49–50.

Jenkins, W. M., Merzenich, M. M., Ochs, M. T., T., A., & Guic-Robles, E. (1990). Functional reorganization of primary somatosensory cortex in adult owl monkeys after behaviorally controlled tactile stimulation. *Journal of Neurophysiology*, **63**, 82–104.

Knapp, H. D., Taub, E., & Berman, A. J. (1958). Effect of deafferentiation on a conditioned avoidance response. *Science*, **128**, 842–843.

Kolb, B. (2003). Overview of cortical plasticity and recovery from brain injury. *Physical Medicine and Rehabilitation Clinics of North America*, **14**, Suppl. 1, S7–S25.

Kopp, B., Kunkel, A., Flor, H. *et al.* (1997). The Arm Motor Ability Test (AMAT): Reliability, validity and sensitivity to change. *Archives of Physical Medicine and Rehabilitation*, **78**, 615–620.

Kopp, B., Kunkel, A., Mühlnickel, W. *et al.* (1999). Plasticity in the motor system correlated with therapy-induced improvement of movement in human stroke patients. *NeuroReport*, **10**, 807–810.

Kunkel, A., Kopp, B., Muller, G. *et al.* (1999). Constraint-induced movement therapy for motor recovery in chronic stroke patients. *Archives of Physical Medicine and Rehabilitation*, **80**, 624–628.

Lashley, K. S. (1924). Studies of cerebral function in learning: V. The retention of motor areas in primates. *Archives of Neurology and Psychiatry*, **12**, 249–276.

Levy, C. E., Nichols, D. S., Schmalbrock, P. M., Keller, P., & Chakers, D. W. (2001). Functional MRI evidence of cortical reorganization in upper-limb stroke hemiplegia treated with constraint-induced movement therapy. *American Journal of Physical Medicine and Rehabilitation*, **80**, 4–12.

Liepert, J., Bauder, H., Sommer, M. *et al.* (1998). Motor cortex plasticity during constraint-induced movement therapy in chronic stroke patients. *Neuroscience Letters*, **250**, 5–8.

Liepert, J., Bauder, H., Miltner, W. H. R., Taub, E., & Weiller, C. (2000). Treatment-induced cortical reorganization after stroke in humans. *Stroke*, **31**, 1210–1216.

Lum, P. S., Taub, E., Schwandt, D. *et al.* (2004). Automated constraint-induced therapy extension (AutoCITE) for movement deficits after stroke. *Journal of Rehabilitation Research and Development*, **41**, 249–257.

Lum, P. S., Uswatte, G., Taub, E., Hardin, P., & Mark, V. W. (2006). A tele-rehabilitation approach to delivery of constraint-induced movement therapy. *Journal of Rehabilitation Research and Development*, **43**, 391–399.

Mark, V. W., & Taub, E. (2004). Constraint-induced movement therapy for chronic stroke hemiparesis and other disabilities. *Restorative Neurology and Neuroscience*, **22**, 317–336.

McCulloch, K., Cook, E. W. I., Fleming, W. C. *et al.* (1988). A reliable test of upper extremity ADL function. *Archives of Physical Medicine and Rehabilitation*, **69**, 755.

Miltner, W. H. R., Bauder, H., Sommer, M., Dettmers, C., & Taub, E. (1999). Effects of constraint-induced movement therapy on patients with chronic motor deficits after stroke: a replication. *Stroke*, **30**, 586–592.

Miltner, W. H. R., Balzer, C., & Taub, E. (submitted). CI therapy treatment outcome tracked by substantial changes in functional magnetic resonance imaging.

Morgan, W. G. (1974). The shaping game: a teaching technique. *Behavior Therapy*, **5**, 271–272.

Morris, D., & Taub, E. (2001). The constraint-induced therapy approach to restoring function after neurological injury. *Topics in Stroke Rehabilitation*, **8**, 16–30.

Morris, D. M., Crago, J. E., DeLuca, S. C., Pidikiti, R. D., & Taub, E. (1997). Constraint-induced (CI) movement therapy for motor recovery after stroke. *Neurorehabitation*, **9**, 29–43.

Morris, D. M., Uswatte, G., Crago, J. E., Cook, E. W. III., & Taub, E. (2001). The reliability of the Wolf Motor Function Test for assessing upper extremity function after stroke. *Archives of Physical Medicine and Rehabilitation*, **82**, 750–755.

Mott, F. W., & Sherrington, C. S. (1895). Experiments upon the influence of sensory nerves upon movement and nutrition of the limbs. *Proceedings of the Royal Society of London*, **57**, 481–488.

Nudo, R. J., Wise, B. M., SiFuentes, F., & Milliken, G. W. (1996). Neural substrates for the effects of rehabilitative training on motor recovery following ischemic infarct. *Science*, **272**, 1791–1794.

Ostendorf, C. G., & Wolf, S. L. (1981). Effect of forced use of the upper extremity of a hemiplegic patient on changes in function. *Physical Therapy*, **61**, 1022–1028.

Panyan, M. V. (1980). *How to use Shaping*. Lawrence, KS: H & H Enterprises.

Pons, T. P., Garraghty, A. K., Ommaya, A. K. *et al.* (1991). Massive cortical reorganization after sensory deafferentation in adult macaques. *Science*, **252**, 1857–1860.

Recanzone, G. H., Jenkins, W. M., & Merzenich, M. M. (1992a). Progressive improvement in discriminative abilities in adult owl monkeys performing a tactile frequency discrimination task. *Journal of Neurophysiology*, **67**, 1015–1030.

Recanzone, G. H., Merzenich, M. M., & Jenkins, W. M. (1992b). Frequency discrimination training engaging a restricted skin surface results in an emergence of a cutaneous response zone in cortical area 3a. *Journal of Neurophysiology*, **67**, 1057–1070.

Recanzone, G. H., Merzenich, M. M., Jenkins, W. M., Grajski, A., & Dinse, H. R. (1992c). Topographic reorganization of the hand representation in area 3b of owl monkeys trained in a frequency discrimination task. *Journal of Neurophysiology*, **67**, 1031–1056.

Skinner, B. F. (1938). *The Behavior of Organisms*. New York, NY: Appleton-Century-Crofts.

Skinner, B. F. (1968). *The Technology of Teaching*. New York, NY: Appleton-Century-Crofts.

Sterr, A., Müller, M. M., Elbert, T. *et al.* (1998). Changed perceptions in Braille readers. *Nature*, **391**, 134–135.

Sterr, A., Elbert, T., Berthold, I. *et al.* (2002). CI therapy in chronic hemiparesis: the more the better? *Archives of Physical Medicine and Rehabilitation*, **83**, 1374–1377.

Taub, E. (1980). Somatosensory deafferentation research with monkeys: implications for rehabilitation medicine. In L. P. Ince (Eds.), *Behavioral Psychology in Rehabilitation Medicine: Clinical Applications* (pp. 371–401). New York, NY: Williams & Wilkins.

Taub, E., Miller, N. E., Novack, T. A. *et al.* (1993). Technique to improve chronic motor deficit after stroke. *Archives of Physical Medicine and Rehabilitation*, **74**, 347–354.

Taub, E., Crago, J. E., Burgio, L. D. *et al.* (1994). An operant approach to rehabilitation medicine: overcoming learned nonuse by shaping. *Journal of the Experimental Analysis of Behavior*, **61**, 281–293.

Taub, E., Crago, J. E., & Uswatte, G. (1998). Constraint-induced movement therapy: a new approach to treatment in physical rehabilitation. *Rehabilitation Psychology*, **43**, 152–170.

Taub, E., Uswatte, G., & Pidikiti, R. (1999). Constraint-induced movement therapy: a new family of techniques with broad application to physical rehabilitation – a clinical review. *Journal of Rehabilitation Research and Development*, **36**, 237–251.

Taub, E., Uswatte, G., & Elbert, T. (2002). New treatments in neurorehabilitation founded on basic research. *Neuroscience*, **3**, 226–236.

Taub, E., Lum, P. S., Hardin, P., Mark, V. W., & Uswatte, G. (2005). AutoCITE: automated delivery of CI therapy with reduced effort by therapists. *Stroke*, **36**, 1301–1304.

Taub, E., Uswatte, G., King, D. K. *et al.* (2006). A placebo controlled trial of constraint-induced movement therapy for upper extremity after stroke. *Stroke*, **37**, 1045–1049.

Twitchell, T. E. (1954). Sensory factors in purposive movement. *Journal of Neurophysiology*, **17**, 239–254.

Uswatte, G., & Taub, E. (1999). Constraint-induced movement therapy: new approaches to outcome measurement in rehabilitation. In D. T. Stuss, G. Winocur, & I. H. Robertson (Eds.), *Cognitive Neurorehabilitation* (pp. 214–229). Cambridge, UK: Cambridge University Press.

Uswatte, G., & Taub, E. (2005). Implications of the learned nonuse formulation for measuring rehabilitation outcomes: lessons from constraint-induced movement therapy. *Rehabilitation Psychology*, **50**, 34–42.

Uswatte, G., Taub, E., Morris, D. M., Vignolo, M., & McCulloch, K. (2005). Reliability and validity of the Upper-extremity Motor Activity Log-14 for measuring real-world arm use. *Stroke*, **36**, 2493–2496.

Uswatte, G., Taub, E., Morris, D. M., Barman, J., & Crago, J. (2006). Contribution of the shaping and restraint components of constraint-induced movement therapy to treatment outcome. *Neurorehabilitation*, **21**, 147–156.

Wittenberg, G. F., Chen, R., Ishii, K. *et al.* (2003). Constraint-induced movement therapy in stroke: magnetic-stimulation motor maps and cerebral activation. *Neurorehabilitation and Neural Repair*, **17**, 48–57.

Wolf, S. L., Lecraw, D. E., Barton, L. A., & Jann, B. B. (1989). Forced use of hemiplegic upper extremities to reverse the effect of learned nonuse among chronic stroke and head-injured patients. *Experimental Neurology*, **104**, 104–132.

Wolf, S. L., Catlin, P. A., Ellis, M. *et al.* (2001). Assessing the Wolf Motor Function Test as an outcome measure for research with patients post-stroke. *Stroke*, **32**, 1635–1639.

Wolf, S. L., Winstein, C., Miller, J. P. *et al.* (2006). The Extremity Constraint Induced Therapy Evaluation (EXCITE) trial for patients with sub-acute stroke. *Journal of the American Medical Association*, **296**, 2095–2104.

24

Effects of physical activity on cognition and brain

Arthur F. Kramer, Kirk I. Erickson and Edward McAuley

Introduction

- There is a growing emphasis on healthy aging, with many services and products being developed to respond to this interest. It is essential to understand the scientific evidence on which such products are based.
- This chapter focuses on the beneficial effects of physical exercise on brain structure and function, with a focus on normal aging.
- The chapter consists of four sections: molecular and cellular mechanisms evidenced in non-human animals; epidemiological studies of the impact of physical activity and exercise on cognition later in life; cross-sectional studies and randomized clinical trial studies; future directions for research.

Given the aging of the population in most industrialized countries (Gokhale & Smetters, 2006) and the fact that the first baby boomers turn 60 in 2006 it is unsurprising that there is an increasing focus on the development of programs and products for healthy aging. This focus has resulted in a dramatic increase in the availability of books, computer programs, nutritional supplements, physical activity programs and other consumer products that claim to provide solutions to the detrimental changes in cognition and brain function that occur during the process of adult aging. For example, a recent search on Amazon.com yielded 175 books that profess to offer successful techniques for maintaining and enhancing memory during aging. An increasing number of computer programs are also available that offer to both track changes in attention, memory, decision making, processing speed and other cognitive processes over time and provide practice and training to ensure maintenance and even enhancement of a variety of cognitive skills and abilities. One recent addition to this rapidly growing field of products to foster healthy aging is a series of games introduced in 2006 by Nintendo. The product *Brain Age*, which has been endorsed in promotional materials by a neuroscientist and cognitive psychologist, provides a variety of tests that purportedly measure users' brain age and offers exercises to reduce "brain age" with practice. Some of these tests include performing math problems, counting, performing Stroop tasks and playing the game Sudoku. According to a recent article in Outside magazine (July, 2006) the first spin-and-learn studio will open in July 2006. Based on the assumption that multimodal training is more effective than uni-modal training, this studio combines spinning (i.e., rapidly riding a stationary bicycle) with learning new skills such as Spanish. However, an important question to ask amidst the flurry of product development is whether these products and programs are based on solid scientific evidence, as well as what gaps exist in the scientific knowledge base concerning factors that influence healthy and successful aging.

In this chapter we focus on the question of whether exercise positively influences cognition and brain function. Consistent with the main focus of this book most of our discussion will concentrate on older organisms, although we will briefly touch

Cognitive Neurorehabilitation, Second Edition: Evidence and Application, ed. Donald T. Stuss, Gordon Winocur and Ian H. Robertson. Published by Cambridge University Press. © Cambridge University Press 2008.

on fitness effects across the lifespan. Additionally, as Chapter 15 by Scherder and Eggermont covers physical activity effects on dementia, we have focused our review, for the most part, on normal or nonpathological older adults. The structure of our chapter is as follows. First, we review the rapidly expanding literature with nonhuman animals that has begun to explicate the molecular and cellular mechanisms which underlie exercise effects on brain structure and function as well as learning and memory. Next, we examine an increasing number of observational or epidemiological studies that explore the question of whether physical activity and exercise at one point in time bestow protective effects on cognition later in life. For the most part these studies examine the influence of exercise across time periods from 5–8 years, although there are some interesting exceptions that range across many decades. Third, we briefly focus on cross-sectional studies of the relation between fitness and cognition and then rapidly shift our exploration to randomized clinical trial studies of exercise training effects on cognition and brain structure and function of older adults. Finally, we suggest several future directions for the research on fitness training effects on brain and cognition.

Animal studies of fitness exercise effects on learning, memory, brain function and structure

- Research in nonhuman animals is important for several reasons: control of environment, cost efficiency and ability to examine cellular and molecular mechanisms.
- Exercise benefits animals at any age.
- Animal models of neurological disease have also reported behavioral benefits of exercise: Parkinson's, Alzheimer's and Huntington's disease.
- Exercise effectively induces angiogenesis (growth of new vasculature) in several brain areas, suggesting this may be an important factor in recovery from stroke.

- Exercise research in animals has also demonstrated the promotion of neurogenesis (development of new neurons) and increase in overall cell survival. There appears to be a complex relationship between neurogenesis, exercise and biological changes with aging.
- Exercise upregulates many neuroprotective molecules that also enhance brain structure and function.

Animal research on exercise training complements research with humans in several important ways. First, the multitude of factors that interact with and likely modify fitness effects in humans, such as social interaction, nutrition and intellectual engagement, can be well controlled (or systematically manipulated) in animal studies. Although some of these factors can be held relatively constant in human clinical trials, issues of cost render it difficult to systematically vary these often confounding factors in human studies. Second, with the rapid development of noninvasive neuroimaging techniques it is now possible to examine fitness effects on human brain structure and function. However, there are clearly limitations on the extent to which the brain can be examined with such techniques. Indeed, the ability to examine cellular and molecular changes as a function of fitness is one of the strongest justifications for animal studies.

Behavior

Behavioral studies with rodents have shown performance benefits of wheel running on a variety of cognitive and motor tasks. For example, in the Morris water maze, animals learn to swim to a platform submerged just beneath the surface of the pool. The platform remains stationary on all trials, but the location that the animal is placed into the pool is altered, so that the animal must learn to use extra-maze cues to learn the location of the submerged platform. This paradigm is thought to assess learning and spatial memory processes and is considered to be a hippocampal-dependent task. In this paradigm, Fordyce & Wehner (1993) reported that exercise produced a 2- to 12-fold increase in the rate of acquisition for learning the placement of the platform. Swimming speeds remained the same for both exercising and sedentary animals. Others have also reported acquisition and retention benefits on this task and other hippocampal dependent tasks in young animals (Adlard *et al.*, 2004; Anderson *et al.*, 2000; Gómez-Pinilla *et al.*, 1998).

More recently, van Praag *et al.* (2005) examined the effect of voluntary exercise on performance in the Morris water maze in aged animals. In this study, aged mice had unlimited access to a running wheel for 45 days and showed similar running rates as young mice. The authors demonstrated that exercising aged animals showed faster acquisition and greater retention on this task than age-matched controls. Thus, exercise offset age-related declines in spatial memory and learning in mice. Similar effects of exercise on Morris water maze performance have been shown in other studies of aging (Albeck *et al.*, 2006).

There are other tasks that have also shown performance benefits associated with wheel running. For example, in the passive avoidance task animals are placed into an apparatus with two chambers, one light and one dark. The animal follows their natural tendency to enter into the dark chamber, but receives a foot shock when entering. Therefore, the rodent learns to suppress the natural tendency to enter into the dark chamber. In young animals, Alaie *et al.* (2006) reported that exercise reduced the amount of time spent in the dark chamber and that retention remained higher than controls for at least one week. Performance on this task is also enhanced in aged running animals. For example, Samorajski *et al.* (1985) reported that middle-aged and older-aged exercising animals performed better than age-matched sedentary controls, and that the effect size was larger for older animals than younger animals. This intriguing finding is some of the only evidence indicating that the benefits of exercise may be greater in aged animals than younger animals.

Models of neurological disease have also reported behavioral benefits of exercise. For example, Parkinson's disease is characterized by dopamine loss in the nigrostriatal pathway and motor and cognitive impairments. In an animal model of Parkinson's disease, injection of 6-hydroxydopamine (6-OHDA), a dopamine toxin, is used to produce nigrostriatal impairments and behavioral and dopamine loss. Using this model, Tillerson *et al.* (2003) reported that 10 days of post-lesion treadmill exercise significantly reduced behavioral loss on a variety of motor tasks. In addition, aged mice who were injected with 6-OHDA and then underwent treadmill running showed behavioral sparing although they showed only moderate dopamine sparing. These effects suggest that exercise may be an effective strategy at reducing neurochemical and motor losses due to Parkinson's disease (however, see Poulton & Muir, 2005).

Alzheimer's disease, a progressive neurodegenerative disease, characterized by loss of neurons in the hippocampus, memory impairments and increases in amyloid plaques, may also be affected by exercise. One study demonstrated in a mouse model of Alzheimer's disease that 5 months of voluntary exercise reduced amyloid plaque formation and spared behavioral deficits on the Morris water maze (Adlard *et al.*, 2005). In addition, a mouse model of Huntington's disease, a disease caused by a genetic mutation and characterized by progressive motor deficits, cognitive deficits and psychiatric problems, showed positive effects of exercise. Pang *et al.* (2006) demonstrated that Huntington's mice showed deficits in T-maze and Y-maze performance, and deficits in motor coordination. However, mice that underwent 10 weeks of voluntary wheel running showed improvements on both maze tasks, indicating that exercise reliably offset the cognitive impairments due to Huntington's disease. Exercise, however, did not affect motor coordination impairments.

Summary

Wheel running in animals has been shown to offset cognitive declines associated with aging as well as spare cognitive and motor deficits in models of Parkinson's, Alzheimer's and Huntington's disease.

These cognitive and behavioral improvements with exercise have been related to exercise-induced increases in angiogenesis and neurogenesis.

Angiogenesis

Black *et al.* (1990) were the first to show that exercise promoted angiogenesis, or the growth of new vasculature, in the brain. In their study, rats were exposed to an acrobatic condition with high motor learning demands, a forced aerobic exercise condition (wheel running), a voluntary aerobic exercise condition, or an inactive control group. Using stereological estimates and camera lucida drawings, the researchers reported that motor learning in the acrobatic condition caused synaptogenesis, or the development of new synapses, whereas, both forced and voluntary exercise produced new vasculature in the cerebellum. These results indicate that motor learning and aerobic exercise produced differential effects on the brain.

New vasculature due to exercise has also been reported in the motor cortex. Kleim *et al.* (2002) demonstrated that 30 days of voluntary exercise resulted in angiogenesis in the forelimb motor cortex compared with sedentary controls. In addition, Swain *et al.* (2003) demonstrated through functional magnetic resonance imaging in rats that 30 days of voluntary exercise resulted in angiogenesis and increased capillary perfusion, or blood volume, in the primary motor cortex. Furthermore, Swain *et al.* (2003) found that resting cerebral blood flow was unaffected by exercise and that blood flow was only increased under high CO_2 demands, suggesting that exercise increases the size of the capillary reserve in the motor cortex.

There is also evidence that exercise can induce angiogenesis in the striatum and frontoparietal cortex in a rat model of stroke. In this model, intraluminal filaments are inserted into the middle cerebral artery in rats, effectively causing a neurological infarct and behavioral deficits similar to the losses seen in stroke patients. Research has found that treadmill exercise before stroke-induction reliably reduces the volume of brain damage caused by the stroke (Ding *et al.*, 2004a; Johansson & Ohlsson, 1996; Stummer *et al.*, 1994, 1995) and reduces mortality rates resulting from stroke (Stummer *et al.*, 1994). It has also been shown that pre-ischemic exercise provided neuroprotection up to 3 weeks post-ischemia with a concomitant increase in new vasculature (Ding *et al.*, 2004b). Importantly, this increase in micro-vessels in the striatum and cortex was paralleled by an increase in mRNA for vascular endothelial growth factor (VEGF) and angiopoietin (Ang), two prominent growth factors involved in the development and growth of new vessels. The authors argued that the induction of angiogenesis by exercise might be one method to reduce brain damage due to stroke.

A recent study has also demonstrated that the induction of angiogenesis by exercise may be dependent on the presence of insulin-like growth factor I (IGF-1), an important growth factor induced by exercise and involved in cognition and neuron proliferation. In this study, Lopez-Lopez *et al.* (2004) found that exercising mice displayed angiogenesis in the cerebellum and hippocampus but mice with low serum levels of IGF-1 failed to induce angiogenesis. They also reported that systemic injection of IGF-1 effectively induced angiogenesis. In cultured tissue, the authors reported that IGF-1 induces the growth of endothelial cells by up regulating VEGF and hypoxia-inducible factor 1α (HIF-1α), two molecular factors involved in vessel growth. Furthermore, they reported that mice with cortical lesions showed increased IGF-1, HIF-1α and VEGF levels around the site of the lesion with a parallel increase in new vasculature. Importantly, blocking IGF-1 also effectively blocked the increase in HIF-1α and VEGF, resulting in an inhibition of angiogenesis around the site of the lesion. Therefore, the authors claim that IGF-1 is an essential component of angiogenesis as a result of enrichment or physical exercise in both normal and brain damaged populations.

Summary

Animal studies have shown that exercise effectively induces angiogenesis in several brain areas. The increase in new vasculature has been related to increased metabolic demands (Isaacs *et al.*, 1992; McCloskey *et al.*, 2001) and increased blood flow (Swain *et al.*, 2003). Induction of new blood vessels is paralleled by increases in growth factors such as VEGF, Ang and HIF-1α, while IGF-1 may be essential for angiogenesis and upregulation of VEGF and HIF-1α in normal and brain-injured mice. Interestingly, both VEGF and IGF-1 have also been related to exercise-induced neuron proliferation. It is possible that one function of angiogenesis is to provide the brain with more nutrients and trophic factors that are necessary for neuroprotection, learning and memory, and cell proliferation.

Neurogenesis

Besides improving cognitive performance, motor performance, and inducing angiogenesis, exercise has been shown to promote neurogenesis, or the development of new neurons, as well as increasing overall cell survival. Van Praag *et al.* (1999a) were the first to show that voluntary exercise increases neurogenesis and cell survival in the hippocampus of mice. In this study, mice were assigned to either a running condition, or one of a few control conditions. The researchers measured cellular proliferation by the injection of bromodeoxyuridine (BrdU), a marker that labels dividing cells. van Praag *et al.* (1999a) found that mice in the running condition showed a doubling of surviving new-born cells and enhanced cell survival. Importantly, cell proliferation in the dentate gyrus of running mice was related to improved performance on the Morris water maze and enhancement of long-term potentiation (LTP), a cellular model of learning and memory (van Praag *et al.*, 1999b). Since the publication of these seminal studies, there have been numerous replications of exercise-induced neurogenesis in the dentate gyrus (Brown *et al.*, 2003; Carro *et al.*, 2000; Eadie *et al.* 2005; Fabel *et al.*, 2003; Rhodes *et al.*, 2003; Trejo *et al.* 2001).

Although hippocampal neurogenesis has been shown to occur throughout adulthood, it is diminished with increasing age (Heine *et al.*, 2004). In addition, a number of neuropathological conditions (e.g., Alzheimer's disease) are related to a loss of cells in the hippocampus. Therefore, it is important to find methods by which neuron proliferation may be enhanced in aged cohorts. In order to examine whether 45 days of voluntary exercise could increase neurogenesis in aged mice, van Praag *et al.* (2005) labeled cells in young and old runners and age-matched sedentary controls with BrdU. The authors reported that wheel running reversed the normal decline in neurogenesis in aged animals and that this was accompanied by improvements in Morris water maze performance. However, they reported that there still remained greater neurogenesis in sedentary young mice than in active aged mice and that aged exercising mice failed to show angiogenesis. In addition, Kronenberg *et al.* (2006) found that 32 days of voluntary exercise reliably prevented age-related declines in precursor cell activity in the dentate gyrus of mice and enhanced cell proliferation, but failed to maintain neurogenesis at the younger aged level. The sum of these results suggests a complex relationship between neurogenesis and exercise in aging populations and argues that short-term exercise may not completely reverse the loss exhibited in older populations.

A number of molecular factors are affected by exercise and have been shown to contribute to neurogenesis in both young and aged animals. For example, administration of IGF-1 induces neurogenesis in the dentate gyrus of young (Anderson *et al.*, 2002) and old animals (Lichtenwalner *et al.*, 2001). In addition, IGF-1 levels are reduced in some neuropathologies such as Alzheimer's (Watanabe *et al.*, 2005) as well as in normal aging (Anderson *et al.*, 2002). In an important set of studies in young animals, Carro *et al.* (2000) and Trejo *et al.* (2001) reported that circulating IGF-1 mediates the positive effects of exercise on the brain and, by blocking IGF-1 influx, exercise-induced neurogenesis was inhibited. Therefore, exercise may be critical in inducing IGF-1 in order to maintain or enhance cell proliferation and may be a potentially important molecule to assess in treatments of neuropathological disease.

Interestingly, as discussed earlier, IGF-1 also promotes angiogenesis in the brain and is a moderator of VEGF. However, VEGF also has cell proliferation properties. In a study examining the effects of exercise-induced VEGF on neurogenesis, Fabel et al. (2003) demonstrated that circulating levels of VEGF were related to exercise-induced neurogenesis in the dentate gyrus, and that by blocking the influx of VEGF into the brain, exercise-induced neurogenesis was abolished. However, blocking VEGF did not affect baseline levels of neurogenesis. This study suggests that VEGF may not be essential in maintaining baseline levels of cell proliferation, but it may be necessary for increased neuron division and development as a result of exercise or environmental enrichment, or treatments that have higher metabolic and cerebral blood flow demands on the brain. However, the way in which VEGF is related to exercise-induced alterations in angiogenesis and other factors such as IGF-1 has yet to be elucidated.

Summary

Exercise has been shown to effectively induce neurogenesis in the dentate gyrus of the hippocampus in both young and aged animals. This effect is accompanied by enhanced spatial learning and memory performance as well as enhanced LTP. Although there is evidence for individual variation in the effects of exercise on neurogenesis (Llorens-Martín et al., 2006), the research conducted thus far provides promising results for pathologies displaying neuronal death. Furthermore, cellular proliferation resulting from exercise is related to levels of circulating growth factors such as VEGF and IGF-1. Additionally, some neurotrophic factors are affected by exercise and are considered to be critically involved in neuroprotection and enhanced learning and memory.

Neurotrophic factors

As has been already discussed, exercise upregulates mRNA and protein levels of certain growth factors that are related to increased angiogenesis and neurogenesis. However, exercise also upregulates other molecules including brain-derived neurotrophic factor (BDNF); BDNF has been shown to be neuroprotective and to promote cell survival, neurite growth and synaptic plasticity (Cotman & Berchtold, 2002; Lu et al., 2005). In an important study by Pang et al. (2004), BDNF was found to be necessary for the elicitation of LTP. They demonstrated that heterozygous BDNF mice showed diminished LTP compared with wild-type mice, and by either blocking the cleavage of BDNF or blocking the binding of BDNF to its tyrosine kinase receptor (TrkB), LTP was effectively eradicated. However, administration of BDNF in vitro rescued the loss of LTP. Other studies have also shown BDNF involvement in neuronal growth and cell proliferation. For example, Mohapel et al. (2005) directly administered BDNF into the striatum of rats with 6-OHDA lesions and using BrdU labeling found that BDNF increased cell proliferation and cell survival in the area of the lesion. Ventricular infusion of BDNF has also been shown to produce neurogenesis in the olfactory bulb (Zigova et al., 1998), while blocking BDNF activity reliably reduced granule cell proliferation (Katoh-Semba et al., 2002). Therefore, BDNF has been shown to be extensively involved in electrophysiological properties of the brain that translate into learning and memory performance as well as neuroprotection, cell proliferation and brain repair.

In a set of early studies, Neeper et al. (1995, 1996) found that voluntary exercise increased mRNA levels of BDNF in the hippocampus and caudal cerebral cortex while transiently increasing levels in the cerebellum and frontal cortex. This effect of exercise on BDNF mRNA and protein has been found extensively in young animals (Berchtold et al., 2001, 2002; Farmer et al., 2004; Gómez-Pinilla et al., 2002; Russo-Neustadt et al., 2001; Vaynman et al., 2004). Importantly, exercise also increases mRNA levels for the TrkB receptor, a high affinity receptor for mature BDNF (e.g., Gómez-Pinilla et al., 2002; Klintsova et al., 2004; Vaynman et al., 2003). In addition, an important study linked BDNF with cognitive benefits of exercise (Vaynman et al., 2004). In this study, the researchers blocked the binding of

BDNF with the TrkB receptor and found that benefits of exercise on the Morris water maze were abolished. Furthermore, the authors reported that those animals displaying the greatest BDNF induction also showed the fastest learning rates, thereby providing an important correlation between BDNF, exercise and learning.

Due to its protective and proliferative properties, BDNF has been suggested to be a key candidate for protecting the brain from disease or damage. Interestingly, patients with Alzheimer's (Murer et al., 2001), Parkinson's (Murer et al., 2001), and Huntington's (Ginés et al., 2006) disease show reduced levels of BDNF and TrkB expression. Although one study failed to find altered exercise-induced BDNF increase in Huntington's mice, BDNF resulting from an exercise regimen has been shown to provide protection against dopamine loss in the nigrostriatal pathway in Parkinson's models (Mohapel et al., 2005). In addition, although there is converging evidence for exercise and BDNF influencing the trajectory of Alzheimer's disease (Adlard et al., 2005; Berchtold et al., 2002), there is no direct evidence that BDNF rescues the cognitive or neural deficits from this disease.

However, a greater number of studies have examined whether BDNF is related to age-related alterations in brain morphology, chemistry and behavior. Many of these studies fail to show age-related reductions in BDNF concentrations (e.g., Silhol et al., 2005). However, it has been found that senescent rats that performed poorly on a learning and memory task had lower levels of BDNF in the hippocampus than age-matched animals that performed well (Schaaf et al., 2001). It is possible that in normal functioning aged animals BDNF levels remain relatively stable, and only when BDNF levels decrease are pathological disturbances detectable. However, aged rats retain the ability to respond to exercise and display alterations in BDNF expression after only one week of exercise (Adlard et al., 2005; Garza et al., 2004). Since reductions in BDNF levels are not dramatically different in aged populations, it is possible that other molecules related to BDNF signaling are affected. For example, there is

evidence that the expression of the TrkB receptor decreases with advancing age (Silhol et al., 2005) suggesting that aging and cognitive deficits may be more attributable to reduced receptor concentration rather than production or secretion of BDNF. However, a study examining whether exercise could rescue depleting levels of TrkB in aged animals has yet to be conducted. In any case, it is plausible that exercise may ameliorate neural and cognitive losses in aged and pathological populations by upregulating expression of BDNF and/or its receptor.

Summary

Brain-derived neurotrophic factor and the TrkB receptor are upregulated with exercise and have been found to influence learning and memory and LTP and are considered to be instrumental in neuroprotection, cell survival, proliferation and brain regeneration and repair. Brain-derived neurotrophic factor and its primary receptor, TrkB, are affected in aging and certain pathologies, and exercise-induced alterations in BDNF or TrkB may prove to be an important method to alter age-related cognitive and neural disturbances.

Observational studies of the relationship between exercise and cognition

- Epidemiological studies provide an opportunity to examine the strength and potential relationship of different variables that might impact cognition. The length of follow-up varies in the different studies; there are a few with longer delays between initial assessment of lifestyle factors and the impact on cognition.
- The studies do imply a beneficial effect of exercise on the presence or severity of subsequent dementia. The relevance of genetic differences has not yet been firmly established.
- Many of these epidemiological studies used self-report. Objective indices are important addenda, and there are not always strong correlations between self-reports and the objective measures.

- The small number of observational studies over much longer time periods have the advantage of controlling for potential undiagnosed disorders that reveal themselves later, and provide an opportunity to truly examine the impact of early levels of physical activity on later cognition.
- Overall, although the observational and epidemiological research suggests a strong relationship between physical activity and later cognitive function that can span several decades, much research needs to be completed with better control and measurement.

Observational studies

A study by Albert and colleagues (1995) typifies the approach of many epidemiological studies that have examined lifestyle choices and other factors which are correlated with successful aging. A set of 22 demographic, physical, psychosocial and cognitive variables were collected from 1192 seventy- to seventy-nine-year-old adults and then 2–2.5 years later cognition was assessed again. The main question under investigation was the extent to which different variables could account for cognitive change over time. A structural equation modeling analysis revealed that four variables accounted for a significant amount of variance in cognitive change in this population – education, strenuous activity, peak pulmonary expiratory flow rate and self efficacy. Strenuous activity was assessed via self-reports of current energy expended in daily activities around the house while peak pulmonary expiratory flow rate was measured with a spirometer. Cognition was measured with a battery of tasks which took approximately 30 minutes to complete and included tests of language, verbal memory, nonverbal memory, conceptualization and visuospatial ability.

Based upon the findings from Albert *et al.* and other similar studies, a number of research groups have further explored the relationship between exercise and physical activity and cognition and dementia. The time course of many of these studies

is relatively short, ranging from 2 to 8 years. However, a small set of prospective and retrospective observational studies have examined much longer delays between initial assessment of lifestyle factors and cognition of older adults. With regard to assessing the effects of physical activity and exercise most of the epidemiological studies have employed self-report instruments of activity.

Larson *et al.* (2006) conducted a study in which 1740 men and women over the age of 65 without cognitive impairment were asked to report the number of times per week that they performed different physical activities (i.e., walking, hiking, bicycling, aerobics or calisthenics, swimming, water aerobics or weight training) for at least 15 minutes per time over the past year. A number of potential confounding factors including self-reported health, a variety of medical conditions, lifestyle factors such as smoking and drinking, and demographic factors were also recorded at the initial assessment. An assessment of genetic risk for Alzheimer's (one or more e4 alleles on the *apoe* gene) was also conducted at this time. After an average follow-up period of 6.2 years 158 individuals had developed Alzheimer's dementia. Following adjustment for the covariates obtained at the initial assessment the incidence rate for Alzheimer's was significantly higher for individuals who exercised fewer than three times per week (19.7 per 1000 person years) as compared to those who exercised more than three times per week (13.0 per 1000 person years). These results were not influenced by a genetic predisposition for Alzheimer's (i.e., one or more e4 alleles on the *apoe* gene). However, the risk reduction for Alzheimer's disease was greater for those participants who initially had the poorest physical performance (e.g., on tests such as a 10-foot timed walk which is considered to be a measure of functional fitness).

Other studies have reported similar effects of exercise on cognition and dementia. Podewils *et al.* (2005) studied the relationship between physical activity and dementia in 3375 men and women over the course of 5.4 years. Physical activity in these individuals over the age of 65 was assessed via the Minnesota Leisure Time questionnaire in which participants are asked about the frequency and duration of 15 types of physical activities over the past 2 weeks. Like the Larson *et al.* study this study found an inverse relationship between Alzheimer's disease and the estimated energy expenditure and number of physical activities performed by the participants. However, unlike the Larson *et al.* study, the present study only found a significant relationship between physical activities and Alzheimer's for the e4 noncarriers, or those people with less of a genetic risk for developing Alzheimer's disease.

Studies have also found an inverse relationship between activity levels and cognitive decline within the normal range of functioning. For example, Yaffe *et al.* (2001) examined 5925 women over 65 years of age over the course of a 6- to 8-year period. They found an inverse relationship between the number of blocks walked per week and energy expended and cognitive decline as assessed by performance on a general test of cognitive function, the Mini Mental State Examination, indicating that cognitive performance increased with increasing levels of reported activity. As part of the Nurses health study, Weuve and colleagues (2004) examined whether physical activity could predict cognitive change across a 2-year period in a cohort of 16 466 women over 70 years of age. A variety of cognitive processes were evaluated in a telephone interview. Extensive health, prescription drug and demographic data were also obtained. Finally, the women were asked to estimate the amount of time per week during the past year that they spent on the activities such as running, jogging, walking or hiking outdoors, racquet sports, lap swimming, bicycling and aerobic dance. The women were also asked to estimate their walking pace in minutes per mile. For purposes of analysis women were divided into quintiles on the basis of the energy that they expended on the set of assessed activities. A significant relationship between energy expended and cognition, across a large set of cognitive measures, was observed and this relationship remained significant after adjusting for medical conditions, prescription

drugs and possessing an e4 allele on the *apoe* gene. Indeed, even for women who did not participate in vigorous activity, those in the highest two quintiles of walking displayed higher cognitive function than women who walked slower or less frequently. Additional analyses also concluded that physical activity levels were not influenced by cognitive or physical disability. Physical activity reports obtained from a subset of the participants ($n = 7907$) when they were younger (i.e., when they were less than 62 years of age) still showed a positive relationship between physical activity and cognition 10 years later.

The studies described thus far have relied on subjective reports of activity and exercise. Although such a procedure is understandable when large populations of subjects are tested, a prospective study by Barnes *et al.* (2003) included both self-report of physical activity and objective (i.e., VO_2 peak) measures of cardiorespiratory fitness in a 6-year study of 349 individuals over the age of 55. Interestingly, whereas a significant inverse relationship was observed for the objective fitness measures and cognitive decline, this was not the case for the self-report activity measures. Although the explanation for this dissociation cannot be unequivocally discerned in these data it is conceivable that it is the aerobic nature of the physical activities, the measures more reliably indexed by the objective than self-report measures, that are more strongly related to spared cognition than nonaerobic activities.

Temporally extended observational studies

A small set of observational studies have examined the relationship between physical activities and cognitive decline or dementia over much more extended time periods. Such studies have several advantages. First, they reduce the likelihood that subjects have undiagnosed dementias or other medical conditions at initial assessment. Second, they enable the determination of whether levels of physical activity earlier in the lifespan have implications for cognition and dementia in later life.

Dik *et al.* (2003) conducted a retrospective study in which they asked 1241 sixty-two- to eighty-five-year-old men and women about their physical activities from 15–25 years of age. Men, but not women, who were active at low or moderate levels when they were young displayed faster processing speed later in life. This relationship was significant after adjustments for a number of lifestyle and demographic characteristics. Interestingly, the most active men did not show cognitive benefits. The authors speculate that this could be due to the fact that high levels of activity for these men were work related and therefore less likely to be aerobic than leisure activities. The failure to find a significant relationship between physical activity and processing speed for women could have been the result of lower intensity activities pursued by women in this cohort.

An examination of the association between leisure time physical activity at midlife and dementia between the ages of 65 and 79 was conducted by Rovio *et al.* (2005). Leisure time physical activity at midlife at least twice a week was associated with a reduced risk of dementia. Interestingly, the association between physical activity and dementia was stronger for *apoe* e4 carriers, that is, those people with the highest genetic risk for developing Alzheimer's.

Finally, Richards *et al.* (2003) examined the influence of self-reported physical exercise and leisure time activities (e.g., playing chess, bridge, going to theatre, playing a musical instrument, etc.) at 36 years of age on memory at 43 years of age as well as memory change from 43 to 53 years of age in a cohort of 1919 males and females. Interestingly, IQ scores were available for these individuals at 15 years of age. This enabled the investigators to control for sex, education and social class as well as cognition at 15 years of age in their examination of exercise and leisure activities on memory performance. Analyses indicated that engagement in physical exercise and other leisure time activities at 36 years of age was associated with higher memory scores at 43. Physical activity at 36 was associated with slower rate of memory decline from 43 to 53 years of age after adjusting for spare time activity and other variables. Interestingly, change in physical activity from 36 to 43 years of age reduced the

relationship between physical activity at 36 and memory change from 43 to 53 years of age. These data suggest little memory protection for those who stopped exercise after 36, but protection for those individuals who began exercise after this time. Other leisure time activity was not associated with change in memory over this interval.

Summary

The studies reviewed above suggest a significant, and sometimes substantial relationship between physical activity and later cognitive function and dementia. Indeed, there is some evidence that this relationship can span several decades. However, it is important to note that other studies (Verghese *et al.*, 2003; Wilson *et al.*, 2002; Yamada *et al.*, 2003) have failed to find such relationships. Clearly, there are many reasons why inconsistent associations might be observed across studies including: the collection of only self-report activity and exercise data, the failure to distinguish between aerobic and nonaerobic activities, the failure to assess duration, intensity and frequency of physical activities, the difficulty of eliminating participants with subclinical signs of dementia, the age of participants at initial and final assessment, and the power of the study to detect significant relationships. The moderating influence of genetic factors on fitness effects on cognition is also intriguing but at present these results are inconsistent for the *apoe* gene. Clearly, additional studies will be necessary which address these issues and also incorporate additional genetic markers which target genes related to particular neurotransmitter system functions and those with neurotrophic effects.

Cross-sectional and longitudinal studies of exercise effects on human cognition and brain structure and function

- Cross-sectional research strongly supports the relationship between fitness and cognition, however, the cross-sectional nature of the studies complicates interpretation.

- Some studies have used randomized longitudinal exercise interventions. In general, these not only support the positive relationship, but suggest that the greatest positive impact is on "executive" functions, those often considered most sensitive to the effects of aging.

- Structural and functional MRI has the potential to examine if exercise has any impact on human brain structure or function. The initial data suggest that exercise does change both structure and function, although the mechanism can only be inferred in these human studies.

Cross-sectional studies

The systematic examination of the relationship between fitness and cognition dates back several decades to the pioneering research of Spirduso and colleagues. For example, in a classic study Spirduso & Clifford (1978) compared young and old racquet sportsmen, runners and sedentary individuals on simple reaction time, choice reaction time and movement time tasks. The older (>60 years of age) athletes' performance on these tasks was substantially better than the older sedentary adults, and indeed was similar to performance exhibited by the young (18–25 years of age) sedentary adults. Other cross-sectional studies have reported similar benefits of exercise on both peripheral and central components of reaction time (Baylor & Spirduso, 1988; Stones & Kozma, 1989) as well as for reasoning, working memory, Stroop, Trails-B, Symbol digit, vigilance and fluid intelligence tests (Abourezk & Toole, 1995; Bunce et al., 1996; Clarkson-Smith & Hartley, 1989; Dustman et al., 1994).

Other cross-sectional studies have examined the relationship between fitness and human brain function and structure. For example, Dustman et al. (1990) examined electroencephalographic activity (EEG), event-related brain potentials (ERP) and behavioral measures of cognition in older and younger adults who differed in fitness level. The latency of some ERP components were shorter in high- than low-fit participants and these differences in latency were exaggerated as a function of adult age for the P300. More recently, Hillman et al. (2006) reported faster P300 latencies for high-fit than for low-fit young and older adults in a task-switching paradigm when subjects were required to switch between two different tasks but not when they performed the same task repeatedly. Such data suggest more rapid information processing particularly in more challenging tasks, for high-fit individuals (see also Bashore & Goddard, 1993).

In a cross-sectional examination of 55 older adults, Colcombe & Kramer (2003) found that, consistent with previous findings, age-related losses in gray and white matter tended to be greatest in the frontal, prefrontal and temporal regions (e.g., O'Sullivan et al., 2001; Raz, 2000). Moreover, consistent with predictions derived from the human and animal literatures, there was a significant reduction of declines in these areas as a function of aerobic fitness. That is, older adults who had better aerobic fitness also tended to retain more tissue in the frontal, parietal and temporal cortices as a function of age. Subsequent analyses, factoring out other potential confounding factors such as hypertension, hormone replacement therapy, caffeine, tobacco and alcohol consumption, confirmed that none of these other variables moderated the effect of aerobic fitness.

Longitudinal studies

Although the studies described above suggest an association between fitness and cognition, the cross-sectional nature of these studies, however, complicates their interpretation. Thus, the positive effects of fitness on perceptual, cognitive and motor processes may reflect a predisposition of the participants towards fast and accurate responding rather than a benefit of aerobic fitness achieved through exercise. A number of researchers have at least partially circumvented the problem of self-selection by employing randomized longitudinal exercise interventions. For example, Dustman et al. (1984) randomized 43 healthy but sedentary 55- to 70-year-olds to three different groups; an aerobic training group who participated in three 1-hour sessions per week for 4 months of walking and slow jogging, an exercise control group who participated in strength and flexibility exercises on the same time schedule as the aerobic training group, and a nonexercise control group. Not surprisingly the aerobic training group showed substantially larger gains in aerobic fitness, as measured in a graded treadmill test, than the other two groups. The aerobic group also showed significant improvements, across the 4-month intervention period, in a variety of different processing speed, inhibitory control and memory tests. This was not the case for the two control groups.

Although the data from the Dustman *et al.* (1994) study are promising in demonstrating a causal link between fitness training and cognition, the data obtained from other longitudinal studies have been more equivocal (see Dustman *et al.*, 1994; Etnier *et al.*, 1997 for reviews of this literature). Clearly, there have been some notable successes in that aerobically trained individuals have outperformed nonaerobic control subjects on a variety of cognitive tasks. On the other hand, other intervention studies have failed to observe such benefits to performance.

In an effort to determine whether a reliable relationship between fitness training and cognition could be observed across the extant literature, Colcombe & Kramer (2003) conducted a meta-analysis on all of the accessible randomised aerobic fitness training studies with control groups, published between 1966 and 2001. The central question examined in the analysis was whether, across the 18 intervention studies in the analysis, fitness training had a positive influence on cognition. The answer was affirmative. A moderate effect size (0.48) for fitness training was obtained in the analysis. Additional analyses examined whether there were significant moderators of the relationship between fitness and cognition. Several significant moderators were revealed. First, although fitness training broadly influenced a variety of cognitive processes, the largest positive effects were observed for executive control processes. Executive control processes include components

of cognition such as planning, scheduling, working memory, inhibitory processes and multi-tasking. Interestingly, these are many of the processes that show substantial age-related decline (Daniels *et al.*, 2006). Second, effects of fitness training were larger when programs of aerobic training were combined with strength and flexibility training. Combinations of different treatment protocols may engender both more varied brain changes (e.g., Black *et al.*, 1990) and serve to further reduce age-associated cardiovascular and muscular skeletal disorders. Third, and perhaps most interestingly, studies that included more women showed larger fitness training benefits than studies with fewer women.

Brain structure and function

Although there is a substantial body of literature which has examined fitness training effects on cognition, thus far there have been very few intervention studies which have examined the influence of fitness training on human brain function or structure. Colcombe and colleagues (2004) randomly assigned older adults to participate in either a walking group, or a stretching and toning control group for a 6-month period. The walking group were continuously monitored by a trained exercise coordinator and walked 3 times a week for 45-minute periods. The control group received the same contact with an exercise coordinator, but instead of participating in a walking regimen, this group participated in nonaerobic stretching and toning exercises 3 times a week for 45-minute periods. All participants performed a focused attention task during an event-related functional magnetic resonance imaging protocol. This task requires participants to focus on a single, central object while ignoring irrelevant distractor objects that flank the target item. Older adults who participated in the walking protocol were better able to ignore the misleading flanking items, but the control older adults were not. Importantly, aerobically trained older adults, but not controls, showed increased activity in the frontal and parietal regions of the brain that are thought to be involved in efficient attentional control and performance on this task, and reduced activity in the dorsal region of the anterior cingulate cortex, a region thought to be sensitive to behavioral conflict, or the need for increased cognitive control.

Kramer and colleagues (2006) used a semi-automated image segmentation technique on high-resolution magnetic resonance imaging data to assess longitudinal changes in the brain structure of older adults who were randomly assigned to participate in either a 6-month aerobic training program, or a nonaerobic control group. This technique provides a means to estimate tissue atrophy on a point-by-point fashion throughout the brain with reasonably high spatial resolution. This allows for regionally specific conclusions about the variables of interest on changes in brain matter. Kramer and colleagues found that older adults who participated in the aerobic training group showed a significant increase in gray matter volume in regions of the frontal and superior temporal lobe, compared with controls. These results suggest that even relatively short exercise interventions can begin to restore some of the losses in brain volume associated with normal aging. However, it should be noted that the limitations of the semi-automated segmentation technique do not allow one to infer precisely what mechanism results in these changes (e.g., increase in cell body size, increased dendritic connections, increased capillary bed volume, increased glial size or number, etc.).

Summary

The human cross-sectional and intervention studies tentatively suggest a moderate relationship between fitness training and improved cognition, brain function and structure. However, additional intervention studies are clearly needed to further examine the relationship between different fitness training protocols and aspects of cognition, brain function and structure, preferably over much more extended time periods than have been previously examined.

Future directions

- The review has indicated that exercise training can have beneficial impact on cognitive functioning throughout the lifespan. However, there are many unanswered questions.
- Future research should continue to address the potential of different factors that might play a role in the relationship between exercise and cognition, such as the type and frequency of exercise, and the importance of individual differences such as age and gender.
- A very important avenue of future research is to examine the potential interplay between different techniques that have been hypothesized to be beneficial, such as diet, exercise, social interaction and intellectual engagement.

The studies that we have examined in our relatively brief review suggest that fitness training can serve an important function in maintaining and enhancing cognitive and brain vitality throughout the adult lifespan. The animal studies have begun to provide important preliminary information concerning the molecular and cellular mechanisms which underlie fitness effects on learning and cognition. Clearly physical activity has a variety of positive morphological and neurochemical effects on the brain that serves both to maintain the performance of older organisms and to protect against age-associated disease.

There are, however, many unanswered questions with regard to the relationship between physical activity, aging, cognition and the brain. For example, although some studies have found a monotonic relationship between activity level and variables such as BDNF (Neeper *et al.*, 1995) other studies have found that high levels of activity can result in increased neuronal loss in response to excitotoxic insult relative to sedentary controls (Ramsden *et al.*, 2003). Human studies have also found variable relationships between fitness level induced by training and the magnitude of cognitive benefits (Colcombe & Kramer, 2003; Etnier *et al.*, 1997). Additional research is necessary to determine the intensity, frequency and type of physical activity that has the most beneficial influence on cognition and the brain. Furthermore, individual differences in age, health, gender and genotype may be important moderators of the fitness–cognition (and brain) relationship.

A number of studies have also begun to examine potential interactive effects of different interventions (or lifestyle choices) on successful cognitive aging. For example, in a study of aging beagles, Milgram *et al.* (2005) found that a combined treatment of enhanced diet and behavioral enrichment had a larger positive influence on learning new skills than either of the treatments in isolation. In a similar vein, Stranahan *et al.* (2006) reported that isolated housing (social isolation) reduced the positive benefits of wheel running on adult neurogenesis in the hippocampus of rats. Molteni *et al.* (2004) have reported that exercise reversed the decrease in BDNF associated with high-fat diets in rats. These fascinating results raise the question of the underlying mechanisms which influence lifestyle interactions as well as the developmental time course of such effects.

To our knowledge there have been only two published studies that have contrasted the separate and joint effects of cognitive and fitness training on performance-based metrics of selective aspects of cognition, and these studies have come to opposite conclusions with regard to whether the effects of these two training modes are additive or interactive (Fabre *et al.*, 1999, 2002). There have also been a small number of multimodal human interventions. For example, Small and colleagues (2006) reported that a group of middle-aged individuals who participated in a 2-week intervention that combined modifications of diet and exercise as well as training in mnemonics and stress reduction showed larger improvements in verbal fluency and activation of dorsolateral prefrontal cortex than control participants. Rebok (2006) reported that older adults who participated in the Experience Corps project, which entailed providing literacy, numeracy, library and other support in kindergarten through 3rd grade in inner city schools for the period of an academic year, enhanced aspects of executive control and

brain function, as indexed in fMRI, in the study participants but not in control subjects. Although the design of these multimodal intervention studies precludes the decomposition of cognitive benefits attributable to specific aspects of the intervention, the results do suggest that follow-up studies are warranted.

Summary

The research reviewed in this chapter describes our current state of knowledge concerning the relationship between fitness training and cognition/ brain. Although more intervention research is needed, in both human and animal studies, to further address questions related to the mechanisms and boundary conditions of exercise effects, the present state of knowledge is sufficient to recommend physical activity and exercise as a means to maintain and enhance cognition throughout the lifespan.

ACKNOWLEDGMENTS

Preparation of this manuscript was supported by research grants R37 AG25667 and RO1 AG25032 from the National Institute of Aging and support from the Institute for the Study of Aging.

REFERENCES

Abourezk, T., & Toole, T. (1995). Effect of task complexity on the relationship between physical fitness and reaction time in older women *Journal of Aging and Physical Activity*, **3**, 251–260.

Adlard, P. A., Perreau, V. M., Engesser-Cesar, C., & Cotman, C. W. (2004). The time course of induction of brain-derived neurotrophic factor mRNA and protein in the rat hippocampus following voluntary exercise. *Neuroscience Letters*, **363**, 43–48.

Adlard, P. A., Perreau, V. M., & Cotman, C. W. (2005). The exercise-induced expression of BDNF within the hippocampus varies across life-span. *Neurobiology of Aging*, **26**, 511–520.

Alaie, H., Borjeian, L., Azizi, M. *et al.* (2006). Treadmill running reverses retention deficit induced by morphine. *European Journal of Pharmacology*, **536**, 138–141.

Albeck, D. S., Sano, K., Prewitt, G. E., & Dalton, L. (2006). Mild forced treadmill exercise enhances spatial learning in the aged rat. *Behavioural Brain Research*, **168**, 345–348.

Albert, M. S., Jones, K., Savage, C. R. *et al.* (1995). Predictors of cognitive change in older persons: MacArthur studies of successful aging. *Psychology and Aging*, **10**, 578–589.

Anderson, B. J., Rapp, D. N., Baek, D. H. *et al.* (2000). Exercise influences spatial learning in the radial arm maze. *Physiology and Behavior*, **70**, 425–429.

Anderson, M. F., Åberg, M. A. I., Nilsson, M., & Eriksson, P. S. (2002). Insulin-like growth factor-I and neurogenesis in the adult mammalian brain. *Developmental Brain Research*, **134**, 115–122.

Barnes, D. E., Yaffe, K., Satariano, W. A., & Tager, I. B. (2003). A longitudinal study of cardiorespiratory fitness and cognitive function in healthy older adults. *Journal of the American Geriatrics Society*, **51**, 459–465.

Bashore, T. R., & Goddard, P. H. (1993). Preservative and restorative effects of aerobic fitness on the age-related slowing of mental processing speed. In J. Cerella, J. M. Rybash, & W. Hoyer (Eds.), *Adult Information Processing: Limits on Loss* (pp. 205–228). San Diego, CA: Academic Press.

Baylor, A. M., & Spirduso, W. W. (1988). Systematic aerobic exercise and components of reaction time in older women. *Journals of Gerontology; Series B; Psychological Sciences and Social Sciences*, **43**, 121–126.

Berchtold, N. C., Kesslak, J. P., Pike, C. J., Adlard, P. A., & Cotman, C. W. (2001). Estrogen and exercise interact to regulate brain-derived neurotrophic factor mRNA and protein expression in the hippocampus. *European Journal of Neuroscience*, **14**, 1992–2002.

Berchtold, N. C., Kesslak, J. P., & Cotman, C. W. (2002). Hippocampal brain-derived neurotrophic factor gene regulation by exercise and the medial septum. *Journal of Neuroscience Research*, **68**, 511–521.

Black, J. E., Isaacs, K. R., Anderson, B. J., Alcantara, A. A., & Greenough, W. T. (1990). Learning causes synaptogenesis, whereas motor activity causes angiogenesis, in cerebellar cortex of adult rats. *Proceedings of the National Academy of Science*, **87**, 5568–5572.

Brown, J., Cooper-Kuhn, C. M., Kempermann, G. *et al.* (2003). Enriched environment and physical activity stimulate hippocampal but not olfactory bulb neurogenesis. *European Journal of Neuroscience*, **17**, 2042–2046.

Bunce, D. J., Barrowclough, A., & Morris, I. (1996). The moderating influence of physical fitness on age gradients in vigilance and serial choice responding tasks. *Psychology and Aging*, **11**, 671–682.

Carro, E., Nunez, A., Busiguina, S., & Torres-Alemán, I. (2000). Circulating insulin-like growth factor I mediates effects of exercise on the brain. *Journal of Neuroscience*, **20**, 2926–2933.

Clarkson-Smith, L., & Hartley, A. (1989). Relationships between physical exercise and cognitive abilities in older adults. *Psychology and Aging*, **4**, 183–189.

Colcombe, S., & Kramer, A. F. (2003). Fitness effects on the cognitive function of older adults: a meta-analytic study. *Psychological Science*, **14**, 125–130.

Colcombe, S. J., Kramer, A. F., Erickson, K. I. *et al.* (2004). Cardiovascular fitness, cortical plasticity, and aging. *Proceedings of the National Academy of Sciences USA*, **101**, 3316–3321.

Cotman, C. W., & Berchtold, N. C. (2002). Exercise: a behavioral intervention to enhance brain health and plasticity. *Trends in Neuroscience*, **25**, 295–301.

Daniels, K., Toth, J., & Jacoby, L. (2006). The aging of executive functions. In E. Bialystok & F. I. M. Craik (Eds.), *Lifespan Cognition: Mechanisms of Change* (pp. 96–111). New York, NY: Oxford University Press.

Dik, M. G., Deeg, D. J. H., Visser, M., & Jonker, C. (2003). Early life physical activity and cognition at old age. *Journal of Clinical and Experimental Neuropsychology*, **25**, 643–653.

Ding, Y., Li, J., Luan, X. *et al.* (2004a). Exercise preconditioning reduces brain damage in ischemic rats that may be associated with regional angiogenesis and cellular overexpression of neurotrophin. *Neuroscience*, **124**, 583–591.

Ding, Y. H., Luan, X. D., Li, J. *et al.* (2004b). Exercise-induced overexpression of angiogenic factors and reduction of ischemia/reperfusion injury in stroke. *Current Neuro-vascular Research*, **1**, 411–120.

Dustman, R. E., Ruhling, R. O., Russell, E. M. *et al.* (1984). Aerobic exercise training and improved neuropsychological function of older individuals. *Neurobiology of Aging*, **5**, 35–42.

Dustman, R. E., Emmerson, R. Y., Ruhling, R. O. *et al.* (1990). Age and fitness effects on EEG, ERPs, visual sensitivity, and cognition. *Neurobiology of Aging*, **11**, 193–200.

Dustman, R., Emmerson, R., & Shearer, D. E. (1994). Physical activity, age, and cognitive neuropsychological function. *Journal of Aging and Physical Activity*, **2**, 143–181.

Eadie, B. D., Redilla, V. A., & Christie, B. R. (2005). Voluntary exercise alters the cytoarchitecture of the adult dentate gyrus by increasing cellular proliferation, dendritic complexity, and spine density. *Journal of Comparative Neurology*, **486**, 39–47.

Etnier, J. L., Salazar, W., Landers, D. M. *et al.* (1997). The influence of physical fitness and exercise upon cognitive functioning: a meta-analysis. *Journal of Sport and Exercise Psychology*, **19**, 249–277.

Fabel, K., Fabel, K., Tam, B. *et al.* (2003). VEGF is necessary for exercise-induced adult hippocampal neurogenesis. *European Journal of Neuroscience*, **18**, 2803–2812.

Fabre, C., Massé-Biron, J., Charmari, K. *et al.* (1999). Evaluation of quality of life in elderly healthy subjects after aerobic and/or mental training. *Archives of Gerontology and Geriatrics*, **28**, 9–22.

Fabre, C., Charmari, K., Mucci, P., Massé-Biron, J., & Préfaut, C. (2002). Improvement of cognitive function and/or individualized aerobic training in healthy elderly subjects. *International Journal of Sports Medicine*, **23**, 415–421.

Farmer, J., Zhao, X., van Praag, H. *et al.* (2004). Effects of voluntary exercise on synaptic plasticity and gene expression in the dentate gyrus of adult male Sprague-Dawley rats *in vivo*. *Neuroscience*, **124**, 71–79.

Fordyce, D. E., & Wehner, J. M. (1993). Physical activity enhances spatial learning performance with an associated alteration in hippocampal protein kinase C activity in C57BL/6 and DBA/2 mice. *Brain Research*, **619**, 111–119.

Garza, A. A., Ha, T. G., Garcia, C., Chen, M. J., & Russo-Neustadt, A. A. (2004). Exercise, antidepressant treatment, and BDNF mRNA expression in the aging brain. *Pharmacology, Biochemistry and Behavior*, **77**, 209–220.

Ginés, S., Bosch, M., Marco, S. *et al.* (2006). Reduced expression of the TrkB receptor in Huntington's disease mouse models and in human brain. *European Journal of Neuroscience*, **23**, 649–658.

Gokhale, J., & Smetters, K. (2006). Measuring social security's financial outlook within an aging society. *Daedalus*, **135**, 91–104.

Gómez-Pinilla, F., So, V., & Kesslak, J. P. (1998). Spatial learning and physical activity contribute to the induction of fibroblast growth factor: neural substrates for increased cognition associated with exercise. *Neuroscience*, **85**, 53–61.

Gómez-Pinilla, F., Ying, Z., Roy, R. R., Molteni, R., & Edgerton, V. R. (2002). Voluntary exercise induces a BDNF-mediated mechanism that promotes neuroplasticity. *Journal of Neurophysiology*, **88**, 2187–2195.

Heine, V. M., Maslan, S., Joëls, M., & Lucassen, P. J. (2004). Prominent decline of newborn cell proliferation, differentiation, and apoptosis in the aging dentate gyrus, in absence of an age-related hypothalamus-pituitary-adrenal axis activation. *Neurobiology of Aging*, **25**, 361–375.

Hillman, C. H., Kramer, A. F., Belopolsky, A. V., & Smith, D. P. (2006). A cross-sectional examination of age and physical activity on performance and event-related brain potentials in a task switching paradigm. *International Journal of Psychophysiology*, **59**, 30–39.

Isaacs, K. R., Anderson, B. J., Alcantara, A. A., Black, J. E., & Greenough, W. T. (1992). Exercise and the brain: angiogenesis in the adult rat cerebellum after vigorous physical activity and motor skill learning. *Journal of Cerebral Blood Flow Metabolism*, **12**, 110–119.

Johansson, B. B., & Ohlsson, A. L. (1996). Environment, social interaction, and physical activity as determinants of functional outcome after cerebral infarction in the rat. *Experimental Neurology*, **139**, 322–327.

Katoh-Semba, R., Asano, T., Ueda, H. *et al.* (2002). Riluzole enhances expression of brain-derived neurotrophic factor with consequent proliferation of granule precursor cells in the rat hippocampus. *FASEB Journal*, **16**, 1328–1330.

Kleim, J. A., Cooper, N. R., & VandenBerg, P. M. (2002). Exercise induces angiogenesis but does not alter movement representations within rat motor cortex. *Brain Research*, **934**, 1–6.

Klintsova, A. Y., Dickson, E., Yoshida, R., & Greenough, W. T. (2004). Altered expression of BDNF and its high-affinity receptor TrkB in response to complex motor learning and moderate exercise. *Brain Research*, **1028**, 92–104.

Kramer, A. F., Colcombe, S. J., Erickson, K. I., & Paige, P. (2006). Fitness training and the brain: From molecules to minds. *Proceedings from the 2006 Cognitive Aging Conference*. Atlanta, Georgia.

Kronenberg, G., Bick-Sander, A., Bunk, E. *et al.* (2006). Physical exercise prevents age-related decline in precursor cell activity in the mouse dentate gyrus. *Neurobiology of Aging*, **27**, 1505–1513.

Larson, E. B., Wang, L., Bowen, J. D. *et al.* (2006). Exercise is associated with reduced risk for incident dementia among persons 65 years of age and older. *Annals of Internal Medicine*, **144**, 73–81.

Lichtenwalner, R. J., Forbes, M. E., Bennet, S. A. *et al.* (2001). Intracerebroventricular infusion of insulin-like growth factor-I ameliorates the age-related decline in hippocampal neurogenesis. *Neuroscience*, **107**, 603–613.

Llorens-Martín, M., Torres-Alemán, I., & Trejo, J. L. (2006). Pronounced individual variation in the response to the stimulatory action of exercise on immature hippocampal neurons. *Hippocampus*, **16**, 480–490.

Lopcz-Lopez, C., LeRoith, D., & Torres-Alemán, I. (2004). Insulin-like growth factor I is required for vessel remodeling in the adult brain. *Proceedings of the National Academy of Sciences USA*, **101**, 9833–9838.

Lu, B., Pang, P. T., & Woo, N. H. (2005). The yin and yang of neurotrophin action. *Nature Reviews Neuroscience*, **6**, 603–614.

McCloskey, D. P., Adamo, D. S., & Anderson, B. J. (2001). Exercise increases metabolic capacity in the motor cortex and striatum, but not in the hippocampus. *Brain Research*, **891**, 168–175.

Milgram, N. W., Head, E., Zicker, S. C. *et al.* (2005). Learning ability in aged beagle dogs is preserved by behavioral enrichment and dietary fortification: a two-year longitudinal study. *Neurobiology of Aging*, **26**, 77–90.

Mohapel, P., Frielingsdorf, H., Häggblad, J., Zachrisson, O., & Brundin, P. (2005). Platelet-derived growth factor (PDGF-BB) and brain derived neurotrophic factor (BDNF) induce striatal neurogenesis in adult rats with 6-hydroxydopamine lesions. *Neuroscience*, **132**, 767–776.

Molteni, R., Wu, A., Vaynman, S. *et al.* (2004). Exercise reverses the harmful effects of consumption of a high-fat diet on synaptic and behavioral plasticity associated to the action of brain-derived neurotrophic factor. *Neuroscience*, **123**, 429–440.

Murer, M. G., Yan, Q., & Raisman-Vozari, R. (2001). Brain-derived neurotrophic factor in the control human brain, and in Alzheimer's disease and Parkinson's disease. *Progress in Neurobiology*, **63**, 71–124.

Neeper, S. A., Gómez-Pinilla, F., Choi, J., & Cotman, C. W. (1995). Exercise and brain neurotrophins. *Nature*, **373**, 109.

Neeper, S. A., Gómez-Pinilla, F., Choi, J., & Cotman, C. W. (1996). Physical activity increases mRNA for brain-derived neurotrophic factor and nerve growth factor in rat brain. *Brain Research*, **726**, 49–56.

O'Sullivan, M., Jones, D. K., Summers, P. E. *et al.* (2001). Evidence for cortical "disconnection" as a mechanism of age-related cognitive decline. *Neurology*, **57**, 632–638.

Pang, P. T., Teng, H. K., Zaitsev, E. *et al.* (2004). Cleavage of proBDNF by tPA/plasmin is essential for long-term hippocampal plasticity. *Science*, **306**, 487–491.

Pang, T. Y. C., Stam, N. C., Nithianantharajah, J., Howard, M. L., & Hannan, A. J. (2006). Differential effects of voluntary physical exercise on behavioral and brain-derived neurotrophic factor expression deficits in Huntington's disease transgenic mice. *Neuroscience*, **141**, 569–584.

Podewils, L. J., Guallar, E., Kuller, L. H. *et al.* (2005). Physical activity, *apoe* genotype, and dementia risk: findings from the Cardiovascular Health Cognition Study. *American Journal of Epidemiology*, **161**, 639–351.

Poulton, N. P., & Muir, G. D. (2005). Treadmill training ameliorates dopamine loss but not behavioral deficits in hemi-Parkinsonian rats. *Experimental Neurology*, **193**, 181–197.

Ramsden, M., Berchtold, N. C., Kesslak, J. P., Cotman, C. W., & Pike, C. J. (2003). Exercise increases the vulnerability of rat hippocampal neurons to kainate lesion. *Brain Research*, **971**, 239–244.

Raz, N. (2000). Aging of the brain and its impact on cognitive performance: integration of structural and functional findings. In F. I. M. Craik & T. A. Salthouse (Eds.), *The Handbook of Aging and Cognition (2nd Edition)* (pp. 1–90). Mahwah, NJ: Lawrence Erlbaum.

Rebok, G. (2006). Paper presented on the Experience Corps project in the Cognitive Activity from Bedside to Bench symposium. *American Geriatrics Society Annual Scientific Meeting*. Chicago, Illinois.

Rhodes, J. S., van Praag, H., Jeffrey, S. *et al.* (2003). Exercise increases hippocampal neurogenesis to high levels but does not improve spatial learning in mice bred for increased voluntary wheel running. *Behavioral Neuroscience*, **117**, 1006–1016.

Richards, M., Hardy, R., & Wadsworth, M. E. J. (2003). Does active leisure protect cognition? Evidence from a national birth cohort. *Social Science and Medicine*, **56**, 785–792.

Rovio, S., Kåreholt, I., Helkala, E.-L. *et al.* (2005). Leisure-time physical activity at midlife and the risk of dementia and Alzheimer's disease. *Lancet Neurology*, **4**, 705–711.

Russo-Neustadt, A., Ha, T., Ramirez, R., & Kesslak, J. P. (2001). Physical activity-antidepressant treatment combination: impact on brain-derived neurotrophic factor and behavior in an animal model. *Behavioural Brain Research*, **120**, 87–95.

Samorajski, T., Delaney, C., Durham, L. *et al.* (1985). Effect of exercise on longevity, body weight, locomotor performance, and passive-avoidance memory of C57BL/6J mice. *Neurobiology of Aging*, **6**, 17–24.

Schaaf, M. J. M., Workel, J. O., Lesscher, H. M. *et al.* (2001). Correlation between hippocampal BDNF mRNA expression and memory performance in senescent rats. *Brain Research*, **915**, 227–233.

Silhol, M., Bonnichon, V., Rage, F., & Tapia-Arancibia, L. (2005). Age-related changes in brain-derived neurotrophic factor and tyrosine kinase receptor isoforms in the hippocampus and hypothalamus in male rats. *Neuroscience*, **132**, 613–624.

Small, G. W., Silverman, D. H. S., Siddarth, P. *et al.* (2006). Effects of a 14-day healthy longevity lifestyle program on cognition and brain function. *American Journal of Geriatric Psychiatry*, **14**, 538–545.

Spirduso, W. W., & Clifford, P. (1978). Replication of age and physical activity effects on reaction and movement time. *Journal of Gerontology*, **33**, 26–30.

Stones, M. I., & Kozma, A. (1989). Age, exercise, and coding performance. *Psychology and Aging*, **4**, 190–194.

Stranahan, A. M., Kahalil, D., & Gould, E. (2006). Social isolation delays the positive effects of running on adult neurogenesis. *Nature Neuroscience*, **9**, 526–533.

Stummer, W., Weber, K., Tranmer, B., Baethmann, A., & Kempski, O. (1994). Reduced mortality and brain damage after locomotor activity in gerbil forebrain ischemia. *Stroke*, **25**, 1862–1868.

Stummer, W., Baethmann, A., Murr, R., Schurer, L., & Kempski, O. S. (1995). Cerebral protection against ischemia by locomotor activity in gerbils: underlying mechanisms. *Stroke*, **26**, 1423–1430.

Swain, R. A., Harris, A. B., Wiener, E. C. *et al.* (2003). Prolonged exercise induces angiogenesis and increases cerebral blood volume in primary motor cortex of the rat. *Neuroscience*, **117**, 1037–1046.

Tillerson, J. L., Caudle, W. M., Reverón, M. E., & Miller, G. W. (2003). Exercise induces behavioral recovery and attenuates neurochemical deficits in rodent models of Parkinson's disease. *Neuroscience*, **119**, 899–911.

Trejo, J. L., Carro, E., & Torres-Alemán, I. (2001). Circulating insulin-like growth factor I mediates exercise-induced increases in the number of new neurons in the adult hippocampus. *Journal of Neuroscience*, **21**, 1628–1634.

van Praag, H., Kempermann, G., & Gage, F. H. (1999a). Running increases cell proliferation and neurogenesis in the adult mouse dentate gyrus. *Nature Neuroscience*, **2**, 266–270.

van Praag, H., Christie, B. R., Sejnowski, T. J., & Gage, F. H. (1999b). Running enhances neurogenesis, learning, and long-term potentiation in mice. *Proceedings of the National Academy of Sciences USA*, **96**, 13427–13431.

van Praag, H., Shubert, T., Zhao, C., & Gage, F. H. (2005). Exercise enhances learning and hippocampal neurogenesis in aged mice. *Journal of Neuroscience*, **25**, 8680–8685.

Vaynman, S., Ying, Z., & Gómez-Pinilla, F. (2003). Interplay between brain-derived neurotrophic factor and signal transduction modulators in the regulation of the effects of exercise on synaptic plasticity. *Neuroscience*, **122**, 647–657.

Vaynman, S., Ying, Z., & Gómez-Pinilla, F. (2004). Hippocampal BDNF mediates the efficacy of exercise on synaptic plasticity and cognition. *European Journal of Neuroscience*, **20**, 2580–2590.

Verghese, J., Lipton, R. B., Katz, M. J. *et al.* (2003). Leisure activities and the risk of dementia in the elderly. *New England Journal of Medicine*, **348**, 2508–2516.

Watanabe, T., Miyazaki, A., Katagiri, T. *et al.* (2005). Relationship between serum insulin-like growth factor-1 levels and Alzheimer's disease and vascular dementia. *Journal of the American Geriatrics Society*, **53**, 1748–1753.

Weuve, J., Kang, J. H., Manson, J. E. *et al.* (2004). Physical activity, including walking, and cognitive function in older women. *Journal of the American Medical Association*, **292**, 1454–1461.

Wilson, R. S., Bennett, D. A., Bienias, J. L. *et al.* (2002). Cognitive activity and incident AD in a population-based sample of older persons. *Neurology*, **59**, 1910–1914.

Yaffe, K., Barnes, D., Nevitt, M., Lui, L.-Y., & Covinsky, K. (2001). A prospective study of physical activity and cognitive decline in elderly women: women who walk. *Archives in Internal Medicine*, **161**, 1703–1708.

Yamada, M., Kasagi, F., Sasaki, H. *et al.* (2003). Association between dementia and midlife risk factors: the radiation effects research foundation adult health study. *Journal of the American Geriatrics Society*, **51**, 410–414.

Zigova, T., Pencea, V., Wiegand, S. J., & Luskin, M. B. (1998). Intraventricular administration of BDNF increases the number of newly generated neurons in the adult olfactory bulb. *Molecular and Cellular Neuroscience*, **11**, 234–245.

25

Aphasia

Susan A. Leon, Stephen E. Nadeau, Michael deRiesthal,
Bruce Crosson, John C. Rosenbek and Leslie J. Gonzalez Rothi

Introduction

- Aphasia is an enduring and common cognitive disorder.
- Aphasia treatment is one of the earliest forms of cognitive rehabilitation.
- Aphasia treatment has been shown to be efficacious.

Although the term "cognitive rehabilitation" is relatively new (Boake, 1991), its roots can be traced to the organized efforts to deal with head injuries in World Wars I and II (Goldstein, 1942; Luria, 1948). From the beginning, treatment of aphasia has had a central role in such endeavors (Goldstein, 1948; Luria, 1947). Indeed, while most other cognitive therapies received sporadic attention between those early attempts and the latter part of the twentieth century, aphasia therapy progressed steadily. Today, aphasia treatment research is driven by an increasing understanding of the cognitive structure of language and its neural substrates. Thus, in the more general context of cognitive rehabilitation, there is much to be learned from the study of aphasia treatments. While cerebral systems underlying language are complex and effective treatment of aphasia requires a full appreciation of this complexity, the goal of this chapter is to give the reader simply a sample of the rich history of aphasia treatment and to provide references to literature that will describe the methods and applications more fully.

Aphasia is a relatively common and enduring disorder of language knowledge or processing resulting from neurological disease or injury, most typically stroke (Orange & Kertesz, 1998). Between 21 and 38% of acute strokes are associated with aphasia (Berthier, 2005). The American Heart Association reports that 700 000 new strokes occur annually in the USA. Thus, each year, 147 000–266 000 newly aphasic persons and their families, friends and communities struggle with the consequences of this communication disorder within the USA (Ferro et al., 1999; Paolucci et al., 2005; Wade et al., 1986). As with most motor, sensory or cognitive deficits resulting from stroke, aphasia evolves in degree and nature during the first year post-onset, with the majority of improvement occurring within the first 3 months (Kertesz, 1979). However, recent review (Ferro et al., 1999) suggests that some degree of aphasia persists in 60% of subjects who display aphasia at stroke onset.

The burden of cognitive disorders such as aphasia is apparent in the findings of Galski et al. (1993) and Lincoln & Blackburn (1989), who showed that cognitive disorders are associated with poorer quality of life and greater risk of institutionalization. As for the impact upon those who live with stroke survivors, Dennis et al. (1998) found that as many as 55% of caregivers expressed "significant emotional distress." Simmons-Mackie (2001) and Lubinski (2001) review the burdens of aphasia on aphasic persons and their environments and describe the influences of burden on aphasia evaluation and treatment.

While aphasia and its underlying mechanisms have been topics of research for centuries, treatment

Cognitive Neurorehabilitation, Second Edition: Evidence and Application, ed. Donald T. Stuss, Gordon Winocur and
Ian H. Robertson. Published by Cambridge University Press. © Cambridge University Press 2008.

of aphasia only came into intense focus more recently in the context of the World Wars and veterans returning home with war-related brain injuries. A number of publications in the 1970s and 1980s involved group comparisons seeking to meet Fred Darley's (1972) challenge to prove the efficacy of aphasia therapy; these various reports did not appear to provide consistent or resounding proof. For example, in three investigations involving a total of 127 subjects receiving various and unspecified aphasia treatments and 95 untreated subjects (Basso *et al.*, 1979; Shewan & Kertesz,1984; Wertz *et al.*, 1986), those receiving treatment were reported to have better language outcomes. In contrast, Lincoln *et al.* (1984) and Sarno *et al.* (1970) each reported that outcomes were not different between those treated (collective total of 263 treated persons) and those untreated (collective total of 282 aphasic persons).

Why the seeming lack of consensus? Wertz & Irwin (2001) would answer that design weaknesses plagued many of these early studies, especially those reporting no evidence of efficacy. Another possibility is that these early studies, designed to answer the question "is aphasia treatment efficacious?," may have been directed at a question that was prematurely posed. That is, they studied the effect of the process of treatment rather than asking what specific treatments were efficacious; in what specific patients and under what therapy conditions. Additionally, these studies were not randomized controlled studies; rather, most of these early studies had relatively small sample sizes with little external controls.

A large number of studies have been reported since the late 1980s that have employed within-subject clinical trial experimental designs. This type of design provides a particularly powerful means for examining theoretically motivated aphasia treatment innovations and the circumstances of their effect, and it is well-suited to address the question of which treatment for which patient. In 1994, Randall Robey reviewed 55 such published reports to determine the circumstances of treatment effect, and, using meta-analytic methods, to confirm that

aphasia treatment was efficacious. He suggested that more intensive treatment (more than 2 hours/ week) might be more effective. Subsequently, extensive reviews of the literature on language rehabilitation have provided further such endorsements, the most extensive having been completed by the Department of Veterans Affairs Taskforce on Aphasia, and the Academy of Neurogenic Communication Disorders and Sciences (ANCDS) writing committee on aphasia. Additionally, the Cochrane review by Greener *et al.* (2005) and the evidence reviews of the Canadian Stroke Network (http://www.canadianstrokenetwork.ca) endorsed the concept that treatment should be delivered early in the recovery interval and at intensive rates (Bhogal *et al.*, 2003).

The earliest classifications of aphasia subtypes led therapists to divide their aphasia rehabilitation efforts into language production and reception therapies. Additionally, language has historically been further divided into levels of phonology, word form, sentence form and discourse, with treatments typically targeting each level and mode (production vs. comprehension) specifically. More recent connectionist views suggest that these subdivisions may not accurately represent the reality of central nervous system neural networks supporting language processing. However, for decades, traditional approaches have provided functional utility in giving therapist and patient a focus to begin reconstructing subcomponents of dysfunctional communication systems. The body of aphasia rehabilitation research that is based upon these historically used subdivisions provides a rich heritage that can serve to inform future efforts.

Our brief review of treatments (see Table 25.1) begins with those focused on the production of language. Starting with the smallest units of language, the sound and the single word, we continue with exemplars of production treatments focused on larger units of language including phrases, sentences and discourse. The treatment section concludes with an overview of language comprehension treatments, a subject of far fewer studies than language production.

Table 25.1. Traditional categories of aphasia rehabilitation methods

Language production
  Word level treatments
  Sentence level treatments
  Verbal fluency, generation and thematic elaboration
    treatments
Language comprehension
  Auditory comprehension treatments

Language production

Word level treatments

- Treatments focusing at the word level are diverse in approach.
- Treatment for naming often uses facilitative strategies such as cueing, which may be provided or self-generated and may target phonemic or semantic levels.
- Manipulation of therapeutic circumstances such as scheduled spacing of retrieval and recruitment of allied cognitive systems may also be used to rehabilitate naming deficits.
- Studies targeting word retrieval have demonstrated therapeutic effect for word level treatments.
- Attributes of the ideal candidate, optimum procedure and dosage, and best outcome measurement instruments remain to be established.

While many treatments for word retrieval are available, this section covers only a subset. Our strategy was to sample from a spectrum of approaches in order to give the reader a sense of the variety. Confrontation naming is in all probability the most common therapeutic focus in language rehabilitation. Difficulties with word finding are pervasive following brain injury, and individuals with both fluent and nonfluent aphasia report this deficit as being the most disruptive in daily communication.

In a number of naming treatments the underlying strategy has been to utilize cueing hierarchies designed to prompt an accurate word production. This strategy provides individuals with aphasia with

cues arranged in hierarchies of most support to least support (or the opposite order depending on the aim of the researcher) in order to enable the individual to produce the name of a given target (Hillis, 1989; Linebaugh & Lehner, 1977; Thompson & Kearns, 1981, among others). Examples of the content of provided cues (hereafter referred to as prompts) include: spoken models (the word is "pond"), sentence completion ("the fish were swimming in the koi …"), or verbal descriptions of the target ("A small body of water").

Another strategy is to encourage individuals with aphasia to create their own cues, rather than providing the cues for them. With "personalization" or self-cueing, the patient develops his or her own personally generated cues (hereafter referred to as self-cues) to help retrieve given targets. For example, if the target was "pond," the patient may create the self-cue "fish in it" to help retrieve the word for pond when presented with that target in a confrontation naming task. The development and use of self-cues has been shown to aid some patients in word retrieval (Freed & Marshall, 1995; Freed et al., 1995; Marshall et al., 2002).

Prompting and self-cueing strategies differ in procedure but are designed to achieve the same goal: the correct production of a target word. A prompt is intended to enable the individual with aphasia to access knowledge that is currently unavailable, either completely or in part. This is done by providing the individual with information that constitutes a feature of the knowledge comprising a target. This feature can be a component of the sound of the target word, an aspect of its appearance, selected semantic attributes, or idiosyncratic episodic knowledge of the target. Self-cueing strategies that encourage the individual to create their own cues are designed to work by forcing the individual with aphasia to recreate the full constellation of features that define a target.

Prompting strategies have been designed to promote attention to the level of the phoneme or phonemic neighborhood of the target. The individual with aphasia is encouraged to focus his or her attention and efforts at the sound level by the use of prompts such as rhyming (e.g., "bond, pond"), repetition (e.g., "say pond"), or the provision of only the first one or two sounds in a given target word, known as phonemic cueing (e.g., "it starts with /pa/"), (Greenwald *et al.*, 1995; Raymer *et al.*, 1993). Prompting at this level has been shown to improve word retrieval/production accuracy in aphasic persons although some studies have shown semantic prompting to be just as effective (Wambaugh, 2003; Wambaugh *et al.*, 2001a).

Both types of cueing strategies (self-cue and prompts) have also focused at the level of the semantic network (Boyle, 2004; Boyle & Coelho, 1995; Coelho *et al.*, 2000; Conley & Coelho, 2003; Lowell *et al.*, 1995). The semantic representation of a word consists of all the features defining the concept corresponding to the word. Producing words that are semantically related to a target word by virtue of shared features may activate sufficient features of the target concept to bring the corresponding word above the threshold for production. Training the naming of a word in the context of semantically related words is thought to sharpen the distinction between the concepts underlying these words and the concept underlying the target, thereby increasing the likelihood that, when the subject seeks to name the target entity, one and only one word – the target name – will be activated, and activated sufficiently for production to occur.

A semantic network strategy that employs prompts is known as semantic cueing treatment (SCT). This treatment employs the semantic features of the target as prompts to aid the individual with aphasia in retrieval. Alternatively, semantic feature analysis (SFA) therapy asks the individual with aphasia to produce the most relevant features of a given target themselves. This type of treatment has shown moderate success in remediation of naming deficits (Boyle & Coelho, 1995; Coelho *et al.*, 2000; Lowell *et al.*, 1995).

No matter whether cues are provided or self-generated, all treatments demand practice of the production of the target. Recently, attention has focused on the structure of the practice. Spaced retrieval (SR) is a memory improvement strategy,

originally designed to help individuals with dementia (Brush & Camp, 1998). It functions by progressively increasing the length of time between presentation of a stimulus and recall. Spaced retrieval has recently been studied as a treatment for naming deficits in aphasia (Fridriksson *et al.*, 2005; Morrow & Fridriksson, 2006). The researchers found that SR was a successful method for improving naming production accuracy in aphasic persons resulting in quicker gains in mastery of items than a more traditional cueing hierarchy treatment.

An alternative strategy to improve word retrieval is to recruit allied cognitive systems that might support the language form system. One such treatment focuses on the use of intentional systems to influence language production. An intentional movement such as a left hand gesture, when paired with a language production task, can presumably cause a shift in neural activity from the left to the right hemisphere during naming tasks (Crosson *et al.*, 2005, 2007). In theory, this either reduces left hemisphere involvement in attentional and intentional processing, thereby permitting more dedicated involvement in language, or it facilitates engagement of the right hemisphere in the linguistic process. As might be predicted from such mechanisms, treatment benefits extend from treated to untreated words.

The ANCDS evidence tables (http://www.u.arizona.edu/~pelagie/ancds/index.html) identify over 100 treatment articles that target word retrieval in aphasia from 1967 to 2006. The majority of treatment studies in the area of word retrieval provide class III evidence for the treatment involving phase I/II trials. Thus, the activity, or therapeutic effect of these treatments has been demonstrated, but data regarding the ideal treatment candidate, optimum treatment procedure and dosage, and best measurement instruments remain to be established.

Phrase/sentence level treatments

- Sentence level treatments are intended to help individuals who have difficulty producing or comprehending sentences.

- Different phrase/sentence components, forms and processes have been targeted in treatments including verb production, production of interrogative question forms, and identification and movement of syntactic structures.
- These treatments have resulted in improvement in sentence use for many individuals with aphasia. However no treatment has been shown to be more effective than others.

Many individuals with aphasia exhibit a deficit in the comprehension or production of sentences that stems from impairment in grammatic function. There are a number of treatments available to remediate deficits in grammatical production. Treatments may focus at the level of the verb, the phrase or the sentence as a whole. This section again aims to present the reader with a wide sample of available treatments.

One treatment, known as cueing verbs treatment (CVT) (Loverso *et al.*, 1988), uses the verb as a "pivot" to aid the individual with aphasia to produce grammatically correct phrases. Target verbs are presented to the individual with aphasia graphically and verbally. The individual is then guided through repetition and prompts to verbally produce the targeted verb with a subject, then with subject plus direct object.

Verb retrieval has also been targeted in some individuals who have demonstrated difficulty in retrieving verb forms but relatively preserved comprehension. Verb retrieval treatment may focus on training confrontation naming of pictures of the verb (Mitchum & Berndt, 1992) or on tasks such as matching a target verb to a picture, or producing the verb based on a spoken scenario (Marshall *et al.*, 1998).

Training individuals to produce wh- questions (e.g., "who", "where") using story completion prompts (Wambaugh & Thompson, 1989) evolved into a commonly used approach in syntactic treatment known as linguistic specific treatment (LST) (Thompson *et al.*, 1993, 1996, 1998). Linguistic specific treatment trains individuals with aphasia to visually identify the components of a sentence (e.g., subject, verb, etc.) and then move those components to create a wh-question form of the given sentence.

Another treatment targeting syntax is the Helm Elicited Program for Syntax Stimulation (HELPSS) (Helm-Estabrooks & Ramsberger, 1986). This is a hierarchically structured treatment using a story completion format combined with question prompts designed to elicit targeted sentence types. As treatment advances, the linguistic difficulty of the targeted sentences is progressively increased.

Mapping therapy is based on the premise that deficits in sentence production and comprehension may result from difficulty identifying the underlying thematic roles within a sentence structure (Caramazza *et al.*, 2005; Chatterjee & Maher, 2000; Nickels *et al.*, 1991; Rochon *et al.*, 2005; Saffran *et al.*, 1980; Schwartz *et al.*, 1980; Wierenga *et al.*, 2006). Mapping therapies address this difficulty in assignment of thematic roles by training individuals with aphasia to recognize thematic elements (i.e., who does what to whom) using visual templates that show where in sentence order a given thematic role usually appears, thereby strengthening the association between thematic roles and word order in sentences (Byng, 1988; Byng *et al.*, 1994; Chatterjee *et al.*, 1995; Maher *et al.*, 1995; Schwartz *et al.*, 1994).

Studies testing treatments for impairment of syntax and sentence production provide class III evidence of efficacy involving phase I/II trials. No particular method has proven generally superior. All of these methods have resulted in improvement for some individuals with aphasia.

Verbal fluency, generation and elaboration treatments

- A variety of treatments targeting discourse and conversational levels of verbal communication are available. These may target:
    Ease of production
    Generativity
    Thematic elaboration.
- Many of these treatments have resulted in improvements in the skill targeted (i.e., fluency or elaboration).

Aphasic persons are commonly referred to as fluent or nonfluent but the definition of this distinction is elusive. Some use this term to refer to the quality of verbal production, which can mean the ease with which one articulates, the amount of words produced, or whether utterances consist predominantly of single words, phrases or sentences. The term fluency might also be used to characterize the quality of discourse, defined by the number of ideas generated and the expansiveness of the discussion of concepts or topics. In most cases these features align, and nonfluent aphasic individuals typically display effortful verbal productions with simplified syntax, grammatical errors, and reduced topical elaboration. Treatments targeting the fluency of production are as varied as the features described above.

One of the most commonly used approaches to treatment of impairments in fluency is melodic intonation therapy (MIT) (Albert *et al.*, 1973). This therapy targets ease of verbal production and was designed for individuals who have nonfluent verbal output but moderately preserved auditory comprehension. The clinician prompts the individual to speak target words or phrases with melodic intonation while concurrently tapping the rhythmic pattern of syllables on the individual's hand. This treatment targets explicit recognition of the melodic line and the rhythmic pattern of normal speech. Treatment with MIT has been shown to produce marked improvements in confrontation naming as well as increases in phrase length (Belin *et al.*, 1996; Sparks *et al.*, 1974). The MIT treatment protocol has been standardized and outcome measures to detect change continue to be developed (Belin *et al.*, 1996).

Other therapies have focused on mitigating sources of nonfluency in the language production of individuals with aphasia. Self-monitoring treatment to reduce speech interruptions has been described by Whitney & Goldstein (1989) and a treatment for verbal perseveration, termed treatment of aphasic perseveration (TAP), has been described by Helm-Estabrooks *et al.* (1987). The TAP program, which encourages the individual with aphasia to give no response or ask for help rather than produce a perseverative response, has been found to reduce perseverations.

Response elaboration training (RET) (Kearns, 1985) was designed to increase thematic elaboration in extended speech. Response elaboration training uses simple pictures as stimuli and a structured questioning technique to guide the individual with aphasia to thematically elaborate. The production of more content and longer utterances is accomplished by modeling and reinforcing of whatever was produced (e.g., "You said boat. You're right, that's a boat."), and by asking wh-questions ("Where is the boat?"). Improvements in the production of treated items have been shown to generalise to novel settings and clinicians (Kearns & Potechin Scher, 1989) and a modified version of the therapy has been shown to result in increased word production in picture description and personal recount tasks (Wambaugh & Martinez, 2000; Wambaugh *et al.*, 2001b). The impact of RET on individuals with different types of aphasia (Kearns & Potechin Scher, 1989) and co-existing apraxia of speech (Wambaugh & Martinez, 2000; Wambaugh *et al.*, 2001b) has also been examined.

Discourse level training targets re-establishing relationships across sentence boundaries in connected speech. This type of therapy is more appropriate for individuals with less severe aphasias and involves various techniques to encourage individuals to produce coherent, conceptually informative connected discourse. One such treatment involves analysing the complexity of the aphasic individual's response to a question, followed by encouragement through targeted questioning to produce a more complex response (Penn *et al.*, 1997). Functional conversational skills have also been targeted wherein individuals with aphasia were trained to produce functionally appropriate statements and questions (Doyle *et al.*, 1991). This therapy was found to improve conversational discourse both with the clinician and with family members (Doyle *et al.*, 1991).

PACE (Davis & Wilcox, 1985) aims to create a "naturalistic" dialogue between a clinician and an individual with aphasia. The focus is less on producing language per se, but rather on encouraging the communicator to seek effective communication using any means available (e.g., gesture, writing and pointing). The therapy is based on four principles: that communication must involve an exchange of new information, that the participation in communication must be equal, that the individual with aphasia may use any communication mode desired, and that feedback given to the individual must be functional. This strategy has been used with different types of aphasias and has been shown to be effective in producing "observable improvement" on confrontation naming and picture description (Li *et al.*, 1988). A modification of this therapy, using card games focusing on requests and bargaining, produced significant improvement in five of eight subjects treated (Pulvermuller & Roth, 1991).

In summary, a variety of treatment approaches have been developed to improve verbal fluency in nonfluent aphasic persons. With few exceptions, published studies provide class III evidence of efficacy. However, several approaches discussed in this section, including response elaboration training (RET) and melodic intonation therapy (MIT), have been tested in randomised controlled trials.

Language comprehension

Auditory comprehension treatments

- Treatments exist to help re-train auditory comprehension of language.
- Treatments range in focus from the level of the single word to sentences and multi-step commands.
- Auditory comprehension treatments have been attempted using nonconventional approaches such as computer-based or telephone training.
- Auditory comprehension treatments are much less common and less evidence exists on effectiveness.

There have been far fewer studies of treatments for disorders of comprehension of language than for disorders of production. One of the earliest forms of auditory comprehension training was based on the Token Test (de Renzi & Vignolo, 1962). The Token Test is a difficult test of auditory comprehension employing stimuli that vary in length and syntactic complexity. West (1973) describes practice starting at less complex levels (e.g., training comprehension of shapes and colors by having subjects repeat the names) and moving onto more complex levels of comprehension that involve increasing memory load or syntactic complexity (e.g., subject verbally instructed to point to several shapes of certain sizes and colors sequentially). While West (1973) showed that this type of training resulted in improvement in performance on the Token Test, the rate of improvement may have correlated with pretreatment functioning, with those at higher pretreatment comprehension levels showing greater gains (Holland & Sonderman, 1974).

Auditory comprehension training programs have also been used to train subjects to distinguish single spoken words through use of picture cards of common nouns and verbs (Czvik, 1976; Kushner & Winitz, 1977; Marshall & Neuberger, 1984). The individual with aphasia is instructed verbally to point to a picture presented within a field of picture distractors. Difficulty is progressively increased by asking the individual to point to a rising number of items sequentially. Spoken word-picture matching and spoken word-printed word matching have also been utilized in a similar program (Hough, 1993) that increased complexity by increasing the field of choices and/or varying the relatedness of the choices.

Sentence level auditory comprehension training has also been used with individuals with aphasia (Hough, 1993; Naeser *et al.*, 1986), although usually as a second or third step of a training program that begins at the single word level. Sentence level training tasks include sentence-picture matching, answering questions, and identifying target words embedded in prerecorded sentences. This type of treatment has been shown to improve auditory comprehension in some patients with chronic aphasia (Naeser *et al.*, 1986).

The auditory comprehension training programs mentioned above all used the standard patient–therapist structure. However, others have been designed that utilize nontraditional treatment frameworks such as telephone therapy (Davidoff & Katz, 1985) or computerized training (Mills, 1982). The telephone-based treatment allowed the individual with aphasia to call in to receive prerecorded sentence and paragraph comprehension tasks to which they were required to give yes/no answers. The computer-based auditory training program allowed individuals with aphasia to complete single word verbal stimulus-picture matching tasks. The computer provided feedback on the accuracy of the response. Studies of both the telephone and computer-based training programs have shown some evidence of efficacy (Davidoff & Katz, 1985; Mills, 1982).

As mentioned previously, relatively few treatments targeting auditory comprehension deficits in aphasia have been published in the literature, despite the fact that most individuals with aphasia have some level of impairment in the ability to comprehend spoken language (Rosenbek *et al.*, 1989). The auditory comprehension treatment approaches described in this chapter provide class III evidence of efficacy.

Functional impact of language treatments

- Many effective treatments for aphasia are in common usage.
- Most treatments do not result in generalization or retention of trained knowledge.
- Generalization may be improved in a number of ways including training more complex rather then less complex structures, activating wider concept representations, activating intentional biases to use spoken language, and training cognitive resources that underlie effective language use.
- Retention may be improved by the use of spaced practice, varied contexts and elaborated encoding of trained items.

This brief review reveals that there is a wide diversity of treatments available to treat language deficits. Many of the treatments we have reviewed approached rehabilitation of the language system by focusing on a particular component of language impairment. This approach is historically the most common method of language rehabilitation, and has yielded important scientific evidence regarding the neural basis of language processes. Importantly, it has shown us that aphasia is treatable, a conclusion supported by meta-analysis (Robey, 1994). Unfortunately, the available treatments also have limitations in that there is often little generalization to untreated language behaviors and performance frequently drops off after therapy has ended. Many treatments have shown improvement in the component of language for which they were developed (e.g., a syntactic treatment results in improvement in sentence use). However, for the vast majority of patients, aphasia treatments have been unable to transform their daily communicative lives.

Generalization is the process by which the effects of a given treatment extend to materials or circumstances that were not explicitly trained in therapy. Generalization is absolutely critical to achieving a real functional impact on the daily lives of individuals with aphasia. Unfortunately, generalization has been somewhat of a mystery in aphasia treatment, in that it has been observed inconsistently and the mechanisms that underlie generalization are still poorly understood (Nadeau *et al.*, in press).

Generalization has been shown to occur within a domain, wherein a treated behavior generalizes to other similar skills in the same domain. Linguistic specific treatment (LST) (Thompson, 1998), has shown promising results in this regard. Linguistic specific treatment is based on the idea that generalization is enhanced when treatment focuses on more complex structures, allowing generalization to less complex structures invoking the same syntactic skill (Thompson *et al.*, 2003). Although this training may generalize both to the simpler structures and to all sentences containing the trained structures, regardless of word content, it will not generalize to structures requiring a fundamentally different syntactic skill. For example, subjects trained to produce who or what questions when given simple declarative sentences are unable to produce when or where questions because this requires a different syntactic skill.

Word retrieval treatments may also produce some generalization when an untreated item shares semantic features with a trained item. For instance, if a treatment focused on training the names of ten types of birds, an individual with aphasia may also improve on naming other types of birds because these words share common semantic features (e.g., has wings, has feathers, can fly, etc.). However, it is unlikely that the individual with aphasia would show substantial improvement in naming types of trees following a treatment training types of birds; these two categories (birds; trees) share few semantic features, and the meaning of words and their phonological representations are arbitrarily related. In order to make more of a functional impact and to encourage the greatest generalization, confrontation naming treatments would need to encompass a large corpus of words essential to daily life, or combine classical confrontation treatments with other tasks that would encourage an individual with aphasia to activate a wider concept representation of the trained items, thus enabling more generalization because of engagement of a much larger semantic feature set during training. Tasks that might help to activate a more elaborate representation include those that combine naming to definition, discussion of semantic features of items (how it feels, how it sounds, etc.), and production of target words in the context of sentences (Nadeau *et al.*, in press).

Another treatment that has shown promise in regards to generalization is constraint-induced language therapy (CILT) (also referred to as constraint-induced aphasia therapy or CIAT by Pulvermuller *et al.*, 2001), which is modeled after an intervention for chronic hemiplegia, known as constraint-induced movement therapy (CIMT) (Kunkle *et al.*, 1999; Miltner *et al.*, 1999; Taub, 2000). Constraint-induced language therapy engages participants in interactive, exclusively spoken-language exchanges

with other individuals, usually also with aphasia, using scripted games, and has shown very promising results in three studies (Maher *et al.*, 2006; Meinzer *et al.*, 2005; Pulvermuller *et al.*, 2001). This treatment is thought to induce generalization through an entirely different means, one that is extrinsic to language processes, which we have termed "mechanistic." Mechanistic generalization involves training a neural resource that, while not a language skill, is essential to language processing (Nadeau *et al.*, in press). The mechanistic resource encouraging generalization in CILT is the development of the intentional bias to use language. The premise is that individuals with aphasia become intimidated by verbal communication following a brain injury and develop habits of avoidance or minimal use of language exchanges. An intentional bias to use spoken language again may allow the individual to use more fully both the skills being trained in a treatment and any language functions remaining after the neural damage.

There are other treatments that could, in theory, produce mechanistic generalization. For example, many subjects with aphasia have impairment of working memory allocation. Improving working memory function could be of considerable value in improving grammatical function, which relies on the ability to maintain multiple concepts simultaneously in mind, and to maintain recall of recent dialogue in order to correctly choose pronouns and articles.

Another reason that treatment might fail to transform the daily communicative lives of individuals with aphasia is lack of retention of the trained language skill once a treatment ends. Retention of learned knowledge is influenced by the quantity of practice, the distribution of practice, and the quality of practice. Quantity of practice is easily understood and already applied in virtually any rehabilitation setting; we know that more practice is better than less. Distribution of practice is less widely understood. It has been known for some time that skills or knowledge that are learned in a temporally distributed fashion are retained better than skills or knowledge learned in massed practice, a phenomenon known as the spacing effect (Baddeley & Longman, 1978; Glenberg, 1979; Glenberg & Lehmann, 1980; Pyle, 1913; Shebilske *et al.*, 1999). However, the spacing effect has not yet been adequately studied in populations of people with brain damage, such as individuals with aphasia. More research is needed to know if spacing of practice will have a potent effect on retention of trained knowledge or skills in rehabilitation. The mechanism underlying the spacing effect is thought to be an increase in the extent of commonality between circumstances during training and circumstances at the time of retention. This increase might be achieved by means other than altering the temporal distribution of practice, for example by providing a richer, more varied treatment context that is more likely to share elements with the subject's circumstances in daily life. Greater spacing of treatment might also improve retention by enabling better consolidation of knowledge. Knowledge consolidation processes are particularly active during sleep (Power, 2004).

Quality of practice may be another powerful factor in retention. Craik & Lockhart (1972) showed that the more "deeply" an item is processed, the better the later recall. Elaboration of trained items may add additional retrieval paths, thus increasing the probability that the trained item will be retrieved at a later time. Elaboration of the representation of an item could be induced using any of a number of approaches, including those mentioned earlier for promoting generalization, and any others that would result in a richer and more variable language context (Nadeau *et al.*, in press). Using a wider variety of contexts to train an item will encourage the individual to activate a multicomponent distributed representation, which may aid retention. An example of this was seen in a recent training paradigm that combined noun and verb naming with a pantomime of the use of the object (Raymer *et al.*, 2006). Learning was improved when naming of a picture was combined with pantomime as opposed to naming of a picture alone.

Conclusions

In summary, we have shown that there are a large number of viable treatments available for the rehabilitation of language deficits. Many of the current treatments focus at a single level of language function (e.g., naming, syntax, etc.) and many have shown treatment effects within their targeted level or with targeted stimuli. However, many thousands of people still suffer from a debilitating loss of communication that language rehabilitation has been unable to mitigate. Two reasons that language rehabilitation may have fallen short in creating a substantial impact on the daily communicative lives of individuals with aphasia are lack of generalization and poor retention of acquired knowledge and skills. Generalisation in language rehabilitation is still poorly understood and needs to be investigated more fully in clinical research as it could be a powerful factor in achieving a functional impact on daily communicative life. Boosting retention is also crucial for individuals with aphasia, and creating a richer and more varied treatment context that captures both spacing effects and levels of processing effects may provide a means to increasing retention.

While there is much yet to be learned about aphasia therapy and its conceptual underpinnings, it is clearly the most developed form of cognitive rehabilitation today. As other forms of cognitive rehabilitation develop, the principles used in aphasia therapy can act as a template for the development of other treatments. In particular, the design of aphasia treatments to target a specific problem suggests that a conceptual understanding of the cognitive structure underlying the target function is essential. Also, the study of generalization of treatment has led to some surprising findings, indicating for example that training more difficult tasks may facilitate generalization to simpler tasks of the same variety. Finally, the emerging questions in aphasia treatment, for example the effects of temporal distribution of treatment and generalization to everyday functioning, are applicable to other cognitive therapies. As the field of cognitive rehabilitation progresses, it is hoped that studies of aphasia therapies and other cognitive treatments will interact in a synergistic fashion.

REFERENCES

Albert, M. L., Sparks, R. W., & Helm, N. A. (1973). Melodic Intonation Therapy for aphasia. *Archives of Neurology*, **29**, 130–131.

Baddeley, A. D., & Longman, D. J. (1978). The influence of length and frequency of training session on the rate of learning to type. *Ergonomics*, **21**, 627–635.

Basso, A., Capitani, E., & Vignolo, L. A. (1979). Influence of rehabilitation on language skills in aphasic patients. A controlled study. *Archives of Neurology*, **36**, 190–196.

Belin, P., van Eckhout, P., Zilbovicus, M. *et al.* (1996). Recovery from nonfluent aphasia after Melodic Intonation Therapy: a PET study. *Neurology*, **47**, 1504–1511.

Berthier, M. L. (2005). Poststroke aphasia: epidemiology, pathophysiology and treatment. *Drugs and Aging*, **22**, 163–182.

Bhogal, S. K., Teasell, R., & Speechley, M. (2003). Intensity of aphasia therapy, impact on recovery. *Stroke*, **34**, 987–993.

Boake, C. (1991). History of cognitive rehabilitation following head injury. In J. S. Kreutzer & P. H. Wehman (Eds.), *Cognitive Rehabilitation for Persons with Traumatic Brain Injury: A Functional Approach*. New York, NY: Paul Brookes Publishing.

Boyle, M. (2004). Semantic Feature Analysis treatment for anomia in two fluent aphasia syndromes. *American Journal of Speech-Language Pathology*, **13**, 236–249.

Boyle, M., & Coelho, C. (1995). Application of Semantic Feature analysis as a treatment for aphasic dysnomia. *American Journal of Speech-Language Pathology*, **4**, 94–98.

Brush, J. A., & Camp, C. J. (1998). Using Spaced Retrieval as an intervention during speech-language therapy. *Clinical Gerontologist*, **19**, 51–64.

Byng, S. (1988). Sentence processing deficits: theory and therapy. *Cognitive Neuropsychology*, 629–676.

Byng, S., Nickels, L., & Black, M. (1994). Replicating therapy for mapping deficits in agrammatism: remapping the deficit? *Aphasiology*, **8**, 315–341.

Caramazza, A., Capasso, R., Capitani, E., & Miceli, G. (2005). Patterns of comprehension performance in agrammatic Broca's aphasia: a test of the Trace Deletion Hypothesis. *Brain and Language*, **94**, 43–53.

Chatterjee, A., & Maher, L. (2000). Grammar and agrammatism. In S. E. Nadeau, L. J. G. Rothi, & B. Crosson (Eds.), *Aphasia and Language: Theory to Practice*. (pp. 133–156). New York, NY: Guilford Press.

Chatterjee, A., Maher, L. M., & Rothi, L. J. G. (1995). Asyntactic thematic role assignment: the use of a temporal-spatial strategy. *Brain and Language*, **49**, 125–139.

Coelho, C. A., Mchugh, R. E., & Boyle, M. (2000). Semantic Feature Analysis as a treatment for aphasic dysnomia: a replication. *Aphasiology*, **14**, 133–142.

Conley, A., & Coelho, C. A. (2003). Treatment of word retrieval impairment in chronic Broca's aphasia. *Aphasiology*, **17**, 203–211.

Craik, F. I. M., & Lockhart, R. S. (1972). Levels of processing: a framework for memory research. *Journal of Verbal Learning and Verbal Behavior*, **11**, 671–684.

Crosson, B., Moore, A. B., Gopinath, K. *et al.* (2005). Role of the right and left hemispheres in recovery of function during treatment of intention in aphasia. *Journal of Cognitive Neuroscience*, **17**, 392–406.

Crosson, B., Fabrizio, K. S., Singletary, F. *et al.* (2007). Treatment of naming in nonfluent aphasia through manipulation of intention and attention: a phase 1 comparison of two novel treatments. *Journal of the International Neuropsychological Society*, **13**, 582–594.

Czvik, P. S. (1976). A preliminary investigation into the application of an auditory approach using non-variable materials in the treatment of aphasia: Two case studies. In R. H. Brookshire (Ed.), *Clinical Aphasiology Conference Proceeding* (pp. 291–301). Minneapolis, MN: BRK.

Darley, F. L. (1972). The efficacy of language rehabilitation in aphasia. *Journal of Speech and Hearing Disorders*, **37**, 3–21.

Davidoff, M., & Katz, R. (1985). Automated telephone therapy for improving auditory comprehension in aphasic adults. *Cognitive Rehabilitation*, **3**, 26–28.

Davis, G. A., & Wilcox, M. J. (1985). *Adult Aphasia Rehabilitation: Applied Pragmatics*. San Diego, CA: College-Hill Press.

de Renzi, E., & Vignolo, L. (1962). The Token Test: a sensitive test to detect receptive disturbances in aphasia. *Brain*, **65**, 665–678.

Dennis, M., O'Rourke, S., Lewis, S., Sharpe, M., & Warlow, C. (1998). A quantitative study of the emotional outcome of people caring for stroke survivors. *Stroke*, **29**, 1867–1872.

Doyle, P. J., Oleyar, K. S., & Goldstein, H. (1991). Facilitating functional conversational skills in aphasia: an experimental analysis of a generalization training procedure. In T. E. Prescott (Ed.), *Clinical Aphasiology* (pp. 229–241). Austin, TX: Pro-Ed.

Ferro, J. M., Mariano, G., & Madureira, S. (1999). Recovery from aphasia and neglect. *Cerebrovascular Diseases*, **9**, Suppl. 5, 6–22.

Freed, D. B., & Marshall, R. C. (1995). The effect of personalized cueing on long-term naming of realistic visual stimuli. *American Journal of Speech-Language Pathology*, **4**, 105–108.

Freed, D. B., Marshall, R. C., & Nippold, M. A. (1995). Comparison of personalized cueing and provided cueing on the facilitation of verbal labeling by aphasic subjects. *Journal of Speech and Hearing Research*, **38**, 1081–1090.

Fridriksson, J., Holland, A. L., Beeson, P., & Morrow, L. (2005). Spaced Retrieval treatment of anomia. *Aphasiology*, **19**, 99–109.

Galski, T., Bruno, R. L., Zorowitz, R., & Walker, J. (1993). Predicting length of stay, functional outcome, and aftercare in the rehabilitation of stroke patients: the dominant role of higher-order cognition. *Stroke*, **24**, 1794–1800.

Glenberg, A. M. (1979). Component-levels theory of the effects of spacing of repetitions on recall and recognition. *Memory and Cognition*, **7**, 95–112.

Glenberg, A. M., & Lehmann, T. S. (1980). Spacing repetitions over 1 week. *Memory and Cognition*, **8**, 528–538.

Goldstein, K. (1942). *After-Effects of Brain Injuries in War.* New York, NY: Grune & Stratton.

Goldstein, K. (1948). *Language and Language Disturbances.* New York, NY: Grune & Stratton.

Greener, J., Enderby, P., & Whurr, R. (2005). Speech and language therapy for aphasia following stroke. The Cochrane Database of Systematic Reviews. *The Cochrane Collaboration, Volume 3.*

Greenwald, M. L., Raymer, A. M., Richardson, M. E., & Rothi, L. J. G. (1995). Contrasting treatments for severe impairments of picture naming. *Neuropsychological Rehabilitation*, **5**, 17–49.

Helm-Estabrooks, N., & Ramsberger, G. (1986). Treatment of agrammatism in long-term Broca's aphasia. *British Journal of Communication Disorders*, **21**, 39–45.

Helm-Estabrooks, N., Emory, P., & Albert, M. L. (1987). Treatment of aphasic perseveration (TAP) program. *Archives of Neurology*, **44**, 1253–1255.

Hillis, A. E. (1989). Efficacy and generalization of treatment for aphasic naming errors. *Archives of Physical Medicine and Rehabilitation*, **70**, 632–636.

Holland, A. L., & Sonderman, J. C. (1974). Effects of a program based on the Token-Test for teaching comprehension skills to aphasics. *Journal of Speech and Hearing Research*, **17**, 589–598.

Hough, M. S. (1993). Treatment of Wernicke's aphasia with jargon: a case study. *Journal of Communication Disorders*, **26**, 101–111.

Kearns, K. P. (1985). Response Elaboration Training for patient initiated utterances. In R. H. Brookshire (Ed.), *Clinical Aphasiology Conference Proceedings* (pp. 196–204). Minneapolis, MN: BRK.

Kearns, K. P., & Potechin Scher, G. (1989). The generalization of Response Elaboration Training. In T. E. Prescott (Ed.), *Clinical Aphasiology* (pp. 223–245). Boston, MA: College-Hill.

Kertesz, A. (1979). *Aphasia and Associated Disorders: Taxonomy, Localization and Recovery.* New York, NY: Grune and Stratton.

Kunkle, A., Kopp, B., Muller, G. *et al.* (1999). Constraint-Induced Movement Therapy for motor recovery in chronic stroke patients. *Archives of Physical Medicine and Rehabilitation*, **80**, 624–628.

Kushner, D., & Winitz, H. (1977). Extended comprehension practice applied to an aphasic patient. *Journal of Speech and Hearing Disorders*, **42**, 296–306.

Li, E. C., Kitselman, K., Dusatko, D., & Spinelli, C. (1988). The efficacy of PACE in the remediation of naming deficits. *Journal of Communication Disorders*, **21**, 111–123.

Lincoln, N. B., & Blackburn, M. (1989). An investigation of factors affecting progress of patients on a stroke unit. *Journal of Neurology, Neurosurgery and Psychiatry*, **52**, 493–496.

Lincoln, N. B., McGuirk, E., Mulley, G. P. *et al.* (1984). Effectiveness of speech therapy for aphasic stroke patients. A randomized controlled trial. *Lancet*, **2**, 1197–1200.

Linebaugh, C. W., & Lehner, L. H. (1977). Cueing hierarchies and word retrieval: a therapy program. In R. H. Brookshire (Ed.), *Clinical Aphasiology Conference Proceedings* (pp. 19–31). Minneapolis, MN: BRK.

Loverso, F. L., Prescott, T. E., & Selinger, M. (1988). Cueing verbs: a treatment strategy for aphasic adults. *Journal of Rehabilitation and Research Development*, **25**, 47–60.

Lowell, S., Beeson, P. M., & Holland, A. L. (1995). The efficacy of semantic cueing procedures on naming performance of adults with aphasia. *American Journal of Speech-Language Pathology*, **4**, 109–114.

Lubinski, R. (2001). Environmental systems approach to adult aphasia. In R. Chapey (Ed.), *Language Intervention Strategies in Aphasia and Related Neurogenic Communication Disorders* (pp. 269–296). Philadelphia, PA: Lippincott Williams & Wilkins.

Luria, A. R. (1947). *Traumatic Aphasia: Its Syndromes, Psychology and Treatment*. (*Translation by D. Bowden, 1947*). Den Haag, Holland: Mouton Publishers.

Luria, A. R. (1948). *Restoration of Function after Brain Injury*. (*Translation by B. Haigh, 1963*). London, UK: Pergamon Press.

Maher, L. M., Chatterjee, A., & Rothi, L. J. G. (1995). Agrammatic sentence production: the use of a temporal-spatial strategy. *Brain and Language*, **49**, 105–124.

Maher, L. M., Kendall, D., Swearengin, J. A. *et al.* (2006). A pilot study of use-dependent learning in the context of Constraint Induced Language Therapy. *Journal of the International Neuropsychological Society*, **12**, 843–852.

Marshall, R. C., & Neuburger, S. I. (1984). Extended comprehension training reconsidered. In R. H. Brookshire (Ed.), *Clinical Aphasiology Conference Proceedings* (pp. 181–187). Minneapolis, MN: BRK.

Marshall, J., Pring, T., & Chiat, S. (1998). Verb retrieval and sentence production in aphasia. *Brain and Language*, **63**, 159–183.

Marshall, R. C., Karow, C. M., Freed, D. B., & Babcock, P. (2002). Effects of personalized cue form on the learning of subordinate category names by aphasic and non-brain damaged subjects. *Aphasiology*, **16**, 763–771.

Meinzer, M., Djundaja, D., Barthel, G., Elbert, T., & Rockstroh, B. (2005). Long-term stability of improved language functions in chronic aphasia after Constraint-Induced Aphasia Therapy. *Stroke*, **36**, 1462–1466.

Mills, R. H. (1982). Microcomputerized auditory comprehension training. In R. H. Brookshire (Ed.), *Clinical Aphasiology Conference Proceedings* (pp. 147–152). Minneapolis, MN: BRK.

Miltner, W., Bauder, H., Sommer, M., Dettmers, C., & Taub, E. (1999). Effects of Constraint-Induced Movement Therapy on patients with chronic motor deficits after stroke: a replication. *Stroke*, **30**, 586–592.

Mitchum, C. C., & Berndt, R. S. (1992). Verb retrieval and sentence construction: Effects of a targeted intervention. In M. J. Riddoch & G. W. Humphreys (Eds.), *Cognitive Neuropsychology and Cognitive Rehabilitation* (pp. 317–348). London, UK: Lawrence Erlbaum.

Morrow, K. L., & Fridriksson, J. (2006). Comparing fixed- and randomized-interval spaced retrieval in anomia treatment. *Journal of Communication Disorders*, **39**, 2–11.

Nadeau, S., Rothi, L. J. G., & Rosenbek, J. (in press). Language rehabilitation from a neural perspective. In R. Chapey (Ed.), *Language Intervention Strategies in Adult Aphasia*. Baltimore, MD: Williams and Wilkins.

Naeser, M. A., Haas, G., Mazurski, P., & Laughlin, S. (1986). Sentence level auditory comprehension treatment program for aphasic adults. *Archives of Physical Medicine and Rehabilitation*, **67**, 393–399.

Nickels, L., Byng, S., & Black, M. (1991). Sentence processing deficits: a replication of therapy. *British Journal of Disorders of Communication*, **26**, 175–199.

Orange, J. B., & Kertesz, A. (1998). Efficacy of language therapy for aphasia. *Physical Medicine and Rehabilitation: State of the Art Reviews*, **12**, 501–517.

Paolucci, S., Matano, A., Bragoni, M. *et al.* (2005). Rehabilitation of left brain-damaged ischemic stroke patients: the role of comprehension language deficits. A matched comparison. *Cerebrovascular Disease*, **20**, 400–406.

Penn, C., Jones, D., & Joffe, V. (1997). Hierarchical discourse therapy: a method for the mild patient. *Aphasiology*, **11**, 601–632.

Power, A. E. (2004). Slow-wave sleep, acetylcholine, and memory consolidation. *Proceedings of the National Academy of Sciences of the United States of America*, **101**, 1795–1796.

Pulvermuller, F., & Roth, V. M. (1991). Communicative aphasia treatment as a further development of PACE therapy. *Aphasiology*, **5**, 39–50.

Pulvermuller, F., Neininger, B., Elbert, T. *et al.* (2001). Constraint-induced therapy of chronic aphasia after stroke. *Stroke*, **32**, 1621–1626.

Pyle, W. H. (1913). Standards of mental efficiency. *Journal of Educational Psychology*, **4**, 61–70.

Raymer, A. M., Thompson, C. K., Jacobs, B., & LeGrand, H. R. (1993). Phonologic treatment of naming deficits in aphasia: model-based generalization analysis. *Aphasiology*, **7**, 27–53.

Raymer, A. M., Singletary, F., Rodriguez, A. *et al.* (2006). Gesture training effects for noun and verb retrieval in aphasia. *Journal of the International Neuropsychological Society*, **12**, 867–882.

Robey, R. R. (1994). The efficacy of treatment for aphasic persons: a meta-analysis. *Brain and Language*, **47**, 582–608.

Rochon, E., Laird, L., Bose, A., & Scofield, J. (2005). Mapping therapy for sentence production impairment in aphasia. *Neuropsychological Rehabilitation*, **15**, 1–36.

Rosenbek, J. C., LaPointe, L. L., & Wertz, R. T. (1989). *Aphasia: A Clinical Approach*. Austin, TX: Pro-Ed, Inc.

Saffran, E. M., Schwartz, M. F., & Marin, O. S. (1980). The word order problem in agrammatism. II. Production. *Brain and Language*, **10**, 263–280.

Sarno, M. T., Silverman, M., & Sands, E. (1970). Speech therapy and language recovery in severe aphasia. *Journal of Speech and Hearing Research*, **13**, 607–623.

Schwartz, M. F., Saffran, E. M., & Marin, O. S. (1980). The word order problem in agrammatism. I. Comprehension. *Brain and Language*, **10**, 249–262.

Schwartz, M. F., Saffran, E. M., Fink, R. B., Myers, J. L., & Martin, N. (1994). Mapping therapy: A treatment programme for agrammatism. *Aphasiology*, **8**, 19–54.

Shebilske, W., Goettl, B., & Regian, J. W. (1999). Executive control of automatic processes as complex skills develop in laboratory and applied settings. In D. Gopher & A. Koriat (Eds.), *Attention and Performance XVII: Cognitive Regulation of Performance: Interaction of Theory and Application* (pp. 401–432). Cambridge, MA: MIT Press.

Shewan, C. M., & Kertesz, A. (1984). Effects of speech and language treatment on recovery from aphasia. *Brain and Language*, **23**, 272–299.

Simmons-Mackie, N. (2001). Social approaches to aphasia rehabilitation. In R. Chapey (Ed.), *Language Intervention Strategies in Aphasia and Related Neurogenic Communication Disorders* (pp. 246–268). Philadelphia, PA: Lippincott Williams & Wilkins.

Sparks, R., Helm, N., & Albert, M. (1974). Aphasia rehabilitation resulting from Melodic Intonation Therapy. *Cortex*, **10**, 303–316.

Taub, E. (2000). Constraint-Induced Movement Therapy and massed practice. *Stroke*, **31**, 986–988.

Thompson, C. K. (1998). Treating sentence production in agrammatic aphasia. In N. Helm-Estabrooks & A. Holland (Eds.), *Approaches to Treatment of Aphasia* (pp. 113–151). San Diego, CA: Singular.

Thompson, C. K., & Kearns, K. P. (1981). An experimental analysis of acquisition, generalization, and maintenance of naming behavior in a patient with anomia. In R. H. Brookshire (Ed.), *Clinical Aphasiology Conference Proceedings* (pp. 19–31). Minneapolis, MN: BRK.

Thompson, C. K., Shapiro, L. P., & Roberts, M. M. (1993). Treatment of sentence production deficits in aphasia: a linguistic-specific approach to wh-interrogative training and generalization. *Aphasiology*, **7**, 111–133.

Thompson, C. K., Shapiro, L. P., Tait, M. E., Jacobs, B. J., & Schneider, S. L. (1996). Training wh-question production in agrammatic aphasia: analysis of argument and adjunct movement. *Brain and Language*, **52**, 175–228.

Thompson, C. K., Ballard, K. J., & Shapiro, L. P. (1998). The role of syntactic complexity in training wh-movement structures in agrammatic aphasia: optimal order for promoting generalization. *Journal of the International Neuropsychological Society*, **4**, 229–244.

Thompson, C. K., Shapiro, L. P., Kiran, S., & Sobecks, J. (2003). The role of syntactic complexity in treatment of sentence deficits in agrammatic aphasia: the complexity account of treatment efficacy (CATE). *Journal of Speech, Language and Hearing Disorders*, **46**, 591–607.

Wade, D. T., Hewer, R. L., David, R. M., & Enderby, P. M. (1986). Aphasia after stroke: natural history and associated deficits. *Journal of Neurology, Neurosurgery and Psychiatry*, **49**, 11–16.

Wambaugh, J. L. (2003). A comparison of the relative effects of phonologic and semantic cueing treatments. *Aphasiology*, **17**, 433–441.

Wambaugh, J. L., & Thompson, C. K. (1989). Training and generalization of agrammatic aphasic adults' WH-interrogative productions. *Journal of Speech and Hearing Disorders*, **54**, 509–525.

Wambaugh, J. L., & Martinez, A. L. (2000). Effects of modified Response Elaboration Training with apraxic and aphasic speakers. *Aphasiology*, **14**, 603–617.

Wambaugh, J. L., Linebaugh, C. W., Doyle, P. J. *et al.* (2001a). Effects of two cueing treatments on lexical retrieval in aphasic speakers with different levels of deficit. *Aphasiology*, **15**, 933–950.

Wambaugh, J. L., Martinez, A. L., & Alegre, M. N. (2001b). Qualitative changes following application of modified response elaboration training with apraxic-aphasic speakers. *Aphasiology*, **15**, 965–976.

Wertz, R. T., & Irwin, W. H. (2001). Darley and the efficacy of language rehabilitation in aphasia. *Aphasiology*, **15**, 231–247.

Wertz, R. T., Weiss, D. G., Aten, J. L. *et al.* (1986). Comparison of clinic, home, and deferred language treatment for aphasia. A Veterans Administration Cooperative Study. *Archives of Neurology*, **43**, 653–658.

West, J. A. (1973). Auditory comprehension in aphasic adults: improvement through training. *Archives of Physical Medicine and Rehabilitation*, **54**, 78–86.

Whitney, J., & Goldstein, H. (1989). Using self-monitoring to reduce disfluencies in speakers with mild aphasia. *Journal of Speech and Hearing Disorders*, **54**, 576–586.

Wierenga, C., Maher, L. M., & Moore, A. B. (2006). Neural substrates of syntactic mapping treatment: an fMRI study of two cases. *Journal of the International Neuropsychological Society*, **12**, 132–146.

26

Rehabilitation of neglect

Victoria Singh-Curry and Masud Husain

Introduction

- The neglect syndrome is associated with a failure to attend to one side of space following unilateral brain injury, most commonly stroke.
- Neglect is a common disorder which can have a negative effect on long-term functional outcome.
- The syndrome is heterogenous, with different patients having varying combinations of underlying cognitive deficits.
- The pattern of cognitive deficits depends upon the areas of brain damaged – and those left intact.
- Both spatial and nonspatial mechanisms contribute to neglect and may represent different targets for treatments aimed at rehabilitating the condition.

The neglect syndrome is a common disorder following unilateral brain injury, particularly prominent after right-hemisphere stroke. It consists of a striking failure to orient towards, report or act upon stimuli – objects, people and even the patient's own body parts – in contralesional space (left side for individuals with right-hemisphere damage and vice versa). This lateralization may result from hemispheric asymmetries that exist for attention functions in the human brain. Many patients are also unaware of their deficits (*anosognosia*) making persistent neglect a disabling syndrome which is particularly difficult to rehabilitate (Robertson & Halligan, 1999). Thus neglect patients generally have poorer functional outcomes compared with other stroke patients with similar physical disabilities.

Neglect is not a unitary disorder, but rather a syndrome. Patients may neglect the contralesional side of their own body (*personal neglect*), near space (*peripersonal neglect*) or distant space (*extrapersonal neglect*). Some patients are primarily deficient in attending to and perceiving objects in contralesional space, even though they may not have any primary sensory disorder. By contrast, others may show little spontaneous use of their contralesional limbs (*motor neglect*), despite being reasonably strong. Different patients may demonstrate different combinations of neglect behavior (Buxbaum *et al.*, 2004), so clinical assessments often consist of a battery of tests (Figure 26.1), designed to take this variation into account (Parton *et al.*, 2004).

Such diversity is likely to be based on the known heterogeneity of brain lesions responsible for the condition. In general, regions in the right inferior parietal and inferior frontal lobe have consistently been implicated in neglect (Mort *et al.*, 2003; Vallar, 2001). However, subcortical strokes too may lead to neglect due to remote effects, e.g., hypoperfusion, of overlying cortical regions, or because of disconnection of parieto-frontal circuits (Doricchi & Tomaiuolo, 2003; Hillis *et al.*, 2005; Karnath *et al.*, 2002). Other studies have also suggested a role for lateral (Karnath *et al.*, 2001) or medial temporal regions in the right hemisphere (Bird *et al.*, 2006; Mort *et al.*, 2003). Even within the classical inferior parietal and frontal areas implicated in neglect, the extent of lesions varies considerably, and because these regions have multiple

Cognitive Neurorehabilitation, Second Edition: Evidence and Application, ed. Donald T. Stuss, Gordon Winocur and Ian H. Robertson. Published by Cambridge University Press. © Cambridge University Press 2008.

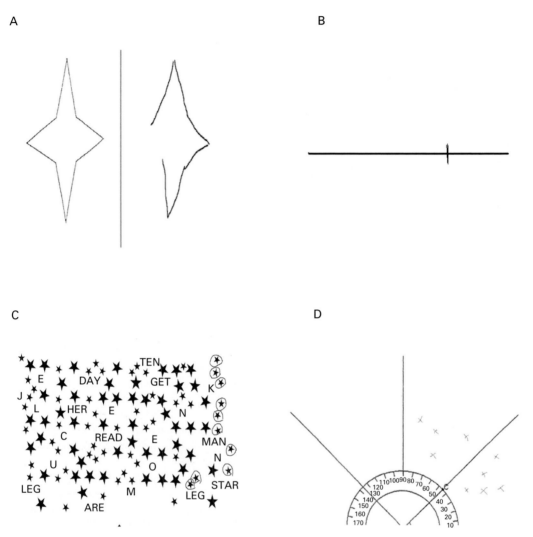

Figure 26.1. Bedside tests of neglect. (A) *Copying objects.* The left side of the star has been omitted. (B) *Line bisection.* When asked to mark the middle of a horizontal line, some patients deviate to the right. (C) *Cancellation tasks.* In this example the patient was asked to circle all of the small stars. Only a few on the far right of the sheet have been circled. (D) *Naming objects around a room.* On this test of extrapersonal neglect, the patient named several objects to the right but none from the left side.

functions, the exact combination of deficits observed in patients is likely to differ according to the distribution of the lesion and its distant effects.

Several cognitive deficits have been postulated to explain the phenomena underlying neglect. Broadly speaking, these can be divided into spatial and nonspatial mechanisms. These are *not* mutually incompatible but instead probably combine to exacerbate the severity of neglect (Husain & Rorden, 2003; Robertson, 2001).

Spatial mechanisms include several types of potential deficit. Some researchers have pointed to evidence for a *spatial gradient of attention* biased towards ipsilesional space (right side for right-hemisphere patients) and away from the contralesional side (Kinsbourne, 1993; Smania *et al.*, 1998). Others have shown that there may be difficulty in *disengaging attention* from stimuli in ipsilesional space and shifting it contralesionally (Posner *et al.*, 1984). More recent theories have also considered a pathological *competitive spatial bias* in which contralesional items lose in the competition for selective attention to ipsilesional items (Duncan *et al.*, 1997). Spatial deficits may play a role too in the *directional motor deficits* that some neglect patients show (Mattingley *et al.*, 1998), while a disorder of keeping track of spatial locations – in *spatial working memory* – is evident in many individuals with the syndrome (Mannan *et al.*, 2005). Finally, all of these impairments may contribute to neglect patients having a disordered *egocentric representation* of the space around them (Bisiach, 1993).

Nonspatial mechanisms have more recently been considered to play an important role in the neglect syndrome (Husain & Rorden, 2003; Robertson, 2001). Deficits in *sustained attention* – even for stimuli that are presented centrally – correlate with the severity of neglect (Robertson *et al.*, 1997). Inferior parietal and frontal regions in the right hemisphere appear to play a critical role in maintaining attention (Husain & Rorden, 2003). In addition to sustained attention deficits, impaired *selective attention* for items presented in either left or right space, or centrally at fixation, is also evident in individuals with neglect (Duncan *et al.*, 1999; Husain *et al.*, 1997). Thus bilateral impairment may be present in neglect despite the most striking aspect of a patient's behavior appearing to be a profound bias towards one side of space. Nonspatial deficits may nevertheless interact with spatial mechanisms to influence the severity of neglect (Husain & Rorden, 2003). For example, a phasic warning sound can reduce the rightward bias of neglect patients on a visual task, even if this sound originates from a rightward location (Robertson *et al.*, 1998b).

Summary

Neglect is a diverse syndrome composed of varying underlying cognitive deficits, which can be discussed in terms of spatial and nonspatial processes. The precise pattern of impairment depends on lesion location and the severity of damage to particular brain regions. We will see in the remainder of this chapter that the functions of undamaged areas of brain are likely to be crucial in predicting the response of particular patients to specific therapies.

Techniques used in the rehabilitation of neglect

- The heterogeneity of the neglect syndrome is related to the variation in location and extent of lesions associated with the disorder.
- Lesion anatomy may therefore be important in determining the most appropriate therapy for patients.
- There are three categories of rehabilitation employed in the treatment of neglect: (1) behavioral techniques, (2) the use of specialized devices and (3) pharmacologic treatments.

Although research on the cognitive processes underlying neglect has guided the development of various rehabilitative methods, few of these techniques have been shown to lead to consistent functional recovery (Luaute *et al.*, 2006; Robertson & Halligan, 1999). In some cases, this may be due to a lack of efficacy of the individual techniques, and in others because of a lack of randomized controlled trials (RCTs). However, another key issue may be the heterogeneity of the syndrome. If different patients have different combinations of deficit, which interact in different ways, one intervention may not be appropriate or effective for everyone. A related concern is that for a particular treatment to be effective it may be crucial that certain brain regions or functions are intact. For example, learning a new strategy may depend upon the integrity of prefrontal regions. Patients who have large parts of such critical brain regions destroyed by their stroke may not be so responsive to that treatment. Thus mapping the lesions of patients involved in trials may be important to understand variations in response to therapy. Finally, it is important to bear in mind when considering treatments that most studies have examined the effects of intervention on neglect as measured using standard neuropsychological tests. It is important also to assess the effects of treatment on more ecologically valid measures as well as on overall functional outcome.

We now discuss some of these rehabilitative techniques, focusing on their efficacy, the underlying mechanisms they may be targeting and the potential for future research. We will divide these therapies as follows:
(1) Purely behavioral interventions.
(2) Treatments involving devices or specialized equipment.
(3) Pharmacological therapies.
Because the rehabilitation of neglect is still in its infancy, there have been few attempts to combine such interventions, but the use of such concurrent treatment might potentially be very powerful if there were synergistic effects.

Behavioral therapies

- Behavioral techniques use *strategies* to help patients orientate attention to the neglected part of space or body.
- Visual scanning or visuospatial training is commonly used but its long-term general efficacy is unclear.
- Feedback, mental imagery, sustained attention training and limb activation have all been reported to be effective but require more extensive testing.

Visual scanning or visuospatial training involves cueing the patient to make leftward eye or head movements. It is used commonly by therapists on stroke and rehabilitation units and involves explicit instructions encouraging these behaviors, e.g., asking the patient to locate the left-hand margin of a page (initially marked with a thick red line) before starting a new line when reading. Although commonly used in clinical practice, there have been

relatively few RCTs demonstrating its efficacy, and where improvements have been shown, these have either been on pen-and-paper tests of neglect rather than behavioral measures, or there has been no follow-up to document whether improvement is maintained (for review see Luaute *et al.*, 2006). Further RCTs are needed, with a prolonged period of follow-up and functional assessment measures. This is critical because early studies of this intervention suggested that there was little generalization of such scanning behavior to tasks outside the training environment (Robertson & Halligan, 1999).

Feedback training attempts to provide information to the patient regarding their impaired performance, originating from the observation that neglect is often accompanied by anosognosia (lack of awareness of deficit). Two methods have been used: (1) visuomotor feedback and (2) video feedback. If a patient is allowed to grasp – rather than point to – the midpoint of a rod, improvement on certain tests of neglect can be obtained over a period of a few days (Harvey *et al.*, 2003; Robertson *et al.*, 1995). However, these tests have all been pen-and-paper tasks. Similarly, providing patients with the opportunity to view their impaired performance on video (with their left side appearing on the right of the screen) combined with discussion of appropriate strategies with a therapist can lead to better subsequent performance of that task – but only that task (Tham & Tegner, 1997). Further study of this technique is needed before any firm conclusions can be drawn.

One matched control trial using functional outcome measures has been conducted to assess *mental imagery training* (Niemeier, 1998). In this study the treatment group was asked to imagine themselves as "lighthouses," sweeping their gaze from left to right. At the end of the treatment period, the experimental group scored significantly better than the control group on standard tests of neglect but also on a functional autonomy rating scale scored by therapists. Reports by family and caregivers, although not formally analyzed, also provided evidence of increased improvement in the treatment group. Unfortunately, the groups were not followed up beyond the end of the treatment period, so very little can be said about the long-term benefit of this technique.

A different strategy has been aimed towards non-spatial deficits by Robertson and colleagues. In their study, neglect patients were required to carry out a variety of tasks that required *sustained attention*, e.g., sorting coins or cards. The investigator would intermittently prompt patients verbally to attend during this. Gradually, patients were trained to prompt themselves subvocally, and were made aware of their sustained attention deficit as well as the importance of this self-alerting process. The eight patients who participated showed considerable improvements 24 hours after training on tests of sustained attention and neglect (Robertson *et al.*, 1995). However, the nature of the intervention requires patients to be aware of their deficit, as well as the situations in which it is necessary to use the alerting procedure. The degree to which patients are able to do this may limit the general applicability of this technique.

Limb activation therapy is based on the idea that making voluntary movements with the contralesional limb in contralesional space can activate poorly attended areas in extrapersonal space and thereby reduce the severity of neglect. There is evidence to suggest that such "spatiomotor cueing" may be effective even if the patient can not see the moving limb (Robertson & North, 1993). An obvious constraint of this technique is that it requires some movement of the often hemiparetic contralesional limb. However, it has been demonstrated that even passive movements of the left arm, if large enough (i.e., of the elbow rather than the wrist), can lead to improvements in neglect (Frassinetti *et al.*, 2001). One randomized-controlled group study has examined the efficacy of this intervention and found that it was associated with reduced inpatient stay, but, although there was a trend towards improved functional outcome, this did not reach conventional levels of statistical significance (Kalra *et al.*, 1997).

Summary

The techniques discussed so far encourage the development of strategies by the patient in order to compensate for their impairment. These strategies are achieved through training sessions with a therapist, which are tailored to the needs of the individual patient. Although in the case of some of these techniques they are the longest established, further trials are needed to properly demonstrate their functional efficacy over a prolonged period of time.

Therapies requiring specialized devices

- A large number of interventions employing devices have been designed to help treat neglect.
- Some of these techniques use devices to extend the behavioral approaches already discussed, whilst others target specific cognitive deficits.

The techniques discussed in this section all have in common the use of devices which have either been taken from other areas of neuroscience research, with the hypothesis that they may have an impact on the signs of neglect, or developed specifically with the aim of producing a new treatment for neglect. Some of these treatments have followed on from behavioral interventions, whilst others seek to target particular underlying cognitive deficits. This section will therefore be further divided as follows:

(1) Treatments using devices to aid in the development of cognitive strategies (i.e., following on from the behavioral interventions discussed above).
(2) Techniques aimed at correcting a disordered egocentric representation of space.
(3) Therapies seeking to alter higher-order spatial representations.
(4) A technique to correct interhemispheric imbalance.

Behavioral therapies incorporating the use of devices

- The neglect alert device phasically alerts the patient as well as acting as a spatiomotor cue to produce a benefit.
- The use of scanning boards has not led to general improvement in neglect.

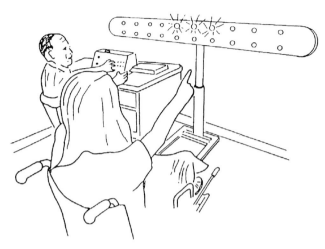

Figure 26.2. Although there is a long history of use of visual scanning therapy, definitive and reliable evidence is lacking regarding its functional efficacy.

● The combination of computerized alertness training with other therapies has considerable potential. Following on from the studies on limb activation, which require the patient to move their contralesional limb, a *neglect alerting device* has been developed. This consists of a light box which emits a loud buzzing noise if its switch is not pressed (by the left hand in left-sided neglect) within a predetermined but variable time limit. A red light also remains on if the switch is not pressed (or activated by movement of the left limb in the case of portable devices attached to the limb) when it should be. These features may in addition help to phasically alert the patient, so the device may potentially improve sustained attention as well as acting as a "spatiomotor cue." It has been shown, in a single patient study, that use of this device can be associated with improvement in peripersonal, but not personal or extrapersonal, neglect (although only one task assessing each of these types of neglect was used). This improvement was maintained at 9 days post-treatment (Robertson *et al.*, 1998a).

A single-blind randomized control trial comparing the use of an alerting device along with standard cognitive training to standard cognitive training alone has since been carried out (Robertson *et al.*, 2002). A total of 32 patients were followed up for 6 months after weekly training sessions administered over 12 weeks. A significant improvement was found in left-sided motor function in neglect patients randomized to limb activation training (with a neglect alert device) in addition to cognitive training, as compared with those receiving cognitive training alone. No significant difference was found between the two groups on the Barthel activities of daily living index or on tests assessing the severity of neglect. Therefore, on the basis of these results, whilst it seems that limb activation using an alerting device is beneficial to neglect patients in terms of their ability to move their affected limbs, it is not clear that this improvement is brought about by a more general amelioration of their neglect symptoms. This issue needs clarification in future work.

Early trials that aimed to improve visual scanning of neglected space also used a *scanning board* (Figure 26.2), a device which allowed the therapist to control a series of lights (Diller & Weinberg, 1977). Patients were asked to point to the lights as they were sequentially turned on further towards the contralesional side. Although this was effective in improving eye movements towards the neglected side on the task, the positive effects did not appear to generalize well outside of this specific testing environment.

In addition to behavioral techniques for improving attention deficits, a series of investigations have been conducted using *computerized training tasks* for alertness and vigilance, as well as selective and divided attention (Sturm *et al.*, 1997). The provision of such training led to significant improvement on standard tests for each domain, whilst nonspecific training of attention problems actually led to deterioration. A more recent investigation (Thimm *et al.*, 2006) assessed the effects of a 3-week computerized alertness training program on seven chronic neglect patients. Following this, the patients performed significantly better on a series of tests assessing alertness and neglect, and these behavioral changes were accompanied by an increase in fMRI activations in right frontoparietal regions associated with alerting and visuospatial attention. Four weeks later, however, most of the behavioral improvement had disappeared, paralleled by a reduction in neural activity on fMRI. While computerized alertness training seems insufficient by itself to induce a lasting improvement in neglect, it is possible that more encouraging results might be obtained if it were to be combined with another rehabilitative technique.

Summary

Limb activation training with the use of a neglect alerting device has shown some encouraging results when combined with traditional cognitive therapy; although further studies are needed to clarify the extent of the benefit obtainable.

Computerized alertness training may also prove to be helpful, if paired with other techniques.

Devices used to correct a disordered egocentric representation of space

- Rotation of the head or trunk has produced some encouraging results. However, the cumbersome nature of some of the devices used has limited its uptake.
- Neck muscle vibration seems very promising, but larger randomized studies are now needed.

- Vestibular stimulation and optokinetic stimulation are unlikely to contribute significantly to the future treatment of neglect.

Rotation of the head or trunk towards the neglected side has often been considered as an alternative way to improve space exploration of the neglected field, by re-centering the egocentric frame of reference (Luaute *et al.*, 2006). One randomised controlled trial used an unusual training device (the Bon Saint Come corset device) which required patients to move a pointer attached to the corset they wore on their trunk to touch targets associated with particular sounds or visual signals. Compared with a control group, patients who used this device were significantly better on a variety of outcome measures including functional scales. This improvement was found to be maintained at 1-month follow-up (Wiart *et al.*, 1997). Despite this encouraging result, no further studies have been carried out with this technique, perhaps due to difficulties in making and maintaining such contraptions.

Neck muscle vibration (NMV) is thought to effect a re-centering of the egocentric frame of reference, by an illusory modification of the afferent information regarding the orientation of the head in space, rather than a real one. Neck muscle vibration is delivered by transcutaneous stimulation with electrodes placed on the posterior left neck muscles. Neck muscle vibration has produced a temporary (up to 30 minute) improvement of neglect on, for example, cancellation tasks (Vallar *et al.*, 1995), mental imagery tests (Guariglia *et al.*, 1998) and postural stability (Perennou *et al.*, 2001). One group did find more permanent effects (stable at 1.4 years). However, these effects were significant only for one of the two pen-and-paper cancellation tests used to measure neglect (Johannsen *et al.*, 2003). A further study investigated the combination of NMV with visual scanning training in a cross-over design. The authors reported that the combination was significantly better than visual scanning training alone. Moreover, this improvement was stable at 2-month follow-up and was also found to affect functional measures of outcome (Schindler *et al.*, 2002).

Left-sided vestibular stimulation (produced by irrigating the left ear with cold water to induce slow phase leftward nystagmus) can alleviate left-sided neglect (Rode & Perenin, 1994; Rubens, 1985). However, it produces only short-lasting effects and is not a particularly pleasant method of rehabilitation! Similarly, although *optokinetic stimulation*, produced by a background of moving dots or lines, is associated with some amelioration of neglect when the direction of movement is to the left, this too is short-lived (Karnath, 1996; Vallar *et al.*, 1997). Neither of these two techniques therefore seems particularly promising for neglect rehabilitation.

Summary

Head or trunk rotation can produce functional improvement in neglect patients. This technique however, is limited by the unwieldy nature of the apparatus used. The device, targeting the egocentric representation of space, which offers the most promise for future rehabilitation programs is neck muscle vibration.

Techniques used to alter higher-order spatial representations

- Prism adaptation has been shown to have long-lasting effects, in some patients.
- Eye patching has not produced any consistent benefit.
- Space remapping training is a new and intriguing technique that requires longer-term evaluation.

Prism adaptation has been used for many years as a tool to explore visuomotor plasticity. It was first shown in 1998 that amelioration of left-sided neglect could *follow* prism adaptation to a rightward optical deviation (Rossetti *et al.*, 1998). Note that the positive effects of prisms occurred after adaptation, not while wearing prisms. When people put on right-deviating prisms, visual targets are displaced to the right. Therefore, when the participant performs pointing movements to such targets, they miss and receive visual feedback that they have reached too far to the right. With successive pointing

movements, this visual feedback leads to motor correction towards the left, a process termed visuomotor adaptation or error reduction (Figure 26.3). When the prisms are removed and visual feedback of limb position is not available or the subject is making rapid, ballistic movements, they usually show a systematic deviation *to the left* when pointing to a visual target (Figure 26.3d). This is the prism after-effect. The process of adapting to such right-deviating prisms appears to lead to improvements in left-sided neglect but the mechanisms underlying this shift in behavior remain controversial (Redding & Wallace, 2006).

The effects of prism adapation have now been shown to be relatively long-lasting and to be associated with an improvement on various tests of neglect, including some behavioral tasks. For example, one study gave a group of seven neglect patients twice-daily training sessions with prisms for 2 weeks and compared them with six control patients matched in terms of neglect severity. All but one of the experimental patients performed significantly better than the control patients on all tests used, with improvement being maintained 5 weeks after treatment ceased (Frassinetti *et al.*, 2002). The duration of neglect amelioration was found to correlate with the length of the after-effect in that study. This has been explained in terms of an effect of prism adaptation on two levels of cognitive function: (1) low-order functions – i.e., sensorimotor coordination and (2) higher-order spatial representations. The authors postulated that the effects of prism adaptation on low-order functions were short lasting, whereas the effects on spatial representation were longer lasting.

Numerous studies have now demonstrated that various aspects of neglect behavior can be ameliorated following prism adaptation. For example, somatosensory deficits (Dijkerman *et al.*, 2004; Maravita *et al.*, 2003), visuoverbal measures (Farne *et al.*, 2002) and postural control (Tilikete *et al.*, 2001) have all been shown to be improved. But not all studies have demonstrated consistent benefits. One recent investigation evaluated the effects of prism adaptation in ten patients, in a repeated

Optical Effect of
Rightward Prism
Induced Shift

Start of Prism
Adaptation Period

End of Prism
Adaptation Period

Post-Adaptation
(After Effect)

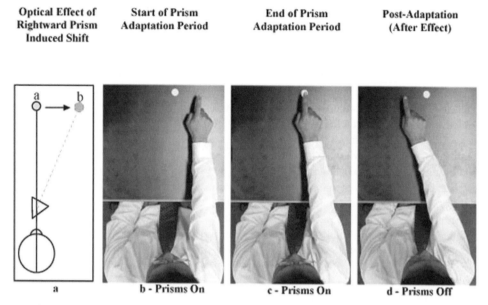

a   b - Prisms On   c - Prisms On   d - Prisms Off

Figure 26.3. The process of adaptation to *rightward* displacing prismatic lenses. When viewing a scene through wedge prisms, all points are displaced horizontally to the right with respect to the optic axis of the eye (see a). Hence, an object at point a will appear to be located at point b. The adaptation process requires the observer to repeatedly reach for targets within the field of view. Misreaching occurs in the early trials (see b). The error quickly improves and disappears completely (*error reduction* or *visuomotor adaptation*) as the participant adapts to the visual shift (see c), although approximately 50 repetitions should be completed for this to fully occur. When the prisms are removed the participant will misreach in the opposite direction to the visual shift (see d), an error referred to as the *after-effect*. In normal observers this after-effect will disappear after only a few minutes, but is much more prolonged in some neglect patients. Adapted from Parton *et al.* (2004) with permission.

measures design. Prismatic lenses or neutral lenses were counterbalanced for order, with a 1-week interval between them. Only partial improvement of neglect was found in the late testing sessions, independent of the type of lens in use, prismatic or neutral (Rousseaux *et al.*, 2006). However, no information is given in this study regarding the size or site of the lesions involved which might be important in determining the capacity for significant improvement.

By contrast, another investigation sought specifically to analyse the behavioral and neuroanatomical predictors of neglect amelioration following prism adaptation (Serino *et al.*, 2006). The treated group, consisting of 16 patients, obtained long-lasting amelioration of their neglect (up to 3 months post-treatment) on a battery of tests which included

some behavioral measures. Following treatment, neglect patients displayed a deviation of their oculomotor responses to the left which was positively correlated with the degree of improvement obtained on neglect tests. These two factors were also found to correlate with the level of visuomotor adaptation obtained whilst wearing the prisms, rather than the after-effect, with patients who were unable to adapt to prisms obtaining little benefit. Lack of benefit from prism adaptation, as well as lack of leftward eye deviation, was found to be associated with large occipital lesions, but not total lesion volume. Large frontal lesions were also associated with poor outcome, perhaps related to the role played by the right frontal lobe in maintaining vigilance and sustaining attention (Husain & Rorden, 2003; Robertson, 2001). Prism adaptation clearly has produced some remarkable long-lasting effects in some patients with neglect. The challenge for the future is to define more precisely those individuals who are most likely to benefit.

Less promising has been the technique of *eye patching*. The rationale for this was based on the theory that each eye has a stronger projection to the contralesional superior colliculus, so patching the ipsilesional eye will reduce input to the contralesional colliculus, thereby allowing the ipsilesional colliculus to initiate more eye movements into the contralesional visual field. It was therefore hypothesized that right eye patching would ameliorate left-sided neglect and left eye patching would increase it. Unfortunately, no consistent improvement was found (Butter & Kirsch, 1992; Walker *et al.*, 1996). *Hemiblinding*, which consists of obscuring vision from the ipsilesional hemifield in both eyes (by wearing "hemianopic" spectacles), has shown more favorable results (Beis *et al.*, 1999; Zeloni *et al.*, 2002). This technique may work by forcing patients to use information from the contralesional visual field and requires further evaluation.

Space remapping training is based on the interesting observation that a stick or tool held by a patient can produce an extension of the body space, such that far space is "remapped" as near space (Berti & Frassinetti, 2000; Farne & Ladavas, 2000). It has also proved possible effectively to "remap" left space as right space (Ackroyd *et al.*, 2002; Castiello *et al.*, 2004). For example, in a virtual reality study, six left-sided neglect patients were asked to reach and grasp a real object. As they did so, they observed the grasping of a virtual object in a virtual environment by a virtual hand – influenced in real time by the movements of their own hand (Castiello *et al.*, 2004). The patients were exposed to a number of trials in which the virtual object appeared on the left side of the virtual space, while they grasped (beneath a screen) a real object located to the right. Following this training, all the patients were able to reach into their left, neglected hemispace, something they had been unable to do prior to training. The mechanism underlying the effect has been proposed to be related to the synthesis of proprioception from the real hand and vision of the virtual hand, by bimodal neurons (responsive to both visual and proprioceptive input) in the parietal cortex. It is suggested that this may act to forge links between neglected and spared space representations (Castiello *et al.*, 2004). Long-term evaluation of this new technique has not been performed.

Summary

A substantial body of the work conducted with devices in neglect rehabilitation has focused on prism adaptation. However, even for this technique, the mechanisms underlying the positive effects remain to be elucidated. Moreover, it is clear that not all patients respond to such treatment, therefore future studies need to consider the causes of variability of response to interventions, including lesion anatomy.

A treatment approach aiming to restore interhemispheric imbalance

- Repetitive transcranial magnetic stimulation is a new and interesting technique that needs further evaluation.

Repetitive transcranial magnetic stimulation (rTMS) is a technique that has been introduced more recently to neglect treatment. The motivation stems from the possibility of restoring balance between the two cerebral hemispheres. Kinsbourne had originally suggested that neglect may result from a pathological hyperactivity of the left hemisphere following right brain damage (Kinsbourne, 1977). When transiently administered over the contralesional parietal lobe (causing short-lasting inhibition), rTMS improves performance of patients on computerised line bisection tasks (Oliveri *et al.*, 2001). Two subsequent studies using this technique (Brighina *et al.*, 2003; Shindo *et al.*, 2006) have demonstrated that low frequency rTMS may be associated with an improvement on a wider range of neglect tasks, including some activities of daily living which are particularly affected by neglect. Moreover, this effect can last for at least 6 weeks (Shindo *et al.*, 2006). Larger, controlled studies are now needed to investigate the potential of this technique further.

Pharmacological therapies

- Several attempts have been made to use dopaminergic drugs but these studies have not been systematic and the effects have been highly variable.
- Noradrenergic agonists have been less well explored but there is some limited evidence of a positive effect using guanfacine, an alpha-2 agonist.

Two different classes of pharmacologic agents have been investigated for potential use in the rehabilitation of neglect. Both target catecholamine systems, either dopaminergic, noradrenergic or possibly both. The rationale for using these compounds comes from animal studies. For example, unilateral injections of the dopaminergic neurotoxin 6-hydroxydopamine into the ventral tegmental area of rats may produce a form of sensory inattention (Marshall, 1979) which is reversible on administration of the dopamine agonist apomorphine (Marshall & Gotthelf, 1979). Similarly, unilateral injections of another dopaminergic neurotoxin, 1-methyl-4-phenyl-1,2,3,6-tetrahydropyridine (MPTP), into the caudate nucleus of monkeys may induce a form of visual inattention (Miyashita *et al.*, 1995). However, it has to be borne in mind that animal models do not mirror the severity or long-lasting nature of the syndrome that is often seen in humans.

Dopaminergic drugs can ameliorate some of the signs of neglect in humans. Bromocriptine given daily for 3–4 weeks led to improvement in line bisection, cancellation tests and reading in two patients with neglect (Fleet *et al.*, 1987). Another study reported that bromocriptine was superior to methylphenidate in causing improvement, but this was in a single patient and the design of the investigation was not ideal (Hurford *et al.*, 1998). Two further studies, one using L-Dopa or levodopa – the precursor of dopamine – (Mukand *et al.*, 2001) and the other apomorphine (Geminiani *et al.*, 1998), have

also demonstrated improvement on standard tests of neglect, but in small groups of patients. However, some reports have not demonstrated a beneficial effect of dopaminergic compounds.

One investigation of seven patients found that, compared with pre-dose testing, visual exploration of the left hemifield on a computerized search task actually worsened after bromocriptine in all but one patient, although target detection in the left hemifield was unaltered (Grujic *et al.*, 1998). All of the patients in this study performed normally on bedside tests of neglect, but clearly demonstrated some neglect on the computerized search task, suggesting that their neglect was relatively mild and that they had perhaps already made substantial recovery, possibly leaving little room for further improvement. Another group also failed to document an improvement of neglect with bromocriptine (Barrett *et al.*, 1999). But, again, this was only a single case study and only one measure of neglect (line bisection) was used. The patient had a lesion which affected both cortical and subcortical structures. It is possible that an appropriately combined cortical and subcortical lesion may disrupt both the mesostriatal and mesocortical dopaminergic systems to such an extent that any exogenous dopaminergic stimulation can only act upon the contralesional hemisphere, thus leading to no improvement or even a deterioration in neglect signs. This is a factor which may need to be considered when assessing neglect patients for participation in future studies.

But how does dopaminergic stimulation affect space exploration in neglect? Studies in primates, including healthy humans, suggest that stimulation of D1 dopamine receptors may improve attention and spatial working memory processes, while D2 agonists can have the opposite effect (Castner & Goldman-Rakic, 2004; Kimberg & D'Esposito, 2003; Muller *et al.*, 1998). However, the relationship and interaction between different dopaminergic receptors is complex. For example, the dose-response curve to dopaminergic stimulation appears to be an inverted U-shape; consequently too little or too much stimulation may be ineffective. In addition, endogenous dopaminergic activity also declines with normal aging and different individuals have different polymorphisms of dopamine metabolizing enzymes. These complexities pose a challenge to future studies using dopaminergic drugs.

Noradrenergic compounds have been even less frequently used. In monkeys, the α2-noradrenergic agonist guanfacine improves performance on spatial delayed response tasks (Franowicz & Arnsten, 1998) by modulating dorsolateral prefrontal cortex (Avery *et al.*, 2000). Guanfacine also improves planning and working memory performance in normal humans (Jakala et al., 1999). A small proof of principle, double-blind cross-over trial has recently been carried out using guanfacine in three neglect patients (Malhotra *et al.*, 2006). An improvement was demonstrated in two of the three patients on pen-and-paper tests of neglect, as well as a computerized visual exploration task. Both the patients who improved were able to sustain attention for signifcantly longer on the space exploration task following guanfacine. The third patient, who did not improve, had a lesion which included the right dorsolateral prefrontal region. Thus it is possible that guanfacine had no effect because of a lack of substrate. Larger trials are now needed, in selected neglect patients, to further investigate the potential of this drug therapy.

Summary

In this section we have discussed two pharmacological modes of treatment for neglect. Studies examining both have yielded some interesting results. However, all the investigations have been small and larger trials with carefully defined patient groups will be required before further advances are likely to be made. Combining pharmacological therapies with other techniques may be particularly beneficial.

Summary and conclusions

Numerous techniques aimed at ameliorating neglect have been developed over the years. However, the syndrome remains difficult to treat effectively for several reasons. First, neglect is heterogenous. There are different subtypes which can dissociate from each other, and different patients may suffer from different combinations of cognitive deficit, so one type of treatment may not be suitable for all individuals. Second, the right hemisphere contains the critical neural circuits responsible for sustaining attention, as well as those necessary for maintaining spatiomotor representations. If a patient is unable to maintain attention, this will have a profound impact on their ability to participate in and benefit from any therapy. Third, lesions of the right hemisphere are often accompanied by depression and anosognosia. If a patient has no motivation to participate in therapy, or does not believe they need any because there is nothing wrong with them, the potential effects of intervention may be limited. Finally, neglect is often associated with extensive lesions of the right hemisphere, affecting cortical and subcortical structures. The larger the area damaged, the less potential there may be for plastic changes and functional reorganization leading to recovery.

Despite all these limitations, it also has to be borne in mind that systematic treatment of neglect is still in its infancy, and though the current literature is highly variable there are reasons to be optimistic. Recent developments in understanding the heterogeneity of the syndrome, its anatomical basis and the range of cognitive deficits underlying it are surely likely to improve the design of treatment trials. Moreover, it may one day be possible to combine interventions, tailored to individual requirements, based on detailed assessments of patients' cognitive deficits and lesion anatomy.

ACKNOWLEDGMENT

This work was funded by The Wellcome Trust.

REFERENCES

Ackroyd, K., Riddoch, M. J., Humphreys, G. W., Nightingale, S., & Townsend, S. (2002). Widening the sphere of influence: using a tool to extend extrapersonal visual space in a patient with severe neglect. *Neurocase*, **8**, 1–12.

Avery, R. A., Franowicz, J. S., Studholme, C., van Dyck, C. H., & Arnsten, A. F. T. (2000). The alpha-2A-adrenoceptor agonist, guanfacine, increases regional cerebral blood flow in dorsolateral prefrontal cortex of monkeys performing a spatial working memory task. *Neuropsychopharmacology*, **23**, 240–249.

Barrett, A. M., Crucian, G. P., Schwartz, R. L., & Heilman, K. M. (1999). Adverse effect of dopamine agonist therapy in a patient with motor-intentional neglect. *Archives of Physical Medicine and Rehabilitation*, **80**, 600–603.

Beis, J. M., Andre, J. M., Baumgarten, A., & Challier, B. (1999). Eye patching in unilateral spatial neglect: efficacy of two methods. *Archives of Physical Medicine and Rehabilitation*, **80**, 71–76.

Berti, A., & Frassinetti, F. (2000). When far becomes near: remapping of space by tool use. *Journal of Cognitive Neuroscience*, **12**, 415–420.

Bird, C. M., Malhotra, P., Parton, A. et al. (2006). Visual neglect following right posterior cerebral artery infarction. *Journal of Neurology, Neurosurgery and Psychiatry*, **77**, 1008–1012.

Bisiach, E. (1993). Mental representation in unilateral neglect and related disorders: the twentieth Bartlett Memorial Lecture. *Quarterly Journal of Experimental Psychology Section A: Human Experimental Psychology*, **46**, 435–461.

Brighina, F., Bisiach, E., Oliveri, M. et al. (2003). 1 Hz repetitive transcranial magnetic stimulation of the unaffected hemisphere ameliorates contralesional visuospatial neglect in humans. *Neuroscience Letters*, **336**, 131–133.

Butter, C. M., & Kirsch, N. (1992). Combined and separate effects of eye patching and visual stimulation on unilateral neglect following stroke. *Archives of Physical Medicine and Rehabilitation*, **73**, 1133–1139.

Buxbaum, L. J., Ferraro, M. K., Veramonti, T. et al. (2004). Hemispatial neglect: subtypes, neuroanatomy, and disability. *Neurology*, **62**, 749–756.

Castiello, U., Lusher, D., Burton, C., Glover, S., & Disler, P. (2004). Improving left hemispatial neglect using virtual reality. *Neurology*, **62**, 1958–1962.

Castner, S. A., & Goldman-Rakic, P. S. (2004). Enhancement of working memory in aged monkeys by a sensitizing regimen of dopamine D1 receptor stimulation. *Journal of Neuroscience*, **24**, 1446–1450.

Dijkerman, H. C., Webeling, M., ter Wal, J. M., Groet, E., & van Zandvoort, M. J. E. (2004). A long-lasting improvement of somatosensory function after prism adaptation, a case study. *Neuropsychologia*, **42**, 1697–1702.

Diller, L., & Weinberg, J. (1977). Hemi-inattention in rehabilitation: the evolution of a rational remediation program. In E. Weinstein & R. P. Friedland (Eds.), *Advances in Neurology* (pp. 63–82). New York, NY: Raven Press.

Doricchi, F., & Tomaiuolo, F. (2003). The anatomy of neglect without hemianopia: a key role for parietal-frontal disconnection? *Neuroreport*, **14**, 2239–2243.

Duncan, J., Humphreys, G., & Ward, R. (1997). Competitive brain activity in visual attention. *Current Opinion in Neurobiology*, **7**, 255–261.

Duncan, J., Bundesen, C., Olson, A. et al. (1999). Systematic analysis of deficits in visual attention. *Journal of Experimental Psychology: General*, **128**, 450–478.

Farne, A., & Ladavas, E. (2000). Dynamic size-change of hand peripersonal space following tool use. *NeuroReport*, **11**, 1645–1649.

Farne, A., Rossetti, Y., Toniolo, S., & Ladavas, E. (2002). Ameliorating neglect with prism adaptation: visuo-manual and visuo-verbal measures. *Neuropsychologia*, **40**, 718–729.

Fleet, W. S., Valenstein, E., Watson, R. T., & Heilman, K. M. (1987). Dopamine agonist therapy for neglect in humans. *Neurology*, **37**, 1765–1770.

Franowicz, J. S., & Arnsten, A. F. T. (1998). The alpha-2a noradrenergic agonist, guanfacine, improves delayed response performance in young adult rhesus monkeys. *Psychopharmacology*, **136**, 8–14.

Frassinetti, F., Rossi, M., & Ladavas, E. (2001). Passive limb movements improve visual neglect. *Neuropsychologia*, **39**, 725–733.

Frassinetti, F., Angeli, V., Meneghello, F., Avanzi, S., & Ladavas, E. (2002). Long-lasting amelioration of visuospatial neglect by prism adaptation. *Brain*, **125**, 608–623.

Geminiani, G., Bottini, G., & Sterzi, R. (1998). Dopaminergic stimulation in unilateral neglect. *Journal of Neurology, Neurosurgery and Psychiatry*, **65**, 344–347.

Grujic, Z., Mapstone, M., Gitelman, D. R. et al. (1998). Dopamine agonists reorient visual exploration away from the neglected hemispace. *Neurology*, **51**, 1395–1398.

Guariglia, C., Lippolis, G., & Pizzamiglio, L. (1998). Somatosensory stimulation improves imagery disorders in neglect. *Cortex*, **34**, 233–241.

Harvey, M., Hood, B., North, A., & Robertson, I. H. (2003). The effects of visuomotor feedback training on the recovery of hemispatial neglect symptoms: assessment of a 2-week and follow-up intervention. *Neuropsychologia*, **41**, 886–893.

Hillis, A. E., Newhart, M., Heidler, J. *et al.* (2005). Anatomy of spatial attention: insights from perfusion imaging and hemispatial neglect in acute stroke. *Journal of Neuroscience*, **25**, 3161–3167.

Hurford, P., Stringer, A. Y., & Jann, B. (1998). Neuropharmacologic treatment of hemineglect: a case report comparing bromocriptine and methylphenidate. *Archives of Physical Medicine and Rehabilitation*, **79**, 346–349.

Husain, M., & Rorden, C. (2003). Non-spatially lateralized mechanisms in hemispatial neglect. *Nature Reviews Neuroscience*, **4**, 26–36.

Husain, M., Shapiro, K., Martin, J., & Kennard, C. (1997). Abnormal temporal dynamics of visual attention in spatial neglect patients. *Nature*, **385**, 154–156.

Johannsen, L., Ackermann, H., & Karnath, H. O. (2003). Lasting amelioration of spatial neglect by treatment with neck muscle vibration even without concurrent training. *Journal of Rehabilitation Medicine*, **35**, 249–253.

Kalra, L., Perez, I., Gupta, S., & Wittink, M. (1997). The influence of visual neglect on stroke rehabilitation. *Stroke*, **28**, 1386–1391.

Karnath, H. O. (1996). Optokinetic stimulation influences the disturbed perception of body orientation in spatial neglect. *Journal of Neurology, Neurosurgery and Psychiatry*, **60**, 217–220.

Karnath, H. O., Ferber, S., & Himmelbach, M. (2001). Spatial awareness is a function of the temporal not the posterior parietal lobe. *Nature*, **411**, 950–953.

Karnath, H. O., Himmelbach, M., & Rorden, C. (2002). The subcortical anatomy of human spatial neglect: putamen, caudate nucleus and pulvinar. *Brain*, **125**, 350–360.

Kimberg, D. Y., & D'Esposito, M. (2003). Cognitive effects of the dopamine receptor agonist pergolide. *Neuropsychologia*, **41**, 1020–1027.

Kinsbourne, M. (1993). Orientational bias model of unilateral neglect: Evidence from attentional gradients within hemispace. In I. H. Robertson & J. C. Marshall (Eds.), *Unilateral Neglect: Clinical and Experimental Studies* (pp. 63–86). Hove, UK: Lawrence Erlbaum.

Luaute, J., Halligan, P., Rode, G., Rossetti, Y., & Boisson, D. (2006). Visuo-spatial neglect: a systematic review of current interventions and their effectiveness. *Neuroscience and Biobehavioural Reviews*, **30**, 961–982.

Malhotra, P. A., Parton, A. D., Greenwood, R., & Husain, M. (2006). Noradrenergic modulation of space exploration in visual neglect. *Annals of Neurology*, **59**, 186–190.

Mannan, S. K., Mort, D., Hodgson, T. L. *et al.* (2005). Revisiting previously searched locations in visual neglect: role of right parietal and frontal lesions in misjudging old locations as new. *Journal of Cognitive Neuroscience*, **17**, 340–354.

Maravita, A., McNeil, J., Malholtra, P. *et al.* (2003). Prism adaptation can improve contralesional tactile perception in neglect. *Neurology*, **60**, 1829–1831.

Marshall, J. F. (1979). Somatosensory inattention after dopamine-depleting intracerebral 6-OHDA injections: spontaneous recovery and pharmacological control. *Brain Research*, **177**, 311–324.

Marshall, J. F., & Gotthelf, T. (1979). Sensory inattention in rats with 6-hydroxydopamine-induced degeneration of ascending dopaminergic neurons: apomorphine-induced reversal of deficits. *Experimental Neurology*, **65**, 398–411.

Mattingley, J. B., Husain, M., Rorden, C., Kennard, C., & Driver, J. (1998). Motor role of human inferior parietal lobe revealed in unilateral neglect patients. *Nature*, **392**, 179–182.

Miyashita, N., Hikosaka, O., & Kato, M. (1995). Visual hemineglect induced by unilateral striatal dopamine deficiency in monkeys. *NeuroReport*, **6**, 1257–1260.

Mort, D. J., Malhotra, P., Mannan, S. K. *et al.* (2003). The anatomy of visual neglect. *Brain*, **126**, 1986–1997.

Mukand, J. A., Guilmette, T. J., Allen, D. G. *et al.* (2001). Dopaminergic therapy with carbidopa L-dopa for left neglect after stroke: a case series. *Archives of Physical Medicine and Rehabilitation*, **82**, 1279–1282.

Muller, U., von Cramon, D. Y., & Pollmann, S. (1998). D1-versus D2-receptor modulation of visuospatial working memory in humans. *Journal of Neuroscience*, **18**, 2720–2728.

Niemeier, J. P. (1998). The Lighthouse Strategy: use of a visual imagery technique to treat visual inattention in stroke patients. *Brain Injury*, **12**, 399–406.

Oliveri, M., Bisiach, E., Brighina, F. *et al.* (2001). rTMS of the unaffected hemisphere transiently reduces contralesional visuospatial hemineglect. *Neurology*, **57**, 1338–1340.

Parton, A. P., Malhotra, P., & Husain, M. (2004). Hemispatial neglect. *Journal of Neurology, Neurosurgery and Psychiatry*, **75**, 13–21.

Perennou, D. A., Leblond, C., Amblard, B. *et al.* (2001). Transcutaneous electric nerve stimulation reduces neglect-related postural instability after stroke. *Archives of Physical Medicine and Rehabilitation*, **82**, 440–448.

Posner, M. I., Walker, J. A., Friedrich, F. J., & Rafal, R. D. (1984). Effects of parietal injury on covert orienting of attention. *Journal of Neuroscience*, **4**, 1863–1874.

Redding, G. M., & Wallace, B. (2006). Prism adaptation and unilateral neglect: review and analysis. *Neuropsychologia*, **44**, 1–20.

Robertson, I. H. (2001). Do we need the "lateral" in unilateral neglect? Spatially nonselective attention deficits in unilateral neglect and their implications for rehabilitation. *Neuroimage*, **14**, S85–S90.

Robertson, I. H., & Halligan, P. W. (1999). *Spatial Neglect: A Clinical Handbook for Diagnosis and Treatment*. Hove, UK: Psychology Press.

Robertson, I. H., & North, N. (1993). Active and passive activation of left limbs: influence on visual and sensory neglect. *Neuropsychologia*, **31**, 293–300.

Robertson, I., Nico, D., & Hood, B. M. (1995). Believing what you feel: using proprioceptive feedback to reduce unilateral neglect. *Neuropsychology*, **11**, 53–58.

Robertson, I. H., Manly, T., Beschin, N. *et al.* (1997). Auditory sustained attention is a marker of unilateral spatial neglect. *Neuropsychologia*, **35**, 1527–1532.

Robertson, I. H., Hogg, K., & McMillan, T. M. (1998a). Rehabilitation of unilateral neglect: improving function by contralesional limb activation. *Neuropsychological Rehabilitation*, **8**, 19–29.

Robertson, I. H., Mattingley, J. B., Rorden, C., & Driver, J. (1998b). Phasic alerting of neglect patients overcomes their spatial deficit in visual awareness. *Nature*, **395**, 169–172.

Robertson, I. H., McMillan, T. M., MacLeod, E., Edgeworth, J., & Brock, D. (2002). Rehabilitation by limb activation training reduces left-sided motor impairment in unilateral neglect patients: a single-blind randomized control trial. *Neuropsychological Rehabilitation*, **12**, 439–454.

Rode, G., & Perenin, M. T. (1994). Temporary remission of representational hemineglect through vestibular stimulation. *NeuroReport*, **5**, 869–872.

Rossetti, Y., Rode, G., Pisella, L. *et al.* (1998). Prism adaptation to a rightward optical deviation rehabilitates left hemispatial neglect. *Nature*, **395**, 166–169.

Rousseaux, M., Bernati, T., Saj, A., & Kozlowski, O. (2006). Ineffectiveness of prism adaptation on spatial neglect signs. *Stroke*, **37**, 542–543.

Rubens, A. B. (1985). Caloric stimulation and unilateral visual neglect. *Neurology*, **35**, 1019–1024.

Schindler, I., Kerkhoff, G., Karnath, H. O., Keller, I., & Goldenberg, G. (2002). Neck muscle vibration induces lasting recovery in spatial neglect. *Journal of Neurology, Neurosurgery and Psychiatry*, **73**, 412–419.

Serino, A., Angeli, V., Frassinetti, F., & Ladavas, E. (2006). Mechanisms underlying neglect recovery after prism adaptation. *Neuropsychologia*, **44**, 1068–1078.

Shindo, K., Sugiyama, K., Huabao, L. *et al.* (2006). Long-term effect of low-frequency repetitive transcranial magnetic stimulation over the unaffected posterior parietal cortex in patients with unilateral spatial neglect. *Journal of Rehabilitation Medicine*, **38**, 65–67.

Smania, N., Martini, M. C., Gambina, G. *et al.* (1998). The spatial distribution of visual attention in hemineglect and extinction patients. *Brain*, **121**, 1759–1770.

Sturm, W., Willmes, K., Orgass, B., & Hartje, W. (1997). Do specific attention deficits need specific training? *Neuropsychological Rehabilitation*, **7**, 81–103.

Tham, K., & Tegner, R. (1997). Video feedback in the rehabilitation of patients with unilateral neglect. *Archives of Physical Medicine and Rehabilitation*, **78**, 410–413.

Thimm, M., Fink, G. R., Kust, J., Karbe, H., & W., S. (2006). Impact of alertness training on spatial neglect: a behavioural and fMRI study. *Neuropsychologia*, **44**, 1230–1246.

Tilikete, C., Rode, G., Rossetti, Y. *et al.* (2001). Prism adaptation to rightward optical deviation improves postural imbalance in left-hemiparetic patients. *Current Biology*, **11**, 524–528.

Vallar, G. (2001). Extrapersonal visual unilateral spatial neglect and its neuroanatomy. *Neuroimage*, **14**, S52–S58.

Vallar, G., Guariglia, C., Nico, D., & Pizzamiglio, L. (1997). Motor deficits and optokinetic stimulation in patients with left hemineglect. *Neurology*, **49**, 1364–1370.

Vallar, G., Rusconi, M. L., Barozzi, S. *et al.* (1995). Improvement of left visuo-spatial hemineglect by left-sided transcutaneous electrical stimulation. *Neuropsychologia*, **33**, 73–82.

Walker, R., Young, A. W., & Lincoln, N. B. (1996). Eye patching and the rehabilitation of visual neglect. *Neuropsychological Rehabilitation*, **6**, 219–231.

Wiart, L., SaintCome, A. B., Debelleix, X. *et al.* (1997). Unilateral neglect syndrome rehabilitation by trunk rotation and scanning training. *Archives of Physical Medicine and Rehabilitation*, **78**, 424–429.

Zeloni, G., Farne, A., & Baccini, M. (2002). Viewing less to see better. *Journal of Neurology, Neurosurgery and Psychiatry*, **73**, 195–198.

27

Rehabilitation of frontal lobe functions

Brian Levine, Gary R. Turner and Donald T. Stuss

Introduction

- Frontal lobe brain damage, which is highly prevalent, can have devastating effects on life quality. Yet the functions of the frontal lobes are difficult to define, variable and pose unique challenges to rehabilitation workers.

The cognitive and behavioral changes subsumed under the labels "the frontal lobe syndrome" or "executive dysfunction" are among the most challenging to rehabilitation workers. These heterogenous capacities are subject to multiple and varying definitions. Their expression varies widely across and within patient groups as well as within a single individual tested on multiple occasions. Rehabilitation of these capacities is hampered by the lack of insight among patients. Many such patients are impaired in real-life situations, but not in the laboratory, further challenging the implementation of interventions specific to patients' true handicaps.

Nonetheless, frontal lobe functions are critical to adaptive functioning, including complex information processing, decision making and social interaction. Indeed, they are considered important in the differentiation of higher from lower species. Deficits in these functions can cause marked handicap, to the point of devastating functional independence. The complexity of these capacities renders them highly sensitive to brain changes. The prevalence of frontal or executive dysfunction is therefore very high, affecting patients' engagement with all forms of rehabilitation.

In this chapter, we begin by clarifying a framework of frontal lobe functions meant to organize existing studies and to pose questions for future research. We also describe the most common causes of frontal dysfunction. We follow with a review of the literature on rehabilitation of these functions, updated from a previous review (Turner & Levine, 2004). We then close with implications for future research and clinical recommendations.

Frontal lobe functions: four functional domains

- The capacities associated with the frontal lobes (more precisely, the prefrontal cortex) are involved in higher-level cognition, behavioral control, attention and social functioning.
- The association of these functions with the frontal lobes is incomplete; posterior, diffuse and nonstructural damage can mimic the effects of frontal damage.
- In focal lesion patients, there is no evidence for a generic frontal lobe, or dysexecutive, syndrome. The term "executive," often used synonymously with "frontal," is reserved for a specific category of frontal lobe functions.
- There are at least four categories of frontal function: energization, executive, self-regulation and metacognition. These are defined by anatomical localization and connectivity as well as function.

Cognitive Neurorehabilitation, Second Edition: Evidence and Application, ed. Donald T. Stuss, Gordon Winocur and Ian H. Robertson. Published by Cambridge University Press. © Cambridge University Press 2008.

- Behavior following diffuse brain damage cannot be easily attributed to a specific lesion location; one or more of the categories of frontal lobe function may be implicated.
- Frontal functions are flexibly assembled over time into different networks within the frontal regions and between frontal and posterior regions, as required by task context and complexity.

"Frontal" functions are diverse capacities involved in higher-level cognition, behavioral control, attention and social functioning. While it may seem a truism that these functions are affected by damage to the frontal lobes (or to be more precise, to the prefrontal cortex anterior to the motor strip), this association is by no means complete. Diffuse damage, posterior damage, or damage to deep structures interconnected with the frontal cortex can mimic the effects of frontal damage. Because frontal functions lie at the apex of cognition, they are also sensitive to changes associated with psychiatric conditions, fatigue, pain, and toxic or metabolic conditions, to name a few. Conversely, frontal damage does not necessarily imply "frontal" dysfunction; it depends on the location of the damage and the specific function in question. While we acknowledge the limitations of defining psychological processes according to anatomy, we nonetheless use the term "frontal" in keeping with historical usage. Furthermore, this nomenclature avoids ambiguity as executive functions can be regarded as a subset of frontal functions (see below).

There are numerous theories of frontal lobe function (Damasio, 1996; Duncan *et al.*, 1996; Goldman-Rakic, 1987; Luria, 1966; Miller, 1999; Shallice & Burgess, 1991; Stuss *et al.*, 1995; for a brief review, see Turner & Levine, 2004), each emphasizing different elements of the frontal lobe syndrome or perspectives on frontal processes. We have adopted a classification delineating four categories of frontal functions (Stuss & Alexander, in press). This system is derived from research on patients with focal prefrontal lesions, incorporating the distinctions previously proposed by major theories of frontal function. Another advantage of this classification is that each function describes a clinical syndrome that is a potential rehabilitation target, allowing for increased precision of interventions. However, as discussed in more detail at the end of this section, we do not regard these functions as discrete or modular. They rather interact in a dynamic manner. Effects of brain damage depend on which system or systems are affected, as well as effects on the systems' interaction through altered connectivity.

The proposal of different functional domains within the frontal lobes is based on principles of anatomical differentiation and connectivity (Pandya & Yeterian, 1996; Sanides, 1970), and secondarily on more recent evidence for functional fractionation within the frontal lobes. The first major division (Stuss & Levine, 2002) is based on the evolution of architectonic development. There are two major functional/anatomical dissociations within the frontal lobes. The first (*executive*), evolving from a hippocampal, archicortical trend, is localized in lateral prefrontal cortical cortex (LPFC), and related to spatial and conceptual reasoning processes. The second (*behavioral/emotional self-regulatory*), evolving from the paleocortical trend and situated in ventral (medial) prefrontal cortex (VPFC), is related to emotional processing. These two major functional divisions within the frontal lobes follow two of the three proposed frontal-subcortical circuits involved in cognitive and/or emotional processing (Alexander *et al.*, 1986; Cummings, 1993). The third frontal-subcortical circuit (the two related to motor functioning are not considered) maps onto another functional division within the frontal cortex, associated with *energization regulating*, related to superior medial regions. The fourth category of frontal functions (*meta-cognitive*) is suggested by recent research on higher order integrative functions of the frontal polar area 10.

Executive cognitive functions

Executive functions are the high-level *cognitive* functions mediated primarily by one region of the frontal lobes, the LPFC, and concerned with the control and direction (e.g., planning, monitoring, activating, switching, inhibiting) of lower level, more automatic functions (Stuss & Alexander, in press; Stuss *et al.*, 2002; Stuss & Levine, 2002). Tests commonly used by many clinicians as measures of frontal lobe "executive" functioning (such as the Wisconsin Card Sorting Test (WCST); Trail Making Test Part B; the Stroop Interference subtest; and specific measures within verbal fluency tasks) are indeed more sensitive in general to focal LPFC (and also not generally to orbitofrontal/ventral medial) pathology (Goldman-Rakic, 1987; Milner, 1963; Petrides & Milner, 1982; for review see Stuss & Levine, 2002). However, the tests are complex and multifactorial, and individuals can fail for many reasons (e.g., Anderson *et al.*, 1991).

A series of simple reaction time tasks have led to dissociations of executive functions within the frontal lobes that appear to be consistent across tasks, with the left ventrolateral prefrontal region involved in task-setting (e.g., bias and false positive errors; Alexander *et al.*, 2003, 2005; Stuss *et al.*, 1995, 2002) and the right lateral prefrontal area important in output monitoring and checking (Stuss *et al.*, 2002, 2005a; Vallesi *et al.*, 2007; Picton *et al.*, 2006; see also Deutsch *et al.*, 1987; Glosser & Goodglass, 1990; Pardo *et al.*, 1991; Rueckert & Grafman, 1996; Wilkins *et al.*, 1987; Woods & Knight, 1986). These same control mechanisms appear to be responsible for the domain general individual variability that is observed in several neurological disorders (Stuss *et al.*, 2003; see also Chapter 3 by Stuss and Binns in this volume).

Behavioral/emotional self-regulatory functions

An important function for the VPFC, because of its involvement in emotional responsiveness (Nauta, 1971; Pandya & Barnes, 1987) and reward processing (Fuster, 1997; Mishkin, 1964; Rolls, 1996, 2000), is behavioral self-regulation. This self-regulation is necessary in situations where cognitive analysis, habit or environmental cues are not sufficient to determine the most adaptive response (Eslinger & Damasio, 1985; Harlow, 1868; Penfield & Evans, 1935).

Affective reversal learning, measuring the acquisition and reversal of stimulus-reward associations, is sensitive to VPFC pathology (Elliott *et al.*, 2000; Rolls, 2000) and is dissociable from attentional (extra-dimensional) set-shifting found after LPFC lesions (Dias *et al.*, 1996, 1997; see also Fellows & Farah, 2005). This dissociation reinforces the distinction between "executive" attentional and affective/emotional behavioral measures. Higher-level decision-making tasks involving reward processing in unstructured situations, such as the gambling task developed by Bechara and colleagues (Bechara *et al.*, 1994), may also be sensitive to damage in this region for obvious reasons; however, these tests may also be multifactorial in nature, requiring other processes such as those we called executive (e.g., planning and monitoring; Levine *et al.*, 2005; for review, see Dunn *et al.*, 2006). The inability to regulate behavior according to internal goals and constraints is also being assessed by naturalistic multiple subgoal tasks (Schwartz *et al.*, 1998, 1999), as well as more structured paper-and-pencil laboratory versions (Burgess *et al.*, 1998, 2000; Levine *et al.*, 1998, 2000a), these tasks also being multifactorial.

Energization regulating functions

The energization function is defined as the capacity to generate and maintain actions important for adequate performance of the other functions. It has been replicably related to the superior medial region of the frontal lobes (Alexander *et al.*, 2005; Stuss *et al.*, 2001a, 2003, 2005a). In its most extreme form, extensive damage to more superior medial (anterior cingulate and superior medial) frontal pathology results in abulia, or severe apathy. However, this diminished energization can be demonstrated even in less clinically obvious cases. Patients with damage in this region are slow in generating lists of words in the absence of a language deficit, particularly in the first 15 seconds (Stuss *et al.*, 1998); have notably slower reaction time (RT) particularly if tasks are more demanding (Alexander *et al.*, 2005; Stuss *et al.*, 2002, 2005a); are deficient in maintaining over time the benefit of a warning stimulus

(Stuss *et al.*, 2005a); and have problems maintaining a selected target such as in the Stroop interference test (Stuss *et al.*, 2001a). The clinical tests, such as verbal fluency and Stroop, lack specificity and tap other cognitive (often executive – see below) abilities. Perhaps the best measures to evaluate impaired activation are demanding reaction time measures.

Metacognitive functions

The fourth frontal lobe functional category is postulated on the basis of recent research (see Burgess *et al.* 2005; Christoff & Gabrieli, 2000; Stuss & Alexander, 1999, 2000; Stuss *et al.*, 2001c for reviews). The frontal polar region Brodmann area 10, possibly more particularly on the right, appears to be maximally involved in the metacognitive aspects of human nature: integrative aspects of personality, social cognition, autonoetic consciousness, theory of mind and humor (Shammi & Stuss, 1999; Stuss *et al.*, 2001b, 2001c; Tulving, 1985; Wheeler *et al.*, 1997). Although this division is not based on the circuitry proposed by Alexander *et al.*, 1986, there is some evidence suggesting that the connectivity within the frontal regions provides it with unique integrative capability (Burgess *et al.*, 2005, 2007; Pandya, personal communication). Because area 10 is among the most recently evolved of human brain regions, it may be uniquely positioned to integrate the higher-level executive cognitive functions, and emotional or drive-related inputs (although seemingly not reducible to these functions; Siegal & Varley, 2002; Shammi & Stuss, 1999; Stuss *et al.*, 2005b) positioning this region for more self-reflective, metacognitive functions (Stuss & Alexander, 1999, 2000). There is also debate as to how much this functional category is associated with damage to a more general area including the anterior medial regions. The neuropsychological assessments in this category of frontal lobe functions are generally experimental.

Functional systems

The evidence for specific functional categories within the frontal lobes does not imply that frontal lobes are simply a series of independent processes. Depending on task demands, there is the fluid recruitment of different processes anywhere in the brain into different networks (Stuss, 2006). For some tasks, only one functional region may be necessary; in others, one or more anatomically distinct frontal processes within the frontal lobes may be recruited (a "within-frontal lobe" network). In some simple repetitive tasks, the more automatic nonfrontal processes may function independently (Shallice & Burgess, 1993); as task demands increase or alter, there may be increased involvement of different frontal (more "strategic") regions, even to the point where it appears all frontal regions are involved (Stuss *et al.*, 1999). Under other conditions the network may function "top-down." In disorders with more diffuse pathology, then, there may well be "executive" dysfunction. However, these should not be made synonymous with frontal lobe dysfunction. Regardless, some of the rehabilitation techniques described in this chapter may be effective in these populations, but perhaps in conjunction with other approaches.

Summary

Frontal lobe functions are heterogenous and centrally involved in higher level cognition, behavioral control, attention and social functioning. Although "frontal" dysfunction can arise from nonfrontal damage, we retain use of this term for simplicity and historical consistency. The use of the term "executive functions" as synonymous with "frontal functions" can be misleading as executive functions are but one class of frontal function. We adopt the following classification system for organizing frontal functions as potential targets for rehabilitation: executive/cognitive functions associated with the lateral prefrontal cortex, behavioral/emotional self-regulatory functions associated with the ventral (medial) frontal cortex, energizing regulating functions associated with the medial prefrontal cortex, behavior and metacognitive functions associated with the frontopolar cortex. Although these functions can be differentially affected by localized brain damage, they interact through extensive inter-connections and can be multiply affected by clinical disorders.

Disorders affecting frontal lobes

- Stroke, tumors and traumatic brain injury (TBI) are the most prevalent forms of acquired brain injury affecting frontal function, although frontal function may be affected by many other conditions.
- Middle cerebral artery strokes affect the lateral prefrontal cortex and thus are maximally expressed via executive/cognitive deficits. Anterior cerebral artery strokes affect the medial prefrontal cortex and thus affect energizing functions. Hemorrhagic infarcts arising from anterior communicating artery (ACoA) aneurysms affect ventromedial prefrontal cortex and basal forebrain, causing self-regulatory and mnemonic dysfunction.
- Tumors affect frontal function through both localised and distal effects. Meningioma effects are fewer relative to faster-growing tumors.
- In terms of prevalence and overall economic impact, TBI is the most important cause of frontal dysfunction, affecting behavior through both diffuse and localized frontal damage, with consequences for all frontal functions, especially self-regulatory.
- Although localization effects are often consistent across etiologies, considering effects of specific etiologies on different frontal functions may increase the specificity of interventions.

As noted above, frontal functions are vulnerable to disruption in any cerebral system, anterior or posterior, cortical or subcortical, as well as to changes in psychological status (e.g., anxiety) and daily fluctuations (e.g., fatigue). Although nearly every neurological or psychiatric disorder can affect frontal function, the most prevalent forms of acquired brain injury that have specific effects on prefrontal systems are strokes tumors, and traumatic brain injury (TBI).

Stroke

Strokes or cerebrovascular accidents (CVAs) occur due to occlusion and hemorrhage, with the former accounting for more than 80% of strokes (Robinson & Starkstein, 1997). Although less prevalent, hemorrhagic events are relevant to the study of frontal lobe dysfunction as 85–95% of aneurysms develop at the anterior portion of the cerebral arterial supply (DeLuca & Diamond, 1995). Strokes involving the distribution of the main trunk or anterior branches of the middle cerebral artery result in unilateral damage to lateral prefrontal brain regions, producing what has been described as a dorsolateral stroke syndrome (Anderson & Damasio, 1995), involving cortical regions across the entirety of the lateral surface of the prefrontal cortex with associated impairments in executive/cognitive functions, often accompanied by unawareness.

Infarcts arising from anterior cerebral artery aneurysms in the superior medial frontal regions produce a dorsomedial frontal-lobe syndrome in which energization is affected. The anterior communicating artery (ACoA) bridges the right and left anterior cerebral arteries (feeding the medial surface of the frontal lobes) as well as sending branches more inferiorly into white matter and basal forebrain regions. It is the source of almost 85% of all ruptured aneurysms within the cerebrum (Anderson & Damasio, 1995). Hemorrhagic damage following ACoA rupture can affect ventral, medial and polar frontal regions as well as basal forebrain regions involved in memory. Thus patients with ruptured ACoA aneurysms can have problems with behavioral self-regulation (Bottger et al., 1998; Mavaddat et al., 2000), self-awareness (Diamond et al., 1997), and memory, including confabulation (DeLuca & Diamond, 1995; Gilboa et al., 2006).

Tumors

Frontal lobe tumors account for one-fifth of all supratentorial tumors (Price et al., 1997). Non-frontal tumors can also cause deficits through diaschisis (i.e., the impairment of neuronal activity in a functionally related but distant region of the brain; von Monakow, 1914) and disconnection of frontal structures from other cerebral regions (Lezak, 1995; Lilja *et al.*, 1992). Neurosurgical approaches through the frontal lobes should also be taken into consideration.

Gliomas and meningiomas are the most common histological classifications of supratentorial tumors (Nakawatase, 1999), with fast-growing glioblastomas resulting in a poorer cognitive profile than a slower growing meningioma (Price *et al.*, 1997). Tumors may produce additional cognitive dysfunction by inducing seizures, increased intracranial pressure, edema and paraneoplastic syndrome. As described earlier, the reliance of frontal function upon extensive neural networks increases the susceptibility of higher cognitive processes to these secondary neuropathological processes (Tucha *et al.*, 2000).

Traumatic brain injury

Owing to its high incidence (80000 to 90000 disabled per year in the USA) and prevalence (5.3 million in the USA disabled by TBI; National Center for Injury Prevention and Control, 1999), and its specific effects on the frontal lobes and their interconnections, TBI is arguably the most important single cause of frontal lobe dysfunction. Although interpretation of TBI effects is complicated by the co-occurrence of physical disability, it is the cognitive and behavioral consequences of TBI that are truly enduring, with a greater impact on outcome than physical symptoms (Brooks *et al.*, 1986; Dikmen *et al.*, 1995; Jennett *et al.*, 1981). The chronic disability of TBI is accentuated by its tendency to take place during early adulthood, affecting behavior for decades.

Traumatic brain injury induces a dizzying array of neuropathologies, the interpretation of which is complicated by time course effects and interaction with noninjury factors (e.g., the psychosocial milieu). For our purposes, a distinction between diffuse and focal injury provides a useful heuristic (Levine *et al.*, 2002). Diffuse axonal injury (DAI) is a crucial neuropathology and cause of coma in TBI (Adams *et al.*, 1982; Gennarelli *et al.*, 1982; Povlishock, 1992; Povlishock *et al.*, 1992; Strich, 1956). It is characterized by disconnection and eventual demise of axons, the result of a complex process studied at the molecular level (Maxwell *et al.*, 1997; Povlishock & Christman, 1995). The behavioral consequences of this widespread disconnection syndrome include impaired arousal, inattention and slowed information processing, particularly on complex tasks (Stuss & Gow, 1992). The otherwise intact environment in which DAI occurs (15 per 1000 axons damaged in a typical motor vehicular accident injury; Povlishock, 1993), is ripe for subsequent neuroplastic changes such as axonal sprouting and synaptogenesis (Christman *et al.*, 1997; Povlishock *et al.*, 1992), as revealed through functional neuroimaging studies of patients with TBI (for review, see Levine *et al.*, 2006).

Focal parenchymal injury in TBI is typically due to contusion resulting from inertial forces causing localized damage in ventral and polar frontal and anterior temporal areas where the brain is confined by bony ridges of the inner skull, regardless of the site of impact (Clifton *et al.*, 1980; Courville, 1937; Gentry *et al.*, 1988; Ommaya & Gennarelli, 1974). There is evidence that focal atrophic damage may exist in these regions even when lesions are not visible on conventional MRI (i.e., localized diffuse injury; Berryhill *et al.*, 1995). The location of focal cortical contusions along the ventral trend corresponds to the self-regulatory and metacognitive deficits known to occur in TBI patients (Levine, 1999; Levine *et al.*, 1998, 2000a).

Summary

Nearly all neurological and psychiatric illnesses can affect frontal function. The most prevalent forms of acquired brain injury affecting frontal function, however, are strokes, tumors and traumatic brain injury. Each etiology can cause specific effects depending on the location and nature of the disease. For example, MCA strokes affect dorsolateral (executive/cognitive) functions, ACA strokes affect energization regulation functions, ACoA strokes affect self-regulatory and mnemonic functions. Tumor effects depend on location and other factors such as distal (diaschisis) effects, neurosurgical approaches and paraneoplastic syndrome. Traumatic brain injury, the most common and costly of these disorders, affects frontal function (especially self-regulation) through diffuse axonal injury and focal ventral frontal contusions.

Rehabilitation of frontal dysfunction

- Fifty-five studies involving rehabilitation of frontal dysfunction were identified.
- Most of the published work involves case studies, regarded as a lesser class of evidence. Only nine studies were identified as randomized control trials, the highest class of evidence.
- Nearly all studies involved patients with acquired brain injury, although details regarding etiology, epoch and lesion location were often not described.
- Most reported interventions for energization regulating functions involved dopamanergic agonists. A small number of case studies used nonpharmacologic interventions.
- Interventions for executive/cognitive functions were divided into those addressing broadly defined problem solving and planning versus those addressing a specific executive cognitive function, usually working memory.
- Interventions for behavioral/emotional self-regulatory functions were designed to train patients to bridge the gap between intention and action. Studies demonstrated efficacy of programmatic goal management training, verbal self-regulation and external cueing techniques.
- Interventions for metacognitive functions attempted to increase awareness of deficits or to more directly increase error monitoring and self-correction, the latter showing case study evidence for improving difficult, impulsive behavior.

We previously reviewed literature on rehabilitation of frontal dysfunction to 2003 (Turner & Levine,

2004). Interventions specifically addressing attention or memory disorders or behavioral dyscontrol were not included, nor were holistic interventions. Forty interventions drawn from 34 papers were identified and tabulated. The papers were organized according to four categories: cognitive control, planning/problem solving/goal direction, initiation/motivation and self-awareness/self-monitoring – corresponding closely to the executive cognitive, self-regulatory, energizing and metacognitive categories described above, which will be used henceforth.

Few of the studies we reviewed contained the design ingredients necessary to draw firm conclusions about treatment effectiveness: control groups, randomization, evidence of real-life generalization and long-term follow-up (Levine & Downey-Lamb, 2002). Furthermore, patient characteristics such as etiology, epoch and lesion location were often not described. Most of the published work involved case studies, which are relevant for forming hypotheses but do not provide sufficient empirical evidence for widespread clinical application.

Of the 15 additional studies identified here, there were five randomized control trials (including a brief rehabilitation probe), four group interventions (two without control groups; two with nonrandomized controls) and six case reports – a distribution similar to that observed in our previous review. Ten of the 15 studies report on TBI samples, with the remaining studies reporting on mixed TBI/CVA, "brain injured" or aging samples.

This updated review incorporates our previous findings with these new reports and builds upon recent reviews of cognitive (Cicerone et al., 2005), executive function (Cicerone et al., 2006) and self-awareness (Lucas & Fleming, 2005) rehabilitation interventions in a number of ways. By framing our review within the four domains of frontal lobe functioning, we were able to broaden our inclusion parameters relative to these earlier reviews (Cicerone, 2000; Cicerone et al., 2005). This was most evident within the domain of "Energization" where we included "apathy" and "abulia" to our search criteria and reviewed reference lists from two recent review papers on the topic (Stuss *et al.*, 2000; van Reekum *et al.*, 2005). In addition to the expanded breadth of the review we were also able to stratify the intervention studies by class of evidence using methods adapted from Cicerone (2000), thereby providing both a comprehensive survey of the rehabilitation interventions specifically targeting frontal dysfunction as well as a qualitative assessment of the state of the literature with respect to empirically validated treatment options.

Executive/cognitive functions

Interventions in this category may be loosely grouped into interventions designed to remediate broadly defined problem-solving and planning skills and those targeted towards improving capacity within a single domain of executive functioning (typically working memory).

Problem solving and planning

The evaluation of problem-solving training (PST; von Cramon *et al.*, 1991) remains the only RCT of problem-solving interventions in the literature. The intervention targeted specific problem-solving goals (e.g., orientation, definition, alternative generation). A control group received memory training. Over an average of 25 sessions, gains for the problem-solving training group were observed on tasks of reasoning, problem solving and experimental planning. However, there was only qualitative evidence of training generalization and no follow-up data were reported. Importantly, length of training was nonstandard across participants with additional training provided for patients demonstrating apathetic or abulic symptomatology. A supplemental single case study (von Cramon & Matthes von Cramon, 1994) also reported success in remediating specific vocational tasks using a variant of this program, but there was no effect on awareness ratings or evidence of generalizability. More recently, interactive strategy modeling training was used to improve problem-solving efficacy in a noncontrolled group study of 20 TBI subjects (Marshall *et al.*, 2004).

Participants were trained in deductive problem-solving techniques to facilitate target picture identification from within a large picture array. Following training to pre-established criteria on 12 training arrays, participants were assessed on novel arrays. Relative to pre-training performance, participants demonstrated a decrease in the number of questions needed to solve the problem, an increase in percentage of constraint questions and an overall increase in question-asking efficiency. Gains were maintained at 1-month follow-up. Soong *et al.* (2005) used an analogy-based approach to problem-solving training in a pilot study with 15 brain-injured persons. Participants were trained to solve everyday life problems over 20 sessions using analogies drawn from successfully solved problems in their own personal histories. Training was delivered across several modalities (i.e., web-based, computer or therapist led) and while results did not vary across mode of intervention, all three groups demonstrated significant change in knowledge of concepts surrounding instrumental activities of daily living, performance on the category test of the Halstead–Reitan Battery and an experimental measure of self-efficacy in problem-solving. There was no comparison group to control for nonspecific effects of the intervention nor were any follow-up assessments reported. Fox *et al.* (1989) reported on the efficacy of specific criterion questions as cues to solve real-life problems in a small controlled study of patients with ABI ($N = 3$) using scenarios and staged interactions. Finally, Park *et al.* (2003) describe a single case of improved functional outcome following a problem-solving intervention involving explicit consideration and strategic evaluation of problem-solving alternatives in real-life situations.

In a brief "rehabilitation probe" experiment (see also Levine *et al.*, 2000b described below), Hewitt *et al.* (2006) theorized that training in explicit retrieval of autobiographical information regarding event planning would aid in overall planning efficacy following TBI. Following 30 min of training on the use of autobiographical memory recollections to aid planning in everyday life situations, patients with TBI ($N = 15$) showed moderate improvements in planning efficacy, number of steps in their plans, and number of autobiographical memories retrieved on an event description task relative to a matched control group of 15 TBI patients who received no training. There was no report of generalization to other measures.

Executive function and working memory

In the only published RCT explicitly targeting the enhancement of remediating deficits within a specific domain of higher cognition, McDowell *et al.* (1998), administered bromocriptine to a group of 24 TBI subjects to aid working memory and executive control performance in a double-blind, crossover, placebo-controlled study. The authors report improvement related to drug administration on an experimental measure of dual-task performance and several neuropsychological measures of executive functioning. More recently, Kraus and colleagues (2005) utilized amantadine to improve executive functioning in a sample of 22 TBI subjects in an open-label, noncontrolled study design. Significant improvement on an index of executive functioning, comprised of performance on a letter fluency task and Trail Making Test, Part B, was reported following a 12-week course of treatment (400 mg daily). Interestingly, there was no evidence of improvement in either attention or memory domains suggesting a domain-specific effect of the intervention. No follow-up or generalization data were reported.

Specific remediation of executive functioning (i.e., working memory) was also addressed in a recent brief report by Serino *et al.* (2006). Nine TBI patients with working memory deficits and six TBI patients without working memory deficits were trained on multiple forms of the Paced Auditory Serial Attention Task (PASAT). Following training, performance improved on tests of working memory, divided attention, executive functioning (letter fluency) and long-term memory. No improvements were observed on tests of speeded processing or vigilance, again supporting the specificity of the intervention. There were no observed differences between the pre- and post-intervention scores for those participants who did not demonstrate working memory deficits, illustrating the importance of defining target groups for rehabilitation. No follow-up or generalization data were reported.

Stablum *et al.* (2000) conducted a controlled group study to assess the feasibility of improving dual-task performance in TBI patients through direct training. Both treatment and control patients improved on the dual-task paradigm, but the rate of improvement was greater for the treatment group. There was evidence of generalization to another working memory task (PASAT) and gains were evident at 3 months on neuropsychological and functional measures. These findings were replicated with a group of ACoA aneurysm rupture patients. Cicerone (2002) utilized a staged training program involving increasingly demanding dual-task paradigms to successfully improve "working attention" (again measured by PASAT) in four mild TBI participants relative to controls. Reduced attentional dysfunction in daily activities was also noted. Deacon & Campbell (1991) successfully used external cuing in a group study of decision-making speed wherein external cueing preferentially improved choice reaction times in TBI patients relative to controls; accuracy was not affected. The effect was carried over into noncued situations, providing some evidence of a generalized enhancement in decision-making speed.

Behavioral/emotional self-regulatory functions

Interventions within this category include those explicitly directed towards bridging the gap between intention and action, a deficit described as "goal neglect" (Duncan, 1986; Luria, 1966) with interventions targeted towards re-establishing endogenous control of behavior. Rath and colleagues (2003) used an RCT design in a cohort of 46 TBI subjects. Treatment consisted of two distinct phases, with the first 12-week phase consisting of emotional self-regulation training. In the second phase, subjects were trained in problem-solving skills in a manner similar to the problem-solving training procedure described above (von Cramon *et al.*, 1991). Controls received a program of conventional cognitive rehabilitation. Improvements specific to treatment included reduced perseverative responding on the WCST and improved problem solving on self-report and role play measures. Treatment gains were stable at 6 months with anecdotal report of generalization to real-life behaviors. The addition of an emotional self-regulation represents a novel approach to self-regulation interventions and was considered essential to facilitating successful problem orientation before progressing to the problem solution phase of the intervention.

Webb & Glueckauf (1994) randomly assigned 16 patients with TBI to a high-involvement goal-setting group (including active strategies for prioritization and goal monitoring) or a low involvement group (including pre-assigned goal lists but no formal monitoring training). Both groups made equivalent gains on ratings of goal attainment and goal change from pre- to post-testing, but maintenance of gains at 2-month follow-up was restricted to the high-involvement group.

Levine and colleagues (2000b) drew upon Duncan's (1986) theory of goal neglect to institute a program of goal management training (GMT) in a brief "rehabilitation probe" in which 30 TBI subjects received GMT or motor skills training (MST). Goal management training consisted of five training stages: stopping (periodic suspension of ongoing behavior), stating the main task, partitioning the task into subgoals, encoding and retention of the goals, and monitoring. The results suggested a beneficial effect of GMT training, measured by experimental planning tests, over and above gains demonstrated in the MST group (due to repeated test administration or contact with the trainer). A more extensive application of GMT was successfully applied in a single case study of a post-encephalitic patient, with training adapted to improve meal preparation (Levine *et al.*, 2000b, experiment 2).

Levine and colleagues (2007) applied GMT within a large-scale cognitive neurorehabilitation program

for aging that also included psychosocial and memory-skills training (Stuss *et al.*, 2007). The training, although expanded in time from the original rehabilitation probe to 4 three-hour sessions, was reduced in complexity by emphasizing the first three stages: (stopping ongoing behavior, stating the main task and splitting the task into subgoals). Outcome measures included desktop simulated real life tasks (SRLTs; e.g., organizing a carpool) videotaped and scored according to the trained concepts. Forty-nine participants were randomized to two groups, one of which received the intervention immediately and the other of which was waitlisted prior to rehabilitation. Results indicated improvements in SRLT performance as well as self-rated executive deficits coinciding with the training in both groups. These gains were maintained at long-term follow-up. However, it was not possible to empirically demonstrate the specificity of these improvements to GMT as the assessment was done before and after the entire cognitive neurorehabilitation program.

In a RCT of 67 healthy older adults with executive complaints randomized to an 11-session version of GMT plus psychosocial training or a waiting-list group, van Hooren and colleagues (2006) found fewer executive complaints, reduced annoyance and reduced anxiety in the intervention group. There was no effect on objective assessment of outcome using the Stroop test, which is not a sensitive measure for this intervention.

The latest version of GMT has an enhanced emphasis on periodic suspension of ongoing activity as a critical prerequisite to on-line evaluation of goal hierarchies, task-splitting and monitoring of performance. Active practice with simulated and real-life complex tasks is incorporated both within and outside of training sessions. Mindfulness practice is also incorporated to bring awareness to the present moment and reduce distractibility. This program has been administered in a 15-hour RCT in groups of patients with mixed-etiology acquired brain injury, with standard outpatient group rehabilitation techniques (e.g., diet, energy conservation, brain health education) as the control treatment. Results indicate positive effects on measures of sustained attention and planning that are sustained at long-term follow-up (O'Connor *et al.*, 2006). Luria & Homskaya (1964) suggested that self-regulation is mediated by covert, "inner speech" that provides a critical bridging mechanism between the general intention to solve a problem and its concrete solution. Arco *et al.* (2004), described a verbal self-regulation procedure to reduce impulsivity in four males who had sustained severe head injury. Impulsivity was reduced and stabilized for two of the four with impulsive behavior rates reduced but unstable after treatment for the other two subjects. A case study by Cicerone & Wood (1987) documented the remediation of a planning deficit in a patient with TBI through the re-establishment of inner-speech to guide behavior. Performance improved on a standardized planning task and gains were maintained at 4-month follow-up. However, generalization required 12 weeks of further training. A follow-up study replicated these findings in a larger sample of six mixed-etiology subjects, with 5/6 showing gains. Two patients who received explicit generalization training spontaneously applied the techniques in novel situations (Cicerone & Giacino, 1992; see also Stuss *et al.*, 1987).

Goal-directed behavior may also be facilitated with external cueing, as suggested by case studies involving verbal instruction and task checklists (Burke *et al.*, 1991; Delazer *et al.*, 1998; Giles & Morgan, 1990; Hux *et al.*, 1994; O'Callaghan & Couvadelli, 1998) and an electronic paging system combined with task-specific checklists (Evans *et al.*, 1998). In this latter study, it was reported that the auditory cueing itself was sufficient to re-establish the connection between intention and action. A similar result is reported in a recent TBI group study in which simulated real-life tasks were administered with and without the provision of random auditory "alerting" cues (Manly *et al.*, 2002). Random auditory cues were used as a prosthetic "marker" to remind patients to monitor ongoing behavior in completing a complex, lifelike planning task. Patients' performance on the cued version of the task was comparable to that of normal controls, suggesting that the auditory alerts higher-order goals into consciousness, facilitating more adaptive

goal-directed behavior. This tone prosthetic has been incorporated into the current version of GMT.

Energization regulating functions

Pharmacologic interventions

Most of the interventions in this category of frontal dysfunction involve pharmacologic treatments with catecholaminergic agents, a literature that has been reviewed more extensively elsewhere (Muller & von Cramon, 1994; van Reekum *et al.*, 2005). In their recent report, Newburn & Newburn (2005) utilized a standardized apathy evaluation scale (AES) to measure the impact of selegeline, a dopaminergic agonist, in four TBI patients presenting with apathetic characteristics but without evidence of depression. All four subjects demonstrated reduced apathy following the start of treatment and improvements were reported both on standardized measures as well as in clinical presentation. There was no report of follow-up after drug cessation. Previously we reviewed a report by Powell (1996), wherein treatment with bromocriptine was related to improvements on measures of active rehabilitation participation, reward responsivity and measures of executive functioning in 11 subjects, with treatment gains stable in eight of the 11 patients 2 weeks after withdrawal of treatment. This finding is similar to that of the first case-controlled report of bromocriptine administration for the treatment of frontal lobe syndrome (Parks *et al.*, 1992) wherein bromocriptine administration ameliorated abulic symptoms. However, their interpretation of improvements in problem-solving and memory domains was complicated by practice effects on neuropsychological measures. A review of bromocriptine administration following acquired brain injury by Muller & von Cramon (1994) concluded that while bromocriptine has been successful in the domain of energizing functions, its utility in treating executive or problem-solving deficits remains unproven (but see 'Executive/Cognitive' section above). Another dopamine agonist, amantadine, was administered in a double-blind placebo-controlled case study in a patient with a severe abulic and apathetic syndrome with positive results (van Reekum *et al.*, 1995). In a recent report, administration of a serotonergic agonist, sertraline, was unsuccessful in raising alertness levels in a group of 11 traumatically brain-injured subjects (Meythaler *et al.*, 2001).

Behavioral interventions

Very few reports of nonpharmacologic treatment of energization deficits were identified, although positive case study evidence has been reported with checklists (Burke *et al.*, 1991) and external cueing systems (Sohlberg *et al.*, 1988).

Metacognitive functions

Within the realm of metacognitive deficits following frontal dysfunction, deficient awareness of one's impairments and their consequences (i.e., the capacity to retain an "objective" view of oneself while maintaining a sense of subjectivity; Prigatano, 1991) is one of the most commonly addressed in the rehabilitation literature. Interventions typically fall within two categories, those addressing awareness of deficits and those more directly targeted at error monitoring and self-correction.

Deficit awareness

Cheng & Man (2006) adopted an RCT design to evaluate the efficacy of their Awareness Intervention Program (AIP). Awareness levels of 11 TBI participants in the treatment group were compared with a control group of 10 matched TBI subjects enrolled in a conventional rehabilitation program. Upon completion of the 32-session AIP, the treatment group scores on the Self-Awareness of Deficits Scale was significantly lower (i.e., greater awareness) than the control group. No between-group differences were observed on the IADL scale or Functional Independence Measure at the end of training, signifying that the increased awareness may not have effected functional change as assessed

by these measures. No follow-up data were reported. Medd & Tate (2000) employed a matched-randomized control design to investigate the efficacy of an anger management and awareness intervention. Traumatic brain injury participants ($N = 16$) were randomly assigned to a 6-hour self-instructional training program or to a waitlist condition. There was some gain in anger management measures post-intervention and at 2-month follow-up. There was no change in awareness measures. Two small group ($N = 3$) studies successfully used awareness board games to improve deficit awareness (Chittum *et al.*, 1996; Zhou *et al.*, 1996). There was only partial evidence, however, that knowledge of these deficits translated into increased awareness.

Several reports describe the use of a more experiential approach, wherein predicted task performance is contrasted with actual performance as a means of increasing deficit awareness in the realm of planning (Cicerone & Giacino, 1992), memory (Rebman & Hannon, 1995; Schlund, 1999), and calculation and verbal recall abilities (Youngjohn & Altman, 1989). Ownsworth & McFarland (2000) used a similar approach to improve deficit awareness and anticipatory awareness of future consequences in a group of 21 ABI subjects. In their sample, improvements in self-regulation and reduction in sickness impact were observed following the intervention and remained stable at 6-month follow-up. DeLuca (1992) has described a "tailored" approach to the remediation of a severe confabulatory disorder following ACoA aneurysm rupture in which the treatment team and family members were provided with explicit direction as to when and how to confront patients with respect to their confabulatory behavior. Improved awareness and reduced confabulation following treatment was reported in two patients.

Error awareness and self-monitoring

Deficient self-monitoring of inappropriate or maladaptive behavior is a common sequelae of brain injury. Such behavioral disorders (e.g., impulsivity, aggression, sexual disinhibition) are highly refractory to treatment and significantly interfere with successful community reintegration (Alderman *et al.*, 1995). Rehabilitation or management of severe behavioral disorders is beyond the scope of this review, but has been reviewed extensively elsewhere (Alderman, 2004). We have limited our review to those interventions where self-monitoring and error correction (as a subcategory of self-awareness) was the primary rehabilitation target.

Targeted remediation programs involving structured feedback, cueing and formal efforts to recognize inappropriate behaviors are often part of interventions to enhance self-monitoring. A recent report by Fleming *et al.* (2006) describes a 10-week intervention program focused on client-centered goals, real-world task performance, error monitoring and multiple feedback mechanisms. Gains in deficit awareness were observed across all participants from pre- to post-intervention; however, these gains were only maintained in 2/4 participants at 4-week follow-up. Moreover, the authors report a link between improved self-awareness and increased emotional distress in all participants, suggesting that emotional stability must be closely monitored throughout any such intervention aimed at increasing deficit awareness. Ownsworth and colleagues (2006) reported a single case report of an error-awareness intervention for a person who had sustained a severe TBI. Using a client-selected target behavior, a system of error monitoring, role reversal and feedback was implemented. Error rates declined and self-corrective behaviors increased over the treatment period. Of note, measures of self-awareness did not improve, suggesting that error monitoring and correction can be improved even though general deficit awareness may remain. Additional case study evidence has been reported for the use of monitoring, feedback, error correction and verbal self-regulation to reduce inappropriate behavior, with some evidence for generalization and maintenance of gains at long-term follow-up (Burke *et al.*, 1991; Cicerone & Tanenbaum, 1997; Lira *et al.*, 1983).

Alderman *et al.* (1995) described the case of a herpes encephalitis patient whose disruptive verbal intrusions were successfully reduced through a formal self-monitoring training (SMT) designed to improve one's ability to attend to one's own behavior and then, through operant conditioning, reduce problem behaviors (Alderman & Burgess, 2003). Self-monitoring training was also successfully employed in a study by Knight and colleagues to reduce problem behaviors in three brain-injured patients (Knight *et al.*, 2002). While operant conditioning methods produced more rapid results (Alderman, 2004), those obtained through SMT were more lasting. More recently, Dayus & van den Broek (2000) used SMT techniques to reduce delusional confabulations in a single patient recovering from subarachnoid hemorrhages. Gains in this patient remained stable at 3-month follow-up. Cicerone & Giacino (1992) described two cases where a verbal reinstatement strategy was used to improve self-monitoring. Improved error monitoring was reported during standardized task performance with evidence of generalization across tasks. However, error rates returned to baseline upon cessation of treatment. In the second case anecdotal evidence indicated that treatment was associated with a reduction in socially inappropriate behavior, even when external prompting was ceased.

Summary and evaluation

- Of 55 published studies on rehabilitation of frontal lobe functions, only 16% meet criteria for Class I evidence sufficient to guide treatment.
- The lack of high-quality evidence reflects the heterogeneity in frontal lobe functions. Researchers tend to focus on clinical observations rather than working from theory.
- Experimental work using rehabilitation probes and carefully described, homogenous patient groups may provide a solid basis for later applications in clinical samples.
- Further work is needed to clarify the importance of metacognitive awareness to rehabilitation outcomes.
- There is a need for validated tasks of real-life function suitable for pre-/post-intervention assessments.

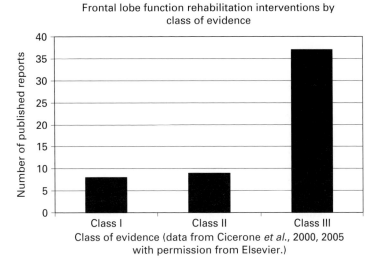

Frontal lobe function rehabilitation interventions by class of evidence

Figure 27.1. Frontal lobe function interventions by class of evidence. Interventions were selected based on criteria described in Turner & Levine (2004) and the revised criteria described in this chapter.

- Increasing numbers, and relative successes, of drug trials for remediating frontal dysfunction point to pharmacology, possibly combined with behavioral interventions, as a promising area of future research.

We identified a total of 55 published studies on rehabilitation of frontal lobe functions (an increment of 15 from our earlier review; Turner & Levine, 2004). As seen in Figure 27.1, only 16% of these meet criteria for Class I evidence sufficient to guide treatment. Significant design limitations, including the lack of control groups, limitations in the selection of outcome measures, lack of follow-up assessment, and lack of generalisation significantly limit the conclusions derived from this literature. In short, there are no standardized, widely accepted methods for rehabilitation of frontal lobe functions.

This deficiency in evidence-based treatments is accentuated when the ubiquity and handicap of frontal lobe dysfunction is taken into consideration. The heterogeneity in definitions of frontal lobe functions is a major source of confusion in the design and reporting of treatments. Although we report interventions in four categories, this classification was a posteriori. It is more common for interventions to use a clinical observation or syndrome as a starting point (e.g., sexual disinhibition, abulia) rather than work top-down from an established theory of frontal lobe function. Notable exceptions include studies specifically addressing working memory (e.g., McDowell et al., 1998; Stablum et al., 2000) and behavioral/emotional self-regulation (e.g., Rath et al., 2003). In this respect, "rehabilitation probes" (Hewitt et al., 2006; Levine et al., 2000b; Manly et al., 2002) – experiments designed as proof-of-principle, provide a good starting point, even if the clinical implications are limited at first.

Even theory-driven interventions, however, are insufficient unless they are applied to the right patient population (see Chapter 3 by Stuss and Binns in this volume, on the importance of minimizing group variability). As defined above, different frontal syndromes arise from different etiologies and lesion locations. As one example, energising regulation functions are closely associated with the medial prefrontal cortex. Although in its early stages, work in patients with energizing regulation deficits suggests that dopaminergic agonists may be effective (e.g., Newburn & Newburn, 2005; Powell, 1996).

The vast majority of patients with frontal dysfunction have complex or diffuse etiologies. While such patients are the ultimate recipients of interventions being developed today, early establishment of the validity of these interventions is well-served by research in well-defined patient populations. Practical considerations, however, limit the number of such patients available for trials. Groups of patients with circumscribed deficits in frontal functions without complicating comorbidity are hard to assemble.

In syndromes with a recovering course, time since injury appears to be a critical factor in treatment planning. Interventions may be most effective at a stage where spontaneous recovery processes can be maximally engaged (Robertson & Murre, 1999). In other words, intervention before basic arousal and attentional mechanisms have recovered, or following the full course of naturalistic recovery, is often less effective than intervention in between these stages.

Recently, functional brain-imaging techniques have been employed to more precisely define brain-based rehabilitation targets and to identify the neural correlates and mechanisms of altered behavioral performance post-intervention (see Chen et al., 2006 for review). Using this approach, neural markers are used to differentiate alterations owing to natural recovery processes from intervention-specific changes and to characterize the relationship between brain function and behavior and/or functional outcome following rehabilitation. These imaging techniques may be of particular importance in the rehabilitation of frontal lobe functions where clear operational definitions and reliable behavioral measures are lacking.

Metacognitive interventions provide an interesting point of reflection on the nature of frontal lobe functions and rehabilitation. Many regard deficit awareness as a necessary prerequisite to behavior change. Yet there is some evidence for dissociations between awareness and behavioral/functional improvement (i.e., in some studies awareness improved without functional change, in others functional change occurred without changes in awareness levels).

A similarly interesting theoretical point relates to generalization: how does one attain generalization in frontal patients, for many of whom the core deficit is a failure to extrapolate rules and principles from one situation (e.g., the clinic) to another (e.g., real-life)? The assessment of real-life behavior, ultimately essential to establish the validity of interventions for frontal dysfunction, is of particular concern. There are few psychometrically validated, performance-based measures of real life functions from which to choose, and none of these have alternate forms for use in pre-/post-intervention assessments.

Finally, although we have segregated pharmacologic and behavioral rehabilitation interventions in our review, a growing literature is beginning to demonstrate the efficacy of a combined drug/behavioral approach to remediate both cognitive and motor disorders (e.g., hemiplegia and aphasia) following brain damage (Walker-Batson et al., 1995; for review, see Phillips et al., 2003). While the mechanisms underlying the efficacy of such a combined approach remain unclear, it is believed that catecholaminergic and cholinergic neuromodulation facilitates neuroplastic change, primarily by altering synaptic strength through long-term potentiation/depression mechanisms, thereby potentiating learning capacity during concurrent behavioral interventions (Floel et al., 2005; Meintzschel & Ziemann, 2006). We did not uncover published reports of combined therapies specifically targeting frontal lobe dysfunction. However, the importance of these neuromodulators in frontal lobe functioning, and the relative success of pharmacologic interventions in the energizing and executive domains we report here, suggest that such combined therapeutic approaches may be a promising area of future research.

Conclusions and recommendations

Frontal lobe functions are critical to adaptive functioning and quality of life. These functions are sensitive to numerous brain diseases, especially strokes, tumors, traumatic brain injury and psychiatric disorders. As these functions are at the apex of cognition, they are sensitive to damage throughout the neuraxis. The true prevalence of handicap owing to frontal lobe dysfunction is inestimable, with societal costs surely in the billions.

Considering the foregoing, it is remarkable that there are no standardized, accepted rehabilitation methods for people with deficits due to frontal lobe damage. In the fields of speech and language or physical therapy, numerous efficacious interventions have been derived from established, validated models. Patients may be classified according to the specific system affected. Outcome measures are available to objectively assess functional changes. These features provide a framework for conducting RCTs, including long-term follow-up. In the case of frontal lobe functions, broadly accepted theoretical frameworks are hard to come by, there is no classification system for patients with heterogenous deficits, and few outcome measures exist by which generalization may be assessed. The framework for conducting high-quality research in rehabilitation of frontal lobe functions has yet to be built.

We have attempted to describe frontal lobe functions and classify interventions according to one model by which four fundamental functions are identified: energization, executive, self-regulation and metacognition. While this model may require modification according to future research, it provides an example of objective classification of deficits required for the appropriate targeting of interventions, just as an analysis of linguistic capacity would influence selection of language rehabilitation.

Rehabilitation of frontal functions is in its infancy. Evidence from a few high-quality studies and carefully conducted clinical group studies shows promise for both behavioral and, increasingly, pharmacologic interventions. Moreover, the application of neuro-imaging techniques will help to better define targets, evaluate and ultimately enhance rehabilitation strategies by integrating neural and behavioral measures both pre- and post-intervention. The questions posed by rehabilitation of frontal functions (e.g., is metacognitive awareness necessary for functional improvement? Can generalization be trained in patients who lack mental flexibility?) concern the highest forms of consciousness in humans. Research on these questions can therefore feed back into theory, ultimately contributing to a foundation necessary for the building of interventions.

ACKNOWLEDGMENTS

We are grateful to all the patients and other individuals who participated in all the projects; to our co-authors on the different papers referenced; and to all the research assistants who assisted in the various studies. The Canadian Institutes of Health Research (CIHR; BL: MOP-108540, MGP-62963; DTS: CIHR 108636), the National Institutes of Health – NICHD (BL: #HD42385-01), the JSF McDonnell Foundation (DTS: JSMF 21002032), the Canadian Foundation for Innovation/Ontario Innovation Trust # 1226, the Heart and Stroke Foundation of Ontario Centre for Stroke Recovery, and the Louis and Leah Posluns Centre for Stroke and Cognition are thanked for financial assistance. D. T. Stuss was supported by the Reva James Leeds Chair in Neuroscience and Research Leadership.

REFERENCES

Adams, J. H., Graham, D. I., Murray, L. S., & Scott, G. (1982). Diffuse axonal injury due to nonmissile head injury in humans: an analysis of 45 cases. *Annals of Neurology*, **12**, 557–563.

Alderman, N. (2004). Disorders of behaviour. In J. Ponsford (Ed.), *Cognitive and Behavioural Rehabilitation* (pp. 269–298). New York, NY: Guilford Publications.

Alderman, N., & Burgess, P. W. (2003). Assessment and rehabilitation of the dysexecutive syndrome. In R. Greenwood, T. M. McMillan, M. P. Barnes, & C. D. Ward (Eds.), *Handbook of Neurological Rehabilitation (2nd Edition)* (pp. 387–402). Hove, UK: Psychology Press.

Alderman, N., Fry, R. K., & Youngson, H. A. (1995). Improvement of self-monitoring skills, reduction of behaviour disturbance and the dysexecutive system. *Neuropsychological Rehabilitation*, **5**, 193–222.

Alexander, G. E., DeLong, M. R., & Strick, P. L. (1986). Parallel organization of functionally segregated circuits linking basal ganglia and cortex. *Annual Review of Neuroscience*, **9**, 357–381.

Alexander, M. P., Stuss, D. T., & Fansabedian, N. (2003). California Verbal Learning Test: performance by patients with focal frontal and non-frontal lesions. *Brain*, **126**, 1493–1503.

Alexander, M. P., Stuss, D. T., Shallice, T., Picton, T. W., & Gillingham, S. (2005). Impaired concentration due to frontal lobe damage from two distinct lesion sites. *Neurology*, **65**, 572–579.

Anderson, S. W., & Damasio, A. R. (1995). Frontal-lobe syndromes. In J. Bogousslavsky & L. Caplan (Eds.), *Stroke Syndromes* (pp. 140–144). New York, NY: Cambridge University Press.

Anderson, S. W., Damasio, H., Jones, R. D., & Tranel, D. (1991). Wisconsin Card Sorting Test performance as a measure of frontal lobe damage. *Journal of Clinical and Experimental Neuropsychology*, **13**, 909–922.

Arco, L., Cohen, L., & Geddes, K. (2004). Verbal self-regulation of impulsive behaviour of persons with frontal lobe injury. *Behavior Therapy*, **35**, 605–619.

Bechara, A., Damasio, A. R., Damasio, H., & Anderson, S. W. (1994). Insensitivity to future consequences following damage to human prefrontal cortex. *Cognition*, **50**, 7–15.

Berryhill, P., Lilly, M. A., Levin, H. S. *et al.* (1995). Frontal lobe changes after severe diffuse closed head injury in children: a volumetric study of magnetic resonance imaging. *Neurosurgery*, **37**, 392–399.

Bottger, S., Prosiegel, M., Steiger, H.-J., & Yassouridis, A. (1998). Neurobehavioural disturbances, rehabilitation outcome, and lesion site in patients after rupture and repair of anterior communicating artery aneurysm. *Journal of Neurology, Neurosurgery and Psychiatry*, **65**, 93–102.

Brooks, N., Campsie, L., Symington, C., Beattie, A., & McKinlay, W. (1986). The five year outcome of severe blunt head injury: a relative's view. *Journal of Neurology, Neurosurgery and Psychiatry*, **49**, 764–770.

Burgess, P. W., Alderman, N., Evans, J., Emslie, H., & Wilson, B. A. (1998). The ecological validity of tests of executive function. *Journal of the International Neuropsychological Society*, **4**, 547–558.

Burgess, P. W., Veitch, E., de Lacy Costello, A., & Shallice, T. (2000). The cognitive and neuroanatomical correlates of multitasking. *Neuropsychologia*, **38**, 848–863.

Burgess, P. W., Simons, J. S., Dumontheil, I., & Gilbert, S. J. (2005). The gateway hypothesis of rostral prefrontal cortex (area 10) function. In L. Duncan, L. Phillips, & P. McLeod (Eds.), *Speed, Control, and Age: In Honour of Patrick Rabbitt* (pp. 217–248). Oxford, UK: Oxford University Press.

Burgess, P. W., Gilbert, S. J., & Dumontheil, I. (2007). Function and localization within rostral prefrontal cortex (area 10). *Philosophical Transactions of the Royal Society of London, Part B*, **362**, 887–899.

Burke, W. H., Zencius, A. H., Wesolowski, M. D., & Doubleday, F. (1991). Improving executive function disorders in brain-injured clients. *Brain Injury*, **5**, 241–252.

Chen, A. J., Abrams, G. M., & D'Esposito, M. (2006). Functional reintegration of prefrontal neural networks for enhancing recovery after brain injury. *Journal of Head Trauma Rehabilitation*, **21**, 107–118.

Cheng, S. K., & Man, D. W. (2006). Management of impaired self-awareness in persons with traumatic brain injury. *Brain Injury*, **20**, 621–628.

Chittum, W. R., Johnson, K., Chittum, J. M., Guercio, J. M., & McMorrow, M. J. (1996). Road to awareness: an individualized training package for increasing knowledge and comprehension of personal deficits in persons with acquired brain injury. *Brain Injury*, **10**, 763–776.

Christman, C. W., Salvant, J. B. J., Walker, S. A., & Povlishock, J. T. (1997). Characterization of a prolonged regenerative attempt by diffusely injured axons following traumatic brain injury in adult cat: a light and electron microscopic immunocytochemical study. *Acta Neuropathologica*, **94**, 329–337.

Christoff, K., & Gabrieli, J. D. E. (2000). The frontopolar cortex and human cognition: evidence for a rostrocaudal hierarchical organization within the human prefrontal cortex. *Psychobiology*, **28**, 168–186.

Cicerone, K. D. (2000). Evidence-based cognitive rehabilitation: Recommendations for clinical practice. *Science*, **290**, 966–969.

Cicerone, K. D., & Giacino, J. T. (1992). Remediation of executive function deficits after traumatic brain injury. *Neurorehabilitation*, **2**, 12–22.

Cicerone, K. D., & Tanenbaum, L. N. (1997). Disturbance of social cognition after traumatic orbitofrontal brain injury. *Archives of Clinical Neuropsychology*, **12**, 173–188.

Cicerone, K. D., & Wood, J. C. (1987). Planning disorder after closed head injury: a case study. *Archives of Physical Medicine and Rehabilitation*, **68**, 111–115.

Cicerone, K. D., Dahlberg, C., Malec, J. F. *et al.* (2005). Evidence-based cognitive rehabilitation: updated review of the literature from 1998 through 2002. *Archives of Physical Medicine and Rehabilitation*, **86**, 1681–1692.

Cicerone, K., Levin, H., Malec, J., Stuss, D., & Whyte, J. (2006). Cognitive rehabilitation interventions for executive function: moving from bench to bedside in patients with traumatic brain injury. *Journal of Cognitive Neuroscience*, **18**, 1–11.

Cicerone, K. W. (2002). The enigma of executive functioning: theoretical contributions to therapeutic interventions. In P. J. Eslinger, M. M. Downey-Lamb, M. L. Glisky, I. Robertson, & S. Ward (Eds.), *Neuropsychological Interventions: Clinical Research and Practice* (pp. 426). New York, NY: Guilford Press.

Clifton, G., Grossman, R., Makela, M. *et al.* (1980). Neurological course and correlated computerized tomography findings after severe closed head injury. *Journal of Neurosurgery*, **52**, 611–624.

Courville, C. B. (1937). *Pathology of the Central Nervous System, Part 4*. Mountain View, CA: Pacific Press Publishing.

Cummings, J. L. (1993). Frontal-subcortical circuits and human behavior. *Archives of Neurology*, **50**, 873–880.

Damasio, A. R. (1996). The somatic marker hypothesis and the possible functions of the prefrontal cortex. *Philosophical Transactions of the Royal Society of London: Biological Sciences*, **351**, 1413–1420.

Dayus, B., & van den Broek, M. D. (2000). Treatment of stable confabulations using self-monitoring training. *Neuropsychological Rehabilitation*, **10**, 415–427.

Deacon, D., & Campbell, K. B. (1991). Decision-making following closed-head injury: can response speed be retrained? *Journal of Clinical and Experimental Neuropsychology*, **13**, 639–651.

Delazer, M., Bodner, T., & Benke, T. (1998). Rehabilitation of arithmetical text problem solving. *Neuropsychological Rehabilitation*, **8**, 401–412.

DeLuca, J. (1992). Cognitive dysfunction after aneurysm of the anterior communicating artery. *Journal of Clinical and Experimental Neuropsychology*, **14**, 924–934.

DeLuca, J., & Diamond, B. J. (1995). Aneurysm of the anterior communicating artery: a review of the neuroanatomical and neuropsychological sequelae. *Journal of Clinical and Experimental Neuropsychology*, **17**, 100–121.

Deutsch, G., Papanicolaou, A. C., Bourbon, W. T., & Eisenberg, H. M. (1987). Cerebral blood flow evidence of right frontal activation in attention demanding tasks. *International Journal of Neuroscience*, **36**, 23–28.

Diamond, B. J., DeLuca, J., & Kelley, S. M. (1997). Memory and executive functions in amnesic and non-amnesic patients with aneurysms of the anterior communicating artery. *Brain*, **120**, 1015–1025.

Dias, R., Robbins, T. W., & Roberts, A. C. (1996). Dissociation in prefrontal cortex of affective and attentional shifts. *Nature*, **380**, 69–72.

Dias, R., Robbins, T. W., & Roberts, A. C. (1997). Dissociable forms of inhibitory control within prefrontal cortex with an analog of the Wisconsin Card Sort Test: restriction to novel situations and independence from "on-line" processing. *Journal of Neuroscience*, **17**, 9285–9297.

Dikmen, S. S., Ross, B. L., Machamer, J. E., & Temkin, N. R. (1995). One year psychosocial outcome in head injury. *Journal of the International Neuropsychological Society*, **1**, 67–77.

Duncan, J. (1986). Disorganization of behavior after frontal lobe damage. *Cognitive Neuropsychology*, **3**, 271–290.

Duncan, J., Emslie, H., Williams, P., Johnson, R., & Freer, C. (1996). Intelligence and the frontal lobe: the organization of goal-directed behavior. *Cognitive Psychology*, **30**, 257–303.

Dunn, B. D., Dalgleish, T., & Lawrence, A. D. (2006). The somatic marker hypothesis: a critical evaluation. *Neuroscience and Biobehavioral Reviews*, **30**, 239–271.

Elliott, R., Dolan, R. J., & Frith, C. D. (2000). Dissociable functions in the medial and lateral orbitofrontal cortex: evidence from human neuroimaging studies. *Cerebral Cortex*, **10**, 308–317.

Eslinger, P. J., & Damasio, A. R. (1985). Severe disturbance of higher cognition after bilateral frontal lobe ablation: Patient EVR. *Neurology*, **35**, 1731–1741.

Evans, J. J., Emslie, H., & Wilson, B. A. (1998). External cueing systems in the rehabilitation of executive impairments of action. *Journal of the International Neuropsychological Society*, **4**, 399–408.

Fellows, L. K., & Farah, M. J. (2005). Different underlying impairments in decision-making following ventromedial and dorsolateral frontal lobe damage in humans. *Cerebral Cortex*, **15**, 58–63.

Fleming, J. M., Lucas, S. E., & Lightbody, S. (2006). Using occupation to facilitate self-awareness in people who have acquired brain injury: a pilot study. *Canadian Journal of Occupational Therapy*, **73**, 44–55.

Floel, A., Breitenstein, C., Hummel, F. *et al.* (2005). Dopaminergic influences on formation of a motor memory. *Annals of Neurology*, **58**, 121–130.

Fox, R. M., Martella, R. C., & Marchand-Martella, N. E. (1989). Acquisition, maintenance and generalization of problem-solving skills by closed head injured adults. *Behaviour Therapy*, **20**, 61–76.

Fuster, J. M. (1997). *The Prefrontal Cortex: Anatomy, Physiology, and Neuropsychology of the Frontal Lobe (3rd Edition)*. New York, NY: Raven Press.

Gennarelli, T. A., Thibault, L. E., Adams, J. H. *et al.* (1982). Diffuse axonal injury and traumatic coma in the primate. *Annals of Neurology*, **12**, 564–572.

Gentry, L. R., Godersky, J. C., & Thompson, B. (1988). MR imaging of head trauma: review of the distribution and radiopathologic features of traumatic lesions. *American Journal of Neuroradiology*, **9**, 101–110.

Gilboa, A., Alain, C., Stuss, D. T. *et al.* (2006). Mechanisms of spontaneous confabulations: a strategic retrieval account. *Brain*, **129**, 1399–1414.

Giles, G. M., & Morgan, J. H. (1990). Self-instruction training of functional skills: a single case study. *British Journal of Occupational Therapy*, **53**, 314–316.

Glosser, G., & Goodglass, H. (1990). Disorders in executive control functions among aphasic and other brain-damaged patients. *Journal of Clinical and Experimental Neuropsychology*, **12**, 485–501.

Goldman-Rakic, P. S. (1987). Circuitry of primate prefrontal cortex and regulation of behavior by representational memory. In F. Plum & V. Mountcastle (Eds.), *Handbook of Physiology: The Nervous System* (pp. 373–417). Bethesda, MD: American Physiological Society.

Harlow, J. M. (1868). Recovery after severe injury to the head. *Publication of the Massachusetts Medical Society*, **2**, 327–346.

Hewitt, J., Evans, J. J., & Dritschel, B. (2006). Theory driven rehabilitation of executive functioning: improving planning skills in people with traumatic brain injury through the use of an autobiographical episodic memory cueing procedure. *Neuropsychologia*, **44**, 1468–1474.

Hux, K., Reid, R., & Lugert, M. (1994). Self-instruction training following neurological injury. *Applied Cognitive Psychology*, **8**, 259–271.

Jennett, B., Snoek, J., Bond, M. R., & Brooks, N. (1981). Disability after severe head injury: observations on the use of the Glasgow Outcome Scale. *Journal of Neurology, Neurosurgery and Psychiatry*, **44**, 285–293.

Knight, C., Rutterford, N. A., Alderman, N., & Swan, L. J. (2002). Is accurate self-monitoring necessary for people with acquired neurological problems to benefit from the use of differential reinforcement methods? *Brain Injury*, **16**, 75–87.

Kraus, M. F., Smith, G. S., Butters, M. *et al.* (2005). Effects of the dopaminergic agent and NMDA receptor antagonist amantadine on cognitive function, cerebral glucose metabolism and D2 receptor availability in chronic traumatic brain injury: a study using positron emission tomography (PET). *Brain Injury*, **19**, 471–479.

Levine, B. (1999). Self-regulation and autonoetic consciousness. In E. Tulving (Ed.), *Memory, Consciousness, and the Brain: The Tallinn Conference* (pp. 200–214). Philadelphia, PA: Psychology Press.

Levine, B., & Downey-Lamb, M. (2002). Design and evaluation of intervention experiments. In P. J. Eslinger (Ed.), *Neuropsychological Interventions: Emerging Treatment and Management Models for Neuropsychological Impairments* (pp. 80–104). New York, NY: Guilford Press.

Levine, B., Stuss, D. T., Milberg, W. P. *et al.* (1998). The effects of focal and diffuse brain damage on strategy application: evidence from focal lesions, traumatic brain injury and normal aging. *Journal of the International Neuropsychological Society*, **4**, 247–264.

Levine, B., Dawson, D., Boutet, I., Schwartz, M. L., & Stuss, D. T. (2000a). Assessment of strategic self-regulation in traumatic brain injury: its relationship to injury severity and psychosocial outcome. *Neuropsychology*, **14**, 491–500.

Levine, B., Robertson, I. H., Clare, L. *et al.* (2000b). Rehabilitation of executive functioning: an experimental-clinical validation of goal management training. *Journal of the International Neuropsychological Society*, **6**, 299–312.

Levine, B., Katz, D., Black, S. E., & Dade, L. (2002). New approaches to brain-behavior assessment in traumatic brain injury. In D. T. Stuss & R. T. Knight (Eds.), *Principles of Frontal Lobe function* (pp. 448–465). New York, NY: Oxford University Press.

Levine, B., Black, S. E., Cheung, G. *et al.* (2005). Gambling task performance in traumatic brain injury: relationships to injury severity, atrophy, lesion location, and cognitive and psychosocial outcome. *Cognitive and Behavioral Neurology*, **18**, 45–54.

Levine, B., Fujiwara, F., O'Connor, C. *et al.* (2006). In vivo characterization of traumatic brain injury neuropathology with structural and functional neuroimaging. *Journal of Neurotrauma*, **23**, 1396–1411.

Levine, B., Stuss, D. T., Winocur, G. *et al.* (2007). Cognitive rehabilitation in the elderly: effects on strategic behavior in relation to goal management. *Journal of the International Neuropsychological Society*, **13**, 143–152.

Lezak, M. D. (1995). *Neuropsychological Assessment (3rd Edition)*. New York, NY: Oxford University Press.

Lilja, A., Salford, L. G., Smith, G. J., & Hagstadius, S. (1992). Neuropsychological indexes of a partial frontal syndrome in patients with nonfrontal gliomas. *Neuropsychology*, **6**, 315–326.

Lira, F. T., Carne, W., & Masri, A. M. (1983). Treatment of anger and impulsivity in a brain damaged patient: a case in applying stress innoculation. *Clinical Neuropsychology*, **5**, 159–160.

Lucas, S. E., & Fleming, J. M. (2005). Interventions for improving self-awareness following acquired brain injury. *Australian Occupational Therapy Journal*, **52**, 160–170.

Luria, A. R. (1966). *Higher Cortical Functions in Man*. New York, NY: Basic Books.

Luria, A. R., & Homskaya, D. (1964). Disturbance in the regulative role of speech with frontal lobe lesions. In J. M. Warren & K. Akert (Eds.), *The Frontal Granular Cortex and Behavior* (pp. 353–371). New York, NY: McGraw-Hill.

Manly, T., Hawkins, K., Evans, J., Woldt, K., & Robertson, I. H. (2002). Rehabilitation of executive function: facilitation of effective goal management on complex tasks using periodic auditory alerts. *Neuropsychologia*, **40**, 271–281.

Marshall, R. C., Karow, C. M., Morelli, C. A. *et al.* (2004). Effects of interactive strategy modelling training on problem-solving by persons with traumatic brain injury. *Aphasiology*, **18**, 659–673.

Mavaddat, N., Kirkpatrick, P. J., Rogers, R. D., & Sahakian, B. J. (2000). Deficits in decision-making in patients with aneurysms of the anterior communicating artery. *Brain*, **123**, 2109–2117.

Maxwell, W. L., Povlishock, J. T., & Graham, D. L. (1997). A mechanistic analysis of nondisruptive axonal injury: a review. *Journal of Neurotrauma*, **14**, 419–440.

McDowell, S., Whyte, J., & D'Esposito, M. (1998). Differential effect of a dopaminergic agonist on prefrontal function in traumatic brain injury patients. *Brain*, **121**, 1155–1164.

Medd, J., & Tate, R. L. (2000). Evaluation of an anger management program following ABI: a preliminary study. *Neuropsychological Rehabilitation*, **10**, 185–201.

Meintzschel, F., & Ziemann, U. (2006). Modification of practice-dependent plasticity in human motor cortex by neuromodulators. *Cerebral Cortex*, **16**, 1106–1115.

Meythaler, J. M., Depalma, L., Devivo, M. J., Guin-Renfroe, S., & Novack, T. A. (2001). Sertraline to improve arousal and alertness in severe traumatic brain injury secondary to motor vehicle crashes. *Brain Injury*, **15**, 321–331.

Miller, E. K. (1999). The prefrontal cortex: complex neural properties for complex behavior. *Neuron*, **22**, 15–17.

Milner, B. (1963). Effects of different brain lesions on card sorting: the role of the frontal lobes. *Archives of Neurology*, **9**, 100–110.

Mishkin, M. (1964). Perseveration of central sets after frontal lesions in monkeys. In K. A. M. Warren (Ed.), *The Frontal Granular Cortex and behavior*. New York, NY: McGraw-Hill.

Monakow, v. (1914). *Localization in the Cerebrum and the Degeneration of Functions through Cortical Sources*. Wiesbaden, Germany: J. F. Bergman.

Muller, U., & von Cramon, D. Y. (1994). The therapeutic potential of bromocriptine in neuropsychological rehabilitation of patients with acquired brain damage. *Progress in Neuro-Psychopharmacology and Biological Psychiatry*, **18**, 1103–1120.

Nakawatase, T. Y. (1999). Frontal lobe tumors. In B. L. Miller & J. L. Cummings (Eds.), *Human Frontal Lobes*. New York, NY: Guilford Press.

National Center for Injury Prevention and Control (1999). *Traumatic Brain Injury in the United States: A Report to Congress*. Atlanta, GA: Centers for Disease Control and Prevention.

Nauta, W. J. (1971). The problem of the frontal lobe: a reinterpretation. *Journal of Psychiatric Research*, **8**, 167–187.

Newburn, G., & Newburn, D. (?005). Selegiline in the management of apathy following traumatic brain injury. *Brain Injury*, **19**, 149–154.

O'Callaghan, M. E., & Couvadelli, B. (1998). Use of self-instructional strategies with three neurologically impaired adults. *Cognitive Therapy and Research*, **22**, 91–107.

O'Connor, C., Turner, G. R., Katerji, S. *et al.* (2006). A randomized control trial of goal management training in adults with neurological damage. *Journal of the International Neuropsychological Society*, **12**, *Suppl. 1*, 93.

Ommaya, A. K., & Gennarelli, T. A. (1974). Cerebral concussion and traumatic unconsciousness. Correlation of experimental and clinical observations of blunt head injuries. *Brain*, **97**, 633–654.

Ownsworth, T., & McFarland, K. (2000). Investigation of psychological and neuropsychological factors associated with clinical outcome following a group rehabilitation programme. *Neuropsychological Rehabilitation*, **14**, 535–562.

Ownsworth, T., Fleming, J., Desbois, J., Strong, J., & Kuipers, P. (2006). A metacognitive contextual intervention to enhance error awareness and functional outcome following traumatic brain injury: a single-case experimental design. *Journal of the International Neuropsychological Society*, **12**, 54–63.

Pandya, D. N., & Barnes, C. L. (1987). Architecture and connections of the frontal lobe. In E. Perecman (Eds.), *The*

Frontal Lobes Revisited (pp. 41–72). New York, NY: IRBN Press.

Pandya, D. N., & Yeterian, E. H. (1996). Morphological correlations of human and monkey frontal lobes. In A. R. Damasio, H. Damasio, & Y. Christen (Eds.), *Neurobiology of Decision Making* (pp. 13–46). New York, NY: Springer Verlag.

Pardo, J. V., Fox, P. T., & Raichle, M. E. (1991). Localization of a human system for sustained attention by positron emission tomography. *Nature*, **349**, 61–64.

Park, N. W., Conrod, B., Hussain, Z. *et al.* (2003). A treatment program for individuals with deficient evaluative processing and consequent impaired social and risk judgement. *Neurocase*, **9**, 51–62.

Parks, R. W., Crockett, D. J., Manji, H. K., & Ammann, W. (1992). Assessment of bromocriptine intervention for the treatment of frontal lobe syndrome: a case study. *Journal of Neuropsychiatry and Clinical Neurosciences*, **4**, 109–111.

Penfield, W., & Evans, J. (1935). The frontal lobe in man: a clinical study of maximum removals. *Brain*, **58**, 115–133.

Petrides, M., & Milner, B. (1982). Deficits on subject-ordered tasks after frontal- and temporal-lobe lesions in man. *Neuropsychologia*, **20**, 249–262.

Phillips, J. P., Devier, D. J., & Feeney, D. M. (2003). Rehabilitation pharmacology: bridging laboratory work to clinical application. *Journal of Head Trauma Rehabilitation*, **18**, 342–356.

Picton, T. W., Stuss, D. T., Shallice, T., Alexander, M. P., & Gillingham, S. (2006). Keeping time: effects of focal frontal lesions. *Neuropsychologia*, **44**, 1195–1209.

Povlishock, J. T. (1992). Traumatically induced axonal injury: pathogenesis and pathobiological implications. *Brain Pathology*, **2**, 1–12.

Povlishock, J. T. (1993). Pathobiology of traumatically induced axonal injury in animals and man. *Annals of Emergency Medicine*, **22**, 980–986.

Povlishock, J. T., & Christman, C. W. (1995). The pathobiology of traumatically induced axonal injury in animals and humans: a review of current thoughts. *Journal of Neurotrauma*, **12**, 555–564.

Povlishock, J. T., Erb, D. E., & Astruc, J. (1992). Axonal response to traumatic brain injury: reactive axonal change, deafferentation, and neuroplasticity. *Journal of Neurotrauma*, **9**, Suppl. 1, S189–S200.

Powell, J. H. (1996). Motivational deficits after brain injury: effects of bromocriptine in 11 patients. *Journal of Neurology, Neurosurgery and Psychiatry*, **60**, 416–421.

Price, R. P., Goetz, K. L., & Lovell, M. R. (1997). Neuropsychiatric aspects of brain tumors. In S. C. Yodofsky & R. E. Hales (Eds.), *American Psychiatric Press Textbook of Neuropsychiatry (3rd Edition)*. (pp. 635–643). Washington, DC: American Psychiatric Press.

Prigatano, G. P. (1991). Disturbances of self-awareness of deficit after traumatic brain injury. In G. Prigatano & D. L. Schacter (Eds.), *Awareness of Deficit after Brain Injury* (pp. 111–126). New York, NY: Oxford University Press.

Rath, J. F., Simon, D., Langenbahn, D. M., Sherr, R. L., & Diller, L. (2003). Group treatment of problem-solving deficits in outpatients with traumatic brain injury: a randomised outcome study. *Neuropsychological Rehabilitation*, **13**, 461–488.

Rebman, M. J., & Hannon, R. (1995). Treatment of unawareness of memory deficits in adults with brain injury. *Rehabilitation Psychology*, **40**, 279–287.

Robertson, I. H., & Murre, J. M. (1999). Rehabilitation of brain damage: brain plasticity and principles of guided recovery. *Psychological Bulletin*, **125**, 544–575.

Robinson, R. G., & Starkstein, S. E. (1997). Neuropsychiatric aspects of cerebrovascular disorders. In S. C. Yodofsky & R. E. Hales (Eds.), *American Psychiatric Press Textbook of Neuropsychiatry (3rd Edition)*. (pp. 607–614). Washington, DC: American Psychiatric Press.

Rolls, E. T. (1996). The orbitofrontal cortex. *Philosophical Transactions of the Royal Society of London, Part B*, **351**, 1433–1444.

Rolls, E. T. (2000). The orbitofrontal cortex and reward. *Cerebral Cortex*, **10**, 284–294.

Rueckert, L., & Grafman, J. (1996). Sustained attention deficits in patients with right frontal lesions. *Neuropsychologia*, **34**, 953–963.

Sanides, F. (1970). Functional architecture of motor and sensory cortices in primates in the light of a new concept of neocortex development. In C. R. Noback & W. Montagna (Eds.), *Advances in Primatology* (pp. 137–208). New York, NY: Appleton-Century-Crofts.

Schlund, M. W. (1999). Case study: Self awareness: effects of feedback and review on verbal self reports and remembering following brain injury. *Brain Injury*, **13**, 375–380.

Schwartz, M. F., Montgomery, M. W., Buxbaum, L. J. *et al.* (1998). Naturalistic action impairment in closed head injury. *Neuropsychology*, **12**, 13–28.

Schwartz, M. F., Buxbaum, L. J., Montgomery, M. W. *et al.* (1999). Naturalistic action production following right hemisphere stroke. *Neuropsychologia*, **37**, 51–66.

Serino, A., Ciaramelli, E., Di Santantonio, A., & Ladavas, E. (2006). A rehabilitative program for central executive deficits after traumatic brain injury. *Brain and Cognition*, **60**, 213–214.

Shallice, T., & Burgess, P. W. (1991). Deficits in strategy application following frontal lobe damage in man. *Brain*, **114**, 727–741.

Shallice, T., & Burgess, P. W. (1993). Supervisory control of action and thought selection. In A. Baddeley & L. Weiskrantz (Eds.), *Attention: Selection, Awareness, and Control. A Tribute to Donald Broadbent* (pp. 171–187). Oxford, UK: Clarendon Press.

Shammi, P., & Stuss, D. T. (1999). Humour appreciation: a role of the right frontal lobe. *Brain*, **122**, 657–666.

Siegal, M., & Varley, R. (2002). Neural systems involved in "theory of mind". *Nature Reviews Neuroscience*, **3**, 463–471.

Sohlberg, M. M., Sprunk, H., & Metzelaar, K. (1988). Efficacy of an external cuing system in an individual with severe frontal lobe damage. *Cognitive Rehabilitation*, **6**, 36–41.

Soong, W., Tam, S. F., Man, W. K., & Hui-Chan, C. (2005). A pilot study on the effectiveness of tele-analogy-based problem-solving training for people with brain injuries. *International Journal of Rehabilitation Research*, **28**, 341–347.

Stablum, F., Umilta, C., Mogentale, C., Carlan, M., & Guerrini, C. (2000). Rehabilitation of executive deficits in closed head injury and anterior communicating artery aneurysm patients. *Psychological Research*, **63**, 265–278.

Strich, S. (1956). Diffuse degeneration of the cerebral white matter in severe dementia following head injury. *Journal of Neurology, Neurosurgery and Psychiatry*, **19**, 163–185.

Stuss, D. T. (2006). Frontal lobes and attention: Processes and networks, fractionation and integration. *Journal of the International Neuropsychological Society*, **12**, 261–271.

Stuss, D. T., & Alexander, M. P. (1999). Affectively burnt in: a proposed role of the right frontal lobe. In E. Tulving (Ed.), *Memory, Consciousness and the Brain: The Tallinn Conference* (pp. 215–227). Philadelphia, PA: Psychology Press.

Stuss, D. T., & Alexander, M. P. (2000). The anatomical basis of affective behavior, emotion and self-awareness: a specific role of the right frontal lobe. In G. Hatano, N. Okada, & H. Tanabe (Eds.), *Affective Minds. The 13th Toyota Conference* (pp. 13–25). Amsterdam, NL: Elsevier.

Stuss, D. T., & Alexander, M. P. (in press). Executive functions: Is there a frontal lobe syndrome? In L. Squire, T. Albright, F. Bloom, F. Gage, & N. Spitzer (Eds.), *New Encyclopedia of Neuroscience*.

Stuss, D. T., & Benson, D. F. (1986). *The Frontal Lobes*. New York, NY: Raven Press.

Stuss, D. T., & Gow, C. A. (1992). "Frontal dysfunction" after traumatic brain injury. *Neuropsychiatry, Neuropsychology, and Behavioral Neurology*, **5**, 272–282.

Stuss, D. T., & Levine, B. (2002). Adult clinical neuropsychology: lessons from studies of the frontal lobes. *Annual Review of Psychology*, **53**, 401–433.

Stuss, D. T., Delgado, M., & Guzman, D. A. (1987). Verbal regulation in the control of motor impersistence: a proposed rehabilitation procedure. *Journal of Neurologic Rehabilitation*, **1**, 19–24.

Stuss, D. T., Shallice, T., Alexander, M. P., & Picton, T. (1995). A multidisciplinary approach to anterior attentional functions. *Annals of the New York Academy of Sciences*, **769**, 191–212.

Stuss, D. T., Alexander, M. P., Hamer, L. *et al.* (1998). The effects of focal anterior and posterior brain lesions on verbal fluency. *Journal of the International Neuropsychological Society*, **4**, 265–278.

Stuss, D. T., Toth, J. P., Franchi, D. *et al.* (1999). Dissociation of attentional processes in patients with focal frontal and posterior lesions. *Neuropsychologia*, **37**, 1005–1027.

Stuss, D. T., van Reekum, R., & Murphy, K. J. (2000). Differentiation of states and causes of apathy. In J. Borod (Ed.), *The Neuropsychology of Emotion* (pp. 340–363). New York, NY: Oxford University Press.

Stuss, D. T., Floden, D., Alexander, M. P., Levine, B., & Katz, D. (2001a). Stroop performance in focal lesion patients: dissociation of processes and frontal lobe lesion location. *Neuropsychologia*, **39**, 771–786.

Stuss, D. T., Gallup, G. G. J., & Alexander, M. P. (2001b). The frontal lobes are necessary for "theory of mind". *Brain*, **124**, 279–286.

Stuss, D. T., Picton, T. W., & Alexander, M. P. (2001c). Consciousness, self-awareness, and the frontal lobes. In S. P. Salloway & P. F. Malloy (Eds.), *The Frontal Lobes and Neuropsychiatric Illness* (pp. 101–109). Washington, DC: American Psychiatric Press.

Stuss, D. T., Binns, M. A., Murphy, K. J., & Alexander, M. P. (2002). Dissociations within the anterior attentional system: effects of task complexity and irrelevant information on reaction time speed and accuracy. *Neuropsychology*, **16**, 500–513.

Stuss, D. T., Murphy, K. J., Binns, M. A., & Alexander, M. P. (2003). Staying on the job: the frontal lobes control individual performance variability. *Brain*, **126**, 2363–2380.

Stuss, D. T., Alexander, M. P., Shallice, T. *et al.* (2005a). Multiple frontal systems controlling response speed. *Neuropsychologia*, **43**, 396–417.

Stuss, D. T., Rosenbaum, R. S., Malcolm, S., Christiana, W., & Keenan, J. P. (2005b). The frontal lobes and self-awareness. In T. E. Feinberg & J. P. Keenan (Eds.), *The Lost Self: Pathologies of the Brain and Identity* (pp. 50–64). London, UK: Oxford University Press.

Stuss, D. T., Robertson, I. H., Craik, F. I. M. *et al.* (2007). Cognitive rehabilitation in the elderly: a randomized trial to evaluate a new protocol. *Journal of the International Neuropsychological Society*, **13**, 120–131.

Tucha, O., Smely, C., Preier, M., & Lange, K. W. (2000). Cognitive deficits before treatment among patients with brain tumors. *Neurosurgery*, **47**, 324–333.

Tulving, E. (1985). Memory and consciousness. *Canadian Psychology*, **26**, 1–12.

Turner, G. R., & Levine, B. (2004). Disorders of executive function and self-awareness. In J. Ponsford (Ed.), *Rehabilitation of Neurobehavioral Disorders* (pp. 224–268). New York, NY: Guilford Press.

Vallesi, A., Shallice, T., & Walsh, V. (2007). Role of the prefrontal cortex in the foreperiod effect. TMS evidence for dual mechanisms in temporal preparation. *Cerebral Cortex*, **17**, 466–474.

van Hooren, S. A., Valentijn, S. A., Bosma, H. *et al.* (2006). Effect of a structured course involving goal management training in older adults: a randomised controlled trial. *Patient Education and Counseling*, **65**, 205–213.

van Reekum, R., Bayley, M., Garner, S. *et al.* (1995). N of 1 study: amantadine for the amotivational syndrome in a patient with traumatic brain injury. *Brain Injury*, **9**, 49–53.

van Reekum, R., Stuss, D. T., & Ostrander, L. (2005). Apathy: Why care? *Journal of Neuropsychiatry and Clinical Neurosciences*, **17**, 7–19.

von Cramon, D. Y., & Matthes von Cramon, G. (1994). Back to work with a chronic dysexecutive syndrome? (A case report). *Neuropsychological Rehabilitation*, **4**, 399–417.

von Cramon, D. Y., Matthes von Cramon, G., & Mai, N. (1991). Problem-solving deficits in brain-injured patients. *Neuropsychological Rehabilitation*, **1**, 45–64.

Walker-Batson, D., Smith, P., Curtis, S., Unwin, H., & Greenlee, R. (1995). Amphetamine paired with physical therapy accelerates motor recovery after stroke. Further evidence. *Stroke*, **26**, 2254–2259.

Webb, P. M., & Glueckauf, R. L. (1994). The effects of direct involvement in goal setting on rehabilitation outcome for persons with traumatic brain injuries. *Rehabilitation Psychology*, **39**, 179–188.

Wheeler, M. A., Stuss, D. T., & Tulving, E. (1997). Toward a theory of episodic memory: the frontal lobes and autonoetic consciousness. *Psychological Bulletin*, **121**, 331–354.

Wilkins, A. J., Shallice, T., & McCarthy, R. (1987). Frontal lesions and sustained attention. *Neuropsychologia*, **25**, 359–365.

Woods, D. L., & Knight, R. T. (1986). Electrophysiologic evidence of increased distractibility after dorsolateral prefrontal lesions. *Neurology*, **36**, 212–216.

Youngjohn, J. F., & Altman, I. M. (1989). A performance-based group approach to the treatment of anosagnosia and denial. *Rehabilitation Psychology*, **34**, 217–222.

Zhou, J., Chittum, R., Johnson, K. *et al.* (1996). The utilization of a game format to increase knowledge of residuals among people with acquired brain injury. *Journal of Head Trauma Rehabilitation*, **11**, 51–61.

28

Executive functioning in children with traumatic brain injury in comparison to developmental ADHD

Gerri Hanten and Harvey S. Levin

Introduction

- Executive functions are defined in cognitive and neuropsychology literature as superordinate, managerial capacity for directing more modular abilities, including language, memory, motor skills and perception in the service of, managing and attaining goals (Shallice & Burgess, 1991).

There is growing recognition that executive function (EF), the superordinate, managerial capacity for directing more modular abilities, is frequently impaired by traumatic brain injury (TBI) in children and mediates the neurobehavioral sequelae exhibited by these patients. Symptoms similar to those that are diagnostic of developmental attention-deficit hyperactivity disorder (ADHD) are among the most ubiquitous and affecting sequelae of TBI, suggesting common mechanisms of neural dysfunction. The unifying theme for this chapter is that the neurobehavioral consequences of TBI in children arise at least in part from maldevelopment of frontally guided, distributed networks (Casey et al., 2002; Diamond, 2002; Miller & Cohen, 2001) mediating the set of higher-order cognitive abilities known as "executive functions," a pattern also reported in children with ADHD (Willcutt et al., 2005).

The neural substrate for EF is described, and the vulnerability of the neural substrate for EF to the pathophysiology of traumatic brain injury is discussed and related to recent findings from brain imaging on children with ADHD. Domains of EFs covered in this review include the basic processes of working memory, inhibition, and shifting response strategy, and more complex processes such as planning, and decision-making. Current and proposed approaches to the rehabilitation of EFs in children with TBI and in children with ADHD are presented.

There is considerable overlap between the concept of EF and *cognitive control*, a term used to denote the capacity to actively maintain goals and the means to achieve them while resisting interference (Miller & Cohen, 2001). Developmental cognitive theorists have proposed that EFs include: maintenance of a problem-solving set for future goals (working memory) (Pennington et al., 1996), inhibition (Miller & Cohen, 2001), set shifting (Diamond, 2002), planning and problem solving (Denckla, 1996; Graham et al., 1996; Shallice, 1982), decision making based on reward and penalty (Bechara et al., 2000; Rolls, 2000), and self-regulation (Borkowski et al., 1996).

The EF literature has traditionally emphasized cognitive skills, whereas emotional self-regulation, motivation and social cognition have been more recently recognized as closely related to EFs. Patient studies (Anderson et al., 1999; Grattan & Eslinger, 1992), and developmental research (Gioia et al., 2000) have also brought to light the role of EFs in everyday activities.

In summary, EF overlaps with the concept of cognitive control, and refers to a set of cognitive and socio-behavioral skills used in correspondence with goal-related activities.

Cognitive Neurorehabilitation, Second Edition: Evidence and Application, ed. Donald T. Stuss, Gordon Winocur and Ian H. Robertson. Published by Cambridge University Press. © Cambridge University Press 2008.

Developmental perspective

- Research on EFs in children is complicated by different developmental trajectories of different EFs.
- Development of underlying fundamental processes must be considered when investigating EFs.

In contrast to assessment of the effects of TBI on fully developed EFs in adults, evaluation of these cognitive skills in children is complicated by both the diversity of processes that are labeled "executive function" and differences in developmental trajectories for the different processes. Apparent insensitivity of a specific measure of EF in young children sustaining TBI could reflect that this skill has not yet developed sufficiently (Goldman, 1974). Although experimental tasks derived from cognitive neuroscience have elucidated the impact of TBI on EFs in children, clinical application of these procedures may be hampered by a lack of age-referenced data from typically developing children. The developmental perspective is important to consider in young children whose EF abilities are undergoing rapid change with age and might be especially sensitive to TBI (Ewing-Cobbs *et al.*, 2004). A further distinction should be made between the presence of executive-level dysfunction, and the mechanism underlying the dysfunction. That is, children with impairments in fundamental processes, such as speed of processing or immediate memory span, will very likely show deficits in the higher-level functions that are supported by those processes. Of particular interest, then, are studies in which fundamental processes have been shown to be intact, but with higher-level executive processes impaired.

Thus, research on EFs in children is complicated by the variety of cognitive skills labeled "EFs" as well as the different developmental trajectory for different skills. In children with TBI, the complications are magnified by the fact that, unlike ADHD, which has a well-defined developmental course, TBI can happen at any time during development, therefore may potentially impact EFs at different stages of maturity.

Development of neural substrate of executive functions

- Executive functions depend on frontal lobe neurocircuitry.
- Advances in neuroimaging techniques facilitate specification of neural substrate supporting EFs and the development and relation to acquired and developmental deficits in EF.

Executive functions are mediated by frontally guided, distributed networks involving prefrontal subregions, posterior cortex and subcortical structures including basal ganglia and ventral striatum (Schultz *et al.*, 2000). Recent studies using volumetric analysis of serial MRI have shown nonlinear growth of cortical gray matter volumes with relatively late maturation of dorsolateral and ventrolateral prefrontal cortex (Gogtay *et al.*, 2004) in conjunction with linear changes in the development of white matter (Giedd *et al.*, 1999). The linear growth of white matter volume with age is also consistent with the concept of more widely distributed networks in older children (Luna *et al.*, 2001), and is consistent with numerous studies demonstrating increasing competence with age on tasks thought to rely on executive-level processes.

Currently a very active area of research is the linking of specific cognitive processes to mediating neural substrates using techniques of functional neuroimaging. Although these techniques are still in development, and results must be viewed cautiously pending replication and reliability studies, some consistent trends have emerged. Based on functional brain-imaging studies of humans and infrahuman primate experiments, dorsolateral and ventrolateral prefrontal cortex and parietal cortex appear to support working memory and related computational aspects of EFs (Collette & van der Linden, 2002). Functional brain-imaging studies have also provided evidence that frontal subregions are involved in mediating strategy applications, concurrent working memory and inhibition, and increased information processing efficiency (Kail, 1991). Processing of reward, which is integral to the motivation component of EF, appears to recruit orbitofrontal cortex, amygdala, thalamus and ventral striatum with evidence for a corticostriatal-thalamocortical loop. However, there is a paucity of data concerning the development of this system in children.

In general, fMRI studies of cognitive control in children have suggested that the lateralization and/or distribution of activation along the neural axis changes with age. However, the direction of change and neuroanatomic regions involved may differ, depending on the task and imaging methodology (Brown *et al.*, 2004; Bunge *et al.*, 2001; Durston *et al.*, 2001; Gaillard *et al.*, 2000; Luna *et al.*, 2001; Rubia *et al.*, 2000).

Neural substrate in children with TBI

In addition to ubiquitous traumatic axonal injury and focal lesions, diffuse injury and secondary brain insult impacts brain development of children following TBI (Bittigau *et al.*, 1999; Kochanek *et al.*, 2000). Exacerbation of the effects of TBI are caused by excitotoxicity associated with post-traumatic stress (De Bellis *et al.*, 1999; Kochanek *et al.*, 2000), other secondary emotional disturbance (Sheline, 2003), and stress related to the child's environment (Yeates *et al.*, 1997). With frontal and extrafrontal regions implicated in EFs (Tong *et al.*, 2004), disruption of the development of frontally guided, distributed networks may be a key mechanism to account for the EF deficits following pediatric TBI. However, we acknowledge that the relation of EF deficit to specific sites of focal lesions in children with TBI has been inconsistent across studies (Slomine *et al.*, 2002), possibly reflecting differences in imaging technique, patient samples and methods of evaluating EF.

Morphometric studies of children with post-acute TBI have revealed reduced brain volumes in the frontal regions (Wilde *et al.*, 2005) and hippocampus Serra-Grabulosa *et al.*, 2005) relative to uninjured children. Advances in diffusion tensor imaging techniques have provided evidence of reduced white matter integrity as a consequence of TBI (Neil *et al.*, 2002; Tasker *et al.*, 2005).

To date there is a notable shortage of functional neuroimaging studies of children after TBI (Munson *et al.*, 2006).

Neural substrate of ADHD

Evidence from several domains has implicated frontostriatal circuitry in the central deficits of ADHD (Durston, 2003). Some theorists have suggested that behavioral subtypes of ADHD may be the consequence of differential dysfunction in the dopaminergic system, with inattention and cognitive impairments hypothesized to be the consequence of a deficit of dopamine in the prefrontal cortex, and hyperactivity resulting from a surfeit of dopamine in the striatum (Solanto, 2002).

Morphometric studies of children with ADHD have revealed reduced volumes in several brain regions, including the cerebellum (Mostofsky *et al.*, 1998), frontostriatal regions (Castellanos *et al.*, 2001; Kates *et al.*, 2002) and regions of the corpus callosum (Giedd *et al.*, 1994; Semrud-Clikeman *et al.*, 1994).

Consistent with the prominence of inhibitory processing impairments in children with ADHD, functional neuroimaging studies of this population using PET (Rosa-Neto *et al.*, 2005), SPECT (Lou *et al.*, 1989), and functional MRI (Durston, 2003) have shown frontal involvement, especially of the frontostriatal region (Vaidya *et al.*, 2005), and the anterior cingulate. However, utility of the functional neuroimaging studies is constrained by the inconsistency of the direction of effects, with some studies reporting hyperactivation and other studies hypoactivation of the region (Mitterschiffthaler *et al.*, 2006).

In summary, structural neuroimaging studies of children have contributed to the body of evidence implicating disruption or dysfunction of frontally guided networks in EF deficits. Findings from structural imaging have been supported by the few studies of functional neuroimaging in children, though consistency remains a concern.

Executive functions in children

- In common with children who have TBI, children diagnosed with developmental ADHD show impairment in areas of executive functioning, including inhibition, working memory (depending on subtype), and error monitoring. Overlap in symptoms is less clear for planning, set shifting and decision making.

In the section following, we present research on specific domains of executive functioning in typically developing children, children with TBI and children with ADHD. A burgeoning body of evidence suggests that the various domains of executive functioning are highly inter-related; for the purpose of discussion, however, we treat the research on these different domains separately, following the general trend in the literature.

Working memory

Working memory, a limited capacity process for the short-term maintenance and manipulation of information (Baddeley, 1992), is age-dependent, and contributes to academic skills such as reading and arithmetic (Bull & Scerif, 2001; Swanson, 1999; Swanson & Sachse-Lee, 2001). In typically developing children, working memory emerges between 7 and 12 months (Diamond, 2002). In school-aged children, studies of nonverbal and spatial working memory have revealed large, age-related improvements in performance between 4 and 8 years, followed by more gradual increments of working memory until around 11 years, which pattern is the typical negatively accelerated trajectory of memory span development in children (Case, 1992; Luciana & Nelson, 1998).

Working memory after TBI in children

Working memory has been studied in children younger than 6 years at the time of TBI (Ewing-Cobbs *et al.*, 2004) with tasks that paralleled the testing methods used with infrahuman primates (Goldman, 1974). Although a subject-ordered self-pointing measure and a delayed response task were sensitive to TBI in preschool children (Ewing-Cobbs *et al.*, 2004), a spatial working memory task did not differentiate their performance from uninjured typically developing children. In older children (ages 6–14 years), using an N-back task in which

memory load varied (Braver *et al.*, 1997), Levin *et al.* (2002) found that working memory was impaired in children with chronic severe TBI. In a longitudinal study with an N-back task administered at 3, 6, 12 and 24 months post-injury, Levin *et al.* (2004a) found that groups of children who had sustained mild, moderate or severe TBI all exhibited improved performance during the first year post-injury. However, the severe TBI group's scores declined from 12 to 24 months, a pattern that was not seen in the less seriously injured children.

Working memory in children with ADHD

Evidence of working memory deficit in ADHD is equivocal (Diamond, 2005; Gathercole & Alloway, 2006). However, some theorists view ADHD as being divisible into two distinct neurological disorders, one of which, the inattentive subtype, is associated with deficits in working memory. In contrast, children diagnosed as the hyperactive subtype show relatively normal working memory, but impaired inhibitory processing (Bauermeister *et al.*, 2005; Diamond, 2005; Pennington & Ozonoff, 1996).

So, although deficits in verbal and nonverbal working memory are common after TBI, they appear to be less so in children with ADHD, possibly reflecting different disorder subtypes.

Inhibition

Empirically and theoretically related to working memory, inhibition is an age-dependent skill closely linked to cognitive control. Forms of inhibition include suppressing a prepotent response (e.g., go/no-go task), stopping a response in progress (e.g., stop signal reaction time; Logan, 1994), and resisting interference (Eriksen & Eriksen, 1974). Inhibition is relevant to academic and psychosocial domains of outcome (Passolunghi & Siegel, 2001; Ylvisaker *et al.*, 1998) in addition to self-regulatory skills in everyday functioning (Gioia *et al.*, 2000). Growth of response inhibition between 3 and 7 years is seen on tasks such as stopping a response

(Williams *et al.*, 1999), verbalizing a semantically incongruent response (Gerstadt *et al.*, 1994), spatial incompatibility tasks (Gerardi-Caulton, 2000) and suppressing recall of information that is no longer relevant (Harnishfeger & Pope, 1996).

Inhibition after TBI

There is a paucity of longitudinal data comparing forms of inhibition and their relationships to outcome in children with TBI. However, such studies that have been done with children have provided evidence of reduced inhibitory processing after TBI. Using a vigilance task, Dennis *et al.* (1995) found resistance to interference was impaired in a sample of children representing a range of TBI severity, with degree of interference inversely related to age at injury and time since injury. Levin *et al.* (1993) reported that go/no-go performance was impaired as a function of TBI severity in children at 2 years post-injury. Konrad *et al.* (2000) found that children at least 6 months after moderate to severe TBI performed poorly on both a go/no-go task and in stopping an ongoing response. In contrast, Schachar *et al.* (2004) noted that impaired stopping at 2 years post-injury was specific to severely injured children who had developed secondary ADHD.

Inhibition in children with ADHD

The most widely cited deficit in ADHD is inhibitory control (Barkley, 1997; Brodeur & Pond, 2001). Recent evidence suggests that inhibition in cognitive processes is not a unitary function, but rather a set of related, but distinct processes that may be differentially impaired (Kipp, 2005). Investigating three forms of inhibition, Scheres *et al.* (2004) found that boys with ADHD showed impairment on inhibition of an ongoing response, and in interference control, but not for inhibition of a prepotent response.

In summary, possibly the most prominent deficit common to children with TBI and ADHD is inhibitory processing. However, a shortage of studies investigating different types of inhibition in these populations impedes a thorough understanding of relative patterns of deficit, which may vary in TBI and ADHD.

Shifting

Cognitive theorists have proposed that the capacity for intermittent switching from one condition to another in a task imposes concurrent demands on working memory and inhibition and has a prolonged developmental trajectory extending through adolescence (Diamond, 2002). For example, the ability to shift from one rule of sorting cards (e.g., color) to another (e.g., shape) emerges by age 4 years (Zelazo *et al.*, 1995) and increases with age. Further age-related improvement in shifting occurs through adolescence (Levin *et al.*, 1991) on the Wisconsin Card Sorting Test (Heaton, 1981), a standardized task that is widely employed to assess EF in clinical settings.

Shifting after TBI

In a sample that included the spectrum of TBI severity studied 1 to 2 years post-injury, Levin *et al.* (1993) reported that the number of categories correctly sorted on the Wisconsin Card Sorting Test was related to TBI severity and to volume of left frontal pathology. However, Ewing-Cobbs *et al.* (2004) did not find an effect of TBI on set shifting in children injured at an early age.

Shifting in children with ADHD

Set shifting on a modified version of the Wisconsin Card Sorting Task was studied in children with combined-type ADHD and inattentive type ADHD with magnetoencephalography. Children with combined type ADHD showed slower reaction times, and impaired set shifting as compared with healthy controls and with the children with inattentive subtype ADHD (Mulas *et al.*, 2006; Rhodes *et al.*, 2005). However, findings from other studies of EF have not found differences between healthy children and children with ADHD on set shifting (Goldberg *et al.*, 2005; O'Driscoll *et al.*, 2005).

So, although set shifting is widely used in the adult literature as an index of EF, the current evidence is equivocal with regard to set shifting deficits in children with TBI and children with ADHD.

Planning

The capacity to "see ahead" during problem solving has been linked by functional brain imaging to dorsolateral prefrontal cortex (Cabeza & Nyberg, 2000) and studied in children using various tasks, including the Tower of London (Shallice, 1982). The Tower of London is thought to engage working memory to retain an overall schema and sequence of planned moves while managing completion of subgoals. By age 4 years children can solve the 2-move problems (Luciana & Nelson, 1998), and age-related improvement in performance continues through to at least age 15 years (Levin *et al.*, 1991).

Planning after TBI

In children sustaining TBI, impairment in the Tower of London task is related to injury severity, with more salience for problems of higher complexity (Levin *et al.*, 1994). Volume of frontal lesions appears to be related to performance, with contributions from orbitofrontal, dorsolateral and frontal white matter subregions (Levin *et al.*, 1994). Impaired planning has also been found in children with TBI using the Porteus Maze Test (Levin *et al.*, 2001b) with total score related to TBI severity and to volume of prefrontal lesion, even when processing speed is controlled. Whether performance on planning tasks such as the Tower of London and Porteus Maze Test is related to planning in daily activities in children is unclear.

Planning in children with ADHD

The literature on planning in children with ADHD is somewhat mixed, though leaning towards deficits of planning, possibly according to subtype.

Impairments in performance on the Tower of London task have been found in children with combined-type ADHD, with less evidence for impairment in inattentive type (Nigg *et al.*, 2002). O'Driscoll *et al.* (2005) used an oculomotor task to look at differences in planning, response inhibition and set shifting in children with either combined type ADHD or with inattentive type ADHD. Children with combined type were impaired on planning and response inhibition (but not set shifting). Children with inattentive ADHD were not impaired on any of these tasks relative to healthy controls (O'Driscoll *et al.*, 2005). Scheres *et al.* (2004) also reported deficient planning in boys with ADHD, in a mixed group of combined and inattentive types. However, when fundamental cognitive processes were controlled (such as speed of processing), the differences diminished or disappeared (Scheres *et al.*, 2004). In contrast, a study of planning in children with ADHD utilising a clock-drawing task found that children with ADHD were impaired on measures of planning as compared with healthy controls, regardless of subtype (Kibby *et al.*, 2002).

The above studies suggest that impairment on neuropsychological tests of planning appears to be associated with TBI. However, as with working memory, the effect of ADHD on planning is less clear.

Decision-making/motivation

Studies with typically developing children have revealed age differences in various aspects of decision-making, including processes that inform the decision (Davidson, 1991), the types of errors committed (Demetre *et al.*, 1992) and individual difference predictors of risk-taking (Levin & Hart, 2003). In particular, younger children appear to have difficulty in discounting information irrelevant to the task.

In addition to cognitive operations involving manipulation of information, some theorists believe that decision-making involving reward and penalty entails an affective valence based on past experience, such as anxiety associated with a risky choice. Based on evidence from a gambling task, Bechara *et al.* (2000) posited that ventromedial frontal cortex is the neural substrate for the linkage between somatic states and representations of current and past events. This methodology for studying decision making has since been recently applied to children using the original Iowa Gambling Task as well as modified versions (Crone & van der Molen, 2004; Kerr & Zelazo, 2004). The results of these studies are varied, and are somewhat hard to interpret insomuch as child-friendly modifications vary from study to study, as do the age ranges, but suggest that factors other than specific response to reward or penalty come into play (Garon & Moore, 2004; Kerr & Zelazo, 2004; Lehto & Elorinne, 2003; Overman, 2004). However, there does appear to be an age-related shift from childhood through young adulthood towards the smaller, but less risky choice (Crone & van der Molen, 2004).

Decision making after TBI

An initial study using the original gambling task in children reported impaired decision making in patients with focal frontal lesions of traumatic and nontraumatic mixed etiology (Anderson *et al.*, 1999). Few studies using this paradigm with children after TBI have been reported. In the single study of which we are aware, Hanten *et al.* (2006) reported impaired decision making on a child version of the Iowa Gambling Task to be related to location of focal brain lesions, such that patients with lesions in the amygdala showed the greatest impairment even when accounting for within-task memory requirements.

Decision making in children with ADHD

Children and adolescents with ADHD showed impaired performance on a child version of the Iowa Gambling Task (Garon *et al.*, 2006; Toplak *et al.*, 2005). Interestingly, in the Garon study, children with comorbid anxiety/depression performed much better than did children who had ADHD

alone, a finding that may relate to the idea that decision making is linked to emotional states (Bechara *et al.*, 2000). However, in a different study in which effects of delay were investigated in relation to reward, children with ADHD responded no differently than children without ADHD (Scheres *et al.*, 2006), indicating that task parameters other than risk and reward may be involved.

In summary, in the complex domain of decision making, firm conclusions about the measurable effects of childhood TBI and ADHD are hampered by the inconsistency within and between tasks. It is clear, however, that in all groups multiple factors inform decision making, and the weight of the factors may vary by age.

Behavioral self-regulation and everyday activities

Performance-based studies of behavioral regulation are sparse, though a number of studies have used observational methods or questionnaires to address issues relating to children's regulation of their own behavior in everyday situations. Recent research has elucidated patterns of behavioral regulation typical of healthy developing children. For example, in very young children, ages 1–4 years, compliance with instructions to initiate or sustain appropriate behavior is more difficult than compliance with instructions to suppress or desist from inappropriate behavior (Kochanska *et al.*, 2001). The relationship between behavioral regulation and various outcome domains is well documented. In young children, emotional and behavioral regulation has been found to predict the number of a child's friends but not acceptance within a group (Walden *et al.*, 1999). Adolescents who report more intense and labile emotions and less effective regulation of these emotions also reported more depressive symptoms and problem behavior (Silk *et al.*, 2003). Eisenberg *et al.* (1995) studied 82 children between the ages of 6 and 16 years using parent questionnaires on emotional intensity, negative affectivity, attentional and behavioral regulation and social functioning. The study revealed that adaptive social functioning was predicted by low negative emotionality and high levels of behavioral regulation. In another study, Eisenberg *et al.* (2000) found that behavioral dysregulation predicted externalizing behavior problems (e.g., conduct disorder) for children regardless of whether their emotionality was primarily positive or negative, whereas prediction of problem behavior from attentional control was significant only for children prone to negative emotionality.

Behavioral self-regulation after TBI

Persons sustaining injury to prefrontal subregions in early childhood show relatively greater behavioral problems than do persons injured in adulthood. This has been hypothesized to reflect the different consequences of damage to well-established rule-guided behavior (in adults) as compared to the disruption of developing socialization processes (in children). Adults who sustained orbitofrontal and ventromedial frontal lesions prior to age 2 years have been found to exhibit disruptive behavior, failure to follow rules, deficient empathy and a lack of moral reasoning, which were refractory to repeated instruction, treatment and punishment (Anderson *et al.*, 1999). In comparison with adults sustaining orbitofrontal and ventromedial frontal lesions acquired in adulthood, early-onset prefrontal lesions are more likely to result in maladaptive behaviors such as theft, violent acts against property, and other blatantly antisocial behavior (Anderson *et al.*, 1999; Price *et al.*, 1990). Although bilateral ventromedial frontal lesions have been frequently noted in pediatric studies of early frontal injury, right frontal cases (Marlowe, 2000) and a child with left frontal lesion (Eslinger & Damasio, 1985) displaying these sequelae have been described (Marlowe, 2000). Anderson *et al.* (1999) inferred that medial prefrontal dysfunction, whether resulting from direct injury or by white matter disconnection, is the key feature. The adverse effects of early prefrontal lesions on psychosocial adjustment may be relevant to TBI occurring later in childhood. School-aged children who sustained a TBI associated with a unilateral prefrontal lesion had poorer psychosocial outcome than a comparison group who had similar severity of TBI without a prefrontal lesion (Levin *et al.*, 2004b). Pertinent to assessment and rehabilitation, these reports indicate that marked disruption of social development and behavioral self-regulation can occur despite relatively normal performance on standard measures of cognition, including some tests of EF.

Behavioral regulation in children with ADHD

Behavioral self-dysregulation is a hallmark of children with ADHD, particularly those of the hyperactive subtype, and, in fact, is central to diagnosis of ADHD (Barkley, 1997). Behavior dysregulation affects outcome in several domains, including academics and social functioning (Hoza *et al.*, 2005; Kessler *et al.*, 2006). Emotional reactivity has been reported to be greater in children with ADHD than typically developing children for negative, but not positive events (Jensen & Rosen, 2004). However, the direct relationship of emotional dysregulation to ADHD is muddied by the very high rate of co-occurring externalizing behaviors (Abikoff *et al.*, 2002; Melnick & Hinshaw, 2000).

As the studies above indicate, profound difficulties in behavioral regulation are a common feature of both childhood TBI and ADHD. Within each group, a particular subgroup is most strongly affected, with prefrontal lesions associated with greater dysregulation in children with TBI, and children with the hyperactive subtype of ADHD showing more dysregulation than inattentive subtypes.

Executive functions in everyday activities after TBI

The ecologic validity of traditional and laboratory-derived measures of EF performance has been questioned because of scant data concerning the relation of the findings to the child's cognitive and self-regulatory behaviors in everyday activities (Gioia & Isquith, 2004). Assessment of EFs in everyday activities has been performed using structured interviews with parents and by rating scales completed by parents and teachers. Utilizing a parent interview to obtain ratings of children who had sustained TBI, Dennis *et al.* (2001) found that difficulties in attentional-inhibitory control (e.g., easily distracted, cannot stay at one task for a long time) and social-behavioral regulation (unaware of effects of behavior on others) were present in children studied at least 6 months post-injury. Performance on measures of intentionality, including making inferences, was related to parental ratings of social regulation. Assessment of EFs in daily activities has been facilitated by the Behavior Rating Inventory of Executive Function (BRIEF: Gioia *et al.*, 2000). Factor analysis of the BRIEF's eight scales initially identified two factors including a Behavioral Regulation Index (Inhibit, Shift, Emotional Control) and a Metacognition Index (Working Memory, Plan/Organise, Organization of Materials, and Monitor), but a three-factor model has also received support (Gioia *et al.*, 2002). The BRIEF has been validated in TBI samples against well-established measures of adaptive functioning (Mangeot *et al.*, 2002). In a different study of children with TBI, however, index scores from the BRIEF showed no correlation with any of the standardized (cognitive) performance measures of EF, including the Wisconsin Card Sort Test, Trail-making B, or verbal fluency (Vriezen & Pigott, 2002).

Executive functions in everyday activities in children with ADHD

Children with ADHD also show areas of elevated dysfunction on the BRIEF, with combined-type ADHD associated with greater impairment on the Inhibition subscales (Gioia *et al.*, 2002). As in children with TBI, studies have shown no correlations of indices of the BRIEF with standardized performance measures (Mahone *et al.*, 2002).

Studies of long-term follow-up of children diagnosed with the hyperactive subtype have shown that the impulsive behavior associated with this diagnosis was predictive of poor maintenance of employment, early parenthood and more treatment of sexually transmitted diseases (Barkley *et al.*, 2006).

In summary, although ample reports indicate that children with TBI and children with ADHD have difficulties in everyday activities that appear to relate to EFs, measurement remains an issue.

Symptom overlap between developmental ADHD and sequelae of TBI

- Bases of diagnoses differ in TBI and ADHD, with some symptom overlap.
- Behavioral features of ADHD are both a risk factor for and consequence of TBI.

Developmental ADHD affects about 6% of children, does not involve acquired brain injury, and has a hereditary component (Thapar *et al.*, 1999). Behavioral symptoms are the basis of diagnosis of ADHD.

In common with children who have moderate to severe TBI, children diagnosed with developmental ADHD show impairment in domains of EF (Pennington *et al.*, 1996; Shallice *et al.*, 2002), including inhibition, working memory (depending on subtype; Berlin *et al.*, 2004) error monitoring (Shallice *et al.*, 2002), and possibly set shifting (Lawrence *et al.*, 2004; Romine *et al.*, 2004). Moreover, developmental theorists have postulated that deficient inhibition is the central feature of developmental ADHD (Barkley, 1997). Although some of the described symptoms of the trauma population are similar, it is important to differentiate children whose symptoms of inattentiveness, impulsivity and restlessness arise following TBI from patients who had developmental ADHD prior to injury. Prospective investigation using a structured interview to identify lifetime psychiatric disorder in children treated for TBI has disclosed that the prevalence of pre-injury ADHD ranges between 10% (Max *et al.*, 2004) and 20% (Gerring *et al.*, 1998). At the same time, the behavioral features of ADHD are also risk factors for traumatic injury in general and are not specific to those children who sustain TBI (Bijur *et al.*, 1988). Setting aside the age criterion for diagnosis of ADHD, approximately 20% of children sustaining TBI first exhibit ADHD (i.e., novel

ADHD) following their injury, a condition that has been identified as secondary ADHD (Gerring *et al.*, 1998; Max *et al.*, 2004; Schachar *et al.*, 2004). When the full spectrum of TBI severity is sampled, secondary ADHD appears to occur primarily with severe TBI. In contrast to developmental ADHD, there is no male predominance and family history is not contributory in secondary ADHD (Max *et al.*, 2004). Reports that secondary ADHD was associated with lesions in right putamen, thalamus and basal ganglia (Gerring *et al.*, 2000; Herskovits *et al.*, 1999) have not been confirmed (Max *et al.*, 2004), but the literature consists of only a few studies.

Comparison of developmental ADHD with sequelae of TBI

Although data are sparse for direct comparison of EFs in children with developmental ADHD and those with secondary ADHD, Konrad *et al.* (2000) compared response inhibition in pediatric TBI patients with performance of children with developmental ADHD and a comparison group of typically developing children. Children were given a stop signal reaction time task and a second task that evaluated the child's capacity to delay a response. In comparison with typically developing children, both patient groups had difficulty stopping a response in progress but the TBI and developmental ADHD patients did not differ in performance. However, reaction time on "go" trials that did not have a stop cue was slower in the TBI patients than the other two groups. Similarly, in the slow speed condition of the delay task, both patient groups had impaired inhibition relative to typically developing children. Within the TBI group, Konrad *et al.* (2000) found no difference in performance on either task related to the presence of secondary ADHD.

However, there is disagreement as to whether poor response inhibition on a stopping task is typically present after TBI (Konrad *et al.*, 2000) or is confined to those severe TBI patients who develop secondary ADHD (Schachar *et al.*, 2004). Schachar *et al.* (2004) found that deficient stopping was confined to those severe TBI patients who had

secondary ADHD. Further investigation of inhibition, including response inhibition and interference mediated by distraction or prior training, is indicated to more fully elucidate the sequelae of pediatric TBI and the contribution of secondary ADHD.

Extrapolation from the separate literatures on pediatric TBI and developmental ADHD suggests distinct patterns of executive dysfunction. Following severe TBI, children show reduced initiation of word finding on measures of verbal fluency (Levin *et al.*, 2001a) a finding which is not characteristic of developmental ADHD (Pennington *et al.*, 1996; Shallice *et al.*, 2002). As noted above, slowing of information processing is a frequent sequel of severe TBI, which together with task complexity contributes to the persistently impaired performance of these patients on measures of attention (Catroppa & Anderson, 2003) that are also sensitive to developmental ADHD (Konrad *et al.*, 2000). Although children with developmental ADHD have been reported to have slowed speed of processing (Fuggetta, 2006), this may vary by subtype (Nigg *et al.*, 2005) and be limited to visual information processing (Weiler *et al.*, 2002).

Executive functioning in everyday activities has been compared for children with TBI and a group of children with developmental ADHD. Using the Behavior Rating Inventory of Executive Function, a parent/teacher rating scale, Gioia *et al.* (2002) found that children with developmental ADHD had higher scores (indicating more severe dysfunction) than children with severe TBI, who in turn had higher scores than children with moderate TBI and uninjured children. A subgroup of children with ADHD who had combined features of inattentiveness and hyperactivity specifically showed deficits in inhibition.

In summary, although there is evidence for the similarity of some symptoms of ADHD and TBI, the overall patterns of deficits may differ considerably, depending on the specific characteristics of each group, such as lesion size and location (in TBI) and diagnostic subgroup in ADHD.

Prefrontal abnormality and the neurocircuitry in developmental ADHD and TBI

As indicated above, the literature regarding the cognitive and behavioral consequences of TBI has revealed significant overlap with the symptoms diagnostic of developmental ADHD, particularly in related domains of inhibition and behavioral dysregulation. These findings suggest common mechanisms of neural dysfunction are related to poor EF.

Structural and functional imaging studies have implicated abnormal prefrontal maturation in developmental ADHD, including reduced prefrontal volume (Hill *et al.*, 2003), diminished right frontostriatal volumes and globally smaller cerebral volumes in children whose developmental ADHD was untreated with stimulants (Castellanos *et al.*, 2002). However, there is variation across studies in the specific brain region volumes that are affected in developmental ADHD, possibly reflecting differences in sampling of ADHD subtypes, and medication effects (Hill *et al.*, 2003; Hynd *et al.*, 1993).

A recent volumetric MRI study of children sustaining severe TBI has disclosed disproportionate reduction of prefrontal and temporal volumes, although both gray and white matter volumes were generally lower than in matched, uninjured children (Wilde *et al.*, 2006). Nonmissile TBI arising from causes such as moving vehicle crashes and vehicular-pedestrian injuries has also been shown in neuropathological and MRI studies to frequently involve contusions of prefrontal cortex and axonal injury which results in reduced white matter volume (Graham *et al.*, 2002; Wilde *et al.*, 2006). Structural MRI has also identified other sites of abnormality such as the corpus callosum in both developmental ADHD (Hill *et al.*, 2003) and TBI (Levin *et al.*, 2000; Mendelsohn *et al.*, 1992). Although lower brain volume is the key finding in both TBI and developmental ADHD, late MRI in children who have sustained severe TBI frequently reveals focal lesions such as gliosis and hemosiderin deposits in addition to volume loss (Levin *et al.*, 2000).

It has been postulated that developmental ADHD arises from corticostriatal dysfunction (Casey *et al.*, 1997) associated with hereditary neurochemical abnormality putatively involving dopamine receptor and transporter genes (Thapar *et al.*, 1999). Diffusion tensor imaging has provided initial evidence for disruption of neurocircuitry in children following TBI (Lee *et al.*, 2003), but these findings are preliminary and no longitudinal study of diffusion tensor imaging has been published in pediatric TBI. A single diffusion tensor imaging study of learning disabled children has suggested that attention disturbance is associated with reduced connectivity (Nagy *et al.*, 2003), but specific investigation of developmental ADHD has not been reported at the time of this review.

To summarize, the symptoms of restlessness, inattentiveness and impulsivity associated with developmental ADHD are frequent sequelae of severe TBI in children. Although deficient inhibition is seen on various tasks following severe TBI and is characteristic of developmental ADHD, its association with secondary ADHD has been reported in one of two studies that have addressed this issue (Konrad *et al.*, 2000; Schachar *et al.*, 2004). Executive dysfunction in performance of daily activities is also common to both TBI and developmental ADHD. In contrast to developmental ADHD, gender and hereditary factors do not appear to be related to the onset of secondary ADHD. Whether dopaminergic or other neurochemical alteration is present in secondary ADHD remains to be demonstrated.

Recovery and treatment

- There are no established cognitive interventions for children with TBI.
- Evidence for successful pharmacological intervention after TBI is sparse and weak.
- Cognitive, social and behaviorally mediated interventions have not been generally efficacious for ADHD.
- Between 50 and 70% of children with ADHD have been successfully treated with pharmacologic intervention.

Interventions for executive function deficit in children after TBI

Cognitive rehabilitation interventions for children following TBI are at an early stage of development. Although there are no controlled clinical trials reported at this time to evaluate rehabilitative interventions in this patient population, the educational psychology and child psychology literature include intervention studies of children with EF deficits associated with other conditions such as learning disability (Kurtz & Borkowski, 1987; Ward & Traweek, 1993). Moreover, rehabilitation psychologists and neuropsychologists have proposed directions for treatment of EF deficit in children with TBI, including methods that could potentially be evaluated in clinical trials (Marlowe, 2000; Ylvisaker et al., 1998).

The proposed approaches to EF deficit in children apply findings from developmental studies of metacognition. For example, Marlowe (2000) proposed a model using successive approximations to teach the child to engage in "executive thinking" through generating and answering questions using an adaptive thinking strategy. This approach segments a task into problem-solving steps including: (1) identifying the goal to be accomplished; (2) identifying the potential strategies to accomplish the goal; (3) formulating an action plan that selects the best strategy; (4) developing a sequential series of steps to accomplish that plan; (5) identifying and collecting the necessary materials; (6) beginning the task; (7) monitoring progress and modifying the approach as necessary; and (8) completion. Based on the metacognitive literature (Koriat & Goldsmith, 1996; Metcalfe & Shimamura, 1994), it would be appropriate to add evaluating the outcome. Implicit in this approach is an emphasis on metacognitive knowledge (e.g., what are the strategies?), monitoring and control (modify the approach as indicated by monitoring). Marlowe advocates teaching these steps as components to facilitate the child gaining mastery in the general approach.

Published drug studies to enhance recovery from TBI in children are sparse and limited to dopaminergic medications, including two randomized cross-over studies (Mahalick et al., 1998) of methylphenidate (MPH), a chart review study of MPH (Hornyak et al., 1997) and a single between-group study of amantadine (Beers et al., 2005). A review of the MPH studies (Jin & Schachar, 2004) identified major methodological shortcomings, including lack of a primary outcome measure, failure to utilize a washout period in a cross-over design, and small sample size. Although secondary ADHD has been reported in a subgroup of children sustaining moderate to severe TBI (Max et al., 2004; Schachar et al., 2004), this diagnosis or associated behaviors were not included in the selection criteria in these pharmacologic studies.

However, the cross-over study by Mahalick et al. ($n = 14$) found that performance on tests of attention and processing speed after taking 0.3 mg/kg of MPH surpassed the placebo condition. In contrast, results reported by Williams et al. (1998) were negative across an array of cognitive measures. Beers et al. (2005) found that children whom they had enrolled at least 3 months after sustaining TBI exhibited a greater improvement on a parent-report measure of executive functions in everyday behavior than children with TBI who received usual treatment. However, there were no group differences on neuropsychological test performance and Beers et al. did not include a placebo condition.

Taken together, the few studies of pharmacological treatment of children following TBI provide limited support to motivate further investigation. At present, there is insufficient evidence to propose that dopaminergic medication for cognitive or behavioral sequelae of TBI in children be a standard of care.

Children with ADHD

Over the last two decades, an abundance of evidence has accumulated to vitiate the belief that childhood ADHD is a transient condition that resolves in adolescence (Kessler et al., 2006). Current views hold that in 50–80% of childhood cases, ADHD persists into adolescence and adulthood. However, symptoms of ADHD in adolescents and young adults may be different than in children, consequent to the emergence of age-related behaviors not present in childhood, such as planning and time management, as well as changing social patterns (Barkley, 2004). The picture is complicated by a high degree of comorbidity with other disorders, especially oppositional defiant and conduct disorder (Angold *et al.*, 1999), which have been found to be much more likely to occur in children with diagnosed ADHD than in the general population.

At this time, ADHD is not curable. Treatments designed to ameliorate the symptoms of ADHD encompass behavioral, social and pharmacological interventions. The results of controlled studies of cognitive, social and behaviorally mediated therapies have been discouraging, though modest improvements have been observed in specific situations (Barkley, 1998; DuPaul & Eckert, 1997).

Long-term generalized conditioned improvements on ADHD symptoms have been reported to be a result of intensive biofeedback using EEG (Monastra, 2004). Although early studies using this approach appear promising, more rigorously controlled studies are needed to ascertain the clinical utility of this approach (Loo & Barkley, 2005).

To date, the most efficacious treatments for developmental ADHD are psychopharmacologic interventions, either alone or in combination with behavioral or family therapies (Mash & Barkley, 2006). However, concerns persist regarding pharmacological treatment, including a high percentage of nonresponders (approx. 30%), patient acceptance due to potential adverse effects, and the inability of stimulants to address specific problem domains such as peer relations. Psychosocial treatments remain an important alternative (Chronis *et al.*, 2006).

Summary

Executive functions encompass cognitive (e.g., decision-making, planning), self-regulative (e.g., motivation, modulation of emotion), metacognitive (e.g., self-appraisal and implementation of self-management strategies) and social cognitive (e.g., processing the intentions of others) domains that have been linked to development of frontally guided, distributed networks, which are vulnerable to TBI. Following moderate to severe TBI in children, clinical neuropsychological assessment should address these EF domains within the context of basic cognitive functioning (i.e., speed of processing, short-term memory), including their utilization in everyday activities. The long-term effects of TBI on development of EFs are under investigation, but deficits persisting for at least 2–3 years have been documented. Although the executive dysfunction following TBI shares some similarity to the features of developmental ADHD and a subgroup of pediatric brain-injured patients exhibit secondary ADHD, the slowing of information processing speed appears to be specific to brain trauma. Volumetric MRI studies implicate low cerebral volume following TBI and in developmental ADHD untreated with stimulant medication, but serial imaging implicates a degenerative process in trauma patients. Based on the progress to date and ongoing studies of EF in children with TBI, it is timely to design and initiate clinical trials of cognitive interventions for this population.

ACKNOWLEDGMENTS

Preparation of this review and the authors' research were supported by grant NS-21889, Neurobehavioral Outcome of Head Injury in Children, and grant NS-42772, Executive Function After Traumatic Brain Injury in Adults. We also acknowledge support by the Baylor College of Medicine General Clinical Research Center at Texas Children's Hospital; the Mental Illness Research, Education, and Clinical Center; and the Michael E. DeBakey Veterans Affairs Medical Center. We are indebted to Stacey Martin for assistance in manuscript preparation.

REFERENCES

Abikoff, H. B., Jensen, P. S., Arnold, L. *et al.* (2002). Observed classroom behavior of children with ADHD: relationship to gender and comorbidity. *Journal of Abnormal Child Psychology*, **30**, 349–359.

Anderson, S. W., Bechara, A., Damasio, H., Tranel, D., & Damasio, A. (1999). Impairment of social and moral behavior related to early damage in human prefrontal cortex. *Nature Neuroscience*, **2**, 1032–1037.

Angold, A., Costello, E. J., & Erkanli, A. (1999). Comorbidity. *Journal of Child Psychology and Psychiatry*, **40**, 57–87.

Baddeley, A. D. (1992). Working memory. *Science*, **255**, 556–559.

Barkley, R. A. (1997). Behavioral inhibition, sustained attention and executive functions: constructing a unifying theory of ADHD. *Psychological Bulletin*, **21**, 65–94.

Barkley, R. A. (1998). Attention-deficit/hyperactivity disorder. In E. J. Mash & R. A. Barkley (Eds.), *Treatment of Childhood Disorders (2nd Edition)*. New York, NY: Guilford Press.

Barkley, R. A. (2004). Adolescents with attention-deficit/ hyperactivity disorder: an overview of empirically based treatments. *Journal of Psychiatric Practice*, **10**, 39–56.

Barkley, R. A., Fischer, M., Smallish, L., & Fletcher, K. (2006). Young adult outcome of hyperactive children: adaptive functioning in major life activities. *Journal of the American Academy of Child and Adolescent Psychiatry*, **45**, 192–202.

Bauermeister, J. J., Matos, M., Reina, G. *et al.* (2005). Comparison of the DSM-IV combined and inattentive types of ADHD in a school-based sample of Latino/ Hispanic children. *Journal of Child Psychology and Psychiatry*, **46**, 166–179.

Bechara, A., Damasio, H., & Damasio, A. R. (2000). Emotion, decision-making and the orbitofrontal cortex. *Cerebral Cortex*, **10**, 295–307.

Beers, S. R., Skold, A., Dixon, C. E., & Adelson, P. D. (2005). Neurobehavioral effects of amantadine after pediatric traumatic brain injury: a preliminary report. *Journal of Head Trauma Rehabilitation*, **20**, 450–463.

Berlin, L., Bohlin, G., Nyberg, L., & Janols, L. (2004). How well do measures of inhibition and other executive functions discriminate between children with ADHD and controls? *Child Neuropsychology*, **10**, 1–13.

Bijur, P., Golding, J., Haslum, M., & Kurzon, M. (1988). Behavioral predictors of injury in school-age children. *American Journal of Diseases of Children*, **142**, 1307–1312.

Bittigau, P., Sifringer, M., Pohl, D. *et al.* (1999). Apoptotic neurodegeneration following trauma is markedly enhanced in the immature brain. *Annals of Neurology*, **45**, 724–735.

Borkowski, J. G., Burke, J. E., Lyon, G. R., & Krasnegor, N. A. (1996). Theories, models, and measurements of executive functioning: an information processing perspective. In G. R. Lyon & N. A. Krasnegor (Eds.), *Attention, Memory, and Executive Function* (pp. 235–262). Baltimore, MD: Paul H. Brookes Publishing Co.

Braver, T. S., Cohen, J. D., Nystrom, L. E. *et al.* (1997). A parametric study of prefrontal cortex involvement in human working memory. *Neuroimage*, **5**, 49–62.

Brodeur, D. A., & Pond, M. (2001). The development of selective attention in children with attention deficit hyperactivity disorder. *Journal of Abnormal Child Psychology*, **29**, 229–239.

Brown, T. T., Lugar, H. M., Coalson, R. S. *et al.* (2004). Developmental changes in human cerebral functional organization for word generation. *Cerebral Cortex*, **15**, 275–290.

Bull, R., & Scerif, G. (2001). Executive functioning as a predictor of children's mathematics ability: inhibition, switching, and working memory. *Developmental Neuropsychology*, **19**, 273–293.

Bunge, S. A., Ochsner, K. N., Desmond, J. E., Glover, G. H., & Gabrieli, J. D. (2001). Prefrontal regions involved in keeping information in and out of mind. *Brain*, **124**, 2074–2086.

Cabeza, R., & Nyberg, L. (2000). Imaging cognition II: an empirical review of 275 PET and fMRI studies. *Journal of Cognitive Neuroscience*, **21**, 1–47.

Case, R. (1992). The role of the frontal lobes in the regulation of cognitive development. *Brain and Cognition*, **20**, 51–73.

Casey, B. J., Castellanos, F. X., Giedd, J. N. *et al.* (1997). Implication of right frontostriatal circuitry in response inhibition and attention-deficit/hyperactivity disorder. *Journal of the American Academy of Child and Adolescent Psychiatry*, **36**, 374–383.

Casey, B. J., Tottenham, N., & Fossella, J. (2002). Clinical, imaging, lesion, and genetic approaches toward a model of cognitive control. *Developmental Psychobiology*, **40**, 237–254.

Castellanos, F. X., Giedd, J. N., & Berquin, P. C. (2001). Quantitative brain magnetic resonance imagining in girls with attention-deficit/hyperactive disorder. *Archives of General Psychiatry*, **58**, 289–295.

Castellanos, F. X., Lee, P. P., Sharp, W. *et al.* (2002). Developmental trajectories of brain volume abnormalities in children and adolescents with attention-deficit/ hyperactivity disorder. *Journal of the American Medical Association*, **288**, 1740–1748.

Catroppa, C., & Anderson, V. (2003). Children's attentional skills 2 years post-traumatic brain injury. *Developmental Neuropsychology*, **23**, 359–373.

Chronis, A. M., Jones, H. A., & Raggi, V. L. (2006). Evidence-based psychosocial treatments for children and adolescents with attention-deficit/hyperactivity disorder. *Clinical Psychology Review*, **26**, 486–502.

Collette, F., & van der Linden, M. (2002). Brain imaging of the central executive component of working memory. *Neuroscience Biobehavior Reviews*, **26**, 105–125.

Crone, E. A., & van der Molen, M. W. (2004). Developmental changes in real life decision making: performance on a gambling task previously shown to depend on the ventromedial prefrontal cortex. *Developmental Neuropsychology*, **25**, 251–279.

Davidson, D. (1991). Children's decision-making examined with an information-board procedure. *Cognitive Development*, **6**, 77–90.

De Bellis, M. D., Keshavan, M. S., Clark, D. B. *et al.* (1999). Bennett research award. Developmental traumatology. Part II: Brain development. *Biological Psychiatry*, **45**, 1271–1284.

Demetre, J. D., Lee, D. N., Pitcairn, T. K., & Grieve, R. (1992). Errors in young children's decisions about traffic gaps: experiments with roadside simulations. *British Journal of Psychology*, **83**, 189–202.

Denckla, M. B. (1996). A theory and model of executive function: a neuropsychological perspective. In G. R. Lyon & N. A. Krasnegor (Eds.), *Attention, Memory, and Executive Function* (pp. 263–278). Baltimore, MD: Paul H. Brookes Publishing Co.

Dennis, M., Wilkinson, M., Koski, L., & Humphreys, R. P. (1995). Attention deficits in the long term after childhood head injury. In S. H. Broman & M. E. Michel (Eds.), *Traumatic Head Injury in Children* (pp. 165–187). New York, NY: Oxford University Press.

Dennis, M., Guger, S., Roncadin, C., Barnes, M., & Schachar, R. (2001). Attentional-inhibitory control and social-behavioral regulation after childhood closed head injury: do biological, developmental, and recovery variables predict outcome? *Journal of the International Neuropsychological Society*, **7**, 683–692.

Diamond, A. (2002). Normal development of prefrontal cortex from birth to young adulthood: cognitive functions, anatomy, and biochemistry. In D. T. Stuss & R. T. Knight (Eds.), *Principles of Frontal Lobe Function*. New York, NY: Oxford University Press.

Diamond, A. (2005). Attention-deficit disorder (attention-deficit/hyperactivity disorder without hyperactivity): a neurobiologically and behaviorally distinct disorder from attention-deficit/hyperactivity disorder (with hyperactivity). *Developmental Psychopathology*, **17**, 807–825.

DuPaul, G. J., & Eckert, T. L. (1997). The effects of school-based interventions for ADHD: a meta-analysis. *School Psychology Digest*, **26**, 5–27.

Durston, S. (2003). A review of the biological bases of ADHD: what have we learned from imaging studies? *Mental Retardation and Developmental Disabilities Research Reviews*, **9**, 184–195.

Durston, S., Hulshoff, P. H. E., Casey, B. J. *et al.* (2001). Anatomical MRI of the developing human brain: what have we learned? *Journal of the American Academy of Child and Adolescent Psychiatry*, **40**, 1012–1020.

Eisenberg, N., Fabes, R. A., Murphy, B., & Maszk, P. (1995). The role of emotionality and regulation in children's social functioning: a longitudinal study. *Child Development*, **66**, 1360–1384.

Eisenberg, N., Guthrie, I. K., Fabes, R. A. *et al.* (2000). Predictions of elementary school children's externalizing problem behaviors from attentional and behavioral regulation and negative emotionality. *Child Development*, **71**, 1367–1382.

Eriksen, B. A., & Eriksen, C. W. (1974). Effects of noise letters upon the identification of a target letter in a non-search task. *Perception and Psychophysics*, **16**, 143–149.

Eslinger, P. J., & Damasio, A. R. (1985). Severe disturbance of higher cognition after bilateral frontal lobe ablation: Patient EVR. *Neurology*, **35**, 1731–1741.

Ewing-Cobbs, L., Prasad, M. R., Landry, S. H., Kramer, L., & DeLeon, R. (2004). Executive functions following traumatic brain injury in young children: a preliminary analysis. *Developmental Neuropsychology*, **26**, 487–512.

Fuggetta, G. P. (2006). Impairment of executive functions in boys with attention deficit/hyperactivity disorder. *Child Neuropsychology*, **12**, 1–21.

Gaillard, W. D., Hertz-Pannier, L., Mott, S. H. *et al.* (2000). Functional anatomy of cognitive development: fMRI of verbal fluency in children and adults. *Neurology*, **54**, 180–185.

Garon, N., & Moore, C. (2004). Complex decision making in early childhood. *Brain and Cognition*, **55**, 158–170.

Garon, N., Moore, C., & Waschbusch, D. A. (2006). Decision making in children with ADHD only, ADHD-anxious/depressed, and control children using a child version of the Iowa Gambling Task. *Journal of Attention Disorders*, **9**, 607–619.

Gathercole, S. E., & Alloway, T. P. (2006). Practitioner review: short-term and working memory impairments in neurodevelopmental disorders: diagnosis and remedial support. *Journal of Child Psychology and Psychiatry*, **47**, 4–15.

Gerardi-Caulton, G. (2000). Sensitivity to spatial conflict and the development of self-regulation in children 24–36 months of age. *Developmental Science*, **3**, 397–404.

Gerring, J. P., Brady, K. D., Chen, A. *et al.* (1998). Premorbid prevalence of ADHD and development of secondary ADHD after closed head injury. *Journal of the American Academy of Child and Adolescent Psychiatry*, **37**, 647–654.

Gerring, J., Brady, K., Chen, A. *et al.* (2000). Neuroimaging variables related to development of secondary attention deficit hyperactivity disorder after closed head injury in children and adolescents. *Brain Injury*, **14**, 205–218.

Gerstadt, C. L., Hong, Y. J., & Diamond, A. (1994). The relationship between cognition and action: performance of children 3 1/2–7 years old on a Stroop-like day-night test. *Cognition*, **53**, 129–153.

Giedd, J. N., Castellanos, F. X., & Casey, B. J. (1994). Quantitative morphology of the corpus callosum in attention deficit hyperactivity disorder. *American Journal of Psychiatry*, **151**, 665–669.

Giedd, J. N., Blumenthal, J., Jeffries, N. O. *et al.* (1999). Brain development during childhood and adolescence: a longitudinal MRI study. *Nature Neuroscience*, **2**, 861–863.

Gioia, G. A., & Isquith, P. K. (2004). Ecological assessment of executive function in traumatic brain injury. *Developmental Neuropsychology*, **25**, 135–158.

Gioia, G. A., Isquith, P. K., Guy, S. C., & Kenworthy, L. (2000). *Behavior Rating Inventory of Executive Function*. Odessa, FL: Psychological Assessment Resources.

Gioia, G. A., Isquith, P. K., Retzlaff, P. D., & Espy, K. A. (2002). Confirmatory factor analysis of the Behavior Rating Inventory of Executive Function (BRIEF) in a clinical sample. *Child Neuropsychology*, **8**, 249–257.

Gogtay, N., Giedd, J. N., Lusk, L. *et al.* (2004). Dynamic mapping of human cortical development during childhood through early adulthood. *Proceedings of the National Academy of Sciences of the United States of America*, **101**, 8174–8179.

Goldberg, M. C., Mostofsky, S. H., Cutting, L. E. *et al.* (2005). Subtle executive impairment in children with autism and children with ADHD. *Journal of Autism and Developmental Disorders*, **35**, 279–293.

Goldman, P. S. (1974). Functional recovery after lesions of the nervous system. 3. Developmental processes in neural plasticity. Recovery of function after CNS lesions in infant monkeys. *Neurosciences Research Program Bulletin*, **12**, 217–222.

Graham, D. I., Gennarelli, T. A., & McIntosh, T. R. (2002). Trauma. In D. I. Graham & P. L. Lantos (Eds.), *Greenfield's Neuropathology (7th Edition)* (pp. 823–897). New York, NY: Oxford University Press.

Graham, S., Harris, K. R., Lyon, G. R., & Krasnegor, N. A. (1996). Addressing problems in attention, memory, and executive functioning: an example from self-regulated strategy development. In G. R. Lyon & N. A. Krasnegor (Eds.), *Attention, Memory, and Executive Function* (pp. 349–366). Baltimore, MD: Paul H. Brookes, Publishing Co.

Grattan, L. M., & Eslinger, P. J. (1992). Long-term psychological consequences of childhood frontal lobe lesion in patient DT. *Brain and Cognition*, **20**, 185–195.

Hanten, G., Scheibel, R. S., Li, X. *et al.* (2006). Decision-making after traumatic brain injury in children: a preliminary study. *Neurocase*, **12**, 247–251.

Harnishfeger, K. K., & Pope, R. S. (1996). Intending to forget: the development of cognitive inhibition in directed forgetting. *Journal of Experimental Child Psychology*, **62**, 292–315.

Heaton, H. K. (1981). *A Manual for the Wisconsin Card Sort Test*. Odessa, FL: Psychological Assessment Resources.

Herskovits, E. H., Megalooikonomou, V., Davatzikos, C. *et al.* (1999). Is the spatial distribution of brain lesions associated with closed-head injury predictive of subsequent development of attention-deficit/hyperactivity disorder? Analysis with brain-image database. *Radiology*, **213**, 389–394.

Hill, D. E., Yeo, R. A., Campbell, R. A. *et al.* (2003). Magnetic resonance imaging correlates of attention-deficit/hyperactivity disorder in children. *Neuropsychology*, **17**, 496–506.

Hornyak, J. E., Nelson, V. S., & Hurvitz, E. A. (1997). The use of methylphenidate in paediatric traumatic brain injury. *Pediatric Rehabilitation*, **1**, 15–17.

Hoza, B., Mrug, S., Gerdes, A. C. *et al.* (2005). What aspects of peer relationships are impaired in children with attention-deficit/hyperactivity disorder? *Journal of Consulting and Clinical Psychology*, **73**, 411–423.

Hynd, G. W., Hern, K. L., Novey, E. S. *et al.* (1993). Attention deficit-hyperactivity disorder and asymmetry of the caudate nucleus. *Journal of Child Neurology*, **8**, 339–347.

Jensen, S., & Rosen, L. A. (2004). Emotional reactivity in children with attention-deficit/hyperactivity disorder. *Journal of Attention Disorders*, **8**, 53–61.

Jin, C., & Schachar, R. (2004). Methylphenidate treatment of attention-deficit/hyperactivity disorder secondary to traumatic brain injury: a critical appraisal of treatment studies. *CNS Spectroscopy*, **9**, 217–226.

Kail, R. (1991). Developmental change in speed of processing during childhood and adolescence. *Psychological Bulletin*, **109**, 490–501.

Kates, W. R., Frederikse, M., Mostofsky, S. H. *et al.* (2002). MRI parcellation of the frontal lobe in boys with attention deficit hyperactivity disorder or Tourette syndrome. *Psychiatry Research*, **116**, 63–81.

Kerr, A., & Zelazo, P. D. (2004). Development of "hot" executive function: the children's gambling task. *Brain and Cognition*, **55**, 148–157.

Kessler, R. C., Adler, L., Barkley, R. *et al.* (2006). The prevalence and correlates of adult ADHD in the United States: results from the national comorbidity survey replication. *American Journal of Psychiatry*, **163**, 716–723.

Kibby, M. Y., Cohen, M. J., & Hynd, G. W. (2002). Clock face drawing in children with attention-deficit/hyperactivity disorder. *Archives of Clinical Neuropsychology*, **17**, 531–546.

Kipp, K. (2005). A developmental perspective on the measurement of cognitive deficits in attention-deficit/hyperactivity disorder. *Biological Psychiatry*, **57**, 1256–1260.

Kochanek, P. M., Clark, R. S. B., Ruppel, R. A. *et al.* (2000). Biochemical, cellular, and molecular mechanisms in the evolution of secondary damage after severe traumatic brain injury in infants and children: lessons learned from the bedside. *Pediatric Critical Care Medicine*, **1**, 4–19.

Kochanska, G., Coy, K. C., & Murray, K. T. (2001). The development of self-regulation in the first four years of life. *Child Development*, **72**, 1091.

Konrad, K., Gauggel, S., Manz, A., & Schoell, M. (2000). Inhibitory control in children with traumatic brain injury (TBI) and children with attention deficit/hyperactivity disorder (ADHD). *Brain Injury*, **14**, 859–875.

Koriat, A., & Goldsmith, M. (1996). Monitoring and control processes in the strategic regulation of memory accuracy. *Psychological Review*, **103**, 490–517.

Kurtz, B. E., & Borkowski, J. G. (1987). Development of strategic skills in impulsive and reflective children: a longitudinal study of metacognition. *Journal of Experimental Child Psychology*, **43**, 129–148.

Lawrence, V., Houghton, S., Douglas, G. *et al.* (2004). Executive function and ADHD: a comparison of children's performance during neuropsychological testing and real-world activities. *Journal of Attention Disorders*, **7**, 137–149.

Lee, Z. I., Byun, W. M., Jang, S. H. *et al.* (2003). Diffusion tensor magnetic resonance imaging of microstructural abnormalities in children with brain injury. *American Journal of Medical Rehabilitation*, **82**, 556–559.

Lehto, J. E., & Elorinne, E. (2003). Gambling as an executive function task. *Applied Neuropsychology*, **10**, 234–238.

Levin, I. P., & Hart, S. (2003). Risk preferences in young children: early evidence of individual differences in reaction to potential gains and losses. *Journal of Behavioral Decision Making*, **16**, 397–413.

Levin, H. S., Culhane, K. A., & Hartmann, J. (1991). Developmental changes in performance on tests of purported frontal lobe functioning. *Developmental Neuropsychology*, **7**, 377–395.

Levin, H. S., Culhane, K. A., Mendelsohn, D. *et al.* (1993). Cognition in relation to MRI in head injured children and adolescents. *Archives of Neurology*, **50**, 897–905.

Levin, H. S., Mendelsohn, D., Lilly, M. *et al.* (1994). Tower of London performance in relation to magnetic resonance imaging following closed head injury in children. *Neuropsychology*, **8**, 171–179.

Levin, H. S., Benavidez, D. A., Verger-Maestre, K. *et al.* (2000). Reduction of corpus callosum growth after severe traumatic brain injury in children. *Neurology*, **54**, 647–653.

Levin, H. S., Song, J. X., Ewing-Cobbs, L., Chapman, S. B., & Mendelsohn, D. (2001a). Word fluency in relation to severity of closed head injury, associated frontal brain lesions, and age at injury in children. *Neuropsychologia*, **39**, 122–131.

Levin, H. S., Song, J. X., Ewing-Cobbs, L., & Roberson, G. (2001b). Porteus maze performance following traumatic brain injury in children. *Neuropsychology*, **4**, 557–567.

Levin, H. S., Hanten, G., Chang, C. C. *et al.* (2002). Working memory after traumatic brain injury in children. *Annals of Neurology*, **52**, 82–88.

Levin, H. S., Hanten, G., Zhang, L. *et al.* (2004a). Changes in working memory after traumatic brain injury in children. *Neuropsychology*, **18**, 240–247.

Levin, H. S., Zhang, L., Dennis, M. *et al.* (2004b). Psychosocial outcome of TBI in children with unilateral frontal lesions. *Journal of the International Neuropsychological Society*, **10**, 305–316.

Logan, G. D. (1994). On the ability to inhibit thought and action: A users' guide to the stop signal paradigm. In D. Dagenbach & T. H. Carr (Eds.), *Inhibitory Processes in Attention, Memory, and Language* (pp. 189–239). San Diego, CA: Academic Press.

Loo, S. K., & Barkley, R. A. (2005). Clinical utility of EEG in attention deficit hyperactivity disorder. *Applied Neuropsychology*, **12**, 64–76.

Lou, H. C., Henriksen, L., Bruhn, P., Borner, H., & Nielsen, J. B. (1989). Striatal dysfunction in attention deficit and hyperkinetic disorder. *Archives of Neurology*, **46**, 48–52.

Luciana, M., & Nelson, C. A. (1998). The functional emergence of prefrontally-guided working memory systems in four- to eight-year-old children. *Neuropsychologia*, **36**, 273–293.

Luna, B., Thulborn, K. R., Munoz, D. P. *et al.* (2001). Maturation of widely distributed brain function subserves cognitive development. *Neuroimage*, **13**, 786–793.

Mahalick, D. M., Carmel, P. W., Greenberg, J. P. *et al.* (1998). Psychopharmacologic treatment of acquired attention disorders in children with brain injury. *Pediatric Neurosurgery*, **29**, 121–126.

Mahone, E., Zabel, T., Levey, E., Verda, M., & Kinsman, S. (2002). Parent and self-report ratings of executive function in adolescents with myelomeningocele and hydrocephalus. *Child Neuropsychology*, **8**, 258–270.

Mangeot, S., Armstrong, K., Colvin, A. N., Yeates, K. O., & Taylor, H. G. (2002). Long-term executive function deficits in children with traumatic brain injuries: assessment using the Behavior Rating Inventory of Executive Function (BRIEF). *Child Neuropsychology*, **8**, 271–284.

Marlowe, W. B. (2000). An intervention for children with disorders of executive functions. *Developmental Neuropsychology*, **18**, 445–454.

Mash, E. J., & Barkley, R. A. (2006). *Treatment of Childhood Disorders (3rd Edition)*. New York, NY: Guilford Press.

Max, J. E., Lansing, A. E., Koele, S. L. *et al.* (2004). Attention deficit hyperactivity disorder in children and adolescents following traumatic brain injury. *Developmental Neuropsychology*, **25**, 159–177.

Melnick, S. M., & Hinshaw, S. P. (2000). Emotion regulation and parenting in AD/HD and comparison boys: linkages with social behaviors and peer preference. *Journal of Abnormal Child Psychology*, **28**, 73–86.

Mendelsohn, D., Levin, H. S., Bruce, D. *et al.* (1992). Late MRI after head injury in children: relationship to clinical features and outcome. *Childs Nervous System*, **8**, 445–452.

Metcalfe, J., & Shimamura, A. P. (1994). *Metacognition: Knowing About Knowing*. Cambridge, MA: MIT Press.

Miller, E. K., & Cohen, J. D. (2001). An integrative theory of prefrontal cortex function. *Annual Review of Neuroscience*, **24**, 167–202.

Mitterschiffthaler, M. T., Ettinger, U., Mehta, M. A., Mataix-Cols, D., & Williams, S. C. (2006). Applications of functional magnetic resonance imaging in psychiatry. *Journal of Magnetic Resonance Imaging*, **23**, 851–861.

Monastra, V. J. (2004). Electroencephalographic biofeedback (neurotherapy) as a treatment for attention deficit hyperactivity disorder: rationale and empirical foundation. *Child and Adolescent Psychiatric Clinics of North America*, **14**, 55–82.

Mostofsky, S. H., Reiss, A. L., Lockhart, P., & Denckla, M. B. (1998). Evaluation of cerebellar size in attention-deficit hyperactivity disorder. *Journal of Child Neurology*, **13**, 434–439.

Mulas, F., Capilla, A., Fernández, S. *et al.* (2006). Shifting-related brain magnetic activity in attention-deficit/hyperactivity disorder. *Biological Psychiatry*, **59**, 373–379.

Munson, S., Schroth, E., & Ernst, M. (2006). The role of functional neuroimaging in pediatric brain injury. *Pediatrics*, **117**, 1372–1381.

Nagy, Z., Westerberg, H., Skare, S. *et al.* (2003). Preterm children have disturbances of white matter at 11 years of age as shown by diffusion tensor imaging. *Pediatric Research*, **54**, 672–679.

Neil, J., Miller, J., Mukherjee, P., & Huppi, P. S. (2002). Diffusion tensor imaging of normal and injured developing human brain: a technical review. *NMR Biomedicine*, **15**, 543–552.

Nigg, J. T., Blaskey, L. G., Huang-Pollock, C. L., & Huang-Pollock, C. L. (2002). Neuropsychological executive functions and DSM-IV ADHD subtypes. *Journal of the American Academy of Child and Adolescent Psychiatry*, **41**, 59–66.

Nigg, J. T., Willcutt, E. G., Doyle, A. E., & Sonuga-Barke, E. J. (2005). Causal heterogeneity in attention-deficit/hyperactivity disorder: do we need neuropsychologically impaired subtypes? *Biological Psychiatry*, **57**, 1224–1230.

O'Driscoll, G. A., Depatie, L., Holahan, A. L. *et al.* (2005). Executive functions and methylphenidate response in subtypes of attention-deficit/hyperactivity disorder. *Biological Psychiatry*, **57**, 1452–1460.

Overman, W. H. (2004). Sex differences in early childhood, adolescence, and adulthood on cognitive tasks that rely on orbital prefrontal cortex. *Brain and Cognition*, **55**, 134–147.

Passolunghi, M. C., & Siegel, L. S. (2001). Short-term memory, working memory, and inhibitory control in children with difficulties in arithmetic problem solving. *Journal of Experimental Child Psychology*, **80**, 44–57.

Pennington, B. F., & Ozonoff, S. (1996). Executive functions and developmental psychopathology. *Journal of Child Psychology and Psychiatry*, **37**, 51–87.

Pennington, B. F., Bennetto, L., McAleer, O. *et al.* (1996). Executive functions and working memory. Theoretical and measurement issues. In G. R. Lyon & N. A. Krasnegor (Eds.), *Attention, Memory, and Executive Function* (pp. 327–348). Baltimore, MD: Paul H. Brookes Publishing Co.

Price, B. H., Daffner, K. R., Stowe, R. M., & Mesulam, M. M. (1990). The comportmental learning disabilities of early frontal lobe damage. *Brain*, **113**, 1383–1393.

Rhodes, S. M., Coghill, D. R., & Matthews, K. (2005). Neuropsychological functioning in stimulant-naive boys with hyperkinetic disorder. *Psychological Medicine*, **35**, 1109–1120.

Rolls, E. T. (2000). The orbitofrontal cortex and reward. *Cerebral Cortex*, **10**, 284–294.

Romine, C. B., Lee, D., Wolfe, M. E. *et al.* (2004). Wisconsin Card Sorting Test with children: a meta-analytic study of sensitivity and specificity. *Archives of Clinical Neuropsychology*, **19**, 1027–1041.

Rosa-Neto, P., Lou, H. C., Cumming, P. *et al.* (2005). Methylphenidate-evoked changes in striatal dopamine correlate with inattention and impulsivity in adolescents with attention deficit hyperactivity disorder. *Neuroimage*, **25**, 868–876.

Rubia, K., Overmeyer, S., Taylor, E. *et al.* (2000). Functional frontalisation with age: mapping neurodevelopmental trajectories with fMRI. *Neuroscience and Biobehavioral Reviews*, **24**, 13–19.

Schachar, R. J., Levin, H. S., Max, J. E., Purvis, K. L., & Chen, S. (2004). Attention deficit hyperactivity disorder symptoms and response inhibition after closed head injury in children: do preinjury behavior and injury severity predict outcome? *Developmental Neuropsychology*, **25**, 179–198.

Scheres, A., Oosterlaan, J., Geurts, H. *et al.* (2004). Executive functioning in boys with ADHD: Primarily an inhibition deficit? *Archives of Clinical Neuropsychology*, **19**, 569–594.

Scheres, A., Dijkstra, M., Ainslie, E. *et al.* (2006). Temporal and probablistic discounting of rewards in children and adolescents effects of age and ADHD symptoms. *Neuropsychologia*, **44**, 2092–2103.

Schultz, W., Tremblay, L., & Hollerman, J. R. (2000). Reward processing in primate orbitofrontal cortex and basal ganglia. *Cerebral Cortex*, **10**, 272–283.

Semrud-Clikeman, M., Steingard, R. J., & Filipek, P. (1994). Attention-deficit hyperactivity disorder: magnetic resonance imaging morphometric analysis of the corpus callosum. *Journal of the American Academy of Child and Adolescent Psychiatry*, **33**, 875–881.

Serra-Grabulosa, J. M., Junque, C., Verger, K. *et al.* (2005). Cerebral correlates of declarative memory dysfunctions in early traumatic brain injury. *Journal of Neurology, Neurosurgery and Psychiatry*, **76**, 129–131.

Shallice, T. (1982). Specific impairments of planning. *Philosophical Transactions of the Royal Society of London*, **298**, 199–209.

Shallice, T., & Burgess, P. W. (1991). Deficits in strategy application following frontal lobe damage in man. *Brain*, **114**, 727–741.

Shallice, T., Marzocchi, G. M., Coser, S. *et al.* (2002). Executive function profile of children with attention deficit hyperactivity disorder. *Developmental Neuropsychology*, **21**, 43–71.

Sheline, Y. I. (2003). Neuroimaging studies of mood disorder effects on the brain. *Biological Psychiatry*, **54**, 338–352.

Silk, J. S., Steinberg, L., & Morris, A. M. (2003). Adolescents' emotion regulation in daily life: links to depressive symptoms and problem behavior. *Child Development*, **74**, 1869.

Slomine, B. S., Gerring, J. P., Grados, M. A. *et al.* (2002). Performance on measures of executive function following pediatric traumatic brain injury. *Brain Injury*, **16**, 759–772.

Solanto, M. V. (2002). Dopamine dysfunction in AD/HD: integrating clinical and basic neuroscience research. *Behavioral Brain Research*, **130**, 65–71.

Swanson, H. L. (1999). What develops in working memory? A life span perspective. *Developmental Psychology*, **35**, 986–1000.

Swanson, H. L., & Sachse-Lee, C. (2001). Mathematical problem solving and working memory in children with learning disabilities: both executive and phonological processes are important. *Journal of Experimental Child Psychology*, **79**, 294–321.

Tasker, R. C., Salmond, C. H., Westland, A. G. *et al.* (2005). Head circumference and brain and hippocampal volume after severe traumatic brain injury in childhood. *Pediatric Research*, **58**, 302–308.

Thapar, A., Holmes, J., Poulton, K., & Harrington, R. (1999). Genetic basis of attention deficit and hyperactivity. *British Journal of Psychiatry*, **174**, 105–111.

Tong, K. A., Ashwal, S., Holshouser, B. A. *et al.* (2004). Diffuse axonal injury in children: clinical correlation with hemorrhagic lesions. *Annals of Neurology*, **56**, 36–50.

Toplak, M. E., Jain, U., & Tannock, R. (2005). Executive and motivational processes in adolescents with attention-deficit-hyperactivity disorder (ADHD). *Behavioral and Brain Functions*, **1**, 1–8.

Vaidya, C. J., Bunge, S. A., Dudukovic, N. M. *et al.* (2005). Altered neural substrates of cognitive control in childhood ADHD: evidence from functional magnetic resonance imaging. *American Journal of Psychiatry*, **162**, 1605–1613.

Vriezen, E. R., & Pigott, S. E. (2002). The relationship between parental report on the BRIEF and performance-based measures of executive function in children with moderate to severe traumatic brain injury. *Child Neuropsychology*, **8**, 296–303.

Walden, T., Lemerise, E., & Smith, M. C. (1999). Friendship and popularity in preschool classrooms. *Early Education and Development*, **10**, 351–371.

Ward, L., & Traweek, D. (1993). Application of a metacognitive strategy to assessment, intervention, and consultation: a think-aloud technique. *Journal of School Psychology*, **31**, 469–485.

Weiler, M. D., Bernstein, J. H., Bellinger, D., & Waber, D. P. (2002). Information processing deficits in children with attention-deficit/hyperactivity disorder, inattentive type, and children with reading disability. *Journal of Learning Disabilities*, **35**, 448–461.

Wilde, E. A., Hunter, J. V., Newsome, M. R. *et al.* (2005). Frontal and temporal morphometric findings on MRI in children after moderate to severe traumatic brain injury. *Journal of Neurotrauma*, **22**, 333–344.

Wilde, E. A., Chu, Z., Bigler, E. D. *et al.* (2006). Diffusion tensor imaging in the corpus callosum in children after moderate to severe traumatic brain injury. *Journal of Neurotrauma*, **23**, 1412–1426.

Willcutt, E. G., Doyle, A. E., Nigg, J. T., Faraone, S. V., & Pennington, B. F. (2005). Validity of the executive function theory of attention-deficit/hyperactivity disorder: a meta-analytic review. *Biological Psychiatry*, **57**, 1336–1346.

Williams, B., Ponesse, J., Schachar, R., Logan, G. D., & Tannock, R. (1999). Development of inhibitory control across the lifespan. *Developmental Psychology*, **33**, 205–213.

Williams, S. E., Ris, M. D., Ayyangar, R., Schefft, B. K., & Berch, D. (1998). Recovery in pediatric brain injury: is psychostimulant medication beneficial? *Journal of Head Trauma Rehabilitation*, **13**, 73–81.

Yeates, K. O., Taylor, H. G., Drotar, D. *et al.* (1997). Preinjury family environment as a determinant of recovery from traumatic brain injuries in school-age children. *Journal of the International Neuropsychological Society*, **3**, 617–630.

Ylvisaker, M., Szekeres, S. F., & Feeney, T. J. (1998). Cognitive rehabilitation: Executive functions. In M. Ylvisaker (Ed.), *Traumatic Brain Injury Rehabilitation: Children and Adolescents (2nd Edition)* (pp. 221–270). Boston, MA: Butterworth-Heinemann.

Zelazo, P. D., Reznick, J. S., & Pinon, D. E. (1995). Response control and the execution of verbal rules. *Developmental Psychology*, **31**, 508–517.

29

Rehabilitation of attention following traumatic brain injury

Jennie Ponsford

Introduction

- Traumatic brain injury results in injury to frontal, temporal, meso-limbic, midbrain reticular formation areas, which are involved in the mediation of aspects of attention.
- Cognitive and behavioral changes following TBI have a significant impact on capacity for work, study, leisure, social activities and relationships.

Traumatic brain injury (TBI) is the leading cause of death and disability in those aged under 40, occurring most frequently in males aged 15–24 years and resulting most commonly from motor vehicle accidents (Kraus & McArthur, 1999; Fortune & Wen, 1999). These predominantly young people are generally in the process of completing their studies or learning vocational skills and establishing important personal and social relationships.

Blunt trauma to the head results in a combination of acceleration-deceleration and rotational forces which may result in cerebral contusion, and diffuse axonal injury, particularly in the frontal and temporal lobes. Shearing strains are created between tissues of different density, causing lesions in areas such as the midbrain reticular formation, cerebellar peduncles, basal ganglia, hypothalamus, fornices and corpus callosum (Gentleman, 1999; Graham, 1999; Povlishock & Katz, 2005). Secondary effects of brain injury, including edema, raised intra-cranial pressure, cerebral hemorrhage, hypotension or respiratory failure, may result in further damage due to pressure effects or hypoxia. The hippocampus and thalamus are particularly vulnerable to the effects of hypoxia. As a result of all these mechanisms, TBI tends to result in diffuse, bilateral injury, affecting many brain regions including the frontal, temporal, meso-limbic, midbrain reticular formation areas. All of these areas are involved in the mediation of aspects of attention. As a consequence of this damage, TBI results in a range of cognitive impairments, particularly in the domains of attention, memory and executive function, as well as behavioral and emotional changes including inflexibility, impulsivity, reduced behavioral control or inhibition, reduced initiative, mood swings and other affective changes. The injured person frequently has a lack of self-awareness of these changes, which tend to be more persistent than physical disabilities (Olver et al., 1996). In many cases, these changes have a significant impact on capacity for work or study, social and leisure activities and personal and social relationships (Boake et al., 2001; Lehtonen et al., 2005; Ponsford et al., 1995b; Tate & Broe, 1999). Less than half of those with moderate to severe injuries are employed 2 years post-injury. The failure to attain important life goals by these young people potentially has a devastating impact on their psychosocial adjustment. Outcome studies have documented high rates of depression and anxiety and reduced self-esteem (Deb et al., 1999; Olver et al., 1996).

Cognitive Neurorehabilitation, Second Edition: Evidence and Application, ed. Donald T. Stuss, Gordon Winocur and Ian H. Robertson. Published by Cambridge University Press. © Cambridge University Press 2008.

The impact of traumatic brain injury on attention

- Subjective reports of attentional problems are common and these impact on outcome.

Numerous TBI outcome studies have documented, on the basis of both subjective reports and objective neuropsychological assessment, the presence of disorders of attention up to 30 years after injury. Indeed, impairment of attention and speed of information processing are amongst the most common cognitive problems associated with TBI, being reported in up to 70% of those with moderate to severe TBI, by their relatives or therapists (Hellawell *et al.*, 1999; Himanen *et al.*, 2006; Hoofien *et al.*, 2001; Olver *et al.*, 1996; Ponsford & Kinsella, 1991; Ponsford *et al.*, 1995a; van Zomeren & van den Burg, 1985; Ziino & Ponsford, 2006a, 2006b). A recent study by Ponsford *et al.* (2006) has documented the presence of attentional deficits as assessed on tests including the Digit Span, Digit Symbol Coding and Symbol Digit Modalities Tests, Sustained Attention and Response Task (SART) and Trail Making Test 10 years post-injury and established a significant association between the presence of these impairments and functional outcome on the Extended Glasgow Outcome Scale.

What is attention?

- Attention is a multidimensional construct, incorporating interactive systems for sensory selective attention, arousal and sustained attention, and intentional control.

It is important to establish from the outset that attention is not a unitary concept, but rather constitutes a set of processes which, according to Cohen (1993, p. 3), interact dynamically to allow the individual to "direct themselves to appropriate aspects of external environmental effects and internal operations. Attention facilitates the selection of salient information and the allocation of cognitive processing appropriate to that information. Therefore, attention acts as a gate for information flow in the brain." Various theories have been put forward to describe the manner in which attentional systems operate and their neuroanatomical correlates (Baddeley, 1993; Cohen, 1993; Norman & Shallice, 1980; Posner & Rothbart, 1992; Shiffrin & Schneider, 1977; Stuss & Benson, 1986). These theoretical explanations are in agreement that there are several multifocal interconnected attentional networks: a *sensory selective attentional system*, mediated by the parieto-temporo-occipital area, responsible for orienting, engaging and disengaging attention and object recognition; a system controlling *arousal, sustained attention and vigilance*, also regulating mood, motivation, the salience of stimuli and readiness to respond, mediated by the midbrain reticular activating system and limbic structures; and an *anterior system for selection and control of responses*, involving intentional control and use of strategies for manipulating information, active switching and inhibition, mediated by the frontal lobes, anterior cingulate gyrus and basal ganglia, with the thalamus acting as the relay station of incoming information and outgoing responses. Finally, the right hemisphere appears to mediate alertness and sustained attention, and the left hemisphere selective or focused attention (Mesulam, 1985; Mottaghy *et al.*, 2006; Robertson *et al.*, 1997b; Sturm & Willmes, 2001)

What aspects of attention are impaired by TBI?

- Traumatic brain injury may impair vigilance, speed of information processing and the ability to allocate attention resources and cause distractibility in complex environments.
- It is important to assess attention in complex environments.

Damage to the parieto-temporo-occipital attentional network is generally manifested as object recognition difficulties and unilateral spatial neglect. These occur relatively rarely following TBI. Rehabilitation of spatial neglect is covered in Chapter 26 by Singh-Curry and Husain in this volume. However, the frequent damage to frontal, temporal, limbic and midbrain-reticular activating system structures would be expected to cause impairments involving the other two systems. These have not always been easy to demonstrate in group studies, possibly due to the heterogeneity of injury in TBI participants.

In the domain of alertness, impaired phasic alertness has been demonstrated on electrophysiological studies (Curry, 1981; Rizzo *et al.*, 1978; Rugg *et al.*, 1989; Segalowitz *et al.*, 1992), but this has not been demonstrated behaviorally (Ponsford & Kinsella, 1992; Whyte *et al.*, 1997a). One possible exception is the demonstration by Dockree *et al.* (2004) of a relative failure by TBI individuals to monitor their responses and thereby prepare for a predictable stimulus on the Sustained Attention to Response Task (Fixed). Although no warning signal is provided prior to target stimuli, the target stimulus is predictable from the sequence of numbers preceding it. Control participants appeared to adjust their responses in anticipation of the forthcoming target stimulus and show associated desynchronization of alpha EEG, which was not evident in the TBI individuals in the study by Dockree *et al.* However, the extent to which this reflects impairment of phasic alertness or executive function would be a matter of debate.

Whilst it has not been possible to demonstrate a consistent vigilance decrement, or decline in accuracy of performance over time, there is a demonstrated reduction in the level of vigilance, in the form of decreased perceptual sensitivity, particularly when stimuli are degraded (Brouwer & van Wolffelaar, 1985; Parasuraman *et al.*, 1991; Ponsford & Kinsella, 1992; Robertson *et al.*, 1997a; Spikman *et al.*, 1996; Whyte *et al.*, 1995; Zoccolotti *et al.*, 2000). Ziino & Ponsford (2006a) found that more errors on a vigilance task were associated with higher subjective fatigue levels and with disproportionate increases in diastolic blood pressure whilst performing the task, suggesting that greater effort is required to maintain performance at some psychophysiological cost. In this study a proportion of TBI individuals did exhibit a decline in performance over time, which was, in turn, associated with greater subjective fatigue (Ziino & Ponsford, 2006a). Greater variability of performance has been evident in some studies

(Stuss *et al.*, 1994; Whyte *et al.*, 1995), although this has again not been a consistent finding (Spikman *et al.*, 1996; van Zomeren & Brouwer, 1987; Ziino & Ponsford, 2006a).

Individuals with TBI are generally slower in performing selective attention tasks (Heinze *et al.*, 1992; Ponsford & Kinsella, 1992; Robertson *et al.*, 1994; Schmitter-Edgecombe & Kibby, 1998). Indeed impairments of speed of information processing have been comprehensively documented on a broad range of tasks following TBI (Gronwall & Sampson, 1974; Ponsford & Kinsella, 1992; Spikman *et al.*, 1996; Stuss *et al.*, 1989; van Zomeren & Brouwer, 1994; Ziino & Ponsford, 2006b). This slowness, may in turn affect capacity for conscious processing of information. Individuals with TBI are significantly slower in sharing their attention between tasks (Brouwer *et al.*, 1989; Cicerone, 1996; Spikman *et al.*, 1996; Stablum *et al.*, 1994; Veltman *et al.*, 1996; Vilkki *et al.*, 1996). However, errors on selective or focused attention, sustained attention or divided attention tasks tend to be made only where there is a significant degree of novelty, complexity and demands on working memory, strategy use and/ or response inhibition associated with the task/s being performed (Azouvi *et al.*, 1996; Bohnen *et al.*, 1992; Couillet *et al.*, 2000; Dockree *et al.*, 2004, 2006; Draper & Ponsford, 2006; McDowell *et al.*, 1997; Park *et al.*, 1999a; Robertson *et al.*, 1997a; Withaar, 2000; Ziino & Ponsford, 2006b). Similarly, susceptibility to distraction is only evident in more complex environments (Whyte *et al.*, 1996, 1998).

Difficulties in applying strategies in the context of changing task demands, reduced mental flexibility and problems with goal-directed allocation of attention across a number of tasks have also been demonstrated on more complex tasks conducted in more naturalistic environments (Boyd & Sautter, 1993; Shallice & Burgess, 1991; Spikman *et al.*, 2000; Stablum *et al.*, 1994; Veltman *et al.*, 1996; Vilkki, 1992). Using functional MRI, McAllister *et al.* (1999) found modified activation in prefrontal and parietal regions during a working memory task one month after mild TBI. Functional MRI studies have also shown the right ventral and left dorsolateral prefrontal cortex, right inferoparietal cortex, rostral anterior cingulate and pre-supplementary motor area to be involved in unpredictable inhibitions, error processing and conflict monitoring on the Sustained Attention to Response Task (SART), another task on which TBI individuals make more errors than controls (Fassbender *et al.*, 2004). McAvinue *et al.* (2005) showed that provision of feedback on errors improved sustained attention performance on the SART. As Leclercq & Azouvi (2002, p. 273) have concluded, "defective activation or modulation of attentional/executive networks including but not limited to the prefrontal cortex" may be associated with attentional impairments following TBI.

Clearly, due to the wide heterogeneity of pathology seen following these injuries, different patterns of attentional difficulty will emerge from one case to the next and each needs to be assessed individually. Moreover it is also clear that many problems emerge only in novel and complex environments, which are typical in everyday life. What this means is that, in a rehabilitation context, assessment of attentional problems should not only utilize standard neuropsychological tests of attention, but should also incorporate observation of performance in novel and complex environments.

Rehabilitation strategies for stimulating alertness, sustained attention and vigilance

- Studies conducted in patients with right hemisphere lesions suggest that external or internal cues may be used to alert patients.
- Brief mindfulness training and other cognitive–behavioral methods have been used with some success to assist TBI individuals to focus their attention and maintain arousal.
- The extent to which cognitive–behavioral methods are effective will depend on the level of self-awareness, motivation and capacity to follow through with instructions in a goal-directed fashion in the injured person.

- Computer training has been shown to enhance alertness or vigilance, as measured neuropsychologically.
- In terms of pharmacological interventions, there is some limited evidence of improved vigilance or sustained attention in response to methylphenidate following TBI. Dopaminergic agents including bromocriptine, levodopa-carbidopa and amantadine have been shown to enhance arousal in individuals with TBI who are vegetative or slow to recover.

The right hemisphere, particularly the right lateral frontal cortex, has been implicated in the maintenance of alertness and sustained attention (Mottaghy *et al.*, 2006; Robertson *et al.*, 1997b). Playing a loud alerting tone has been shown to remove the spatial bias of patients with left-sided neglect, suggesting a direct link between neglect and alertness (Robertson *et al.*, 1998). Thimm *et al.* (2006) found that 3 weeks of computerized alertness training in seven patients with right hemisphere stroke resulted in improved alertness and reduced neglect relative to a baseline phase, with an associated increase in neural activity in the right frontal cortex, although performances had returned to baseline at 3-week follow-up.

Self-alerting

Robertson *et al.* (1995) evaluated the impact of self-alerting training, using a cognitive–behavioral approach, in alleviating neglect. Following external prompting by a therapist to "Attend!" eight patients were cued to use covert self-instruction to alert themselves at regular intervals. Improvements were evident on measures of both visual neglect and sustained attention. However there was no follow-up as to whether patients were able to continue using the self-alerting procedure or whether it improved their visual scanning beyond the therapy setting. These findings raise the possibility that self-alerting or alertness training might be applied to patients with TBI who may have impaired alertness or sustained attention, in the absence of neglect.

Brief mindfulness training

McMillan *et al.* (2002) evaluated the impact of a *brief mindfulness meditation* technique on sustained attention following TBI. This involved training TBI participants, using an audiotape, to control their attention by concentrating on breathing over extended periods. Unfortunately the training, which was conducted over a 4-week period, did not result in a reduction in cognitive failures or improvement on a range of attentional and memory tasks and psychological adjustment measures relative to the two control groups, which received either physical fitness training or no treatment. Whilst the authors considered that more intensive training by skilled therapists may have been more effective, this was not felt to be feasible within the existing healthcare system.

Arguably, training of this nature is likely to be more effective if it is intensive and focused on specific attentional difficulties manifested in daily activities. Wilson & Robertson (1992) carried out an intervention with a head-injured man, who was bothered by involuntary slips of attention whilst reading, which affected his ability to complete accountancy homework. The intervention focused on helping him understand how his difficulties came about, relaxation training and strategies for dealing with internal and external distractions. He was instructed to monitor involuntary slips of attention when reading, defined as when he needed to reread a word or sentence or when his mind wandered from the text to a different train of thought. Over 39 days he gradually increased time reading without an attentional slip from 50 to 325 seconds. More modest gains were achieved when background noise was introduced. The intervention resulted in a significant reduction in attentional slips while reading an accountancy text over a 15-minute period.

Webster & Scott (1983) used a similar self-instructional technique to train a constructional worker 2 years post head injury to focus attention during reading or listening. He was taught self-instructional statements to prepare himself to listen and ask for repetition if attention had strayed, initially repeated aloud and then subvocalized. Results showed significant gains in recall of stories and improvement was noted in other settings. Effects were reportedly still evident 18 months later.

The extent to which self-instructional techniques may be used to increase arousal and improve the ability to sustain attention will depend on the level of self-awareness, motivation and capacity to follow through with instructions in a goal-directed fashion in the injured person. For some TBI individuals this will be difficult. Nevertheless, cognitive–behavioral techniques may be useful as a means of providing these individuals with strategies to focus their attention and maintain arousal.

Computer training of alertness and vigilance

Sturm *et al.* (1997) designed a hierarchical series of computer-mediated tasks, some of which were designed to enhance intensity aspects of attention (alertness and vigilance), whilst others focused on selective and divided attention. They demonstrated gains on neuropsychological measures of alertness and vigilance in response to both training modules, each of which was conducted over 14 one-hour sessions. For selectivity aspects of attention, reaction time also improved after training of basic attentional domains. The authors concluded that attentional processes were hierarchical, and that training the most basic aspects (alertness and vigilance) could have a positive impact upon higher aspects (SAS–dual task or selective attention tasks). As is argued below, these gains were, however, confined to neuropsychological tests which bore some resemblance to the training tasks and there was no attempt to measure the generalization or maintenance of gains.

Pharmacologic interventions for arousal and vigilance

Pharmacologic interventions present an alternative means of enhancing arousal and sustained attention. There is some evidence of improved vigilance or sustained attention in response to methylpheni-date following TBI (Mahalick *et al.*, 1998; Plenger *et al.*, 1996). After 30 days of drug treatment, and a 30-day drug-free follow-up, subjects treated with methylphenidate demonstrated better vigilance per-formance than a placebo control group on the Continuous Performance Task (Plenger *et al.*, 1996). Speech *et al.* (1993) found no statistically significant drug effects on a vigilance task from the Gordon Diagnostic System (GDS) after 1 week of treatment with methylphenidate. However, Mahalick *et al.* (1998) found significant drug treatment effects in a pediatric sample on the same measure (GDS-delayed efficiency ratio, distractibility commission, vigilance commission). Whyte (2003; Whyte *et al.* 1997b, 2002) did not find any impact of treatment with methyl-phenidate on arousal or vigilance performances, but did find an increase in speed of processing.

Dopaminergic agents such as bromocriptine and levodopa-carbidopa have been used to augment arousal in patients in a vegetative state. In an unblinded, uncontrolled study, Lal *et al.* (1988) report improvements in alertness, sustained atten-tion and concentration following treatment with levodopa-carbidopa. Subjective reports of increased arousal have also followed treatment with amanta-dine (Gualtieri *et al.*, 1989), and improvements in general outcome with amantadine have been found to be independent of natural recovery (Meythaler *et al.*, 2002). McDowell *et al.* (1998) found that low-dose bromocriptine improved performance on the Trail Making Test, the Wisconsin Card Sorting Test, the Controlled Oral Word Association Test, and a computerised dual-task in 24 TBI subjects, conclud-ing that the drug effect was primarily upon dual-task performance and executive processes.

Rehabilitation of selective attention

- Attentional training results in gains on trained tasks and similar neuropsychological measures.
- Application of training directly to functional daily tasks or tasks resembling these is more likely to result in meaningful gains.

Most research studies aimed at improving selective attention following TBI have utilized computer-mediated training, whereby the injured person undertakes repeated practice on tasks requiring them to respond selectively to stimuli on the screen according to instructions, or analogous tasks using paper and pencil or tape-recorded tasks. The speed of presentation, complexity of the task or the amount of cueing or feedback provided may be altered systematically to shape the development of particular skills with the aim of restoring attentional functions (Ben Yishay *et al.*, 1987; Boman *et al.*, 2004; Gansler & McCaffrey, 1991; Gray *et al.*, 1992; Gray & Robertson, 1989; Malec *et al.*, 1984; Niemann *et al.*, 1990; Novack *et al.*, 1996; Palmese & Raskin, 2000; Park *et al.*, 1999b; Penkman & Mateer, 2004; Ponsford & Kinsella, 1988; Ruff *et al.*, 1994; Sohlberg *et al.*, 2000; Sohlberg & Mateer, 1987; Stablum *et al.*, 2000; Sturm *et al.*, 1997; Sturm & Willmes, 1991; Wood & Fussey, 1987). Most of the studies evaluat-ing these approaches have demonstrated improve-ment on the trained tasks, where this was measured. The 11 studies listed first, from Ben Yishay *et al.* (1987) to Penkman & Mateer (2004) have also dem-onstrated gains on some neuropsychological meas-ures and in some cases, as reported by those treated. In all of these studies the training tasks involved elements similar to these measures. However, there has been no evidence of generalization to everyday activity or participation measures.

Park *et al.* (1999b) have argued that the mecha-nism underlying these improvements is one of spe-cific skill training, which generalizes to tasks of a similar nature (neuropsychological measures), rather than actually bringing about recovery of underlying damaged attentional functions. Support for this contention came from a meta-anal-ysis of 30 studies by Park & Ingles (2001) which found that performance improvements were only evident in pre-post studies, but not in studies employing controls. The single exception was a study by Kewman *et al.* (1985), which focused more directly on specific skills of functional signifi-cance involved in driving (keeping track of more than one thing at once or shifting the focus of attention from one activity to another), providing the training on a small electric-powered vehicle. Such training resulted in better on-road driving performance than that of a control group which simply practiced driving. This suggests that it may be possible to make functional gains by focusing training more directly on the functional activities.

Results of a study by Schmitter-Edgecombe & Beglinger (2001) have suggested that skill training using consistent mapping techniques may result in development of automatic attention responses, which are not affected by TBI. Since the ultimate goal of rehabilitation is to improve the ability to perform functional activities, it is arguably preferable to focus training or massed practice on elements of those activities directly, until they become automatic and no longer place demands on the capacity-limited controlled processing system. Schmitter-Edgecombe & Beglinger (2001) suggest that such training should be provided in a manner whereby responses to the same class of stimuli are always the same. As they point out (p. 628), "studies with non head-injured participants have shown that complex multiple-task performances can improve to a skilled level when one of the tasks is first practised alone and becomes 'automatic' (e.g., Schneider & Fisk, 1982)."

In summary, whilst some studies have shown that individuals with TBI can benefit from skill training in the domain of selective attention, there is limited evidence that such training generalizes beyond tasks of a very similar nature to those on which the individual is trained. In light of this, it is arguably more likely to be effective to focus training or massed practice on elements of those activities which have to be performed in everyday life, rather than abstract tasks such as those utilized in most computer-mediated attentional training modules.

Recent studies have suggested the importance of incorporating generalization training into remedial interventions, with practice in applying compensatory strategies to specific difficulties experienced being a recommended component of intervention (Boman et al., 2004; Cicerone et al., 2005). The importance of this cannot be over-emphasized.

Even in individuals with high levels of self-awareness, executive function and motivation, without this important link being made explicitly the impact of such training will rarely be lasting. It is absolutely vital that a detailed task analysis be performed of tasks performed by the injured person in their daily life to identify aspects on which attentional difficulties are likely to impinge, so that strategies can be applied to these directly. Ideally, involvement of close others, work colleagues or school buddies can assist in reinforcing the use of the strategies. Many hours of practice will usually be required to establish the routine use of strategies, with follow-up being particularly important. Even with such intensive intervention the extent of ongoing use of strategies will depend on the level of self-awareness and self-monitoring capability of the injured person and those around them. These benefits are not easily achieved!

Rose et al. (2005) have highlighted the possible use of Virtual Reality Technology for training of individuals with attentional disturbance in real world environments. However, although some tasks have been developed for assessment purposes, this technology has not yet been used and evaluated for treatment.

Strategies for mental slowness

- Time pressure monitoring may enhance compensatory coping with slowed information processing.

Given the frequency of slowed information processing following TBI and its potential impact on vocational and social activities, the development of coping strategies for this problem is particularly important. In one of only two Class I studies of attention rehabilitation published since 1998, Fasotti et al. (2000) evaluated specific compensatory strategies for dealing with reduced speed of information processing following TBI, termed time pressure management (TPM). Time pressure management training involved three steps: (i) increasing the person's awareness of the relationship between their mental slowness and their performance on the tasks, and their ability to discriminate between effective and ineffective performance on the task; (ii) acceptance and acquisition of the TPM strategy, using guided self-instruction: recognizing the sources of time pressure in the task at hand, planning ways to reduce time pressure before starting the task, developing "managing steps" to deal with time pressure problems experienced whilst performing the task as quickly as possible (e.g., turning off the tape, asking for repetition or asking the person to slow down the delivery of information) and monitoring the implementation of the TPM strategies; (iii) the final stage involved application and maintenance of strategies under more distracting and difficult conditions, for example with a radio playing in the background.

Fasotti *et al.* (2000) compared the effectiveness of TPM training with more general instructions to concentrate on video-taped instructions as to how to get somewhere, and how to use a computer program. Both treatments improved task performance. However, following training the experimental group took significantly more TPM "managing steps" than controls, resulting in greater and more durable gains in task performance, which also generalized to other measures of speed and memory function. There was no change in measures of psychosocial well-being. Some responded better to the training than others. Factors influencing the success of the training included self-awareness (subjects must see the sense in using strategy if they are to use it) and assertiveness to take managing steps in social situations.

Interventions for divided attention or working memory

- Strategies for dividing attention across tasks should be taught and applied directly to real world activities.

The allocation of attentional resources across more than one task can pose a significant challenge for many individuals with TBI. Cicerone (2002) trained four participants with mild TBI and "working

attentional" difficulties to more effectively allocate their attentional resources when performing tasks requiring divided attention. Training was conducted over 11–27 weeks on increasingly demanding dual-task paradigms (n-back, random generation and dual-task procedures), along with tasks similar to work-related tasks in their daily lives, with encouragement to develop and employ strategies for more effectively allocating their attentional resources and managing the rate of information during task performance and in everyday situations. Gains were evident on attentional measures including the PASAT and continuous performance tasks and improvements in coping with everyday attentional demands were also reported. These were attributed to the discussion of management strategies for allocating working attentional resources. The extent to which management strategies are able to be implemented will again depend on the level of self-awareness and goal-directed behavior of the injured individual.

Role of psychotherapeutic input in alleviating attentional disturbance

- The success of rehabilitation requires assessment and treatment of all possible causes of attentional disturbance, including pain, medication, post-traumatic stress, anxiety, depression or other psychological issues.

Several recent papers have highlighted the difficulties in differentiating symptoms directly associated with the head injury from those due to other factors such as pain, associated with neck, back or other injuries, medication effects, post-traumatic stress, anxiety, depression, pre-accident personality issues, individual coping styles or the presence of other stressors and/or litigation/compensation (Carroll *et al.*, 2004; Mateer *et al.*, 2005; Rose, 2005; Ruff, 2005; Wood, 2004). Previous studies have identified these factors as being associated with the presence of ongoing disability following mild TBI (Carroll *et al.*, 2004; Ponsford *et al.*, 2000). Since all of these conditions may contribute to attentional difficulties following TBI it is clearly important to assess the relative contribution of each of these factors and apply intervention accordingly (Ponsford, 2005).

There is now evidence to suggest that psychotherapeutic input may also have beneficial effects on attention (Palmese & Raskin, 2000; Penkman & Mateer, 2004) although its specific impact on outcome has not been evaluated. Studies of mild TBI suggest that at least a proportion of those experiencing ongoing symptomatology also have depression, anxiety disorders including post-traumatic stress which may exacerbate or even primarily underlie their attentional and memory difficulties (Mooney & Speed, 2001; Parker, 1996; Ponsford et al., 2000). In such cases psychotherapeutic intervention is likely to be efficacious and indeed will represent a vital component of treatment.

Mateer et al. (2005) and Ruff (2005) recommend a cognitive–behavioral (CBT) approach to therapy which aims to demonstrate to patients that their symptoms are common following mild TBI and that their inner dialogue may be increasing stress levels, and to equip them with strategies to manage and have a sense of mastery over symptoms and take control of their lifestyle. Cognitive remedial interventions may also be offered to assist in overcoming or managing cognitive difficulties. As Ruff (2005) points out, for some, experiencing a traumatic injury may unearth the effects of earlier traumatic experiences which require much more intensive psychotherapy. Although there have been few evaluations of such interventions, a recent randomized controlled trial by Tiersky et al. (2005) demonstrated significantly improved emotional functioning, including lessened anxiety and depression, as well as improved performance on a measure of divided attention (PASAT), following a combined program of individual cognitive–behavior therapy designed to increase coping skills and decrease stress, and cognitive remediation 3 times a week for 11 weeks.

Goal management training

- Periodic auditory stimuli may assist self-monitoring.

- Goal management training has been used with some success to assist with planning, self-monitoring and execution of complex tasks, although further evidence is required to demonstrate how and with whom this should be implemented.

A number of studies have also focused on the facilitation of self-monitoring in patients with executive dysfunction, who have difficulty planning and following through with a course of action, generally secondary to frontal lobe impairment. For example, Manly et al. (2002) demonstrated that provision of a brief auditory stimulus, acting as a cue to consider the overall goal of the activity, assisted brain-injured individuals to monitor their performance and make fewer errors. These patients may also exhibit problems with efficient allocation of attentional resources where controlled processing is required, difficulty switching, or paying attention to more than one thing at a time and difficulty holding in working memory instructions to guide performance of a task or tasks. As discussed above, compensatory strategies may be taught to assist in compensating for these problems in certain cases, although the effectiveness of such training may be limited by awareness and monitoring capacity. Another approach which may assist with planning, self-monitoring and execution of complex tasks is goal management training. However, further evidence is required to examine how and with whom this can be most effectively implemented. This is comprehensively discussed by Levine, Turner and Stuss in Chapter 27 in this volume, which focuses on rehabilitation of executive function.

Environmental manipulation to maximize attentional performance

- For those with limited awareness, self-monitoring capacity and executive function, modification of the environment or the tasks the person performs is more likely to achieve better attentional performance.

Clearly the use of any of these compensatory strategies to overcome attentional difficulties presupposes some level of self-awareness and some capacity for verbal self-regulation of behavior. In those with extensive injuries, particularly involving the frontal lobes, this may not be present and there is likely to be minimal potential for the use of compensatory strategies. Moreover, those with extensive injuries are less likely to show recovery and regeneration with or without intervention (Kolb & Cioe, 2004).

The environment can, however, be manipulated to minimise the impact of attentional problems. As suggested by Sloan & Ponsford (1995), the work environment might be altered to reduce distractions (e.g., work in a quiet room, facing a wall, reduce interruptions and background noise, clear workspace). Tasks may be modified to reduce speed demands or the amount of information to be processed.

Incorporating rest breaks into activities is important. Verbal prompts or cues may be provided to encourage the person to re-focus on the task or to assist the person to move from one component of the task to the next. Removal of unstructured periods reduces opportunity for distraction. Frequent changes of activities may also assist in maintaining interest. Material to be remembered, such as instructions, should be repeated, and in work or study environments a dictaphone may be useful to record and replay important material.

Allowing a realistic time-frame for completion of tasks will reduce time pressure and associated stress. More complex tasks may be scheduled at the time of day when fatigue levels are lower and there are few competing demands. Learning to identify the signs of fatigue and take appropriate action is important. Stress management, relaxation or meditation techniques may also be helpful.

Conclusions

Traumatic brain injury may have a significant impact on a number of aspects of attention, including vigilance, speed of information processing and the ability to allocate attention resources and avoid distraction in complex environments. Despite the large number of attention rehabilitation studies conducted to date, there is still limited evidence of their success. A number of methods have been shown to be effective in alleviating attentional problems, at least in some cases. However, careful assessment as to the ways in which the problem is manifested in complex everyday activities should precede intervention. Although training may initially be given in the rehabilitation setting, this should be applied to activities resembling the demands of the individual's daily life. The training will only be effective if it is applied directly and repeatedly in everyday settings. Where there is some degree of self-awareness and self-monitoring capability, compensatory strategies may be applied. Cognitive–behavioral approaches may be used to train these strategies to enhance alertness, attention to tasks such as reading or the ability to divide attention across several tasks simultaneously. Where psychological factors such as anxiety, depression or pain are thought to be contributing to attentional problems these should also be addressed using cognitive–behavioral strategies. This is particularly important in cases of mild head injury. In those cases where there is extensive injury particularly involving the frontal lobes, manipulation of the environment or task demands is likely to be more effective. Whatever approach is taken, objective evaluation of the impact of interventions on the injured person's daily functioning represents a vital component of the rehabilitation process.

REFERENCES

Azouvi, P., Jokic, C., van der Linden, M., Marlier, N., & Bussel, B. (1996). Working memory and supervisory control after severe closed head injury. A study of dual task performance and random generation. *Journal of Clinical and Experimental Neuropsychology*, **18**, 317–337.

Baddeley A. D. (1993). Working memory or working attention? In A. D. Baddeley & L. Weiskrantz (Eds.), *Attention: Selection, Awareness and Control. A Tribute to Donald Broadbent* (pp. 152–170). Oxford: Oxford University Press.

Ben-Yishay, Y., Piasetsky, E. B., & Rattock, J. (1987). A systematic method for ameliorating disorders in basic attention. In M. J. Meier, A. L. Benton, & L. Diller (Eds.), *Neuropsychological Rehabilitation* (pp. 165–181). New York, NY: Churchill Livingstone.

Boake, C., Millis, S. R., High, W. M. *et al.* (2001). Using early neuropsychologic testing to predict long-term productivity outcome from traumatic brain injury. *Archives of Physical Medicine and Rehabilitation*, **82**, 761–768.

Bohnen, N., Jolles, J., & Twijnstra, A. (1992). Modification of the Stroop Color Word Test improves differentiation between patients with mild head injury and matched controls. *Clinical Neuropsychologist*, **6**, 178–184.

Boman, I.-L., Lindsted, M., Hemmingsted, H., & Bartfai, A. (2004). Cognitive training in the home environment. *Brain Injury*, **18**, 985–995.

Boyd, T. M., & Sautter, S. W. (1993). Route-finding: a measure of everyday executive functioning in the head-injured adult. *Applied Cognitive Psychology*, **7**, 171–181.

Brouwer, W. H., & van Wolffelaar, P. C. (1985). Sustained attention and sustained effort after closed head injury. *Cortex*, **21**, 111–119.

Brouwer, W. H., Ponds, R. W., van Wolffelaar, P. C., & van Zomeren, A. H. (1989). Divided attention 5 to 10 years after severe closed head injury. *Cortex*, **25**, 219–230.

Carroll, L., Cassidy, J. D., Peloso, P. *et al.* (2004). Prognosis for mild traumatic brain injury: results of the WHO Collaborating Centre Task Force on Mild Traumatic Brain Injury. *Journal of Rehabilitation Medicine*, **36,** Suppl. 43, 84–105.

Cicerone, K. D. (1996). Attention deficits and dual task demands after mild traumatic brain injury. *Brain Injury*, **10**, 79–90.

Cicerone, K. D. (2002). Remediation of "working attention" in mild traumatic brain injury. *Brain Injury*, **16**, 185–195.

Cicerone, K. D., Dahlberg, C., Malec, J. F. *et al.* (2005). Evidence-based cognitive rehabilitation: updated review of the literature from 1998 through 2002. *Archives of Physical Medicine and Rehabilitation*, **86**, 1681–1692.

Cohen, R. A. (1993). *The Neuropsychology of Attention*. New York: Plenum Press.

Couillet, J., Leclercq, M., Martin, Y., Rousseaux, M., & Azouvi, P. (2000). Divided attention after severe diffuse traumatic brain injury. *European Brain Injury Association Meeting*. Paris.

Curry, S. H. (1981). Event-related potentials as indicants of structural and functional damage in closed head injury. *Progress in Brain Research*, **54**, 507–515.

Deb, S., Lyons, I., Koutzoukis, C., Ali, I., & McCarthy, G. (1999). Rate of psychiatric illness 1 year after traumatic brain injury. *American Journal of Psychiatry*, **156**, 374–378.

Dockree, P. M., Kelly, S. P., Roche, R. A. P. *et al.* (2004). Behavioral and physiological impairments of sustained attention after traumatic brain injury. *Cognitive Brain Research*, **20**, 403–414.

Dockree, P. M., Bellgrove, M. A., O'Keefe, F. M. *et al.* (2006). Sustained attention in traumatic brain injury and healthy controls: enhanced sensitivity with dual-task load. *Experimental Brain Research*, **168**, 218–229.

Fasotti, L., Kovacs, F., Eling, P. A. T. M., & Brouwer, W. H. (2000). Time pressure management as a compensatory strategy training after closed head injury. *Neuropsychological Rehabilitation*, **10**, 47–65.

Fassbender, C., Murphy, K., Foxe, J. J. *et al.* (2004). A topography of executive functions and their interactions revealed by functional magnetic resonance imaging. *Cognitive Brain Research*, **20**, 132–143.

Fortune, N., & Wen, X. (1999). *The Definition, Incidence and Prevalence of Acquired Brain Injury in Australia*. Canberra: Australian Institute of Health and Welfare.

Gansler, D. A., & McCaffrey, R. J. (1991). Remediation of chronic attention deficits in traumatic brain-injured patients. *Archives of Clinical Neuropsychology*, **6**, 335–353.

Gentleman, D. (1999). Improving outcome after traumatic brain injury – progress and challenges. *British Medical Bulletin*, **55**, 910–926.

Graham, D. I. (1999). Pathophysiological aspects of injury and mechanisms of recovery. In M. Rosenthal, J. S. Kreutzer, E. R. Griffith, & B. Pentland (Eds.), *Rehabilitation of the Adult and Child with Traumatic Brain Injury (3rd Edition)* (pp. 19–41). Philadelphia: Davis.

Gray, J. M., & Robertson, I. (1989). Remediation of attentional difficulties following brain injury: three experimental case studies. *Brain Injury*, **3**, 163–170.

Gray, J. M., Robertson, I. H., Pentland, B., & Anderson, S. J. (1992). Microcomputer based cognitive rehabilitation for brain damage: a randomized group controlled trial. *Neuropsychological Rehabilitation*, **2**, 97–116.

Gronwall, D., & Sampson, H. (1974). *The Psychological Effects of Concussion*. Auckland, New Zealand: Auckland University Press/Oxford University Press.

Gualtieri, T., Chandler, M., Coons, T. B., & Brown, L. T. (1989). Amantadine: a new clinical profile for traumatic brain injury. *Clinical Neuropharmacology*, **12**, 258–270.

Heinze, H.-J., Münte, T. F., Gobiet, W., Niemann, H., & Ruff, R. M. (1992). Parallel and serial visual search after closed head injury: electrophysiological evidence for perceptual dysfunctions. *Neuropsychologia*, **30**, 495–514.

Hellawell, D. J., Taylor, R., & Pentland, B. (1999). Cognitive and psychosocial outcome following moderate to severe traumatic brain injury. *Brain Injury*, **13**, 489–504.

Himanen, L., Portin, R., Isoniemi, H. *et al.* (2006). Longitudinal cognitive changes in traumatic brain injury: a 30-year follow-up study. *Neurology*, **66**, 187–192.

Hoofien, D., Gilboa, A., Vakil, E., & Donovick, P. J. (2001). Traumatic brain injury (TBI) 10–20 years later: a comprehensive outcome study of psychiatric symptomatology, cognitive abilities and psychosocial functioning. *Brain Injury*, **15**, 189–209.

Kewman, D. G., Seigerman, C., Kintner, H. *et al.* (1985). Simulation training of psychomotor skills: teaching the brain-injured to drive. *Rehabilitation Psychology*, **30**, 11–27.

Kolb, B., & Cioe, J. (2004). Neuronal organization and change after neuronal injury. In J. Ponsford (Ed.), *Cognitive and Behavioral Rehabilitation: From Neurobiology to Clinical Practice* (pp. 30–58). New York, NY: Guilford Press.

Kraus, J. F., & McArthur, D. L. (1999). Incidence and prevalence of and costs associated with traumatic brain injury. In M. Rosenthal, E. R. Griffith, J. S. Kreutzer, & B. Pentland (Eds.), *Rehabilitation of the Adult and Child with Traumatic Brain Injury (3rd Edition)* (pp. 3–17). Philadelphia, PA: Davis.

Lal, S., Merbitz, C. P., & Grip, J. C. (1988). Modification of function in head-injured patients with sinemet. *Brain Injury*, **2**, 225–233.

Leclercq, M., & Azouvi, P. (2002). Attention after traumatic brain injury. In M. Leclercq & P. Zimmerman (Eds.), *Applied Neuropsychology of Attention* (pp. 257–279). London: Psychology Press.

Lehtonen, S., Stringer, A. Y., Millis, S. *et al.* (2005). Neuropsychological outcome and community re-integration following traumatic brain injury: the impact of frontal and non-frontal lesions. *Brain Injury*, **19**, 239–256.

Mahalick, D. M., Carmel, P. W., Greenberg, J. P. *et al.* (1998). Psychopharmacologic treatment of acquired attention disorders in children with brain injury. *Pediatric Neurosurgery*, **29**, 121–126.

Malec, J., Jones, R., Rao, N., & Stubbs, K. (1984). Video-game practice effects on sustained attention in patients with cranio-cerebral trauma. *Cognitive Rehabilitation*, **2**, 18–23.

Manly, T., Hawkins, K., Evans, J., Woldt, K., & Robertson, I. H. (2002). Rehabilitation of executive function: facilitation of effective goal management on complex tasks using periodic auditory alerts. *Neuropsychologia*, **40**, 271–281.

Mateer, C. A., Sira, C. S., & O'Connell, M. E. (2005). Putting Humpty Dumpty together again: the importance of integrating cognitive and emotional interventions. *Journal of Head Trauma Rehabilitation*, **20**, 62–75.

McAllister, T. W., Saykin, A. J., Flashman, L. A. *et al.* (1999). Brain activation during working memory 1 month after mild traumatic brain injury. A functional MRI study. *Neurology*, **53**, 1300–1308.

McAvinue, L., O'Keefe, F., McMackin, D., & Robertson, I. H. (2005). Impaired sustained attention and error awareness in traumatic brain injury: implications for insight. *Neuropsychological Rehabilitation*, **15**, 569–587.

McDowell, S., Whyte, J., & D'Esposito, M. (1997). Working memory impairments in traumatic brain injury: evidence from a dual-task paradigm. *Neuropsychologia*, **35**, 1341–1353.

McDowell, S., Whyte, J., & D'Esposito, M. (1998). Differential effect of a dopaminergic agonist on prefrontal function in traumatic brain injury patients. *Brain*, **121**, 1155–1164.

McMillan, T., Robertson, I. H., Brock, D., & Chorlton, L. (2002). Brief mindfulness training for attentional problems after traumatic brain injury: a randomised control treatment trial. *Neuropsychological Rehabilitation*, **12**, 117–125.

Mesulam, M.-M. (1985). *Principles of Behavioral Neurology*. Philadelphia, PA: F. A. Davis.

Meythaler, J. M., Brunner, R. C., Johnson, A., & Novack, T. A. (2002). Amantadine to improve neurorecovery in traumatic brain injury-associated diffuse axonal injury: a pilot double-blind randomized trial. *Journal of Head Trauma Rehabilitation*, **17**, 300–313.

Mooney, G., & Speed, J. (2001). The association between mild traumatic brain injury and psychiatric conditions. *Brain Injury*, **15**, 865–877.

Mottaghy, F. M., Willmes, K., Horwitz, B. *et al.* (2006). Systems level modeling of a neuronal network subserving intrinsic alertness. *Neuroimage*, **29**, 225–233.

Niemann, H., Ruff, R. M., & Baser, C. A. (1990). Computer-assisted attention retraining in head-injured individuals: a controlled efficacy study of an outpatient program. *Journal of Consulting and Clinical Psychology*, **58**, 811–817.

Norman, D. A., & Shallice, T. (1980). Attention to action: willed and automatic control of behaviour.

Center for Human Information Processing Technical Report No. 99.

Novack, T. A., Caldwell, S. G., Duke, L. W., Bergquist, T. F., & Gage, R. J. (1996). Focused versus unstructured intervention for attention deficits after traumatic brain injury. *Journal of Head Trauma Rehabilitation*, **11**, 52–60.

Olver, J. H., Ponsford, J. L., & Curran, C. A. (1996). Outcome following traumatic brain injury: a comparison between 2 and 5 years after injury. *Brain Injury*, **10**, 841–848.

Palmese, C. A., & Raskin, S. A. (2000). The rehabilitation of attention in individuals with mild traumatic brain injury, using the APT-II programme. *Brain Injury*, **14**, 535–548.

Parasuraman, R., Mutter, S. A., & Molloy, R. (1991). Sustained attention following mild closed-head injury. *Journal of Clinical and Experimental Neuropsychology*, **13**, 789–811.

Park, N. W., & Ingles, J. L. (2001). Effectiveness of attention rehabilitation after an acquired brain injury: a meta-analysis. *Neuropsychology*, **15**, 199–210.

Park, N. W., Moscovitch, M., & Robertson, I. H. (1999a). Divided attention impairments after traumatic brain injury. *Neuropsychologia*, **37**, 1119–1133.

Park, N. W., Proulx, G.-B., & Towers, W. M. (1999b). Evaluation of the Attention Process training programme. *Neuropsychological Rehabilitation*, **9**, 135–154.

Parker, R. S. (1996). The spectrum of emotional distress and personality changes after minor head injury incurred in a motor vehicle accident. *Brain Injury*, **10**, 287–302.

Penkman, L., & Mateer, C. A. (2004). The specificity of attention retraining in traumatic brain injury. *Journal of Cognitive Rehabilitation, Spring*, 13–26.

Plenger, P. M., Dixon, C. E., Castillo, R. M. *et al.* (1996). Subacute methylphenidate treatment for moderate to moderately severe traumatic brain injury: a preliminary double-blind placebo-controlled study. *Archives of Physical Medicine and Rehabilitation*, **77**, 536–540.

Ponsford, J. (2005). Rehabilitation interventions after mild head injury. *Current Opinion in Neurology*, **18**, 692–697.

Ponsford, J. L., & Kinsella, G. (1988). Evaluation of a remedial programme for attentional deficits following closed head injury. *Journal of Clinical and Experimental Neuropsychology*, **10**, 693–708.

Ponsford, J. L., & Kinsella, G. (1991). The use of a rating scale of attentional behaviour. *Neuropsychological Rehabilitation*, **1**, 241–257.

Ponsford, J. L., & Kinsella, G. (1992). Attentional deficits following closed-head injury. *Journal of Clinical and Experimental Neuropsychology*, **14**, 822–838.

Ponsford, J. L., Olver, J. H., & Curran, C. (1995a). A profile of outcome: two years after traumatic brain injury. *Brain Injury*, **9**, 1–10.

Ponsford, J. L., Sloan, S., & Snow, P. (1995b). *Traumatic Brain Injury: Rehabilitation for Everyday Living.* London, UK: Lawrence Erlbaum.

Ponsford, J., Willmott, C., Rothwell, A. *et al.* (2000). Factors influencing outcome following mild traumatic brain injury in adults. *Journal of the International Neuropsychological Society*, **6**, 568–579.

Ponsford, J., Draper, K., & Schanberger, M. (in press). Predictors of functional outcome on the GOSE 10 years following traumatic brain injury. *Journal of the International Neuropsychological Society.*

Posner, M. I., & Rothbart, M. K. (1992). Attentional mechanisms and conscious experience. In A. D. Milner & M. D. Rugg (Eds.), *The Neuropsychology of Consciousness* (pp. 91–112). London: Academic Press.

Povlishock, J. T., & Katz, D. I. (2005). Update of neuropathology and neurological recovery after traumatic brain injury. *Journal of Head Trauma Rehabilitation*, **20**, 76–94.

Rizzo, P., Amabile, G., Caporali, M. *et al.* (1978). A CNV study in a group of patients with traumatic head injuries. *Electroencephalography and Clinical Neurophysiology*, **45**, 281–285.

Robertson, I. H., Ward, T., Ridgeway, V., & Nimmo-Smith, I. (1994). *The Test of Everyday Attention.* Cambridge, UK: MRC Applied Psychology Unit.

Robertson, I. H., Tegner, R., Tham, K., Lo, A., & Nimmo-Smith, I. (1995). Sustained attention training for unilateral neglect: theoretical and rehabilitation implications. *Journal of Clinical and Experimental Neuropsychology*, **17**, 416–430.

Robertson, I. H., Manly, T., Andrade, J., Baddeley, B. T., & Yiend, J. (1997a). 'Oops!': Performance correlates of everyday attentional failures in traumatic brain injured and normal subjects. *Neuropsychologia*, **35**, 747–758.

Robertson, I. H., Manly, T., Beschin, N. *et al.* (1997b). Auditory sustained attention is a marker of unilateral spatial neglect. *Neuropsychologia*, **35**, 1527–1532.

Robertson, I. H., Mattingley, J. M., Rorden, C., & Driver, J. (1998). Phasic alerting of neglect patients overcomes their spatial deficit in visual awareness. *Nature*, **395**, 169–172.

Rose, F. D., Brooks, B. M., & Rizzo, A. A. (2005). Virtual reality in brain damage rehabilitation: review. *CyberPsychology and Behavior*, **8**, 241–262.

Rose, J. M. (2005). Continuum of care model for managing mild traumatic brain injury in a workers' compensation context: a description of the model and its development. *Brain Injury*, **19**, 29–39.

Ruff, R. (2005). Two decades of advances in understanding of mild traumatic brain injury. *Journal of Head Trauma Rehabilitation*, **20**, 5–18.

Ruff, R., Mahaffey, R., Engel, J. *et al.* (1994). Efficacy study of THINKable in the attention and memory retraining of traumatically head-injured patients. *Brain Injury*, **8**, 3–14.

Rugg, M. D., Cowan, C. P., Nagy, M. E. *et al.* (1989). CNV abnormalities following closed head injury. *Brain Injury*, **112**, 489–506.

Schmitter-Edgecombe, M., & Beglinger, L. (2001). Acquisition of skilled visual search performance following severe closed-head injury. *Journal of the International Neuropsychological Society*, **7**, 615–630.

Schmitter-Edgecombe, M., & Kibby, M. K. (1998). Visual selective attention after severe closed head injury. *Journal of the International Neuropsychological Society*, **4**, 144–159.

Schneider, W., & Fisk, A. D. (1982). Degree of consistent training: improvements in search performance and automatic process development. *Perception and Psychophysics*, **31**, 160–168.

Segalowitz, S. J., Unsal, A., & Dywan, J. (1992). CNV evidence for the distinctiveness of frontal and posterior neural processes in a traumatic brain-injured population. *Journal of Clinical and Experimental Neuropsychology*, **14**, 545–565.

Shallice, T., & Burgess, P. W. (1991). Deficits in strategy application following frontal lobe damage in man. *Brain*, **114**, 727–741.

Shiffrin, R. M., & Schneider, W. (1977). Controlled and automatic human information processing: II. Perceptual learning, automatic attending and a general theory. *Psychological Review*, **84**, 127–190.

Sloan, S., & Ponsford, J. L. (1995). Managing cognitive problems. In J. L. Ponsford, S. Sloan & P. Snow (Eds.), *Traumatic Brain Injury: Rehabilitation for Everyday Adaptive Living*. London, UK: Lawrence Erlbaum.

Sohlberg, M. M., & Mateer, C. A. (1987). Effectiveness of an attention-training program. *Journal of Clinical and Experimental Neuropsychology*, **9**, 117–130.

Sohlberg, M. M., McLaughlin, K. A., Pavese, A., Heidrich, A., & Posner, M. I. (2000). Evaluation of attention process training and brain injury education in persons with acquired brain injury. *Journal of Clinical and Experimental Neuropsychology*, **22**, 656–676.

Speech, T. J., Rao, S. M., Osmon, D. C., & Sperry, L. T. (1993). A double-blind controlled study of methylphenidate treatment in closed head injury. *Brain Injury*, **7**, 333–338.

Spikman, J. M., van Zomeren, A. H., & Deelman, B. G. (1996). Deficits of attention after closed-head injury:

Slowness only? *Journal of Clinical and Experimental Neuropsychology*, **18**, 755–767.

Spikman, J. M., Deelman, B. G., & van Zomeren, A. H. (2000). Executive functioning, attention and frontal lesions in patients with chronic CHI. *Journal of Clinical and Experimental Neuropsychology*, **22**, 325–338.

Stablum, F., Leonardi, G., Mazzoldi, M., Umiltà, C., & Morra, S. (1994). Attention and control deficits following closed head injury. *Cortex*, **30**, 603–618.

Stablum, F., Umiltà, C., Mogentale, C., Carlan, M., & Guerrini, C. (2000). Rehabilitation of executive deficits in closed head injury and anterior communicating artery aneurysm patients. *Psychological Research*, **63**, 265–278.

Sturm, W., & Willmes, K. (1991). Efficacy of a reaction training on various attentional and cognitive functions in stroke patients. *Neuropsychological Rehabilitation*, **1**, 259–280.

Sturm, W., & Willmes, K. (2001). On the functional neuroanatomy of intrinsic and phasic alertness. *Neuroimage*, **14**, S76–S84.

Sturm, W., Willmes, K., Orgass, B., & Hartje, W. (1997). Do specific attention deficits need specific training. *Neuropsychological Rehabilitation*, **7**, 81–103.

Stuss, D. T., & Benson, D. F. (1986). *The Frontal Lobes*. New York, NY: Raven Press.

Stuss, D. T., Stethem, L. L., Hugenholtz, H. *et al.* (1989). Reaction time after head injury: fatigue, divided and focused attention, and consistency of performance. *Journal of Neurology, Neurosurgery, and Psychiatry*, **52**, 742–748.

Stuss, D. T., Pogue, J., Buckle, L., & Bondar, J. (1994). Characterization of stability of performance in patients with traumatic brain injury: variability and consistency on reaction time tests. *Neuropsychology*, **8**, 316–324.

Tate, R. L., & Broe, G. A. (1999). Psychosocial adjustment after traumatic brain injury: what are the important variables? *Psychological Medicine*, **29**, 713–725.

Thimm, M., Fink, G. R., Küst, J., Karbe, H., & Sturm, W. (2006). Impact of alertness training on spatial neglect: a behavioural and fMRI study. *Neuropsychologia*, **44**, 1230–1246.

Tiersky, L. A., Anselmi, V., Johnston, M. V. *et al.* (2005). A trial of neuropsychologic rehabilitation in mild-spectrum traumatic brain injury. *Archives of Physical Medicine and Rehabilitation*, **86**, 1565–1574.

van Zomeren, A. H., & Brouwer, W. H. (1987). Head injury and concepts of attention. In H. S. Levin, J. Grafman, & H. M. Eisenberg (Eds.), *Neurobehavioral Recovery from Head Injury* (pp. 398–415). New York, NY: Oxford University Press.

van Zomeren, A. H., & Brouwer, W. H. (1994). *Clinical Neuropsychology of Attention*. New York, NY: Oxford University Press.

van Zomeren, A. H., & van den Burg, W. (1985). Residual complaints of patients two years after severe head injury. *Journal of Neurology, Neurosurgery, and Psychiatry*, **48**, 21–28.

Veltman, J. C., Brouwer, W. H., van Zomeren, A. H., & van Wolffelaar, P. C. (1996). Central executive aspects of attention in subacute severe and very severe closed head injury patients: planning, inhibition, flexibility, and divided attention. *Neuropsychology*, **10**, 357–367.

Vilkki, J. (1992). Cognitive flexibility and mental programming after closed head injuries and anterior or posterior cerebral excisions. *Neuropsychologia*, **30**, 807–814.

Vilkki, J., Virtanen, S., Surma-Aho, O., & Servo, A. (1996). Dual task performance after focal cerebral lesions and closed head injuries. *Neuropsychologia*, **34**, 1051–1056.

Webster, J. S., & Scott, R. R. (1983). The effects of self-instructional training on attentional deficits following head injury. *Clinical Neuropsychology*, **5**, 69–74.

Whyte, J. (2003). Pharmacological treatment of attention deficits after traumatic brain injury: results of a randomized placebo trial of methylphenidate. *26th Annual Brain Impairment Conference*. Sydney, Australia.

Whyte, J., Polansky, M., Fleming, M., Coslett, H. B., & Cavallucci, C. (1995). Sustained arousal and attention after traumatic brain injury. *Neuropsychologia*, **33**, 797–813.

Whyte, J., Polansky, M., Cavallucci, C. *et al.* (1996). Inattentive behavior after traumatic brain injury. *Journal of the International Neuropsychological Society*, **2**, 274–281.

Whyte, J., Fleming, M., Polansky, M., Cavallucci, C., & Coslett, H. B. (1997a). Phasic arousal in response to auditory warnings after traumatic brain injury. *Neuropsychologia*, **35**, 313–324.

Whyte, J., Hart, T., Schuster, K. *et al.* (1997b). Effects of methylphenidate on attentional function after traumatic brain injury: a randomized, placebo-controlled trial. *American Journal of Physical Medicine and Rehabilitation*, **76**, 440–450.

Whyte, J., Fleming, M., Polansky, M., Cavallucci, C., & Coslett, H. B. (1998). The effects of visual distraction following traumatic brain injury. *Journal of the International Neuropsychological Society*, **4**, 127–136.

Whyte, J., Vaccaro, M., Grieb-Neff, P., & Hart, T. (2002). Psychostimulant use in the rehabilitation of individuals with traumatic brain injury. *Journal of Head Trauma Rehabilitation*, **17**, 284–299.

Wilson, C., & Robertson, I. H. (1992). A home-based intervention for attentional slips during reading following head injury: a single case study. *Neuropsychological Rehabilitation*, **2**, 193–205.

Withaar, F. K. (2000). Divided attention and driving: the effects of aging and brain injury. Unpublished Doctoral Dissertation, Riiksuniversiteit Groningen.

Wood, R. L. (2004). Understanding the "miserable minority": a diasthesis-stress paradigm for post-concussional syndrome. *Brain Injury*, **18**, 1135–1153.

Wood, R. L., & Fussey, I. (1987). Computer-based cognitive retraining: a controlled study. *International Disability Studies*, **9**, 149–153.

Ziino, C., & Ponsford, J. (2006a). Vigilance and fatigue following traumatic brain injury. *Journal of the International Neuropsychological Society*, **12**, 100–110.

Ziino, C., & Ponsford, J. (2006b). Selective attention deficits and subjective fatigue following traumatic brain injury. *Neuropsychology*, **20**, 383–390.

Zoccolotti, P., Matano, A., Deloche, G. *et al.* (2000). Patterns of attentional impairment following closed head injury: A collaborative European study. *Cortex*, **36**, 93–107.

30

Memory rehabilitation for people with brain injury

Barbara A. Wilson and Narinder Kapur

Introduction

- Handicaps in everyday memory functioning cross neurological boundaries and represent a major burden on the health of any nation.
- Restoration of memory functioning to pre-injury levels is unlikely, but much can be done to enable memory-impaired people and their families and carers to come to terms with and compensate for everyday problems.
- Environmental modifications can be of considerable help in reducing everyday memory difficulties.
- New technology has an increasingly important part to play in helping memory-impaired people to compensate for their problems.
- Structured teaching is often required to help memory-impaired individuals to use memory aids.
- Internal strategies such as mnemonics and rehearsal techniques can be employed to teach new information although most memory-impaired people will not use these spontaneously.
- Errorless learning is usually more effective than trial-and-error learning for those with memory difficulties.
- In addition to memory problems, many brain-injured people will have other cognitive and emotional problems which will need to be addressed.
- Anxiety, depression and other emotional difficulties should be treated together with the memory problems.

Since the first edition of this book appeared in 1999, a number of developments have occurred in brain-injury rehabilitation particularly in the field of cognitive rehabilitation. Technological advances to help people compensate for their difficulties have moved forward at a considerable pace and continue to do so (Kapur *et al.*, 2004). It is now well recognized that we need to address the emotional consequences of cognitive impairment in rehabilitation (Williams & Evans, 2003) and there is a widespread acceptance that rehabilitation is a partnership between patients, families and professional staff so that the aims and goals of rehabilitation are negotiated between these parties rather than dictated by professionals (Wilson, 2003). Thus, the picture is brighter than it was in 1999 when much was written about theoretical aspects of memory but much less about tangible help for those with everyday memory deficits. Several practical books have appeared in the last decade including *Coping with Memory Problems: A Practical Guide for People with Memory Impairments, Relatives, Friends and Carers* (Clare & Wilson, 1997); *Managing your Memory* (Kapur, 2001); and *Compensating for Memory Deficits: Using a Systematic Approach* (Kime, 2006). Other books have included practical topics set in a wider context. The most notable of these are *The Essential Handbook of Memory Disorders for Clinicians* (Baddeley *et al.*, 2004) and *Case Studies in Neuropsychological Rehabilitation* (Wilson, 1999).

This chapter will describe the main approaches to the rehabilitation of memory disorders, discuss

Cognitive Neurorehabilitation, Second Edition: Evidence and Application, ed. Donald T. Stuss, Gordon Winocur and Ian H. Robertson. Published by Cambridge University Press. © Cambridge University Press 2008.

evidence supporting the efficacy of these approaches, and provide guidelines for implementing rehabilitation for people with memory disorders. We consider the following: (1) environmental adaptations, (2) new learning, (3) emerging technologies including virtual reality, (4) treatment of semantic memory disorders, (5) emotional aspects of memory impairment and (6) memory therapy in practice. Although it will not be possible to provide exhaustive coverage, we nevertheless hope to provide the reader with an understanding of active topics in the field of memory rehabilitation. We have not included a separate section on external memory aids as there is comprehensive coverage of this elsewhere (Kapur *et al.*, 2004; Sohlberg, 2005).

The rehabilitation of patients with memory impairment following acquired brain injury/illness is similar to, and also different from, memory rehabilitation that is focused on elderly populations such as those described by Glisky and Glisky (see Chapter 31 in this volume). In the case of patients who are in the early stages of Alzheimer's disease, or who have a diagnosis of "mild cognitive impairment," there may be some overlap in the types of memory rehabilitation interventions used with these individuals and those individuals with acquired brain injury, since both samples may have mild–moderate memory impairment in the context of relatively preserved general cognitive functioning. In most other instances, however, memory rehabilitation for the two populations may differ to a significant degree – elderly patients are less likely to use electronic compensatory devices, they are less likely to adopt cognitive strategies such as complex mnemonics and they are more likely to respond to environmental cues or reminders. Issues such as "cognitive reserve" may perhaps be more relevant to elderly patients, since there will usually have been greater opportunities for knowledge and experience to have been acquired and formed as a part of such reserve. Memory rehabilitation interventions will of necessity be somewhat time-limited in patients with dementia, whereas those individuals with acquired brain injury may often remain stable in their needs,

once they have passed the early stages of recovery from a brain insult.

Environmental adaptations

- Environmental memory aids may be classified into three types – proximal environmental memory aids, distal environmental memory aids and object-integrated memory aids.
- Environmental memory aids may help memory-impaired individuals in a variety of ways, such as remembering to do things, and remembering where items are located.
- Environmental memory aids may be passive (e.g., labels on cupboards) or active (e.g., alarms that are built into objects in the environment).
- Carers can also be considered as a key environmental memory aid.

Introduction

Use of the term "environment" in public discussions has enjoyed a revival in recent years, with people and governments professing to be more aware of the importance of environmental factors in determining the quality of life, and even our survival. A recent textbook on environmental psychology (Bell *et al.*, 2001, p. 506) defines "environment" as – "one's surroundings; the word is frequently used to refer to a specific part of one's surroundings, as in social environment (referring to the people and groups among whom one lives), physical environment (all of the nonanimal elements of one's surroundings, such as cities, wilderness, or farmland), natural (nonhuman) environment, or built environment (referring specifically to that part of the environment built by humans)". Theoretically, "environment" could refer to the involvement of any of the five senses, but in most instances reference is made to the visual environment, as human beings are essentially visual creatures, with visual processing of one form or another taking over by far the largest combined area of the human brain compared to the other four senses.

Environmental memory aids

Features of our environment shape our behavior, both consciously and unconsciously. We respond (often automatically) to cues in our environment for many of our daily activities. Contextual support from environmental cues may be more critical for those with failing memory (Craik & Jennings, 1992). It makes sense to consider how our environment may be better designed and organized to enhance memory functioning. As in the case of visuospatial functions, where a distinction has been made between personal, peripersonal and extrapersonal space (Robertson & Halligan, 1999), it may be useful to divide environmental memory aids into three categories – proximal environmental memory aids, distal environmental memory aids and object-integrated memory aids. By *proximal environmental memory aids*, we include features such as the design and contents of a room. We would also briefly refer to items, such as clocks, calendars and white-boards, that are usually fixed to parts of a room and which exert their value in part by virtue of their location within the room. By *distal environmental memory aids*, we mean settings such as the layout of a building, shopping centers, the design of streets and towns, and the design of transportation networks. Within *object-integrated memory aids*, we would include devices such as reminder-alarms in kitchen equipment or in automobiles that help prevent memory lapses. Since objects can be animate or inanimate, it may be appropriate to include people within this type of memory aid.

Proximal environmental memory aids

A proximal environment, well-structured and organized, is less likely to result in memory lapses such as forgetting where something has been put (Fulton & Hatch, 1991). As a basic principle, the items to be stored for later retrieval should be categorized, and separate shelves or storage units allocated to each category. Categories should be meaningful to the individual in question, and may have a number of subcategories, possibly reflected in the structure of the storage unit. Distinctive storage units should differ in features such as size, shape, color and/or spatial position. They should be clearly labeled, and containers within the storage units should also be labeled. Writing on labels should be in large print (with lower-case, non-serif font usually easiest to read at a distance). While the print may be of different colors to match any other color-coding system in place, black-against-white is often best for elderly or neurologically disabled people. If the storage units have to be retrieved according to sequence, then some form of alpha-numeric labeling will be of value. The prominence of a storage unit in a room will depend on how frequently the stored items are used, how important they are, and how often they tend to be forgotten. If possible, there should be some relationship between the contents and the visual features of the unit, e.g., a brown container for storing coffee, a white one for storing sugar, etc. Transparent storage boxes are preferable, as the person can see at a glance what is inside and whether the contents need replenishing.

Orientation for time, place and current events will be helped by the presence of items such as clocks that display the day of the week/month/year, orientation boards, large windows at ground level to allow individuals to see the trees and therefore cues to indicate the time of year, etc. Regularity of routine activities may help improve knowledge such as orientation for time, e.g., if the tea trolley always comes at 11 am, this may provide an anchor point for "confused" patients who are disoriented for time. White-boards can act as a "knowledge board" to display important information, such as emergency telephone numbers. Moffat (1989) described the display of a simple flow chart of likely places to search to help a man who frequently lost items around the home.

Providing familiar items, such as photographs or mementos of people, holidays/trips, etc. and having in place natural surroundings that include plants, flowers, animals, birds, etc. may help to cue remote memories and may indirectly help to reduce disruptive behaviors (Bell *et al.*, 2001, pp. 426–429).

Items such as calendars and white-boards may not only act as knowledge storage/retrieval aids, but also as prospective memory aids, reminding individuals to do certain things at certain times. White-boards need to be kept in a prominent place, so that they can readily grab the attention of the individual with memory lapses. Magnetic white-boards allow for the possibility of magnetic colored markers to denote specific types of events/information. White-boards may form the focus of a family "memory centre"/"message centre."

Changes to a work-place or home environment can be engineered to minimize prospective memory lapses. Examples include leaving something beside the front door, attaching a Post-it note to a mirror in the hallway, and keeping in a visible place an empty carton of something that needs to be replaced. Simple changes to the design of an environment may act as a catalyst for such memory aids, e.g., items one has to take when leaving home or leaving the office could be located on an appropriate shelf near the exit itself. The shelf should be clearly labeled and within the horizontal and vertical limits of the person's visual field. Putting together two items may act as a visual reminder to carry out a particular action, e.g., a pill-bottle next to a toothbrush may remind a patient to take his medicine before cleaning his teeth.

Distal environmental memory aids

As mentioned above, by distal environmental memory aids we mean settings such as the layout of a building, shopping centers, the design of streets and towns, and the design of transportation networks. Most distal environmental memory aids are intended to help people retrieve knowledge, simple rules, etc. rather than act to improve prospective memory functioning. Many distal memory aids may be determined by governments/local authorities and thus be beyond intervention by rehabilitation professionals. It may be useful for the therapist to carry out a "site visit" to a patient's home to obtain a first-hand perspective of environmental features and how best to modify the environment so as to enhance everyday memory functioning. Alternatively, patients may bring to the clinic photographs of the layout of relevant parts of their home, perhaps using cameras on their mobile phones, to enable the clinician to obtain a better understanding of how the home environment may best be modified to help improve everyday memory functioning.

Dogu & Erkip (2000) point to some design features to be kept in mind if spatial orientation in a shopping complex is to be maximized. For similar observations relating to more general navigational activities, such as route finding, see Canter (1996), and for those relating to the specific needs of patients with dementia, see Passini et al. (1998, 2000), Warner (2000) and Zeisel (2006).

The carefully planned use of signs can be of benefit as preventative measures, e.g., warning signs near stairs in homes for elderly people, road traffic warning signs, etc. Other forms of visual cues may also help, such as cues on steps to alert someone who is visually impaired. In residential homes or hospitals for memory-impaired people, wall or floor markers indicating the direction to somewhere, together with clearly marked rooms (color coded, icons, written labels, etc.), may help residents to find their way about (cf. Elmstahl et al., 1997; Olsen et al., 1999). Simple measures, such as having the name and photograph of the resident on his/her door, may help in locating the room, and may also help to promote identity/self-esteem (Gross et al., 2004). The interior design of a residential home should be distinctive rather than monotonous, with landmarks, as these may help way-finding among residents. Alarms fitted to doors that activate when the door is opened help provide information to care workers on patients who are likely to wander out of the premises. Use of elevators can pose particular problems for some patients with dementia – either they should be out of bounds, or some residents may need to be accompanied when using them. If elevators have to be used, the control panel needs to be distinctive, easy to understand and easy to use. Since residential homes vary in their design, significant changes to the environment intended to support everyday memory functioning should be evidence-based, and include information from staff and observations of residents' way-finding behaviors.

Object-integrated memory aids

Simple labels help people know what to do in certain settings. As Norman (1988) has pointed out, we are all aware of doors where there is no indication whether to PULL or to PUSH. In-built alarms or cut-off devices, as are found in some domestic appliances, help prevent memory lapses such as forgetting to carry out a certain activity. Where a device needs to be turned on and off at certain times, and does not have an inbuilt timer, timer-plugs are readily available in most DIY stores. Voice-based messages to accompany or replace the actual alarm signal are sometimes helpful in order to tell the individual what the alarm means when it is activated. If, as is often the case, switches of a similar design are in close proximity, or are particularly important to locate, it may be useful to attach a distinctive tactile cue, such as a velcro pad on to one of the switches. Similar application may arise in other settings, such as finding switches in a room in the dark.

While reminders that are built into objects may form useful cues for those with memory lapses, reminders that emanate from carers are probably the most common form of cue that patients tend to rely on, and symptoms such as repetitive questioning or locating lost items may be particularly amenable to support from those who are looking after a memory-impaired individual.

Summary

Environmental memory aids are valuable for a number of reasons, not least of all that many of them require little in the way of active concentration or memory on the part of the user for them to be noticed and effectively used. Keeping environments simple and well-organized, with reminder cues in prominent places, should form a key feature of any compensatory memory system. It is important to use a range of reminder cues, including those that may be passive, such as labels on cupboards, and those that are active, such as inbuilt devices which give alarm signals or people who give verbal reminders. It is therefore critical that the clinician has a clear picture of the patient's home environment (and, if relevant, work environment), and make suggested modifications as appropriate.

New learning

- The main strategies for enhancing new learning are expanded rehearsal (also known as spaced retrieval), mnemonics and errorless learning.
- Expanded rehearsal/spaced retrieval involves the gradual increase of the retention interval once the information to be learned has been presented.
- Mnemonics are systems to help people organize, store and retrieve new information more efficiently.
- Guidelines are provided for the use of mnemonics with memory-impaired people.
- Errorless learning is a teaching technique whereby errors are avoided or reduced during the learning process.
- In order to benefit from our mistakes we need to remember them; as memory-impaired people tend to forget their mistakes, these should be avoided as far as possible during learning.

Introduction

Although external aids and environmental adaptations can be of great assistance to memory-impaired people, it is unlikely that they will offer sufficient support for all the demands of daily living. Memory-impaired people need to learn new information on certain occasions. For example, although people's names can be written down in a notebook, reference to the notebook would not help in a normal social setting when people need to be greeted by name. Referring to a notebook in such a situation would seriously affect natural communication and also be

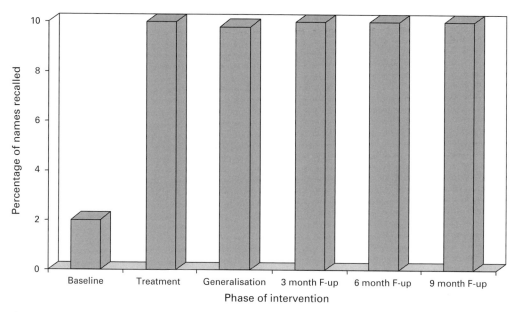

Figure 30.1. Name recall: VJ.

embarrassing. While it is true that learning names is particularly difficult for people with organic memory impairment, there are a number of studies showing that it is possible to teach names to amnesic people using strategies that enhance learning. Wilson (1987) evaluated the strategy of visual imagery to teach names and demonstrated that it is virtually always superior to rote repetition. Thoene & Glisky (1995) also found visual imagery superior to other methods for teaching people's names to amnesic subjects. Clare *et al.* (1999) were able to teach a 74-year-old man (VJ) in the early stages of Alzheimer's disease, the names of his colleagues at a social club. They used a combination of strategies, which included finding a distinctive feature of the face, backward chaining and expanding rehearsal. For example, one of the subject's colleagues was named Sylvia and this name was learned using a combination of all three methods described above. The distinctive feature selected was her silvery hair, which the subject was asked to associate with the name Sylvia. At the same time, backward chaining was employed so that the subject was given written versions of his colleague's name with progressively more letters omitted, as in the following

example: SYLVIA, SYLVI_, SYLV_, and so on. The patient completed the missing letters and eventually learned the name without any cues. These two strategies were combined with expanding rehearsal otherwise known as spaced retrieval, in which the information to be remembered is first presented, then tested immediately, tested again after a very brief delay, tested again after a slightly longer delay and so on. This is a form of distributed practice and is a fairly powerful learning strategy in memory rehabilitation (Baddeley & Longman, 1978). The method of expanding rehearsal owes much to the work of Landauer & Bjork (1978). Clare *et al.*'s patient learned the names of his colleagues using photographs in his memory therapy sessions, and demonstrated generalization by greeting his colleagues by name at a social club. The results can be seen in Figure 30.1.

The use of mnemonics in memory rehabilitation

Mnemonics are systems that enable people to organize, store and retrieve information more efficiently. Some people use the term mnemonics to refer to anything that helps people remember, including external aids. In memory rehabilitation, however, the term is used for methods involving the mental manipulation of material. For example, in order to remember how many days there are in each month, most people use a system of mnemonics. In the UK and much of the USA, people recite a rhyme: "Thirty days hath September . . ." In other parts of the world, people use their knuckles to refer to "long" months and the dips between the knuckles to refer to the "short" months. Mnemonics are often employed to learn the names of cranial nerves, notes of music, colors of the rainbow and other ordered material. (See Wilson (1987) and Moffat (1989) for further discussion of mnemonics in memory rehabilitation, and West (1995) for the use of these strategies in people with age-related memory impairment.)

The following suggestions are offered to those wishing to employ mnemonics with memory-impaired people.

(1) Mnemonics are sometimes useful for teaching new information. However, most brain-injured people will not use them spontaneously.
(2) Dual coding, i.e., using verbal and pictorial encoding strategies, will probably result in more efficient learning than the use of one method alone.
(3) Information or the component skills of a new task should be taught one step at a time.
(4) If visual imagery is employed, i.e., transforming a name or word to be learned into a picture (such as remembering Barbara as a barber), it is better for the memory-impaired person to see a drawing of the image on paper or card rather than to rely on a mental image.
(5) Information to be learned should be realistic and relevant to the everyday needs of patients or clients. Thus, it is better to teach people things they really need to know rather than material from a workbook that might not be relevant to their real lives.
(6) Individual styles, needs and preferences should be recognized. Not everyone will benefit from the same strategy.

(7) Generalization issues need to be addressed. If a patient learns to use a notebook in the psychology department or ward setting, this does not necessarily mean the book will be used when they are discharged to the community unless such usage is specifically taught.
(8) Although some memory-impaired people can use mnemonics in new situations, most find it difficult to use them spontaneously. In fact, the real value of mnemonics is that they are useful for *teaching* memory-impaired people new information, and they almost invariably lead to faster learning than rote rehearsal.

Errorless learning

One series of potentially important studies in recent years has involved errorless learning. This is a method for teaching new skills to people with learning difficulties (Jones & Eayrs, 1992; Sidman & Stoddard, 1967), but until quite recently its principles had not been applied to any great extent to neurologically impaired adults. As the name implies, errorless learning involves learning without errors or mistakes. Most of us can learn or benefit from our errors because we can remember and thus avoid them in our future efforts to learn. However, people with impaired episodic memory are more likely to forget their mistakes, so fail to correct them. Furthermore, the very fact of engaging in a behavior may strengthen or reinforce it even though that behavior is errorful. Consequently, for someone with a severe memory impairment, it makes sense to ensure that any behavior that is going to be reinforced is correct rather than incorrect.

Work on errorless learning in memory-impaired adults has been influenced by studies of implicit learning from the field of cognitive neuropsychology as well as by earlier studies from the field of learning disability. There have been numerous studies showing that amnesic subjects can learn some things normally or almost normally, even though they may have no conscious recollection of learning anything at all (Brooks & Baddeley, 1976; Glisky & Schacter, 1987; Graf & Schacter, 1985). Glisky &

Schacter tried to use the implicit learning abilities of amnesic subjects to teach them computer technology, and although some success was achieved this was at considerable expense of time and effort. These attempts, and others that try to build on the relatively intact skills of memory-impaired people, have, on the whole, been disappointing. One reason for failures and anomalies could be that implicit learning is poor at eliminating errors. Error elimination is a function of explicit not implicit memory and consequently, when subjects are forced to rely upon implicit memory (as amnesic subjects are), the subsequent trial-and-error learning becomes a slow and laborious procedure.

In 1994, Baddeley and Wilson published the first study demonstrating that amnesic subjects learn better when they are prevented from making mistakes during the learning process. The conclusions of this study were (1) errorless learning appears to be superior to trial-and-error learning; (2) the effect is greater for amnesic subjects than it is for controls; and (3) amnesic subjects show less forgetting with errorless learning. Since then, several studies have been conducted with memory-impaired patients, comparing errorful and errorless learning for teaching practical, everyday information (Squires et al., 1996; Wilson et al., 1994, Wilson & Evans, 1996). The latter paper also discusses some of the potential problems connected with errorless learning.

Results from recent work (Evans et al., 2000) involving ten errorless learning experiments suggest that tasks and situations that depend upon implicit memory (such as stem completion or retrieving a name from a first letter cue) are more likely to benefit from errorless learning methods than tasks requiring explicit recall of new situations. Nevertheless, Wilson et al. (1994) demonstrated new explicit learning in a memory-impaired, head-injured patient. Clare et al. (1999), mentioned above, also demonstrated explicit learning in a man with Alzheimer's disease. The Evans et al. (2000) studies found that the more severely amnesic patients benefited to a greater extent from errorless learning methods than did those who were less severely impaired, although this may only apply when the interval between learning and recall is relatively short, i.e. within an hour or so, which was the length of the individual experimental session. How long the errorless learning advantage is maintained has not yet been tested. One of the implications from this finding is that errorless learning should be combined with expanding rehearsal to enhance its effectiveness. The studies of Clare et al. (1999, 2000, 2001) support this view.

A recent paper by Page et al. (2006) claims that preserved implicit memory in the absence of explicit memory is sufficient for errorless memory to occur. Page et al. describe two experiments with patients with severe and moderate memory deficits. In addition to errorful and errorless learning for stem completion tasks, patients were given recognition and source memory tasks. Both those with severe and moderate deficits were good at the recognition tasks provided their own errors were not included. When asked to distinguish between their own mistakes and genuine target words they were unable to do this. Source memory was absent for those with severe deficits and poor for those with moderate deficits. Thus memory-impaired people showed an advantage of errorless over errorful learning that did not depend on whether they were asked for implicit or explicit recall; they could not distinguish their own errors from genuine targets and they could not tell from which source the information had been obtained. All this suggests that implicit memory can explain why people with no or very little explicit recall can learn under certain conditions such as errorless learning.

Summary

Although external aids and environmental adaptations are very important in reducing everyday problems, there are times when memory-impaired people need to learn new information. Expanded rehearsal/spaced retrieval can be a fairly powerful learning strategy. Mnemonics also enable people to organise, store and retrieve information more efficiently and thus can enhance learning. As memory-impaired people often find it difficult to employ mnemonics spontaneously, therapists, teachers or relatives may have to work together with the person to ensure that learning occurs. A series of studies have demonstrated the value of errorless learning when teaching new skills or information to those with everyday memory problems. If we are unable to remember our mistakes we cannot benefit from them and the fact of making an incorrect response may strengthen the erroneous response. For this reason, the reduction or elimination of errors during learning is recommended for people with poor episodic memory.

Emerging technologies

- Emerging technologies hold considerable promise for producing devices that may be of benefit as compensatory memory aids.
- Mobile phone technology provides users with an increasing number of facilities that may help everyday memory functioning.
- Paging systems have already been shown to be of benefit to memory-impaired patients.
- Advanced brain imaging and virtual reality technologies hold out the promise of impacting positively on memory rehabilitation.

Introduction

Wilson & Evans (2000) and Cheek *et al.* (2005) noted the emergence of "smart houses," where appliances are centrally controlled and include reminder functions that help prevent memory lapses, e.g., ensuring equipment is turned on or off. Future domestic and work environments may include electronic reminder and knowledge systems as integral parts of the environment. Refrigerators, one of the most commonly visited sites in a typical household, are already on the market with inbuilt reminder and internet facilities on the door.

Mobile phones

Mobile phones have become more sophisticated in terms of the range of functions that they perform, and also in the degree to which they can integrate with other devices, such as computers. Most mobile phones now have personal digital assistant (PDA) features, and these may include a voice recorder, a diary, various alarm features, a camera, etc. Although few mobile phones appear to have been designed with the memory-impaired or the neurologically disabled in mind, there are some with real or virtual QWERTY keyboards that may be easier to use for text entry purposes (Wright *et al.*, 2000). Teaching memory-impaired patients to use mobile phones requires some thought and planning (Lekeu *et al.*, 2002). The use of mobile phones to receive text message reminders has been shown to improve clinic attendance rates (Leong *et al.*, 2006).

Cameras

Devices which automatically keep a photographic record of activities during the day, such as a device produced by Microsoft called SenseCam (Berry *et al.*, 2007), may help to act as a pictorial diary to enable events to be reviewed and rehearsed at regular intervals, after downloading onto a computer. The images may also act as cues to help retrieve forgotten memories. The advantages over general photographic devices is the automaticity of image production, and the ability to readily categorise and retrieve images that are subsequently stored on a computer. More generally, there may be developments in software that will enable video and other photographic records to be easily archived and readily retrieved, and thus allow "blogging" to be interfaced with sophisticated data retrieval systems.

Location detection devices

Location detection devices, for helping to find lost items at home, have become more sophisticated in recent years, with radio frequency and radar-technology based devices now available in the market. It is possible that in the future radio frequency identification devices may become miniaturized to the extent that they can be attached to items such as glasses which are easily lost, or to household items in general, so that the owner can instantly locate the item in question.

Paging systems

Paging technologies are also emerging as potentially useful memory aids. NeuroPage (Hersh & Treadgold, 1994) has been evaluated in the UK since 1994. The first study involved 15 people with everyday memory and/or planning problems. Each client selected target behaviors they wanted to remember each day, for example "Take medication;" "Feed the dog;" "Turn on the central heating." During a 6-week baseline, an independent observer (usually a relative) monitored whether or not the targets had been achieved.

Clients were then given NeuroPage for 12 weeks. The pager reminded them of the target behaviors and these were monitored as before in the baseline phase. Following the treatment phase, clients returned their pagers and were monitored for a further 4 weeks. The group as a whole improved from a success rate of 37% in the baseline phase to over 85% in the treatment phase. Furthermore, every one of the 15 clients showed a statistically significant improvement between baseline and treatment. When the pagers were returned, performance for the group as a whole fell slightly to 74%, still a considerable improvement over baseline (Wilson et al. 1997).

Two single case studies showed how NeuroPage increased independence (Evans et al., 1998; Wilson et al., 1999). A larger randomized control cross-over design study comprising 143 clients confirmed the earlier results (Wilson et al. 2001). Following a 2-week baseline, clients were randomly allocated to "pager first" or "waiting list" first. After 7 weeks with NeuroPage or 7 weeks on the waiting list, those with the pager returned it and those on the waiting list received a pager. Targets were monitored as described in the earlier study. Over 80% of the clients were more successful in achieving their everyday targets with the pager in comparison with the baseline period. When we just look at the subgroup of 63 patients with traumatic brain injury (Wilson

et al., 2005) we see that the same pattern emerges. Wilson & Evans (2002) discuss the cost implications of NeuroPage. For at least some clients, NeuroPage saves money for the health and social services.

As a result of these research studies, the local National Health Service trust set up a commercial service offering NeuroPage to people throughout the UK. Wilson et al. (2003) report on the first 40 people to be recruited to the service. The age range was 14–81 years, the majority of clients were men and the most frequent diagnosis was TBI although different diagnostic groups were represented. The most frequent messages sent each week were those reminding people to take their medication. Orientation messages reminding people about the day, date and time were the second most frequent, followed in order by reminders about food, hygiene, chores, family responsibilities, rest, hobbies, work/study, exercise, other (mostly one-off reminders), appointments, contacts with family or friends, NeuroPage itself, transport and finance. It would appear that the majority of people enrolled in the service benefit from the pager. The cost of £60/$90 per month is relatively inexpensive when one considers that some of these clients no longer require healthcare/social service staff (or require these staff for less hours). In addition, less medication is being wasted and less stress is placed on families or care staff.

Virtual reality

Virtual reality procedures are beginning to impact on the discipline of neurorehabilitation (e.g., Merians et al., 2006), and in the field of cognitive rehabilitation virtual reality software is being increasingly used to help bridge the gap between treatments that take place in the clinic setting and activities which take place in the patient's home environment. Such software may also have a role in providing more ecologically valid assessments of areas such as prospective memory functioning. A few promising pilot studies have been carried out (Rose et al., 1999, 2005; Schultheis & Rizzo, 2001; Zhang et al., 2003), but more work needs to be done before the full benefits of virtual reality are to be ascertained.

Advanced brain imaging

In general, advances in brain imaging and advances in memory rehabilitation have travelled along separate paths, with little in the way of cross-fertilization of data or ideas. There is, however, every reason to try and promote such interactions, and to expect that they may occur in the future (cf. Strangman *et al.*, 2005). Advanced structural and functional brain-imaging procedures may help to identify those individuals who might benefit from certain forms of memory rehabilitation. Structural imaging, both in the form of gray matter status and fiber tract integrity, may provide a detailed profile of brain pathology and sparing, and it is possible, for example, that comprehensive measures of frontal lobe or limbic-diencephalic integrity will help to predict which patients could benefit from mnemonic strategy training as opposed to external memory aids. As in the case of language rehabilitation (Peck *et al.*, 2004), functional brain-imaging paradigms before and after a period of memory rehabilitation may provide useful information on the neural mechanisms underlying any changes that have taken place as the result of treatment (cf. Behrmann *et al.*, 2005). More speculatively, there is the prospect of on-line fMRI-mediated teaching of encoding and retrieval strategies, if we can generalize from some recent developments in neuroimaging (Weiskopf *et al.*, 2004; Yoo *et al.*, 2006).

Summary

Emerging technologies hold out the prospect of providing a valuable resource for therapists who are exploring the use of compensatory devices for memory rehabilitation. Mobile phone technology is now in such widespread use, by all age groups, that it may often be one of the first options in the form of external memory aids to be harnessed by therapists. Brain-imaging findings may help to provide a solid foundation for certain interventions in memory rehabilitation, and virtual reality procedures may help to tackle the ever-present issue of transfer of rehabilitation benefits from the clinic to the community.

Treatment of semantic memory disorders

- Few studies have reported treatments for semantic disorders and these few typically describe patients with progressive semantic memory loss.
- Intensive rehearsal of forgotten words can result in improvement but the words are lost again once the intensive rehearsal ceases.
- Treatments using a combination of strategies (mnemonics, expanded rehearsal, errorless learning and vanishing cues) have been effective both for patients with progressive and with nonprogressive disorders.
- Maintenance and generalization of new learning have been reported in two patients with encephalitis.

Introduction

Semantic memory refers to our general knowledge about the world such as the meanings of words, the recognition of faces and objects, what things are used for, what things feel, smell and taste like, the colors of things, geographical facts, etc. The term semantic memory was first used by Tulving (1972) when he categorized memory into two main systems, namely semantic and episodic memory. Semantic memory is independent of context and is generally acquired through multiple exposure to or rehearsal of the material.

Semantic relearning studies

Few studies have tried to teach lost semantic knowledge to people with a damaged semantic memory system. Of those few, Graham *et al.* (2001) have possibly carried out the most systematic work. They note that the predominant, and most socially isolating, symptom typically seen in semantic dementia is anomia or word-finding difficulties. They demonstrated that repeated rehearsal of the names of concepts paired with pictures of them and/or real items resulted in a dramatic improvement in the ability of a patient, DM with semantic dementia, to produce previously difficult-to-retrieve words on tests of word production. Although the substantial improvement shown by DM suggests that home rehearsal with pictorial and verbal stimuli could be a useful rehabilitative strategy for word-finding difficulties in semantic dementia, the experiment also revealed that constant exposure to items was necessary in order to prevent the observed decline in performance once DM's daily drill was stopped.

Snowden & Neary (2002) also looked at the relearning of object names in two patients with severe anomia associated with semantic dementia. They found that some relearning of lost vocabulary is possible in semantic dementia. In both these studies, however, the patients' learning was confounded by deterioration in their condition.

Given the difficulty of measuring new learning in people who are deteriorating, Dewar *et al.* (2006) looked at the learning and the generalization of new semantic information in people with semantic memory problems following nonprogressive brain damage. They taught the names of 10 famous people to two patients who had survived herpes simplex encephalitis. Stimuli comprised 10 photographs and 10 semantic facts. Mnemonics were used following an errorless learning procedure incorporating vanishing cues and expanded rehearsal in much the same way as the procedure used by Clare *et al.* (1999). The patients also practiced each day at home. Recall of all items was tested at the beginning of each session. Maintenance and generalization were assessed at the end of training. Both subjects improved relative to baseline in naming of the photographs but recall of the semantic facts was less robust. There was some evidence of subsequent maintenance of learning following cessation of practice and one patient demonstrated some generalization to new photographs of the famous people used in training. Another patient with

prosopagnosia (an inability to recognize familiar faces) was also taught to recognize the faces of family and friends using a similar procedure (Dewar *et al.*, 2006). Following multiple baselines to ensure that practice alone was not causing improvement, eight faces were selected for training. Two faces were trained at weekly sessions, in addition to home practice. Recall of all faces was tested at the beginning of each session. Maintenance and generalisation of learning were also assessed. The patient was able to correctly name the faces following training. There was evidence of generalization of learning to different (profile) photographs and learning was maintained in the absence of practice. Although many questions remain to be answered in this area, there is evidence to support the view that people with semantic memory deficits can relearn some new information.

Summary

Although most memory rehabilitation programs are concerned with the reduction of episodic memory deficits, patients with semantic memory difficulties are sometimes seen. Semantic memory refers to our knowledge about the world such as the meanings of words, recognition of faces and objects, geographical facts and other general knowledge. The few studies reported which try to improve semantic memory have been, for the most part, with patients with progressive semantic dementia. Graham *et al.* (2001) showed that repeated rehearsal of words paired with pictures and/or real objects enabled one man to produce previously difficult-to-retrieve words. However, constant exposure was necessary in order to prevent decline and once the daily drill was stopped the man's word retrieval performance dropped. Dewar *et al.* (2006) treated two patients with semantic memory deficits following herpes simplex encephalitis. These patients were taught the names of ten famous people and ten semantic facts about these people. Maintenance and generalization were also assessed. Both subjects learned the name but had greater difficulty with the facts. Another patient with prosopagnosia was taught to recognize photographs of her family and friends using the same procedure.

Emotional aspects of memory impairment

- Emotional consequences of memory impairment are common and should be included in treatment and rehabilitation programs.
- Holistic programs address both cognitive and emotional issues.
- There is evidence of increased self-esteem and reduced anxiety and depression in patients who are treated in holistic programs.
- Cognitive–behavioral therapy is one of the most widely used methods to address emotional difficulties, at least in the UK.

Introduction

Although cognitive problems are among the most handicapping for brain-injured people, they are generally not seen in isolation. Emotional and behavioral problems are also common, and may indeed worsen over time. Depression, anxiety, irritability and aggression may all occur. Social isolation is frequently reported by patients and families (Talbott, 1989; Wilson, 1991), as are mood disorders. Kopelman & Crawford (1996) found that 40% of 200 consecutive referrals to a memory clinic were suffering from clinical depression. Evans & Wilson (1992) found anxiety common in people attending a memory group. Fleminger et al. (2003) looking at the frequency of depression after TBI found studies ranging from a low of 18% to a high of 39%. Different personality characteristics and premorbid lifestyles may exacerbate or diminish the relevance of current problems for everyday functioning, and may influence the effectiveness of rehabilitation.

Holistic approaches

Holistic rehabilitation programs attempt to deal with the "whole person" and try to deal with the multitude of problems following brain injury. The original holistic neuropsychological rehabilitation regime for brain-injured people appears to be that of Ben Yishay and his colleagues in Israel in 1974 (Prigatano et al., 1986). Major themes of these programs include the development of increased awareness, acceptance and understanding, cognitive retraining, development of compensatory skills and vocational counselling. Evidence is provided of increased self-esteem among patients, reduction in anxiety and depression, and greater social interaction (Ben Yishay & Prigatano, 1990). A special issue of the journal *Neuropsychological Rehabilitation* (Williams & Evans, 2003) was devoted to the biopsychosocial aspects of rehabilitation and addressed the assessment and management of neuropsychiatric, mood and behavioral disorders following brain injury.

Cognitive–behavioral therapy

Clinical psychologists working in brain-injury rehabilitation have a range of methods to deal with the emotional sequelae of memory impairment with cognitive–behavioral therapy (CBT) being one of the most important. Since Beck's influential book *Cognitive Therapy and the Emotional Disorders* appeared in 1976, CBT has become one of the most important and best validated psychological treatments for emotional disorders for people without organic brain damage (Salkovskis 1996). One of its major strengths has been its derivation from clinically relevant theoretical frameworks. There are several theories not only for depression and anxiety but also for panic, obsessive-compulsive disorder and phobias (Salkovskis 1996). In recent years CBT has been increasingly employed in neuropsychological rehabilitation (Williams et al., 1999). Prigatano (1995, 1999) believes that dealing with the emotional effects of brain injury is essential to rehabilitation success. At present, it is certainly an integral component in the programs of many rehabilitation centers. Wilson et al. (2006) found that CBT is the most commonly used model for British clinical neuropsychologists working in adult brain injury rehabilitation.

Summary

Cognitive problems are among the most handicapping for people with brain injury but they are generally not seen in isolation. Depression, anxiety, social isolation and mood disorders are all common. Holistic programs such as those advocated by Ben-Yishay & Prigatano (1990) would appear to lead to improved self-esteem and reduced anxiety and depression. Clinical psychologists working in brain injury rehabilitation have a range of methods to deal with the emotional consequences of memory impairment and CBT is the most popular among British clinical neuropsychologists working in adult brain injury rehabilitation.

Memory therapy in practice

- Significant improvement in memory functioning is unlikely to occur once the period of natural recovery is over.
- Nevertheless, people can be taught to avoid problems, how to compensate for their difficulties and how to learn more efficiently.
- Providing written information for patients and families can also help.
- Brain-injured people may have other deficits in addition to their memory problems all of which should be targeted in rehabilitation programs.

Although some recovery of memory functioning can be expected during the early stages following head injury and other nonprogressive brain damage, memory-impaired people and their families should not be led to believe that significant improvement will occur once the period of natural recovery is over. However, this does not mean that nothing can be done to help. As indicated above, people can be taught to avoid problems, compensate for their difficulties and learn more efficiently. Their distress can be reduced and awareness and understanding can be increased. "Memory rehabilitation does not occur in a vacuum" (Prigatano, 1995). Personality factors, awareness, motivation, levels of anxiety, depression, lifestyle and additional cognitive problems may all affect the way memory problems are experienced and subsequently dealt with in everyday life. Prigatano (1995) suggested that patients with low motivation and low awareness after brain injury were the most difficult to treat.

Listening to what families have to say and providing straightforward information or explanations are therapeutic in themselves. Family members commonly ask why it is that their memory-impaired relative can remember what happened 20 years earlier but cannot remember what happened an hour before, or variations on that theme. They should be given simple explanations such as the fact that old memories are stored differently in the brain. For some relatives, this will not be enough and they will demand a fairly detailed anatomical or biochemical explanation. When such demands occur, the therapist should be sufficiently knowledgeable and confident to be able to provide an explanation.

Anxiety in family members can be reduced by offering reassurance that their relative is experiencing a typical pattern of difficulties found in most memory-impaired people. Written information is also appreciated by families. There are useful pamphlets and books available and these are described in the introduction to this chapter. A useful reference on the topic of self-help and support groups for memory-impaired people and their carers is by Wearing (1992).

Relaxation therapy can be helpful in reducing anxiety, and its benefits may last even though treatment sessions have been forgotten. Relaxation audio-cassette tapes can be bought or made for patients so that they do not need to rely upon memory in order to carry out exercises. One word of caution here, though. When tense-and-release exercises (Bernstein & Borkovec, 1973) are employed for relaxation, therapists need to be aware that some brain-injured people, particularly those with motor difficulties, may have problems. Tensing muscles can cause a spasm or increase spasticity. It is best, therefore, to discuss the advisability of such exercises with a physiotherapist treating the particular patient or, alternatively, to look for another form of relaxation such as that recommended by Ost (1987) or those described by Clark (1989).

Memory functioning can be impaired by depression in those without brain injury (Watts, 1995), probably because of diminished resources available as a result of emotional preoccupations. For similar reasons, depression may well exacerbate difficulties in people with organic memory impairment. Cognitive–behavioral therapy approaches such as those employed by Beck (1976) are appropriate for some brain-injured patients (Williams & Evans, 2003). Psychotherapy is a well-established intervention with brain-injured people. Prigatano *et al.* (1986) firmly believe in group and individual psychotherapy with brain-injured patients, and use principles from the school of Jung. Jackson & Gouvier (1992) provide descriptions and guidelines for group psychotherapy with brain-injured adults and their families.

Brain-injured people may well have multiple cognitive problems that will need to be tackled in rehabilitation in addition to the memory problems and any emotional difficulties. People with a pure amnesic syndrome are relatively rare, and most patients present with attentional deficits, word-finding problems or executive difficulties of planning and organization. Memory problems may, in fact, be secondary to other cognitive deficits. Detailed neuropsychological assessment will probably be necessary to obtain an accurate picture of a person's cognitive strengths and weaknesses before a coherent and sensible memory therapy program can be designed. More detailed information on the neuropsychological assessment of memory can be found in Howieson & Lezak (1995) and Wilson (2002). Information from detailed neuropsychological assessment needs to be supplemented with a behavioral assessment defining the real-life, everyday problems to be targeted for treatment.

Summary and conclusions

Since handicaps in everyday memory functioning cut across neurological disease boundaries, and also occur as part of the aging process, they represent a major burden on the health of any nation, and form the focus of a wide range of attempts at therapeutic

intervention. In addition to the types of intervention discussed in this chapter, such treatments may encompass novel drug compounds, gene therapy, brain stimulation, transcranial magnetic stimulation, tissue implant procedures, vagal nerve stimulation, etc. It may well be that the optimal intervention for improving everyday memory functioning will consist of a combination of procedures. Just as in cancer treatment, particular combinations of drugs, with or without radiotherapy, may form the best intervention, or in the field of mental health, psychological and pharmacologic interventions in the right combination may often provide maximum benefit. There remains scope for multidisciplinary approaches to the treatment of human memory disorder, and we would hope that when the next edition of this book is written, data will have been gathered in relation to such integrated approaches to treatment so as to allow evidence-based interventions to be implemented.

Although restoration of memory functioning to pre-injury levels is unlikely to occur, and attempts to apply constraint-induced therapy principles to improve memory functioning need to be treated with caution (Lillie & Mateer, 2006), there is a considerable amount that can be done to enable memory-impaired people and their relatives to come to terms with their difficulties and surmount a number of them by using various strategies and aids.

Environmental modifications can be of considerable help to people whose memory functioning is impaired, and new technology has an increasingly important role to play in the future management of memory problems. As discussed, some technological aids such as pagers and electronic reminders are proving to be beneficial. When a variety of technological aids are set to work cooperatively in the same building, we have what has become known as a "smart" house, and it is possible that such dwellings will be developed in increasing numbers and greater sophistication for the benefit of elderly and cognitively impaired people in the future.

Non-electronic external memory aids such as diaries, notebooks etc. are widely used but are often problematic for memory-impaired people simply because reliance upon them demands exercising memory. However, the successful use of these aids is possible through carefully structured teaching, particularly with people who are younger, have less severe memory problems or have fewer additional cognitive impairments. Others may need more intensive therapy or rehabilitation to ensure efficient usage. As Sohlberg (2005) has pointed out, there is a pressing need for well-designed research studies to evaluate both the efficacy of external memory aids and also the instructional strategies that are used to train their use by neurological patients.

Internal strategies such as mnemonics and rehearsal techniques can be employed to teach new information, and although they almost always lead to faster learning than rote repetition, it must be recognized that most memory-impaired people will be unable or unwilling to use mnemonics spontaneously. Instead, relatives, carers and therapists will have to employ mnemonics to encourage learning among memory-impaired people.

Errorless learning is usually more effective than trial-and-error learning for most memory-impaired people. This is because, in order to benefit from our mistakes, we need to be able to remember them, and this is something which most memory-impaired people will not be able to do. In the absence of episodic memory, making an error may strengthen or reinforce the erroneous response.

In addition to poor memory, many brain-injured people will have other cognitive problems which will need to be addressed. The emotional sequelae of memory impairment such as anxiety, depression and loneliness will also have to be reduced by counselling, anxiety-management techniques and treatment in memory or psychotherapy groups.

Although we cannot restore lost memory functioning, we can help people to bypass problems and compensate for their difficulties. We can help them learn more efficiently and we can reduce the effects of their problems in their daily lives. We can also help to educate society so that there is a greater understanding of what it means to have severe memory impairment.

REFERENCES

Baddeley, A. D., & Longman, D. J. A. (1978). The influence of length and frequency on training sessions on the rate of learning to type. *Ergonomics*, **21**, 627–635.

Baddeley, A. D., Kopelman, M. D., & Wilson, B. A. (2004). *The Essential Handbook of Memory Disorders for Clinicians*. Chichester, UK: John Wiley & Sons Ltd.

Beck, A. T. (1976). *Cognitive Therapy and Emotional Disorders*. New York, NY: International Universities Press.

Behrmann, M., Marotta, J. J., Gauthier, I., Tarr, M. J., & McKeeff, T. J. (2005). Behavioural change and its neural correlates in visual agnosia after expertise training. *Journal of Cognitive Neuroscience*, **17**, 554–568.

Bell, P. A., Greene, T. C., Fisher, J. D., & Baum, A. (2001). *Environmental Psychology (5th Edition)*. Belmont, CA: Thomson Wadsworth.

Ben-Yishay, Y., & Prigatano, G. P. (1990). Cognitive remediation. In E. Griffith, M. Rosenthal, M. R. Bond, & J. D. Miller (Eds.), *Rehabilitation of the Adult and Child with Traumatic Brain Injury* (pp. 393–409). Philadelphia, PA: F. W. Davis.

Bernstein, D. A., & Borkovec, R. D. (1973). *Progressive Relaxation Training: A Manual for the Helping Professions*. Champaign, IL: Research Press.

Berry, E., Kapur, N., Williams, L. *et al.* (2007). The use of a wearable camera, Sensecam, as a pictorial diary to improve autobiographical memory in a patient with limbic encephalitis: a preliminary report. *Neuropsychological Rehabilitation*, **17**, 582–601.

Brooks, D. N., & Baddeley, A. D. (1976). What can amnesic patients learn? *Neuropsychologia*, **14**, 111–122.

Canter, D. (1996). Wayfinding and signposting: penance or prosthesis? In D. Canter (Ed.), *Psychology in Action* (pp. 139–155). San Diego, CA: Academic Press.

Cheek, P., Nikpour, L., & Nowlin, H. D. (2005). Aging well with smart technology. *Nursing Administration Quarterly*, **29**, 329–338.

Clare, L., & Wilson, B. A. (1997). *Coping with Memory Problems. A Practical Guide for People with Memory Impairments, Relatives, Friends and Carers*. Bury St Edmunds, UK: Thames Valley Test Company.

Clare, L., Wilson, B. A., Breen, K., & Hodges, J. R. (1999). Errorless learning of face-name associations in early Alzheimer's disease. *Neurocase*, **5**, 37–46.

Clare, L., Wilson, B. A., Carter, G. *et al.* (2000). Intervening with everyday memory problems in dementia of Alzheimer type: an errorless learning approach. *Journal of Clinical and Experimental Neuropsychology*, **22**, 132–146.

Clare, L., Wilson, B. A., Carter, G., Hodges, J. R., & Adams, M. (2001). Long-term maintenance of treatment gains following a cognitive rehabilitation intervention in early dementia of Alzheimer type: a single case study. *Neuropsychological Rehabilitation*, **11**, 477–494.

Clark, D. M. (1989). Anxiety states: panic and generalised anxiety. In K. Hawton, P. M. Salkovskis, J. Kirk, & D. M. Clark (Eds.), *Cognitive Behaviour Therapy for Psychiatric Problems* (pp. 52–97). Oxford, UK: Oxford Medical Publications.

Craik, F. I. M., & Jennings, J. M. (1992). Human memory. In F. I. M. Craik & T. A. Salthouse (Eds.), *Handbook of Aging and Cognition* (pp. 51–110). Mahwah, NJ: Lawrence Erlbaum.

Dewar, B.-K., Wilson, B. A., Patterson, K., & Graham, K. S. (2006). Can people with semantic memory deficits relearn information? *Journal of the International Neuropsychological Society*, **12** (S2), 21.

Dogu, U., & Erkip, F. (2000). Spatial factors affecting way-finding and orientation. A case study in a shopping mall. *Environment and Behaviour*, **32**, 731–755.

Elmstahl, S., Annerstedt, L., & Ahlund, O. (1997). How should a group living unit for demented elderly be designed to decrease psychiatric symptoms? *Alzheimer Disease and Related Disorders*, **11**, 47–52.

Evans, J. J., & Wilson, B. A. (1992). A memory group for individuals with brain injury. *Clinical Rehabilitation*, **6**, 75–81.

Evans, J. J., Emslie, H., & Wilson, B. A. (1998). External cueing systems in the rehabilitation of executive impairments of action. *Journal of the International Neuropsychological Society*, **4**, 399–408.

Evans, J. J., Wilson, B. A., Schuri, U. *et al.* (2000). A comparison of "errorless" and "trial-and-error" learning methods for teaching individuals with acquired memory deficits. *Neuropsychological Rehabilitation*, **10**, 67–101.

Fleminger, S., Oliver, D., Williams, W. H., & Evans, J. (2003). The neuropsychiatry of depression after brain injury. *Neuropsychological Rehabilitation*, **13**, 65–87.

Fulton, A., & Hatch, P. (1991). *It's Here. . . . . . .Somewhere.* Cincinnati, OH: Writers Digest Books.

Glisky, E. L., & Schacter, D. L. (1987). Acquisition of domain-specific knowledge in organic amnesia: training for computer-related work. *Neuropsychologia*, **25**, 893–906.

Graf, P., & Schacter, D. L. (1985). Implicit and explicit memory for new associations in normal and amnesic subjects. *Journal of Experimental Psychology: Learning, Memory and Cognition*, **11**, 501–518.

Graham, K. S., Patterson, K., Pratt, K. H., & Hodges, J. R. (2001). Can repeated exposure to 'forgotten' vocabulary help alleviate word-finding difficulties in semantic dementia? An illustrative case study. *Neuropsychological Rehabilitation*, **11**, 429–454.

Gross, J., Harmon, M. E., Myers, R. *et al.* (2004). Recognition of self among persons with dementia. *Environment and Behaviour*, **36**, 424–454.

Hersch, N., & Treadgold, L. (1994). NeuroPage: the rehabilitation of memory dysfunction by prosthetic memory and cueing. *NeuroRehabilitation*, **4**, 187–197.

Howieson, D. B., & Lezak, M. D. (1995). Separating memory from other cognitive problems. In A. D. Baddeley, B. A. Wilson, & F. N. Watts (Eds.), *Handbook of Memory Disorders* (pp. 411–426). Chichester, UK: John Wiley.

Jackson, W. T., & Gouvier, W. D. (1992). Group psychotherapy with brain-damaged adults and their families. In C. J. Long, & L. K. Ross (Eds.), *Handbook of Head Trauma: Acute Care to Recovery* (pp. 309–327). New York, NY: Plenum Press.

Jones, R. S. P., & Eayrs, C. B. (1992). The use of errorless learning procedures in teaching people with a learning disability. *Mental Handicap Research*, **5**, 304–312.

Kapur, N. (2001). *Managing Your Memory (2nd Edition)*. Cambridge, UK: Addenbrooke's Hospital.

Kapur, N., Glisky, G. L., & Wilson, B. A. (2004). Technological memory aids for people with memory deficits. *Neuropsychological Rehabilitation*, **14**, 41–60.

Kime, S. K. (2006). *Compensating for Memory Deficits: Using a Systematic Approach*. Bethesda, MD: AOTA Press.

Kopelman, M., & Crawford, S. (1996). Not all memory clinics are dementia clinics. *Neuropsychological Rehabilitation*, **6**, 187–202.

Landauer, T. K., & Bjork, R. A. (1978). Optimum rehearsal patterns and name learning. In M. M. Gruneberg, P. E. Morris, & R. N. Sykes (Eds.), *Practical Aspects of Memory* (pp. 625–632). London, UK: Academic Press.

Lekeu, F., Wojtasik, V., van der Linden, M., & E., S. (2002). Training early Alzheimer patients to use a mobile phone. *Acta Neurologica Belgica*, **102**, 114–121.

Leong, K. C., Chen, W., Leong, K. W. *et al.* (2006). The use of text messaging to improve attendance in primary care: a randomised controlled trial. *Family Practice*, **23**, 699–705.

Lillie, R., & Mateer, C. A. (2006). Constraint-based therapies as a proposed model for cognitive rehabilitation. *Journal of Head Trauma and Rehabilitation*, **21**, 119–130.

Merians, A. S., Poizner, H., Boian, R., Burdea, G., & Adamovich, S. (2006). Sensimotor training in a virtual reality environment: does it improve functional recovery post-stroke? *Neurorehabilitation and Neural Repair*, **20**, 252–267.

Moffat, N. (1989). Home based cognitive rehabilitation with the elderly. In L. W. Poon, D. C. Rubin, & B. A. Wilson (Eds.), *Everyday Cognition in Adulthood and Late Life* (pp. 659–680). Cambridge, UK: Cambridge University Press.

Norman, D. A. (1988). *The Psychology of Everyday Things*. New York, NY: Basic Books.

Olsen, R., Hutchings, B., & Ehrenkrantz, E. (1999). The physical design of the home as a caregiving support: an environment for persons with dementia. *Care Management Journals*, **1**, 125–131.

Ost, L. G. (1987). Applied relaxation: description of a coping technique and review of controlled studies. *Behaviour Research and Therapy*, **25**, 397–410.

Page, M., Wilson, B. A., Shiel, A., Carter, G., & Norris, D. (2006). What is the locus of the errorless-learning advantage? *Neuropsychologia*, **44**, 90–100.

Passini, R., Rainville, C., Marchand, N., & Joanette, Y. (1998). Wayfinding and dementia: some research findings and a new look at design. *Journal of Architecture and Planning Research*, **15**, 133–151.

Passini, R., Pigot, H., Rainville, C., & Tetreault, M.-H. (2000). Wayfinding in a nursing home for advanced dementia of the Alzheimer-type. *Environment and Behaviour*, **32**, 684–710.

Peck, K. K., Moore, A. B., Crosson, B. A. *et al.* (2004). Functional magnetic resonance imaging before and after aphasia therapy. *Stroke*, **35**, 554–559.

Prigatano, G. P. (1995). Personality and social aspects of memory rehabilitation. In A. D. Baddeley, B. A. Wilson, & F. N. Watts (Eds.), *Handbook of Memory Disorders* (pp. 603–614). Chichester, UK: John Wiley & Sons.

Prigatano, G. P. (1999). *Principles of Neuropsychological Rehabilitation*. New York, NY: Oxford University Press.

Prigatano, G. P., Fordyce, D. J., Zeiner, H. K. *et al.* (1986). *Neuropsychological Rehabilitation after Brain Injury*. Baltimore, MD: The Johns Hopkins University Press.

Robertson, I. H., & Halligan, P. W. (1999). *Spatial Neglect. A Clinical Handbook for Diagnosis and Treatment*. Hove, UK: Psychology Press.

Rose, F. D., Brooks, B. M., Attree, E. A. *et al.* (1999). A preliminary investigation into the use of virtual environments in memory retraining after vascular brain injury: indications for future strategy. *Disability and Rehabilitation*, **21**, 548–554.

Rose, F. D., Brooks, B. M., & Rizzo, A. A. (2005). Virtual reality in brain damage rehabilitation: a review. *Cyberpsychology and Behavior*, **8**, 241–262.

Salkovskis, P. M. (1996). *Frontiers of Cognitive Therapy*. New York, NY: Guilford Press.

Schultheis, M. T., & Rizzo, A. (2001). The application of virtual reality technology in rehabilitation. *Rehabilitation Psychology*, **46**, 296–311.

Sidman, M., & Stoddard, L. T. (1967). The effectiveness of fading in programming simultaneous form discrimination for retarded children. *Journal of Experimental Analysis of Behavior*, **10**, 3–15.

Snowden, J. S., & Neary, D. (2002). Relearning of verbal labels in semantic dementia. *Neuropsychologia*, **40**, 1715–1728.

Sohlberg, M. M. (2005). External aids for management of memory impairment. In W. M. J. High, A. M. Sander, M. A. Struchen, & K. A. Hart (Eds.), *Rehabilitation for Traumatic Brain Injury* (pp. 47–70). New York, NY: Oxford University Press.

Squires, E. J., Hunkin, N. M., & Parkin, A. J. (1996). Memory notebook training in a case of severe amnesia: generalising from paired associate learning to real life. *Neuropsychological Rehabilitation*, **6**, 55–65.

Strangman, G., O'Neil-Pirozzi, T. M., Burke, D. *et al.* (2005). Functional neuroimaging and cognitive rehabilitation for people with traumatic brain injury. *American Journal of Physical Medicine and Rehabilitation*, **84**, 62–75.

Talbott, R. (1989). The brain injured person and the family. In R. L. Wood & P. Eames (Eds.), *Models of Brain Injury Rehabilitation* (pp. 3–16). London, UK: Chapman and Hall.

Thoene, A. I. T., & Glisky, E. L. (1995). Learning of name-face associations in memory impaired patients: a comparison of different training procedures. *Journal of the International Neuropsychological Society*, **1**, 29–38.

Tulving, E. (1972). Episodic and semantic memory. In E. Tulving & W. Donaldson (Eds.), *Organization of Memory* (pp. 381–403). New York, NY: Academic Press.

Warner, M. L. (2000). *The Complete Guide to Alzheimer's Proofing your Home*. Indiana: Purdue University Press.

Watts, F. N. (1995). Depression and anxiety. In A. D. Baddeley, B. A. Wilson, & F. N. Watts (Eds.), *Handbook of Memory Disorders* (pp. 293–317). Chichester, UK: John Wiley & Sons.

Wearing, D. (1992). Self help groups. In B. A. Wilson & N. Moffat (Eds.), *Clinical Management of Memory Problems* (pp. 271–301). London, UK: Chapman and Hall.

Weiskopf, N., Scharnowski, F., Veit, R. *et al.* (2004). Self-regulation of local brain activity using real-time functional magnetic resonance imaging (fMRI). *Journal of Physiology Paris*, **98**, 357–373.

West, R. L. (1995). Compensatory strategies for age-associated memory impairment. In A. D. Baddeley, F. N. Watts, & B. A. Wilson (Eds.), *Handbook of Memory Disorders* (pp. 481–500). Chichester, UK: Wiley and Sons.

Williams, W. H., & Evans, J. J. (2003). *Biopsychosocial Approaches in Neurorehabilitation: Assessment and Management of Neuropsychiatric, Mood and Behaviour Disorders*. Oxford, UK: Taylor & Francis.

Williams, W. H., Evans, J. J., & Wilson, B. A. (1999). Outcome measures for survivors of acquired brain injury in day and outpatient neurorehabilitation programmes. *Neuropsychological Rehabilitation*, **9**, 421–436.

Wilson, B. A. (1987). *Rehabilitation of Memory*. New York, NY: Guilford Press.

Wilson, B. A. (1991). Long term prognosis of patients with severe memory disorders. *Neuropsychological Rehabilitation*, **1**, 117–134.

Wilson, B. A. (1999). *Case Studies in Neuropsychological Rehabilitation*. New York, NY: Oxford University Press.

Wilson, B. A. (2002). Assessment of memory disorders. In A. D. Baddeley, M. D. Kopelman, & B. A. Wilson (Eds.), *The Handbook of Memory Disorders (2nd Edition)* (pp. 617–636). Chichester, UK: John Wiley.

Wilson, B. A. (2003). Goal planning rather than neuropsychological tests should be used to structure and evaluate cognitive rehabilitation. *Brain Impairment*, **4**, 25–30.

Wilson, B. A., & Evans, J. J. (1996). Error free learning in the rehabilitation of individuals with memory impairments. *Journal of Head Trauma Rehabilitation*, **11**, 54–64.

Wilson, B. A., & Evans, J. J. (2000). Practical management of memory problems. In G. E. Berrios & J. R. Hodges (Eds.), *Memory Disorders in Psychiatric Practice* (pp. 291–310). Cambridge, UK: Cambridge University Press.

Wilson, B. A., & Evans, J. J. (2002). Does cognitive rehabilitation work? Clinical and economic considerations and outcomes. In G. Prigatano & N. H. Pliskin (Eds.), *Clinical Neuropsychology and Cost-outcome Research: An Introduction* (pp. 329–349). Hove, UK: Psychology Press.

Wilson, B. A., Baddeley, A. D., Evans, J., & S., S. A. (1994). Errorless learning in the rehabilitation of memory impaired people. *Neuropsychological Rehabilitation*, **4**, 307–326.

Wilson, B. A., Evans, J. J., Emslie, H., & Malinek, V. (1997). Evaluation of NeuroPage: a new memory aid. *Journal of Neurology, Neurosurgery and Psychiatry*, **63**, 113–115.

Wilson, B. A., Emslie, H., Quirk, K., & Evans, J. (1999). George: learning to live independently with NeuroPage. *Rehabilitation Psychology*, **44**, 284–296.

Wilson, B. A., Emslie, H. C., Quirk, K., & Evans, J. J. (2001). Reducing everyday memory and planning problems by means of a paging system: a randomised control cross-over study. *Journal of Neurology, Neurosurgery and Psychiatry*, **70**, 477–482.

Wilson, B. A., H., S., Evans, J., & Emslie, H. (2003). Preliminary report of a NeuroPage service within a health care system. *Neurorehabilitation*, **18**, 3–9.

Wilson, B. A., Emslie, H., Quirk, K., Evans, J., & Watson, P. (2005). A randomised control trial to evaluate a paging system for people with traumatic brain injury. *Brain Injury*, **19**, 891–894.

Wilson, B. A., Rous, R., & Sopena, S. (2006). The influence of models and theories on the clinical practice of neuropsychologists working in brain injury rehabilitation. *European Neuropsychological Societies*. Toulouse, France.

Wright, P., Bartram, C., Rogers, N. *et al.* (2000). Text entry on handheld computers by older users. *Ergonomics*, **43**, 702–716.

Yoo, S., O'Leary, H., Fairneny, T. *et al.* (2006). Increased cortical activity in auditory areas through neurofeedback functional magnetic resonance imaging. *NeuroReport*, **17**, 1273–1278.

Zeisel, J. (2006). *Inquiry by Design, Revised Edition*. New York, NY: Norton.

Zhang, L., Abreu, B. C., Seale, G. S. *et al.* (2003). A virtual reality environment for evaluation of a daily living skill in brain injury rehabilitation: reliability and validity. *Archives of Physical Medicine and Rehabilitation*, **84**, 1118–1124.

31

Memory rehabilitation in older adults

Elizabeth L. Glisky and Martha L. Glisky

Introduction

- The adult brain is plastic and learning continues into the oldest ages.
- The aging population is heterogenous.
- Good memory function will depend on a complex interaction of biological, psychological and social variables.

The past decade has seen an explosion of research on the aging brain and its cognitive correlates, which has opened up new avenues for intervention that might reduce the negative effects of aging on memory. Increasing evidence of plasticity in the brain of older adults indicates that learning continues into the oldest ages and that there is considerable potential to modify the downward trajectories in memory function that have been associated with normal aging. Yet the field has lagged behind in the translation of the science into practical application. Nevertheless, there are some promising new developments emerging from a range of perspectives – biological, cognitive, neuropsychological and psychosocial – that, although not yet definitive, suggest directions in which memory rehabilitation might proceed.

One of the difficulties in providing a set of principles on which to base memory interventions for older adults lies in the heterogeneity of the aging population (Glisky *et al.*, 1995). Some individuals are vigorous and cognitively competent at age 80, while others are struggling to maintain function at age 60. Moreover, some abilities seem to hold up well or even increase with age while others diminish. How aging affects memory likely depends on a complex interaction of biological, psychological, environmental and lifestyle variables, and interventions might target any of these areas.

The focus of the present chapter is on changes in memory that occur in normal aging and the kinds of interventions appropriate for this population. Much less is known about how to reduce the more serious memory deficits associated with a progressive dementia such as Alzheimer's disease (AD), and there is reason to believe that techniques most likely to be successful in normal aging will not be appropriate for this group. However, those cognitive interventions that have been directed specifically at individuals with AD are also included in this chapter. The reader is referred in addition to the previous chapter (Chapter 30 by Wilson and Kapur in this volume) for methods that also may be appropriate for individuals with AD.

The following section outlines the nature of the memory problems in aging that rehabilitation must address, noting also the kinds of memory that are relatively preserved with age and thus might serve an assistive or compensatory role in reducing the impact of deficits.

Memory changes in aging

- In normal aging, declines are evident in episodic memory, source memory, working memory and prospective memory, but not in semantic, implicit or procedural memory.

Cognitive Neurorehabilitation, Second Edition: Evidence and Application, ed. Donald T. Stuss, Gordon Winocur and Ian H. Robertson. Published by Cambridge University Press. © Cambridge University Press 2008.

- In AD, deficits in episodic memory appear early and are severe and semantic memory is also affected.

Normal aging

Although considerable variability exists in the memory performance of older adults, episodic memory – memory for relatively recent personally experienced events or episodes – generally causes the most difficulty for people as they age, beginning to show declines when individuals enter their late 40s and 50s and dropping precipitously beyond the early to mid 70s (Albert *et al.*, 1987; Salthouse, 1991). Nevertheless, even within the episodic memory domain, not all kinds of memory are equally affected (for reviews, see Craik & Jennings, 1992; McDaniel *et al.*, 2008; Zacks & Hasher, 2006). For example, age decrements tend to be largest in tasks that require free recall of unrelated words or memory for novel information and least in tasks that require recognition or retrieval of familiar events. Older adults also have more difficulty than young adults remembering contextual details or source information although they usually retain focal or gist information.

Craik (1986, 2002) has proposed that older people are impaired on memory tasks that require self-initiation of encoding or retrieval processes. For example, older people may fail to initiate elaborate semantic encoding processes, thus creating memory traces that are impoverished and difficult to retrieve. In addition, they may not integrate contextual aspects of an experience with central content during encoding, and they may fail to initiate strategic search or monitoring processes at retrieval. Initiation of effortful encoding or retrieval strategies may require a greater infusion of mental energy, a resource that may decline with age or be allocated less efficiently (Craik, 1983). Memory tasks that are more effortful or resource-demanding such as free recall are therefore more likely to show deficits. In a similar vein, older adults tend to have little difficulty when information merely has to be passively held in short-term memory (e.g., forward digit span), although they have problems when that information has to be actively manipulated or reorganized in some way (e.g., backward digit span or mental arithmetic) – what is referred to as working memory. Finally, older adults might be expected to have problems with prospective memory – remembering to do things in the future such as keeping appointments or paying bills on time – because these tasks require the kinds of self-initiated activities that present problems for many older adults (Craik, 1986; Einstein *et al.*, 1995). However, older adults often do surprisingly well at real-world prospective tasks because they take advantage of external aids such as calendars and notebooks to remember their appointments and other daily tasks (Moscovitch, 1982). Nevertheless, on complex laboratory tasks where such aids are not available and cues are not salient, older individuals show the expected impairments in prospective memory (Mäntylä, 1994; Maylor, 1996; Maylor *et al.*, 2002).

In contrast to the declines in memory that are found in the episodic domain, information that has been accumulated over the years, including such things as vocabulary and general world knowledge, is well-retained in old age, and indeed older people often outshine their younger counterparts in what is called semantic memory. One exception to this generality, however, concerns the increased difficulty that many older people have retrieving familiar names. Craik (2002) suggests that the problem with proper names may be another example of the difficulty that older people have with the retrieval of specific details. They are often able to retrieve the more generic or conceptual information about people that they know, but the specifics, such as the name, sometimes elude them. Other kinds of memory that hold up well with age include procedural memory and priming: well-learned skills are usually maintained into the upper years and older adults are as able as young adults to acquire new procedures and skills; and older people show minimal declines on implicit memory tasks such as word fragment completion and tachistoscopic identification of recently presented materials.

Alzheimer's disease

The picture in AD is somewhat different. Episodic memory is often the first kind of memory affected but the severity of the impairment is much greater in AD than in normal aging, with performance falling more than two standard deviations below the normative average on standardised tests. Individuals with AD also have increasing difficulty producing words to conceptual cues and even understanding the meanings of words, symptoms that are indicative of the progression of the disease into the semantic memory realm. Although some word-finding difficulties are also common in normal aging, most older adults are skilled conversationalists and easily find appropriate semantic substitutions. This intrusion of the disease into semantic memory is also observed in impaired conceptual and semantic priming – relatively automatic responses to meaning-based cues – although perceptual priming holds up reasonably well as do many procedural memory tasks.

In summary, normally aging older adults tend to have problems in memory tasks that are particularly resource-demanding, requiring self-initiation of encoding and retrieval processes and retrieval of specific details. Retrieval of well-learned general knowledge and skills, however, is largely preserved. Alzheimer's disease, on the other hand, is associated with a severe and global impairment in episodic memory, and a gradually increasing decline in semantic memory as the disease progresses.

Neural correlates of memory and aging

- In normal aging, changes in prefrontal cortex and hippocampus account for memory declines.
- In AD, neuropathology appears in entorhinal cortex and hippocampus early in the disease, accounting for episodic memory declines, and then spreads to other neocortical regions, implicating semantic memory.
- White matter declines are evident in normal aging as well as in AD.

The memory deficiencies that are observed in normal aging are likely attributable to atrophy or shrinkage in medial temporal and/or prefrontal regions of the brain and in the white matter tracts that connect them (for reviews, see Raz, 2000, 2005). Whereas evidence suggests that the changes in normal aging are most marked in prefrontal cortex (Resnick et al., 2003), those in AD appear earliest in medial temporal regions, specifically in entorhinal cortex (Braak & Braak, 1991) and then gradually spread to other brain regions including parietal, lateral temporal and prefrontal cortex. Little change has been observed in entorhinal cortex in normal aging (Raz et al., 2004), but changes in the hippocampus, particularly in the dentate gyrus and subiculum, have been reported (Small et al., 2002).

Although episodic memory processes have been linked to both medial temporal and prefrontal cortices, the exact mapping between neuroanatomical structures and specific mnemonic functions is still being constructed, but there are a few emerging patterns. First, considerable evidence from functional neuroimaging studies suggests that prefrontal regions are implicated in executive functions and in the more strategic aspects of memory processing. Encoding into episodic memory and retrieval from semantic memory have been associated with left prefrontal cortex suggesting that this region is involved in meaningful and elaborate processing during encoding of episodic memories (Tulving et al., 1994). Right prefrontal cortex has been associated with episodic retrieval processes and has been variously hypothesized to reflect retrieval mode, retrieval effort, search processes and monitoring of performance (Tulving et al., 1994; see Cabeza & Nyberg, 2000 for review). Medial temporal brain regions including the hippocampus and surrounding neocortical structures have been implicated at both encoding and retrieval. The hippocampus in particular is thought to play a role in consolidation, by binding the various elements of an experience together and to its spatiotemporal context, and maintaining an index to these various components for purposes of retrieval. Regions outside these areas are involved in other kinds of memory – lateral temporal cortex in semantic memory, which becomes increasingly affected in AD, and basal ganglia and cerebellum in procedural memory, which are less affected by normal aging and AD.

Findings from functional neuroimaging studies of memory in normally aging older adults have revealed a variety of patterns of activation in memory studies, probably reflective of the variability that exists in this population (for reviews, see Hedden & Gabrieli, 2004; Park & Gutchess, 2005). Several studies have found reductions in activations in older adults compared to young adults during episodic encoding in medial temporal lobe regions (e.g., Grady *et al.*, 1995) and in prefrontal cortex (e.g., Stebbins *et al.*, 2002). Such reductions have been associated with reduced performance in older adults. However, other studies have observed the opposite pattern, namely increased activations in older compared with younger adults particularly in prefrontal cortex during retrieval (e.g., Bäckman *et al.*, 1997; Cabeza *et al.*, 2000; Grady *et al.*, 2002). These increases have typically involved bilateral activation in older adults compared to unilateral activation in young and have been observed mainly in a subgroup of high-performing older adults (e.g., Cabeza *et al.*, 2002). Although a number of interpretations of these findings have been proposed, one possibility is that the increased activity represents a form of compensation that may indicate the recruitment of complementary processes from the other hemisphere or functional reorganization of the brain in those individuals who are aging most successfully (for further discussion, see Colcombe *et al.*, 2005; Daselaar & Cabeza, 2005). The ability to make use of these additional brain regions may depend on high levels of cognitive reserve available to those individuals in the highest functioning groups (Stern, 2002).

White matter declines have also been observed in normal aging, in volumetric measures, in the increase in the number of white matter hyperintensities with age, and in increased diffusion of water molecules in white matter tracts, suggesting a loss of the integrity of white matter (Raz, 2005). Although there are relatively few studies of the effects of white matter decline in older adults, there is initial evidence that such declines are associated with reduced memory and executive function (e.g., Van Petten *et al.*, 2004), highlighting the importance of connectivity among the different brain regions necessary for good memory performance.

In summary, shrinkage in prefrontal cortex, hippocampus and in the white matter tracts that connect them likely accounts for the episodic memory declines observed in normal aging. Compensation for such declines may be possible, however, particularly in the highest functioning older adults, either through recruitment of intact, complementary processes or through functional reorganization.

Goals and methods of rehabilitation

As life expectancy has increased and evidence for substantial plasticity in the aging brain has been uncovered (see Kolb & Gibb, Chapter 1 this volume), greater numbers of studies have focused on finding ways to enhance memory performance in older adults. The following sections outline several of these methods. The methods are organized according to three broad goals, which are differentially attainable depending on the severity of the memory problem: (1) optimization of existing or residual memory function, (2) substitution of intact function for declining or lost function and (3) external compensation for lost or reduced function (see Table 31.1). Included in each section are descriptions of the remedial techniques associated with that goal, the theoretical rationale and empirical findings that support the techniques, the strengths and weaknesses of the methodologies, and the individual difference variables that might moderate the effectiveness of each intervention.

Optimization of existing or residual function

- These methods are appropriate for those with considerable residual memory function, but not for those with severe impairment, as in AD.

Table 31.1. Goals and methods of rehabilitation

Optimization of residual function	Substitution of intact function	Compensation for lost function
Encoding strategies	Spaced retrieval	External memory aids
Visual imagery		Diaries, notebooks, lists
Semantic elaboration	Vanishing cues	Calendars, alarm watches
Self-generated strategies		PDAs, pagers
Generation of materials	Errorless learning	Environmental support
Self-referential processing		Cues
Integrative encoding	Skills and expertise	Past learning
Retrieval processes		
Recollection		
Non-mnemonic methods		
Practice, study time, experience, schooling		
Leisure activity, exercise, fitness		
Time of day		
Pharmacological		

- Many older adults do not spontaneously engage effective encoding or retrieval processes, but can be trained to use such residual mnemonic processes more efficiently.
- Training can focus on encoding strategies such as visual imagery, semantic elaboration, generation, self-referential processing, and integrative encoding, or on retrieval processes such as recollection.
- Improvement or maintenance of memory function may also be achieved through general non-mnemonic methods such as practice, aerobic exercise, stimulating lifestyles and nonprescription drugs.

Considerable evidence suggests that many older adults do not engage in appropriate mnemonic activities when confronted with memory tasks although they are capable of learning the strategies and benefiting from them – what has been called a production deficit. Whereas young adults appear to use at least some encoding and retrieval strategies spontaneously, older adults appear to find many strategies quite resource-demanding and so often fail to initiate them. This age-related difference may be attributable to reduced processing resources in older adults and/or to the greater amount of experience or practice that young people have with memorization tasks. In either case, it suggests that practice in using mnemonic strategies may benefit older adults selectively.

The methods that fall within this approach assume that older people have the processing capabilities to carry out the mnemonic activities and that re-training and practice will essentially revive previously used strategic processes and brain circuits, enabling them to be used more efficiently. Because these methods rely on pre-existing or residual memory and brain function, they are likely to be most effective for relatively high functioning older adults. Older people who are experiencing significant problems with memory, those with mild cognitive impairment (MCI) and individuals with AD are less likely to benefit.

Training encoding strategies

Most mnemonic strategies focus on creating encodings that are meaningful and elaborate and on establishing potential cues that will be readily available at time of retrieval. The techniques that have been used most often with older adults involve visual imagery although verbally based strategies have also been suggested.

Visual imagery

These techniques require the formation of distinctive visual images of material-to-be-remembered, which are then linked to some easily retrievable cues such as well-learned locations in the method of loci, a set of keywords in the peg-word method, or features of a face for learning name/face associations. Visual imagery mnemonics have been found to be effective for remembering names, lists and locations, but little in the way of long-term maintenance or generalization of the strategies has been demonstrated (Verhaeghen *et al.*, 1992; West, 1995). In an attempt to improve the effectiveness of imaging methods, Stigsdotter Neely & Bäckman (1993a, 1993b) used a multifactorial memory training program combining interactive imagery and the method of loci with attentional and relaxation training (Yesavage, 1984; Yesavage & Rose, 1983). They reported significant memory improvements on the trained tasks, which were maintained up to 3.5 years later, although the training effects were relatively task-specific (Stigsdotter Neely & Bäckman, 1995; see also Ball *et al.*, 2002 for long-term maintenance of training effects). However, those individuals receiving mnemonic instruction without attention and relaxation training showed equivalent benefits, suggesting that learning how to encode, using visual imagery and the method of loci was the critical component in the success of this training, not the multifactorial aspect (see Stigsdotter Neely, 2000).

Whether people use mnemonic strategies spontaneously may depend on the amount of practice they have using them. Woolverton *et al.* (2001) found that a 24-hour self-taught practice program that included 111 practice exercises using five different mnemonic strategies including visual imagery was more effective, particularly for recall of people's names, than a shorter version of the same program that included 13 hours and 47 practice exercises focusing on just two techniques including visual imagery. This work highlights not only the importance of practice but also the considerable investment of time and energy needed to make these strategies less resource-demanding and more likely to be implemented. Because such training is very time-consuming, it is unlikely to be acceptable to large numbers of older adults, as suggested by the high drop-out rates (~40%) in the Woolverton *et al.* study.

In summary, although older adults can benefit from training in the use of visual imagery mnemonics after extensive practice, benefits are usually task-specific and show little evidence of generalization to untrained tasks or real-world contexts. Further, it has been demonstrated that even though some older adults benefit from imagery training, the benefits achieved by young adults are sometimes greater, suggesting that some older people may have a processing deficit in addition to their production deficit (Nyberg, 2005; Verhaeghen & Marcoen, 1996).

Semantic elaboration

Because many older adults retain excellent verbal skills well into the upper years, strategies that take advantage of this preserved ability may well be less resource-demanding and more acceptable to older people than visual imagery mnemonics. Semantic elaboration and organizational strategies have been explored in older adults in the laboratory and, like other kinds of memory strategies, they seem not to be engaged spontaneously by older people. Early studies of the levels of processing effects (Craik, 1977) indicated that older adults improved their recognition memory when given deep processing instructions relative to intentional learning instructions, whereas young people performed as well or better in the intentional learning condition. A similar finding was recently reported in a study in which participants attempted to learn the names of people (Troyer *et al.*, 2006). Here again, recognition of names was impaired in older adults in the learning condition, but when semantic processing of the names was induced, age differences were eliminated. These findings imply that young people engage semantic processes relatively automatically when trying to learn and remember new material, whereas older adults may not, and suggest that training in semantic elaboration strategies might benefit older adults selectively. Providing deep processing instructions does not always eliminate the age deficit, however, again suggesting that a production deficit may not account for all of the age effects (Craik, 2002; Craik & Kester, 2000).

Self-generated strategies

In a series of experiments with older adults that examined memory for number sequences, Derwinger and colleagues (Derwinger *et al.*, 2003, 2005) demonstrated that practice in a number-consonant mnemonic and practice at generating and remembering numbers using one's own strategies were equally effective in improving recall of number sequences and this benefit was maintained over 8 months. Interestingly, the findings indicated that self-generated strategies were somewhat better for long-term maintenance. These results support the claim that older adults have knowledge of mnemonic strategies and can generate them appropriately, but may need practice to increase their efficient use. Self-generated strategies may also have the advantage that they are based on prior knowledge and do not have to be learned, and they are more likely to be compatible with an individual's cognitive style or preferences.

Generation of materials-to-be-remembered

In numerous experiments, active generation of materials-to-be remembered as opposed to passive reading has been shown to provide memorial benefits across a range of conditions (e.g., Glisky & Rabinowitz, 1985; Slamecka & Graf, 1978). This effect may depend, at least partly, on the increased semantic processing that is usually required for generation. Early experiments demonstrated that generation effects were of approximately equal magnitude in older and younger adults (Rabinowitz, 1989), and more recent studies have found that these

advantages extend to individuals in early stages of Alzheimer's disease (Multhaup & Balota, 1997). Beyond the mild stage of AD, however, generation effects are generally not found (e.g., Dick *et al.*, 1989). These observations are consistent with the notion that the generation effect relies partly on a preserved semantic memory, which remains relatively intact in the early stages of AD but becomes increasingly compromised as the disease progresses.

In a related vein, it has been found that performing an action (Cohen, 1981) compared to reading an action sentence (e.g., break the toothpick) provides memory benefits for both older and younger adults. This self-enactment effect has sometimes been found to be equivalent in older and younger adults (e.g., Rönnlund *et al.*, 2003) but at other times has appeared greater in older adults, thus reducing the age differences relative to a non-action condition (e.g., Bäckman, 1985). The selective benefit to older adults in some studies may occur because young adults spontaneously generate meaningful elaborative encoding processes and so attain no further benefit from enactment. Older adults, on the other hand, may fail to initiate effective encoding processes, and so benefit from the requirement to perform the specified action.

Self-referential processing

Processing information in relation to the self has long been known to provide memory benefits in young people (Rogers *et al.*, 1977), but few studies have investigated this effect in older adults. In a recent experiment in our lab (Glisky & Marquine, in press), normally aging older adults showed a beneficial effect of self-referential processing on subsequent memory for trait adjectives, relative to a shallow encoding condition. In this case, the benefit was greatest (and equal to that observed in young people) in older individuals whose overall memories were above average. For those with poorer memories, the benefit of self-referential processing was still evident but reduced. These findings highlight the individual differences that exist within a normally aging cohort and again point out that the success of some interventions depends on the degree of residual memory function.

Integrative encoding

Considerable evidence suggests that older adults have particular difficulty remembering arbitrary associations such as unrelated paired associates, name/face pairings, and contextual or source information (e.g., Glisky *et al.*, 1995; Naveh-Benjamin, 2000). Interactive visual imagery strategies (as outlined above), which have been used effectively for the learning of name/face pairings, often involve creating a meaningful link between a name and a feature of the face (Troyer *et al.*, 2006; Yesavage *et al.*, 1983). Similarly, it has been shown that source memory deficits in older adults can be eliminated when the item and its source are integrated at encoding. For example, Glisky *et al.* (2001) demonstrated that when older adults were required to answer an encoding question such as "How well does this particular chair fit in this room?" subsequent memory for the contextual information (i.e., the location of the chair) was improved selectively in older adults, completely eliminating the normal age-related source memory deficit. Interestingly, in this study, the benefit was specific to those individuals with below-average executive function, suggesting that it is this subgroup of people that have difficulty initiating integrative encoding processes. These findings again suggest that older adults are capable of carrying out the processing necessary for good memory performance but do not always do so unless given appropriate task instructions.

Training of an integrative encoding strategy was also attempted by Schmidt *et al.* (2001) in a prospective memory task in older adults. In this study, people were taught to associate an intended future action with retrieval cues that were expected to be present when the action had to be performed. Findings indicated a small advantage for the training group relative to a control group, but the advantage was not maintained at a 3-month follow-up. Only 6 hours of training were provided in this study, however, which may have been insufficient to produce long-term benefits.

Summary of encoding strategies

The majority of encoding strategies involve the creation and generation of meaningful links to prior knowledge or the integration of content to context, and their initiation appears to be resource-demanding for older people. Under most conditions, older adults do not initiate these strategies spontaneously but do benefit from instruction and training, although long-term gains and generalization have been demonstrated infrequently. To increase long-term gains, extensive practice is probably necessary so that demands on limited resources are reduced and strategy implementation becomes more automatic. Also of note are the considerable individual differences that exist among older adults such that strategies will not benefit everyone. Because these methods rely on residual memory ability, they are likely to be most effective in older adults who retain substantial memory and/or executive function.

Training retrieval processes

Recollection

Relatively few studies have focused on improving retrieval aspects of remembering. One notable exception is the work of Jennings & Jacoby (2003; Jennings *et al.*, 2005). These studies are based on findings that older adults are impaired in the controlled process of recollecting specific details of prior memory experiences but have no deficits in making the more automatic familiarity judgments of prior occurrence (Jacoby *et al.*, 1996; Jennings & Jacoby, 1993). In a recent training study, Jennings & Jacoby (2003) demonstrated that older adults can be trained to overcome their tendency to base decisions on familiarity (which in their paradigm would lead to an error) and instead base memory judgments on recollection. Specifically, people were trained, using a modified spaced retrieval technique, to increase their ability to detect and reject repetitions of distractors in a recognition test across gradually increasing delays extending from an initial lag of two items up to a lag of as many as 28 intervening items. Lags increased systematically as a function of performance, and materials changed across sessions, suggesting that a strategy had been learned rather than a specific set of items. In addition, this incremented difficulty approach was twice as effective as simple practice at random lags. In a follow-up study (Jennings *et al.*, 2005), recollection-based training was shown to transfer to a rather different set of laboratory memory tasks (e.g., source memory, self-ordered pointing). This finding is consistent with the notion that recollection, like source memory and other working memory tasks, is at least partly dependent on prefrontal function (e.g., Davidson & Glisky, 2002). Recollection-based training is therefore most likely to be beneficial for individuals with substantially preserved residual executive as well as memory abilities.

Non-mnemonic methods

Practice, study time, experience, schooling

Extensive practice regimens (Woolverton *et al.*, 2001) and greater amounts of study time (Wahlin *et al.*, 1995) usually result in improved memory performance in older adults, but do not usually eliminate age differences. At the same time, minimal age effects are observed in memory for information that is highly familiar or within one's area of expertise. For example, Shimamura *et al.* (1995) found no differences among university professors in text recall, a task in which professors are more or less continuously engaged, although age deficits were observed in memory for unrelated paired associates, reflecting the usual age-related deficits in memory for arbitrary associations. These findings suggest that continued schooling into the upper years might reduce age-related memory decline by enabling use or practice of memory-relevant activities, although the benefits of such activity are likely to be relatively task-specific. Evidence supporting the

beneficial effects of current schooling is mixed, however (Parks *et al.*, 1986; Zivian & Darjes, 1983), although several studies have shown that educational and occupational attainment is positively correlated with good memory function in old age (e.g., Albert *et al.*, 1995; Hill *et al.*, 1995; Zelinski *et al.*, 1993) and is associated with reduced incidence of AD (Stern, 2002).

Leisure activity, exercise and physical fitness

There is mounting evidence from population-based longitudinal studies to suggest that a more cognitively, socially and physically active lifestyle is associated with better cognitive outcomes (for reviews, see Colcombe & Kramer, 2003; Fratiglioni *et al.*, 2004; see also Chapters 15, by Scherder and Eggermont, and 24, by Kramer, Erickson and McAuley in this volume). For example, the Bronx Aging Study (Verghese *et al.*, 2003, 2006) and the Chongqing Aging Study (Wang *et al.*, 2006) examined large groups of older adults across more than 5 years and found that engaging in cognitively stimulating leisure activities, such as reading and playing board games, helped preserve memory functions and decreased the risk of developing amnestic MCI and Alzheimer's disease. Other studies have reported a consistent positive association between physical exercise and cognitive functioning (e.g., Colcombe & Kramer, 2003; Lautenschlager & Almeida, 2006) with the largest effects observed in executive control tasks (including working memory), particularly when exercise is aerobic (but see Lachman *et al.*, 2006 for positive non-aerobic finding). Most studies have controlled for the effects of potentially confounding variables, such as education, intellectual function, health status and baseline performance levels, increasing the likelihood that activity or physical fitness is the causal variable. In addition, benefits have been found both for lifetime levels of fitness and exercise participation, as well as for short-term exercise regimens introduced to sedentary older individuals as interventions (e.g., Colcombe *et al.*, 2004).

The mechanism by which activity influences cognitive functioning is not well understood. Possible psychological explanations have included increasing cognitive reserve, reducing chronic stress, promoting a generally healthy lifestyle, and increasing feelings of well-being (e.g., Stevens *et al.*, 2001). At a neurophysiological level, fMRI studies have reported differences in brain activity in physically fit individuals and in those who participated in an aerobic training intervention (Colcombe *et al.*, 2004). Animal studies have suggested that aerobic training increases levels of various neurochemicals, including brain-derived neurotrophic factor, which in turn can increase plasticity, neuronal survival and the development of new neurons and synapses. Other findings have suggested that aerobic exercise increases neurogenesis in the hippocampus in particular (e.g., van Praag *et al.*, 1999). Whatever the mechanism, an active lifestyle appears to be associated with higher levels of cognitive function and lower incidence of AD, and may also delay the onset of clinical symptoms associated with AD (e.g., Andel *et al.*, 2006; Karp *et al.*, 2006; Scarmeas & Stern, 2003).

Time of day

Studies have shown that older and younger adults experience peak circadian arousal levels at different times of day: most older people are at their peak early in the day whereas most young adults experience their peak in the late afternoon (May *et al.*, 1993). Moreover, the effectiveness of certain cognitive processes is correlated with circadian arousal levels. For example, in a difficult test of recognition memory, May *et al.* (1993) found that older adults (as well as young) performed significantly more accurately when tested in their preferred time of day and there were no age-related deficits when testing occurred in the morning (i.e., in the optimal time of day for the older people). Hasher *et al.* (1999) have since shown that time of day may be particularly important for cognitive tasks that require inhibitory control and may have relatively little if any effect on tasks that require the relatively automatic retrieval of well-learned information. Because inhibitory processes appear to be important for the efficient operation of working memory (Hasher & Zacks, 1988), any cognitive activities that require working memory are likely to show deficits when attempted at off-peak times.

Pharmacologic interventions

Pharmacologic interventions (see also Chapters 17–19 in this volume) including the use of cholinesterase inhibitors have been extensively studied in AD, where they have been found to provide some symptomatic relief in patients in the early stages of the disease. Use of these drugs in older adults with memory complaints that are insufficient to warrant a diagnosis of probable AD is just beginning, but early results suggest that treatment with cholinergic drugs in preclinical phases of AD may have positive effects on hippocampal function and hippocampally dependent memory tasks (Grön *et al.*, 2006).

There are also a number of readily available nonprescription substances that have been shown to have positive effects on memory. Ingestion of glucose (relative to saccharin), for example, has been found to increase free recall performance in older adults (Manning *et al.*, 1997) as well as in people with AD (Manning *et al.*, 1993), but not in young people. Although the exact mechanism of this effect is uncertain, older adults show poorer regulation of glucose, which may account for its age-specific memory benefits. Further, the beneficial effects of glucose appear to be selective to hippocampally dependent memory tasks (Winocur, 1995), consistent with findings of increased levels of acetylcholine following glucose injection in the hippocampus of rats when they are performing a memory task (Ragozzino *et al.*, 1996).

Caffeine is another easily obtainable substance that has been shown to have positive effects on memory in older adults. Ryan *et al.* (2002) demonstrated that giving older adults caffeine in the afternoon at their nonoptimal time of day substantially improved their performance relative to a noncaffeine control. They suggested that the increased arousal provided by the caffeine offset the decreasing circadian arousal levels experienced by most older people in the afternoon.

Summary of optimization methods

Training in the use of explicit encoding and retrieval processes such as visual imagery, semantic and generative strategies, and the use of recollection at retrieval is likely to provide benefits to older adults with residual explicit memory function. Because many of these strategies are resource-demanding, however, extensive amounts of practice are required so that initiation and use of the strategies becomes more efficient. Without such practice, strategies are unlikely to be maintained over time or transfer to untrained tasks or real-world situations. More general mnemonic benefits may also be achieved through aerobic exercise, active lifestyles and continued education, and these activities have also been shown to reduce the incidence and symptoms of AD.

Substitution of intact function for declining or lost function

- These methods use alternative intact processes and brain regions to accomplish memory activities, particularly those associated with implicit and procedural memory.
- Methods are appropriate for those with more serious memory deficits including those with MCI and AD.
- Methods include spaced retrieval, vanishing cues, errorless learning and the use of previously learned skills or expertise.

This approach to rehabilitation assumes that memory processes normally used in younger years may no longer be available to older adults or may be sufficiently compromised as to be nonfunctional. To overcome these deficits, other intact processes, not normally used in the performance of episodic memory tasks, may have to be recruited. This reorganization of function at the cognitive level is assumed to be supported by a reorganization of

function at the neural level (Luria, 1963; Woodruff-Pak & Hanson, 1995). The methods subsumed under this approach are appropriate for a broader range of older adults including those with mild to moderate Alzheimer's disease (for reviews, see De Vreese *et al.*, 2001; Grandmaison & Simard, 2003). These techniques generally will not benefit normal young adults without declining memory function as these individuals have no need to recruit alternative processes.

Implicit and procedural memory

Numerous studies have demonstrated that implicit and procedural memory hold up well with age, suggesting that a reasonable strategy for intervention might be to recruit these intact implicit memory processes to compensate for explicit memory functions that may have been compromised by age (Howard, 1996). Although this tactic has been used with some success among brain-damaged patients (for reviews, see Glisky, 2004; Glisky & Glisky, 2002), relatively little is known about its potential for use among normally aging older adults. Descriptions of some methods that tap implicit processes are outlined below.

Spaced retrieval

The spaced retrieval technique (Landauer & Bjork, 1978) is a relatively simple rehearsal method in which to-be-learned information is retrieved repeatedly at gradually increasing delays. Although the effects of spaced practice compared to massed practice are well-documented in young people, relatively few studies have investigated the spacing effect or the effects of spaced retrieval in normally aging older adults. In a recent study in older people, Craik (2006) reported that successful retrieval of information was found to be more effective than simple repetition and the benefits were greater at longer lags (8 items) when retrieval was most demanding. Similarly, Balota *et al.* (2006) found large benefits of spaced versus massed practice in healthy older adults and in individuals with mild

AD, but did not find an advantage for expanding lags relative to fixed intervals. Retrieval at long lags, however, is unlikely to be successful initially in people with memory impairments, and so the standard spaced retrieval technique with gradually increasing lags is recommended.

A number of studies have demonstrated the effectiveness of the spaced retrieval technique in individuals with AD, who were able to learn the names of familiar people in their environment, the locations of objects and daily calendar use (Camp, 1989; Camp et al., 1996; Camp & McKitrick, 1992), and retain them over a period of several weeks (for review, see Camp et al., 2000). In these studies, only a single stimulus was trained at a time, feedback was provided, and lags were adjusted downward when retrieval was unsuccessful. In a more recent study, Hawley & Cherry (2004) demonstrated that patients could also learn a novel name-face association using this method, and that such learning was transferable from a photograph to the real person in about half of the studied cases. There was little evidence in this study for long-term retention (i.e., beyond 6 minutes), however. Camp and colleagues have speculated that this relatively effortless retrieval method, in which retention intervals are increased only when success is achieved at a shorter interval, may rely on relatively automatic and effortless implicit memory processes. However, findings of positive effects in normal young and old people suggest that explicit memory may also benefit from this method (for discussion, see Camp et al., 2000). Note also that the technique as used here to teach specific pieces of information differs from the previously described modified version of spaced retrieval used by Jennings and colleagues (Jennings & Jacoby, 2003; Jennings et al., 2005), in which older adults were taught an explicit recollective strategy that could be applied to new materials.

Vanishing cues

The method of vanishing cues (Glisky et al., 1986) was designed specifically to take advantage of preserved implicit memory processes in amnesic patients. The technique involves the use of partial cue information, which is gradually withdrawn or faded across learning trials until a target is produced in the absence of cues (e.g., save, sav_, sa__, s___, ____). It has been used successfully to teach memory-impaired individuals, including those with AD, specific pieces of meaningful information relevant to a variety of everyday tasks, although it appears to be less useful for the learning of arbitrary associations such as name-face pairs, which cannot be learned implicitly (Thöne & Glisky, 1995). Normally aging older adults, however, seem not to benefit from this method; in two studies in our lab exploring the learning of new vocabulary in older people, no advantage was observed for the vanishing cues procedure relative to an anticipation procedure. These findings are consistent with the view that the method of vanishing cues depends primarily on implicit memory processes, and is useful only for individuals with severe impairments in explicit memory. For people with only mild memory deficits, such as those that occur in normal aging, using implicit processes may be less reliable than using residual explicit memory function.

Errorless learning

Errorless learning (Baddeley, 1992; Baddeley & Wilson, 1994) is a training method that relies on eliminating or minimizing errors, and is thought to be particularly effective for individuals with severe memory impairment (Evans et al., 2000; Wilson et al., 1994), who must depend on implicit memory processes in order to acquire new information (Page et al., 2006). It has not been found to be consistently effective for normally aging older adults (Baddeley & Wilson, 1994), who do not use implicit memory processes for most memory tasks. Nevertheless, under some difficult testing circumstances, older adults may rely on less demanding implicit processes such as familiarity rather than use an explicit controlled process such as recollection. In a recent paper using the process dissociation procedure (Jacoby, 1991), Anderson & Craik (2006) found that errorless learning had a positive effect on memory in older adults by reducing familiarity-based errors, but had a negative effect in young adults by reducing recollection. The authors suggested that errorless learning reduces errors in those individuals relying on implicit memory, but also prevents elaboration during encoding, thus reducing the likelihood of explicit retrieval.

Errorless learning has also been used effectively with people who have AD. In these individuals, the method has been used primarily for the re-learning of previously known information, such as the names of friends or famous people (Clare *et al.*, 1999, 2002; Winter & Hunkin, 1999), and has been most effective when combined with other techniques such as vanishing cues and spaced retrieval (e.g., Clare *et al.*, 1999, 2002). For example, Clare and colleagues (1999) taught a 72-year-old man in the early stages of AD, the names of 11 members of his support group, using spaced retrieval and vanishing cues to ensure errorless learning, along with an elaborative mnemonic strategy. Learning transferred from photographs to the faces in the real-world environment and was largely (70%) maintained 2 years later (Clare *et al.*, 2001). Given the combination of strategies, however, it is difficult to assess the contribution of errorless learning per se. Nevertheless, these studies provide some indication that patients in the early stages of AD are able to re-learn information of personal relevance and thus enhance their quality of life.

Skills and expertise

There is considerable evidence that procedural memory and skill learning are preserved as people age and that people with domain-specific expertise continue to maintain high levels of performance across the lifespan. For example, Salthouse (1984) found that expert typists maintained typing speed into their 70s, despite the fact that the component skills required for typing, such as finger tapping speed and choice reaction time declined. Salthouse determined that skilled typists maintained overall performance levels by looking further ahead at material to be typed, thus substituting an intact function to compensate for age-related declines in other functions. Similarly, Charness (1989) reported that older chess experts were as accurate as young experts in selecting the best move in a chess game despite declining working memory capacities. Charness suggested that older experts developed more efficient chunking and search strategies, which reduced working memory demands and enabled them to maintain high levels of performance.

There are few studies that have attempted to capitalise on procedural memory to alleviate memory problems in normal older adults or those with AD. One such study (Zanetti *et al.*, 2001) demonstrated that people with mild to moderate AD were able to improve their performance on several activities of daily living (e.g., washing face, using the telephone) by means of a behavioral shaping procedure with cues and reinforcement, along with modeling of the task. The authors suggested that this success was attributable to preservation of procedural memory, which could be recruited to retrain or reactivate previously learned skills.

Summary of substitution methods

These findings have clear-cut implications for rehabilitation. First, deficits in some processes may be offset by the substitution of alternative processes that are less affected by age. Second, knowledge, which increases in normal aging, may be able to compensate for age-related deficits in encoding, retrieval or other speeded processes. Third, in a practical sense, older people with extensive experience in a particular field (e.g., a job) may be able to maintain performance in that domain, despite declining function in other domains (Park, 1994). Finally, in people with AD, one may be able to take advantage of preserved procedural memory to teach skills that are relevant in their daily lives (see Glisky, 1995 for demonstration of computer training in an individual with amnesia).

External compensation for lost or reduced function

- External memory aids and environmental support can benefit even those with severe memory impairments.
- External aids such as diaries, notebooks, calendars, alarm watches, PDAs and pagers are all appropriate, but may require considerable training in their use, particularly for those individuals with AD.
- Use of environmental cues and prior knowledge may also be helpful.

Another way that older adults may compensate for declining memory abilities is through the use of external aids or environmental support. To a large extent these external compensations can benefit all older adults, even those with severe memory deficits, because they do not depend on memory ability or internal mnemonic processes. Instead, they provide a way to achieve desired functional outcomes while placing minimal cognitive demands on the user.

External memory aids

External aids can take a variety of forms and serve a variety of purposes (for review, see Kapur *et al.*, 2002). Diaries, notebooks and lists can be used to record and store information so that it is easily retrievable when needed. Calendars, appointment books, alarm watches and timers can provide prompts and reminders for future actions. Older adults, particularly those in the younger 65–75 age range, are also becoming increasingly computer literate and are more comfortable with a variety of electronic devices (e.g., PDAs) that might be used to keep track of appointments and other personal information. For those not familiar with electronic aids, however, training in their use may be required and may be successful only for those without serious memory impairment. Training may also be needed even for the more familiar memory aids, particularly for individuals with AD. For example, Clare *et al.* (2000) used an errorless learning approach to train an individual with AD to use a calendar to keep track of his appointments. The training significantly reduced the number of repeated questions directed towards his caregiver. Attempts to train another patient with AD in the use of an electronic paging device – NeuroPage – however, were unsuccessful. Wilson and colleagues (2001) have had considerable success with NeuroPage in patients with nonprogressive memory disorders and so this remains a possibility particularly with those in the earliest stages of the disease.

Environmental support

Craik (1986, 2005) has argued that memory involves an interaction between internal mnemonic processes and external environmental influences. As people age, they become increasingly less able to initiate effortful encoding and retrieval processes and are therefore increasingly more reliant on environmental support. Tasks such as free recall that provide no cues at retrieval tend to show large age-related declines, whereas tasks such as recognition show less or no decline particularly if support is also provided at encoding. Age differences are also often reduced or eliminated when the studied materials themselves seem to drive meaningful processing such as when complex pictures are studied (Park *et al.*, 1986). Recently, Craik (2005) has suggested that "schematic support" from past learning can also be used to compensate for memory decline. For example, in a study in which the relatedness of word pairs was varied, older adults achieved a greater benefit from the relatedness than young adults. In this case, prior semantic knowledge appeared to automatically engage meaningful processing, thus creating a more elaborate memory trace of the related pairs. Such schematic support may be available to people in the early stages of AD but is likely to erode as semantic memory is increasingly affected by the disease.

Conclusions

In recent years, as the population has aged, there has been increasing interest in finding ways to enhance life experiences at the upper end of the lifespan. Maintenance of good memory function has been at the forefront of these efforts. This chapter has outlined the major methods of memory rehabilitation that have been attempted to date and has suggested some boundary conditions for their use. First, methods that involve the training of strategies are likely to be useful only for people who have substantial residual memory function that can be reactivated and trained to be used more efficiently. For those individuals with more compromised memory function including those with AD, alternative processes or brain regions will have to be recruited to enable learning of new information. For those with very severe memory deficits, only external compensations are likely to be useful. Second, semantic memory and prior knowledge, which remain largely accessible in normal aging and in the early stages of AD, and active lifestyles including continuing education and aerobic exercise, may help to moderate the negative effects of aging on memory and other cognitive functions. Third, considerable individual differences exist in cognitive and brain aging, even among those who appear to be aging normally, and so all strategies will likely not suit all individuals. Recent neuroimaging studies, which have focused on individual differences, have suggested that the aging brain retains considerable plasticity although compensatory processes seem to be more available to some people than others. What accounts for these individual differences is unclear, but a reasonable hypothesis is that those people that have considerable cognitive reserve, acquired perhaps as a result of education, occupation or active lifestyle, may be more able to adapt to or compensate for age-related changes (Stern, 2002). As yet, there are few studies documenting changes in brain activation patterns as a result of interventions (but see Colcombe et al., 2004), and this would seem to be an important direction for future research.

REFERENCES

Albert, M., Duffy, F. H., & Naeser, M. (1987). Nonlinear changes in cognition with age and their neuropsychologic correlates. *Canadian Journal of Psychology*, **41**, 141–157.

Albert, M. S., Jones, K. S., Savage, C. R., & Berkman, L. (1995). Predictors of cognitive change in older persons: MacArthur studies of successful aging. *Psychology and Aging*, **10**, 578–589.

Andel, R., Vigen, C., Mack, W. J., Clark, L. J., & Gatz, M. (2006). The effect of education and occupational complexity on rate of cognitive decline in Alzheimer's patients. *Journal of the International Neuropsychological Society*, **12**, 147–152.

Anderson, N. D., & Craik, F. I. M. (2006). The mnemonic mechanisms of errorless learning. *Neuropsychologia*, **44**, 2806–2813.

Bäckman, L. (1985). Further evidence for the lack of adult age differences on free recall of subject-performed tasks: the importance of motor action. *Human Learning: Journal of Practical Research and Applications*, **4**, 79–87.

Bäckman, L., Almkvist, O., Andersson, J. et al. (1997). Brain activation in young and older adults during implicit and explicit retrieval. *Journal of Cognitive Neuroscience*, **9**, 378–391.

Baddeley, A. D. (1992). Implicit memory and errorless learning: a link between cognitive theory and neuropsychological rehabilitation. In L. R. Squire & N. Butters (Eds.), *Neuropsychology of Memory* (pp. 309–321). New York, NY: Guilford Press.

Baddeley, A. D., & Wilson, B. A. (1994). When implicit learning fails: amnesia and the problem of error elimination. *Neuropsychologia*, **32**, 53–68.

Ball, K., Berch, D. B., & Helmers, K. F. (2002). Effects of cognitive training interventions with older adults: a randomized controlled trial. *Journal of the American Medical Association*, **288**, 2271–2281.

Balota, D. A., Duchek, J. M., Sergent-Marshall, S. D., & Roediger III, H. L. (2006). Does expanded retrieval produce benefits over equal-interval spacing? Explorations of spacing effects in healthy aging and early stage Alzheimer's disease. *Psychology and Aging*, **21**, 19–31.

Braak, H., & Braak, E. (1991). Neuropathological staging of Alzheimer-related changes. *Acta Neuropathologica*, **82**, 239–259.

Cabeza, R., & Nyberg, L. (2000). Imaging cognition II: an empirical review of 275 PET and fMRI studies. *Journal of Cognitive Neuroscience*, **12**, 1–47.

Cabeza, R., Anderson, N. D., Houle, S., Mangels, J. A., & Nyberg, L. (2000). Age-related differences in neural activity during item and temporal-order memory retrieval: a positron emission tomography study. *Journal of Cognitive Neuroscience*, **12**, 197–206.

Cabeza, R., Anderson, N. D., Locantore, J. K., & McIntosh, A. R. (2002). Aging gracefully: compensatory brain activity in high-performing older adults. *Neuroimage*, **17**, 1394–1402.

Camp, C. J. (1989). Facilitation of new learning in Alzheimer's disease. In G. C. Gilmore, P. J. Whitehouse, & M. L. Wykle (Eds.), *Memory, Aging, and Dementia* (pp. 212–225). New York, NY: Springer.

Camp, C. J., & McKitrick, L. A. (1992). Memory interventions in Alzheimer's-type dementia populations: methodological and theoretical issues. In R. L. West & J. D. Sinnott (Eds.), *Everyday Memory and Aging: Current Research and Methodology* (pp. 155–172). New York, NY: Springer.

Camp, C. J., Foss, J. W., Stevens, A. B., & O'Hanlon, A. M. (1996). Improving prospective memory task performance in persons with Alzheimer's disease. In M. Brandimonte, G. O. Einstein, & M. A. McDaniel (Eds.), *Prospective Memory: Theory and Applications* (pp. 351–367). Mahwah, NJ: Lawrence Erlbaum.

Camp, C. J., Bird, M. J., & Cherry, K. E. (2000). Retrieval strategies as a rehabilitation aid for cognitive loss in pathological aging. In R. D. Hill, L. Bäckman, & A. Stigsdotter Neely (Eds.), *Cognitive Rehabilitation in Old Age* (pp. 224–248). Oxford, UK: Oxford University Press.

Charness, N. (1989). Age and expertise: Responding to Talland's challenge. In L. W. Poon, D. C. Rubin, & B. A. Wilson (Eds.), *Everyday Cognition in Adulthood and Late Life* (pp. 437–456). Cambridge, UK: Cambridge University Press.

Clare, L., Wilson, B. A., Breen, K., & Hodges, J. R. (1999). Errorless learning of face-name associations in early Alzheimer's disease. *Neurocase*, **5**, 37–46.

Clare, L., Wilson, B. A., Carter, G. *et al.* (2000). Intervening with everyday memory problems in dementia of Alzheimer type: an errorless learning approach. *Journal of Clinical and Experimental Neuropsychology*, **22**, 132–146.

Clare, L., Wilson, B. A., Carter, G., Hodges, J. R., & Adams, M. (2001). Long-term maintenance of treatment gains following a cognitive rehabilitation intervention in early dementia of Alzheimer type: a single case study. *Neuropsychological Rehabilitation*, **11**, 477–494.

Clare, L., Wilson, B. A., Carter, G., Roth, I., & Hodges, J. R. (2002). Relearning face-name associations in early Alzheimer's disease. *Neuropsychology*, **16**, 538–547.

Cohen, R. L. (1981). On the generality of some memory laws. *Scandinavian Journal of Psychology*, **22**, 267–281.

Colcombe, S., & Kramer, A. F. (2003). Fitness effects on the cognitive function of older adults: a meta-analytic study. *Psychological Science*, **14**, 125–130.

Colcombe, S. J., Kramer, A. F., Erickson, K. I. *et al.* (2004). Cardiovascular fitness, cortical plasticity, and aging. *Proceedings of the National Academy of Sciences of the United States of America*, **101**, 3316–3321.

Colcombe, S. J., Kramer, A. F., Erickson, K. I., & Scalf, P. (2005). The implications of cortical recruitment and brain morphology for individual differences in inhibitory function in aging humans. *Psychology and Aging*, **20**, 363–375.

Craik, F. I. M. (1977). Age differences in human memory. In J. E. Birren & W. Schaie (Eds.), *Handbook of the Psychology of Aging* (pp. 384–420). New York, NY: Van Nostrand Reinhold.

Craik, F. I. M. (1983). On the transfer of information from temporary to permanent memory. *Philosophical Transactions of the Royal Society of London, Series B*, **302**, 341–359.

Craik, F. I. M. (1986). A functional account of age differences in memory. In F. Klix, & H. Hagendorf (Eds.), *Human Memory and Cognitive Capabilities, Mechanisms and Performances* (pp. 409–422). Amsterdam, NL: Elsevier.

Craik, F. I. M. (2002). Human memory and aging. In L. Bäckman, & C. von Hofsten (Eds.), *Psychology at the Turn of the Millennium* (pp. 261–280). Hove, UK: Psychology Press.

Craik, F. I. M. (2005). On reducing age-related declines in memory and executive control. In J. Duncan, P. McLeod, & L. Phillips (Eds.), *Measuring the Mind: Speed, Control and Age* (pp. 273–290). Oxford, UK: Oxford University Press.

Craik, F. I. M. (2006). Age-related changes in human memory: Practical consequences. In L.-G. Nilsson, & N. Ohta (Eds.), *Memory and Society: Psychological Perspectives* (pp. 181–197). New York, NY: Psychology Press.

Craik, F. I. M., & Jennings, J. M. (1992). Human memory. In F. I. M. Craik, & T. A. Salthouse (Eds.), *The Handbook of Aging and Cognition* (pp. 51–110). Hillsdale, NJ: Lawrence Erlbaum.

Craik, F. I. M., & Kester, J. D. (2000). Divided attention and memory: impairment of processing or consolidation? In E. Tulving (Ed.), *Memory, Consciousness, and the Brain* (pp. 38–51). Philadelphia, PA: Psychology Press.

Daselaar, S., & Cabeza, R. (2005). Age-related changes in hemispheric organization. In R. Cabeza, L. Nyberg, & D. Park (Eds.), *Cognitive Neuroscience of Aging* (pp. 186–217). Oxford, UK: Oxford University Press.

Davidson, P. S. R., & Glisky, E. L. (2002). Neuropsychological correlates of recollection and familiarity in normal aging. *Cognitive, Affective and Behavioral Neuroscience*, **2**, 174–186.

De Vreese, L. P., Neri, M., Fioravanti, M., Belloi, L., & Zanetti, O. (2001). Memory rehabilitation in Alzheimer's disease: a review of progress. *International Journal of Geriatric Psychiatry*, **16**, 794–809.

Derwinger, A., Stigsdotter Neely, A., Persson, M., Hill, R. D., & Bäckman, L. (2003). Remembering numbers in old age: mnemonic training versus self-generated strategy training. *Aging, Neuropsychology, and Cognition*, **10**, 202–214.

Derwinger, A., Stigsdotter Neely, A., & Bäckman, L. (2005). Design your own memory strategies! Self-generated strategy training versus mnemonic training in old age: an 8-month follow-up. *Neuropsychological Rehabilitation*, **15**, 37–54.

Dick, M. B., Kean, M.-L., & Sands, D. (1989). Memory for internally generated words in Alzheimer-type dementia: breakdown in encoding and semantic memory. *Brain and Cognition*, **9**, 88–108.

Einstein, G. O., McDaniel, M. A., Richardson, S. L., Guynn, M. J., & Cunfer, A. R. (1995). Aging and prospective memory: examining the influences of self-initiated retrieval processes. *Journal of Experimental Psychology: Learning, Memory, and Cognition*, **21**, 996–1007.

Evans, J. J., Wilson, B. A., Schuri, U. *et al.* (2000). A comparison of "errorless" and "trial-and-error" learning methods for teaching individuals with acquired memory deficits. *Neuropsychological Rehabilitation*, **10**, 67–101.

Fratiglioni, L., Paillard-Borg, S., & Winblad, B. (2004). An active and socially integrated lifestyle in late life might protect against dementia. *Lancet Neurology*, **3**, 343–353.

Glisky, E. L. (1995). Acquisition and transfer of word processing skill by an amnesic patient. *Neuropsychological Rehabilitation*, **5**, 299–318.

Glisky, E. L. (2004). Disorders of memory. In J. Ponsford (Eds.), *Cognitive and Behavioral Rehabilitation* (pp. 100–128). New York, NY: Guilford Press.

Glisky, E. L., & Glisky, M. L. (2002). Learning and memory impairments. In P. J. Eslinger (Eds.), *Neuropsychological Interventions* (pp. 137–162). New York, NY: Guilford Press.

Glisky, E. L., & Marquine, M. J. (in press). Semantic and self-referential processing of positive and negative trait adjectives in older adults. *Memory*.

Glisky, E. L., & Rabinowitz, J. C. (1985). Enhancing the generation effect through repetition of operations. *Journal of Experimental Psychology: Learning, Memory, and Cognition*, **11**, 193–205.

Glisky, E. L., Schacter, D. L., & Tulving, E. (1986). Learning and retention of computer related vocabulary in memory-impaired patients: method of vanishing cues. *Journal of Clinical and Experimental Neuropsychology*, **8**, 292–312.

Glisky, E. L., Polster, M. R., & Routhieaux, B. C. (1995). Double dissociation between item and source memory. *Neuropsychology*, **9**, 229–235.

Glisky, E. L., Rubin, S. R., & Davidson, P. S. R. (2001). Source memory in older adults: an encoding or retrieval problem? *Journal of Experimental Psychology: Learning, Memory, and Cognition*, **27**, 1131–1146.

Grady, C. L., McIntosh, A. R., Horwitz, B. *et al.* (1995). Age-related reductions in human recognition memory due to impaired encoding. *Science*, **269**, 218–221.

Grady, C. L., Bernstein, L., Beig, S., & Siegenthaler, A. (2002). The effects of encoding task on age-related differences in the functional neuroanatomy of face memory. *Psychology and Aging*, **17**, 7–23.

Grandmaison, E., & Simard, M. (2003). A critical review of memory stimulation programs in Alzheimer's disease. *Journal of Neuropsychiatry and Clinical Neuroscience*, **15**, 130–144.

Grön, G., Brandenburg, I., Wunderlich, A. P., & Riepe, M. W. (2006). Inhibition of hippocampal function in mild cognitive impairment: targeting the cholinergic hypothesis. *Neurobiology of Aging*, **27**, 78–87.

Hasher, L., & Zacks, R. T. (1988). Working memory, comprehension, and aging: a review and a new view. In G. H. Bower (Ed.), *The Psychology of Learning and Motivation* (pp. 193–225). New York, NY: Academic Press.

Hasher, L., Zacks, R. T., & May, C. P. (1999). Inhibitory control, circadian arousal, and age. In D. Golpher & A. Koriat (Eds.), *Attention and Performance XVII* (pp. 653–675). Cambridge, MA: MIT Press.

Hawley, K. S., & Cherry, K. E. (2004). Spaced-retrieval effects on name-face recognition in older adults with probably Alzheimer's disease. *Behavior Modification*, **28**, 276–296.

Hedden, T., & Gabrieli, J. D. E. (2004). Insights into the ageing mind: a view from cognitive neuroscience. *Nature Reviews Neuroscience*, **5**, 87–96.

Hill, R. D., Wahlin, A., Winblad, B., & Bäckman, L. (1995). The role of demographic and life style variables in utilizing cognitive support for episodic remembering among very old adults. *Journals of Gerontology, Series B: Psychological Sciences and Social Sciences*, **50**, 219–227.

Howard, D. V. (1996). The aging of implicit and explicit memory. In F. Blanchard-Fields & T. M. Hess (Eds.), *Perspectives on Cognitive Change in Adulthood and Aging* (pp. 221–254). New York, NY: McGraw-Hill.

Jacoby, L. L. (1991). A process dissociation framework: separating automatic from intentional uses of memory. *Journal of Memory and Language*, **30**, 513–541.

Jacoby, L. L., Jennings, J. M., & Hay, J. F. (1996). Dissociating automatic and consciously controlled processes: implications for diagnosis and rehabilitation of memory deficits. In D. J. Herrmann, C. McEvoy, C. Hertzog, P. Hertel, & M. K. Johnson (Eds.), *Basic and Applied Memory Research: Theory in Context* (pp. 161–193). Mahwah, NJ: Lawrence Erlbaum.

Jennings, J. M., & Jacoby, L. L. (1993). Automatic versus intentional uses of memory: aging, attention, and control. *Psychology and Aging*, **8**, 283–293.

Jennings, J. M., & Jacoby, L. L. (2003). Improving memory in older adults: training recollection. *Neuropsychological Rehabilitation*, **13**, 417–440.

Jennings, J. M., Webster, L. M., Kleykamp, B. A., & Dagenbach, D. (2005). Recollection training and transfer effects in older adults: successful use of a repetition-lag procedure. *Aging, Neuropsychology, and Cognition*, **12**, 278–298.

Kapur, N., Glisky, E. L., & Wilson, B. A. (2002). External memory aids and computers in memory rehabilitation. In A. D. Baddeley, M. D. Kopelman, & B. A. Wilson (Eds.), *Handbook of Memory Disorders* (pp. 757–783). Chichester, UK: Wiley.

Karp, A., Paillard-Borg, S., Wang, H.-X. *et al.* (2006). Mental, physical and social components in leisure activities equally contribute to decreased dementia risk. *Dementia and Geriatric Cognitive Disorders*, **21**, 65–73.

Lachman, M. E., Neupert, S. D., Bertrand, R., & Jette, A. M. (2006). The effects of strength training on memory in older adults. *Journal of Aging and Physical Activity*, **14**, 59–73.

Landauer, T. K., & Bjork, R. A. (1978). Optimum rehearsal patterns and name learning. In M. M. Gruneberg, P. E. Morris, & R. N. Sykes (Eds.), *Practical Aspects of Memory* (pp. 625–632). London, UK: Academic Press.

Lautenschlager, N. T., & Almeida, O. P. (2006). Physical activity and cognition in old age. *Current Opinion in Psychiatry*, **19**, 190–193.

Luria, A. R. (1963). *Restoration of Function after Brain Injury*. New York, NY: Macmillan.

Manning, C. A., Ragozzino, M. E., & Gold, P. E. (1993). Glucose enhancement of memory in patients with probable senile dementia of the Alzheimer's type. *Neurobiology of Aging*, **14**, 523–528.

Manning, C. A., Parsons, M. W., Cotter, E. M., & Gold, P. E. (1997). Glucose effects on declarative and nondeclarative memory in healthy elderly and young adults. *Psychobiology*, **25**, 103–108.

Mäntylä, T. (1994). Remembering to remember: adult age differences in prospective memory. *Journals of Gerontology, Series B: Psychological Sciences and Social Sciences*, **49**, 276–282.

May, C. P., Hasher, L., & Stoltzfus, E. R. (1993). Optimal time of day and the magnitude of age differences in memory. *Psychological Science*, **4**, 326–330.

Maylor, E. (1996). Age-related impairment in an event-based prospective-memory task. *Psychology and Aging*, **11**, 74–78.

Maylor, E. A., Smith, G. E., Della Sala, S., & Logie, R. H. (2002). Prospective and retrospective memory in normal aging and dementia: an experimental study. *Memory and Cognition*, **30**, 871–884.

McDaniel, M. A., Einstein, G. O., & Jacoby, L. L. (2008). New considerations in aging and memory: the glass may be all full. In F. I. M. Craik & T. A. Salthouse (Eds.), *The Handbook of Aging and Cognition*. 3rd edn. (pp. 251–310). Hove, UK: Psychology Press.

Moscovitch, M. (1982). A neuropsychological approach to perception and memory in normal and pathological aging. In F. I. M. Craik & S. Trehub (Eds.), *Aging and Cognitive Processes* (pp. 55–79). New York, NY: Plenum Press.

Multhaup, K. S., & Balota, D. A. (1997). Generation effects and source memory in healthy older adults and in adults with dementia of the Alzheimer type. *Neuropsychology*, **11**, 382–391.

Naveh-Benjamin, M. (2000). Adult age differences in memory performance: tests of an associative deficit hypothesis. *Journal of Experimental Psychology: Learning, Memory, and Cognition*, **26**, 1170–1187.

Nyberg, L. (2005). Cognitive training in healthy aging: A cognitive neuroscience perspective. In R. Cabeza, L. Nyberg, & D. Park (Eds.), *Cognitive Neuroscience of Aging* (pp. 309–321). Oxford, UK: Oxford: Oxford University Press.

Page, M., Wilson, B. A., Shiel, A., Carter, G., & Norris, D. (2006). What is the locus of the errorless-learning advantage? *Neuropsychologia*, **44**, 90–100.

Park, D. C. (1994). Aging, cognition, and work. *Human Performance*, **7**, 181–205.

Park, D. C., & Gutchess, A. H. (2005). Long-term memory and aging: a cognitive neuroscience perspective. In R. Cabeza, L. Nyberg, & D. Park (Eds.), *Cognitive Neuroscience of Aging* (pp. 218–245). Oxford, UK: Oxford University Press.

Park, D. D., Puglisi, J. T., & Smith, A. D. (1986). Memory for pictures: does an age-related decline exist? *Psychology and Aging*, **1**, 11–17.

Parks, C. W. J., Mitchell, D. B., & Perlmutter, M. (1986). Cognitive and social functioning across adulthood: age or student status differences? *Psychology and Aging*, **1**, 248–254.

Rabinowitz, J. C. (1989). Judgments of origin and generation effects: comparisons between young and elderly adults. *Psychology and Aging*, **4**, 259–268.

Ragozzino, M. E., Unick, K. E., & Gold, P. E. (1996). Hippocampal acetylcholine release during memory testing in rats: augmentation by glucose. *Proceedings of the National Academy of Sciences of the United States of America*, **93**, 4693–4698.

Raz, N. (2000). Aging of the brain and its impact on cognitive performance: integration of structural and functional findings. In F. I. M. Craik & T. A. Salthouse (Eds.), *The Handbook of Aging and Cognition* (pp. 1–90). Mahwah, NJ: Lawrence Erlbaum.

Raz, N. (2005). The aging brain observed in vivo: differential changes and their modifiers. In R. Cabeza, L. Nyberg, & D. Park (Eds.), *Cognitive Neuroscience of Aging* (pp. 19–57). Oxford, UK: Oxford University Press.

Raz, N., Rodrigue, K. M., & Head, D. (2004). Differential aging of the medial temporal lobe: a study of a five-year change. *Neurology*, **62**, 433–438.

Resnick, S. M., Pham, D. L., Kraut, M. A., Zonderman, A. B., & Davatzikos, C. (2003). Longitudinal magnetic resonance imaging studies of older adults: a shrinking brain. *Journal of Neuroscience*, **23**, 3295–3301.

Rogers, T. B., Kuiper, N. A., & Kirker, W. S. (1977). Self reference and the encoding of personal information. *Journal of Personality and Social Psychology*, **35**, 677–688.

Rönnlund, M., Nyberg, L., Bäckman, L., & Nilsson, L.-G. (2003). Recall of subject-performed tasks, verbal tasks, and cognitive activities across the adult life span: parallel age-related deficits. *Aging, Neuropsychology, and Cognition*, **10**, 182–201.

Ryan, L., Hatfield, C., & Hofstetter, M. (2002). Caffeine reduces time-of-day effects on memory performance in older adults. *Psychological Science*, **13**, 68–71.

Salthouse, T. A. (1984). Effects of age and skill in typing. *Journal of Experimental Psychology: General*, **113**, 345–371.

Salthouse, T. A. (1991). *Theoretical Perspectives on Cognitive Aging*. Hillsdale, NJ: Lawrence Erlbaum.

Scarmeas, N., & Stern, Y. (2003). Cognitive reserve and lifestyle. *Journal of Clinical and Experimental Neuropsychology*, **25**, 625–633.

Schmidt, I. W., Berg, I. J., & Deelman, B. G. (2001). Prospective memory training in older adults. *Educational Gerontology*, **27**, 455–478.

Shimamura, A. P., Berry, J. M., Mangels, J. A., Rusting, C. L., & Jurica, P. J. (1995). Memory and cognitive abilities in university professors: evidence for successful aging. *Psychological Science*, **6**, 271–277.

Slamecka, N. J., & Graf, P. (1978). The generation effect: delineation of a phenomenon. *Journal of Experimental Psychology: Human Learning and Memory*, **4**, 592–604.

Small, S. A., Tsai, W. Y., De LaPaz, R., Mayeux, R., & Stern, Y. (2002). Imaging hippocampal function across the human life span: is memory decline normal or not? *Annals of Neurology*, **51**, 290–295.

Stebbins, G. T., Carillo, M. C., Dorfman, J. *et al.* (2002). Aging effects on memory encoding in the frontal lobes. *Psychology and Aging*, **17**, 44–55.

Stern, Y. (2002). What is cognitive reserve? Theory and research application of the reserve concept. *Journal of the International Neuropsychological Society*, **8**, 448–460.

Stevens, F. C., Kaplan, C. D., Ponds, R., & Jolles, J. (2001). The importance of active lifestyles for memory performance and memory self-knowledge. *Basic Applied Social Psychology*, **23**, 137–145.

Stigsdotter Neely, A. (2000). Multifactorial memory training in normal aging: in search of memory improvement beyond the ordinary. In R. D. Hill, L. Bäckman, & A. Stigsdotter Neely (Eds.), *Cognitive Rehabilitation in Old Age* (pp. 63–80). Oxford, UK: Oxford University Press.

Stigsdotter Neely, A., & Bäckman, L. (1993a). Long-term maintenance of gains from memory training in older adults: two 3 1/2-year follow-up studies. *Journals of Gerontology, Series B: Psychological Sciences and Social Sciences*, **48**, 233–237.

Stigsdotter Neely, A., & Bäckman, L. (1993b). Maintenance of gains following multifactorial and unifactorial memory training in late adulthood. *Educational Gerontology*, **19**, 105–117.

Stigsdotter Neely, A., & Bäckman, L. (1995). Effects of multifactorial memory training in old age: generalizability across tasks and individuals. *Journals of Gerontology, Series B: Psychological Sciences and Social Sciences*, **50**, 134–140.

Thöne, A. I. T., & Glisky, E. L. (1995). Learning of name-face associations in memory impaired patients: a comparison of different training procedures. *Journal of the International Neuropsychological Society*, **1**, 29–38.

Troyer, A. K., Häfliger, A., Cadieux, M. J., & Craik, F. I. M. (2006). Name and face learning in older adults: the effects of level of processing, self-generation, and intention to learn. *Journals of Gerontology, Series B: Psychological Sciences and Social Sciences*, **61**, 67–74.

Tulving, E., Kapur, S., Craik, F. I. M., Moscovitch, M., & Houle, S. (1994). Hemispheric encoding/retrieval asymmetry in episodic memory: positron emission tomography findings. *Proceedings of the National Academy of Sciences of the United States of America*, **91**, 2016–2020.

Van Petten, C., Plante, E., Davidson, P. S. R. *et al.* (2004). Memory and executive function in older adults: relationships with temporal and prefrontal gray matter volumes. *Neuropsychologia*, **42**, 1313–1335.

van Praag, H., Christie, B. R., Sejnowski, T. J., & Gage, F. H. (1999). Running enhances neurogenesis, learning, and long-term potentiation in mice. *Proceedings of the National Academy of Sciences of the United States of America*, **96**, 13427–13431.

Verghese, J., Lipton, R. B., Katz, M. J. *et al.* (2003). Leisure activities and the risk of dementia in the elderly. *New England Journal of Medicine*, **348**, 2508–2516.

Verghese, J., LeValley, A., Derby, C. *et al.* (2006). Leisure activities and the risk of amnestic mild cognitive impairment in the elderly. *Neurology*, **66**, 821–827.

Verhaeghen, P., & Marcoen, A. (1996). On the mechanisms of plasticity in young and older adults after instruction in the method of loci: evidence for an amplification model. *Psychology and Aging*, **11**, 164–178.

Verhaeghen, P., Marcoen, A., & Goosens, L. (1992). Improving memory performance in the aged through mnemonic training: a meta-analytic study. *Psychology and Aging*, **7**, 242–251.

Wahlin, A., Bäckman, L., & Winblad, B. (1995). Free recall and recognition of slowly and rapidly presented words in very old age: a community-based study. *Experimental Aging Research*, **21**, 251–271.

Wang, J. J., Zhou, D., Li, J. *et al.* (2006). Leisure activity and risk of cognitive impairment: the Chongqing aging study. *Neurology*, **66**, 911–913.

West, R. L. (1995). Compensatory strategies for age-associated memory impairment. In A. D. Baddeley, B. A. Wilson, & F. M. Watts (Eds.), *Handbook of Memory Disorders* (pp. 481–500). Chichester, UK: John Wiley & Sons.

Wilson, B. A., Baddeley, A. D., Evans, J., & Shiel, A. (1994). Errorless learning in the rehabilitation of memory impaired people. *Neuropsychological Rehabilitation*, **4**, 307–326.

Wilson, B. A., Emslie, H. C., Quirk, K., & Evans, J. J. (2001). Reducing everyday memory and planning problems by means of a paging system: a randomised control crossover study. *Journal of Neurology, Neurosurgery and Psychiatry*, **70**, 477–482.

Winocur, G. (1995). Glucose-enhanced performance by aged rats on a test of conditional discrimination learning. *Psychobiology*, **23**, 270–276.

Winter, J., & Hunkin, N. M. (1999). Re-learning in Alzheimer's disease. *International Journal of Geriatric Psychiatry*, **14**, 983–990.

Woodruff-Pak, D. S., & Hanson, C. (1995). Plasticity and compensation in brain memory systems in aging. In R. A. Dixon & L. Bäckman (Eds.), *Compensating for Psychological Deficits and Declines* (pp. 191–217). Mahwah, NJ: Lawrence Erlbaum.

Woolverton, M., Scogin, F., Shackelford, J., Black, S. E., & Duke, L. (2001). Probel-targeted memory training for older adults. *Aging, Neuropsychology, and Cognition*, **8**, 241–255.

Yesavage, J. A. (1984). Relaxation and memory training in the elderly. *American Journal of Psychiatry*, **141**, 778–781.

Yesavage, J. A., & Rose, T. L. (1983). Concentration and mnemonic training in elderly with memory complaints: a study of combined therapy and order effects. *Psychiatry Research*, **9**, 157–167.

Yesavage, J. A., Rose, T. L., & Bower, G. H. (1983). Interactive imagery and affective judgments improve face-name learning in the elderly. *Journals of Gerontology, Series B: Psychological Sciences and Social Sciences*, **38**, 197–203.

Zacks, R. T., & Hasher, L. (2006). Aging and long-term memory: deficits are not inevitable. In F. I. M. Craik &

E. Bialystok (Eds.), *Lifespan Cognition* (pp. 162–177). Oxford: Oxford University Press.

Zanetti, O., Zanieri, G., Di Giovanni, G. *et al.* (2001). Effectiveness of procedural memory stimulation in mild Alzheimer's disease patients: a controlled study. *Neuropsychological Rehabilitation*, **11**, 263–272.

Zelinski, E. M., Gilewski, M. J., & Schaie, K. W. (1993). Individual differences in cross-section and 3-year longitudinal memory performance across the adult life span. *Psychology and Aging*, **8**, 176–186.

Zivian, M. T., & Darjes, R. W. (1983). Free recall by in-school and out-of-school adults: performance and memory. *Developmental Psychology*, **19**, 513–520.

SECTION 6

Overview

32

The future of cognitive neurorehabilitation

Ian H. Robertson and Susan M. Fitzpatrick

The future of cognitive neurorehabilitation

In this chapter we will attempt to set out the opportunities and challenges facing the development of an integrated science of cognitive neurorehabilitation, in the context of the impressive range of clinical, methodological and theoretical advances outlined in the previous chapters. We will begin by considering a possible working definition of cognitive neurorehabilitation. This may at first sight seem to be strange – defining the concept in the last chapter of a book on the subject. Neurorehabilitation is such a bewilderingly varied enterprise, however, and in such an early stage of development, that we believe it to have been better to set out the table first of the rich diversity of the field, and in that context try to hew out a possible working definition. We leave it to the readers to assess the usefulness of this definition, which underpins the rest of the chapter, in its attempt to assess the future of cognitive neurorehabilitation.

Definition

Cognitive neurorehabilitation can be defined in terms of the following elements:
- Structured, planned experience;
- derived from an understanding of brain function;
- which ameliorates dysfunctional cognitive and brain function;
- and improves everyday life function.

For the purposes of this chapter, we will define successful cognitive neurorehabilitation as follows:

Structured, planned experience derived from an understanding of brain function which ameliorates dysfunctional cognitive and brain processes caused by disease or injury and improves everyday life function.

By this definition, cognitive neurorehabilitation is a subset of what might be considered the more broadly defined field of general rehabilitation. General rehabilitation may focus on goals that do not attempt to change brain function – for instance on altering family processes to facilitate better adjustment and improved quality of life, eliminating socially constructed barriers that hinder participation such as inaccessible buildings, transportation, or leisure activities, or providing assistive technologies. While these activities may change brain function as a result of experience, altering brain function is not usually the stated goal, as is the case for cognitive neurorehabilitation.

Furthermore, principles derived from cognitive neurorehabilitation (attending, learning, practice, goal-setting) may be necessary to help people – even individuals without brain-damage or cognitive loss – achieve general rehabilitation goals. For instance cognitive demands must be addressed when learning to use a wheelchair, achieving standing balance, acquiring skilled use of a prosthetic device or implementing strategies for independence in everyday life.

We will return to our definition later in this chapter, after a brief assessment of the progress that has been made creating a science of cognitive neurorehabilitation over the last few decades.

Cognitive Neurorehabilitation, Second Edition: Evidence and Application, ed. Donald T. Stuss, Gordon Winocur and Ian H. Robertson. Published by Cambridge University Press. © Cambridge University Press 2008.

An assessment

- Cognitive neurorehabilitation increasingly calls on theoretical, methodological and practical advances made in neuroscience, cognitive neuroscience, pharmacology and medical imaging.
- A major challenge for the future of cognitive neurorehabilitation is integrating across the behavioral and cognitive changes observed in recovery and neurorehabilitation with the underlying neural systems, cellular and molecular alterations resulting from neurological insults. Cognitive impairment presents an enormous health challenge far beyond disorders more conventionally associated with brain damage such as stroke and traumatic brain injury.
- Validated outcome measurements that could be used to demonstrate effectiveness across the entire spectrum of interventional approaches must become a priority for cognitive neurorehabilitation.
- The successful delivery of "smart" prosthetics, cellular transplantation and nanotechnology will rely on the ability to retrain neural function and provide correct experiences in optimal learning environments via the science of cognitive neurorehabilitation.
- Improving neural function through the use of pharmaceutical interventions will also most likely require pairing with behaviorally based neurorehabilitation interventions to achieve the desired goals.
- In the "translational continuum" for cognitive neurorehabilitation, cognitive neuroscience (itself a multidisciplinary endeavor) represents the basic science much as basic biomedical research is the foundation of medicine.

Considerable progress has been made during the last 20 years in developing a scientific basis of cognitive neurorehabilitation, as readers of the excellent series of chapters of this book can attest. Two developments are particularly striking. One is the emergence of a "basic science" of cognitive neurorehabilitation. By calling on theoretical, methodological and practical advances made in neuroscience, cognitive neuroscience, pharmacology, medical imaging and other related fields, cognitive neurorehabilitation is now the province of a community of researchers and clinicians covering the full breadth of the translational continuum. Particular areas where progress can be highlighted include those outlined below.

Brain imaging

The availability of a variety of clinical imaging tools that can be used to monitor the extent and location of brain tissue disruption resulting from injury or disease, including restoration of blood flow and metabolism, increasingly allows treatment to be based on the underlying neurological nature and cause of dysfunction. Diagnostic scans should accompany patients and guide treatment from the initial clinical episode through neurorehabilitation.

The use of functional brain imaging in evaluating possible mechanisms of recovery of function, and more rarely in evaluating the effects of therapy, is a major advance. Functional brain imaging need not, or indeed should not, replace the use of robust behavioral outcome measurements in the clinical rehabilitation setting but imaging can and should be used to develop and validate interventions. Functional brain imaging is likely to play its most important role in the research setting or in the study of small patient groups, aiding the development of neurorehabilitation methods more closely tied to theoretical models of cognitive function.

Multilevel integration

A major challenge for the future of cognitive neurorehabilitation is integrating across the behavioral and cognitive changes observed in recovery and neurorehabilitation with the underlying neural systems, cellular and molecular alterations resulting from neurological insults. Such integration is a major scientific challenge, as attempts at integration across levels of analysis are in their infancy even within basic neuroscience. One goal for the future of cognitive neurorehabilitation could be a more explicit attempt at a multilevel description of interventional approaches (see Stickland, Weiss and Kolb, Chapter 22, this volume). It occurs to us that the science of cognitive neurorehabilitation, precisely because it requires serious attempts at such integration, could actually lead the field of neuroscience in this effort. The ability to design successful cognitive neurorehabilitation strategies is, to some degree, the ultimate test that theories and models of nervous system function, particularly the dynamic nature of its organization, function and response to experience, are correct.

The science of complex systems provides the theoretical and mathematical tools needed for taking a multilevel approach to the study of neurorehabilitation. Gene expression, cellular functions, neural circuits, functional networks, and behavioral outputs are linked such that changes at any one level can alter functional characteristics at many other levels (see Chapter 2 by Dixon, Garrett and Bäckman and Chapter 10 by Corbetta, in this volume). For example, it is possible to affect brain function and the resulting behavioral readouts by using pharmacologic interventions whose mechanisms of action are to alter neurotransmitter actions at the synapse. The converse is also true – altering behavior can affect neurotransmitter function, gene expression, cellular properties and so on. A more sophisticated understanding of such interlevel dynamics should be a fundamental component of a mature science of cognitive neurorehabilitation.

A multilevel systems approach also provides a way to rationally incorporate findings from animal research. To some extent, animal research has both contributed to, and hindered, cognitive neurorehabilitation research. Species similarities and differences must be carefully catalogued. The current controversy over whether or not neocortical neurogenesis occurs in human brain is one example of how extrapolation from animal models to humans must be done carefully lest animal results mislead efforts to design neurorehabilitation strategies. Most often, animal research is too far removed from patient needs to provide clinically useful findings immediately. The similarity of genetic background, environmental experiences and rigidly controlled experimental protocols stand in stark contrast to the variability characterizing human patients in a clinic. How might animal research contribute meaningfully to a science of cognitive neurorehabilitation? Animal models can be used for evaluating how interventions and perturbations at one level of analysis, for example the molecular (e.g., pharmaceutical), affect neural systems, cognitive function and behavior. Too often, causal relationships have been assumed and offered as explanations without the required evidence. Perturbations at the circuit or network level may or may not result in changes at the functional level. Similarly, interventions aimed at altering neuronal properties may very well have their intended effect at the level of the neuron but may or may not alter the behavioral output of a circuit or a network. Rather than being assumed, a deeper understanding of these relationships requires empirical study. Studies with animal models, where invasive procedures can be used, may make it possible to identify and validate noninvasive imaging biomarkers or behavioral outcome markers amenable to use with human subjects that are diagnostic or predictive of neural change and recovery. What are needed are animal models that are more reflective and predictive of human neurological dysfunction and recovery.

The challenge for the future is to build the required translational linkages (we will turn to this topic again later in the chapter). Carefully designed animal studies can play an important role in advancing the science of cognitive neurorehabilitation, particularly in the development of small-scale neurorehabilitation research studies whereby the animal studies are a component of converging evidence models. Results from diverse experimental systems, including findings from animal models and computational models, when integrated with data acquired from human subjects, could achieve a goal of extracting principles of brain function that, in turn, can be used to develop research studies with patient populations and, ultimately, clinical trials.

- Understanding how attentional demands interact with function.

The need for a science of cognitive neurorehabilitation

It is possible that impairment of brain function resulting in cognitive impairments (CI) may be one of the most common and disabling categories of health problem in the world today. While no comprehensive review of the prevalence of cognitive deficits has been carried out, this conclusion has support from the range of diseases and injuries that impair brain function. For example, aging: 16–24% of the aging population have mild cognitive impairment and dementia; schizophrenia: 85% of schizophrenics with impaired memory; traumatic brain injury (virtually all with CI); stroke (high prevalence of CI); substance and alcohol abuse (significant levels of CI); diabetes (significant levels of CI); multiple sclerosis (high levels of CI); depression (significant levels of CI).

This is an enormous health, social and personal burden, and cognitive neurorehabilitation may be indicated for all, or at least a majority, of these conditions. Yet the investment in research and services for cognitive neurorehabilitation does not reflect the size of the problem. Why is this?

Without an effort to develop a research-based, clinically relevant science, the delivery of cognitive neurorehabilitation and the development of new research-based clinical interventions are likely to persist as somewhat marginal endeavors against the backdrop of the enormous investment made in providing patients with acute medical services. It is important that those committed to cognitive neurorehabilitation explicitly ask why it is we are willing to invest so heavily in acute medical care and so sparingly in the neurorehabilitation needed to make good on that investment. Altering the future course for cognitive neurorehabilitation requires that there be an international effort to demonstrate that the field is rooted in and grows strongly from clear models of brain and mental functioning, with links from the cognitive to the molecular level informing both research and practice. If the research progress on new models of nervous system structure-function relationships made over the last 20 years

continues, or hopefully quickens its pace over the next two decades, we can be cautiously optimistic that our vision for the future will happen. Achieving our scientifically optimistic projections is, of course, subject to economic realities. All healthcare delivery systems are going to become increasingly financially challenged (a) by the increased demands of aging populations and (b) by the development of new and very expensive therapies for a range of diseases and injuries arising from molecular medicine, nanobiology and the medical devices industry. Treatments and therapies that cannot demonstrate efficacy will not survive in the healthcare marketplace.

We do not believe that a true economics of health-care inherently values technology-based or molecular/cellular-based treatments over ostensibly less glamorous behaviorally based treatments, but we do believe the development of validated outcome measurements that could be used to demonstrate effectiveness across the entire spectrum of interventional approaches must become a priority for cognitive neurorehabilitation. Effective cognitive neurorehabilitation programs, allowing individuals with cognitive impairments and/or their caregivers to resume participation in important life activities will figure substantially in medical and social economic analysis. Over time, it is likely that pharmacological and technical interventions will also be held to rigorous standards and also be required to demonstrate efficacy in terms of real world functional outcomes. A true complex systems approach to healthcare may, in fact, lead to more rather than fewer behavioral interventions. It is not controversial to state that our eventual efforts to make good on the promissory notes currently offered by the development of "smart" prosthetics, cellular transplantation and nanotechnology will rely on the ability to retrain neural function and provide correct experiences in optimal learning environments via the science of cognitive neurorehabilitation.

Improving neural function through the use of pharmaceutical interventions designed to alter neurotransmitter and neuromodulator actions will also most likely require pairing with behaviorally based neurorehabilitation interventions to achieve the desired goals. The widening use of cognitive therapy for the treatment of individuals diagnosed with depression provides a good illustration. Research shows that cognitive, behavioral-based treatments can, for certain subgroups, be as effective or even more effective than pharmacologic treatments. Combining cognitive therapy with the use of pharmacologic agents may offer another alternative approach for some patients. These conclusions have been arrived at after a number of trials of a consistently applied, protocol-based therapy, which in turn grew out of a broad base of basic research characterising cognitive mechanisms of depression and its recovery. Cognitive therapy treatments for depression are now widely accepted and used in relatively standardized ways worldwide. The standardization of the therapy is important. Standardization not only makes it possible to assess efficacy, it allows for continuous improvement and refinement. New theoretically motivated, testable hypotheses can be generated, new protocols can be developed, and better outcome measures can be field-tested. Cognitive therapy for depression stands in marked contrast to the rather fragmented way many interventions in cognitive neurorehabilitation are conceived, implemented and evaluated.

Building a true science of cognitive neurorehabilitation could also serve as a model for how to accomplish the much sought-after biomedical "translational research." How is it possible to create a continuum balancing the tenets of research (often focused on identifying the differences among groups) with the needs of clinicians faced with the responsibility for delivery care to individual patients? At the moment, cognitive neurorehabilitation services are designed to address an individual patient's needs but the interventions have often been devised in isolation of current neuroscience and cognitive neuroscience research. The neurorehabilitation protocols often arise from the desire of well-intentioned and caring therapists to provide something to desperate patients seeking treatment.

Often, the therapist providing the therapy is also responsible for monitoring the patient's progress, making objective evaluation difficult. Evaluating efficacy is further confounded by using the same tasks for both the training paradigms and the outcome measurement. Conversely, researchers are often not particularly interested in developing treatments but rather in pursuing projects that may yield scientifically interesting results. Effects achieved in the research setting may be statistically significant on highly selected subjects. Validating effects, scaling up studies for large clinical trials, and developing protocols amenable to clinical settings offers researchers few academic rewards. Unfortunately, too often the magnitude of the effect seen in a controlled research setting is small and may not be sufficiently robust to withstand the variability introduced in real-world clinical environments where neither the skill of the therapist nor patient individuality is controllable. Efficiency could be gained if the science of cognitive neurorehabilitation can establish a shared language that facilitates two-way communication between academic research centers and the non-academic clinics where much of patient services are provided.

We are proposing that in the "translational continuum" for cognitive neurorehabilitation cognitive neuroscience (itself a multidisciplinary endeavor) represents the basic science much as basic biomedical research is the foundation of medicine. Clinicians might question the need for a science of cognitive neurorehabilitation based on an understanding of brain function. A convincing argument could be put forward that cognitive neurorehabilitation might be best served by a highly individualized, idiosyncratic approach (see Chapter 7 by Cicerone in this volume). Wilson and Kapur's chapter (Chapter 30, this volume) presents practical, empirically tested interventions derived from a performance perspective that relies very little on basic science research. However, we think cognitive neuroscience research could make real contributions in determining why a particular intervention is effective, which aspects of an intervention are essential for the desired effect, and for which patients the treatment is indicated. It is important to know how treatment effects could be maximized, what the proper dose-response relationship is, and how to structure the learning environment so that behaviorally based strategies become less effortful and more automatic over time. We believe we can get better at matching treatment strategies to patients using an understanding of both the anatomical and functional deficit. It may seem counterintuitive – but it is likely a scientifically motivated approach to cognitive neurorehabilitation will result in more, rather than less, personalised care.

Examples of a cognitive neuroscience approach to cognitive neurorehabilitation

- Cognitive neurorehabilitation methods should be instantiated in detailed protocols, with or without assistive technologies, which allow for replication of evaluation studies.
- There should be at least some theoretically articulated and empirically supported model underlying the intervention.
- Effective cognitive neurorehabilitation should be able to demonstrate changes both in cognitive function and in brain function as measured by one or more imaging or associated methods.
- Cognitive neurorehabilitation should be able to demonstrate effects in the everyday life of the individual.
- There are very few examples of cognitive neurorehabilitation which meet these criteria: constraint-induced therapy may be one of the few.

Constraint-induced therapy (CIT; see Chapter 23, this volume, by Morris and Taub) is based on years of research carried out by Edward Taub and colleagues. It focuses on loss of motor function, which is of course a complex, cognitive-controlled process. Taub's initiating model proposed that injury to a limb results in neural shock and initial depression of function, leading to a learned non-use of that limb even when movements could potentially be made. Taub demonstrated, first in a nonhuman primate model and later with human subjects, that learned non-use can be overcome. In cases where there is a minimum of residual function, restricting movement of the intact limb can induce use of the deafferented limb.

Constraint-induced therapy occupies a special importance in the development of cognitiveneurorehabilitation. In addition to its theoretical grounding in neuroscientific principles, the therapy design is articulated into a coherent and replicable protocol which allows for a degree of assessment and replication notably lacking in a landscape littered with protocols of uncertain efficacy. The fact that CIT has been evaluated in over 400 patients (see Chapter 23) worldwide in multicenter clinical trials is a mark of the maturity and critical importance of this milestone in neurorehabilitation. The theoretical principles, the feedback from clinical use, and validated outcomes provide a blueprint that should encourage the design and testing of new interventions extending the CIT approach.

Perhaps one of the important lessons learned from CIT derives from its somewhat counterintuitive nature – *stopping* patients from doing something that may interfere with, or inhibit, behavioral recovery. One of us (IR) remembers clearly attending a workshop by the advocate of an internationally used physiotherapy method where it was categorically stated that rehabilitation of hemiplegia *must* be "symmetrically based," namely with repeated bilateral movements – if necessary with the hemiplegic arm lifted by the unimpaired arm – being an essential component of treatment. While of course this may be a valid approach under *some* conditions (Staines *et al.*, 2000), it is clearly not a panacea to be advocated in a blanket fashion. Similarly, the belief that interventions can not be assessed until *after* natural recovery has plateaued needs to be empirically investigated. Intuition-based treatment is an understandable consequence of having a practice-led rather than a research-led culture of developing therapies, and cognitive neurorehabilitation is still beset by this type of approach, though this is changing slowly.

Nevertheless, if one considers the costs – to the patient in terms of time, effort and discomfort devoted to a significantly suboptimal treatment – and to the health provider in terms of precious and expensive therapist time – then the dangers of not developing a strong scientific base for therapies can not be justified. We need to know to whom which treatment should be delivered, when, and how intensively for how long. The functional organization of the nervous system and the principles of recovery and plasticity should guide cognitive neurorehabilitation.

There are other examples of relatively nonintuitive methods of neurorehabilitation. As we have seen in Chapter 26 by Singh-Curry and Husain, a wide range of such methods have arisen out of largely theoretically derived cognitive neuroscience research into spatial neglect. Schindler *et al.* (2002), for instance, showed that applying a standard electromechanical vibrator to the left neck muscles of patients while they engage in visual search exercises produces marked and enduring clinical and real-life benefits. This treatment arose out of basic research into the brain mechanisms of sensory integration and higher level perception. Neglect patients were studied because of what their damaged brains revealed about the functional architecture of the intact brain. Neck vibration was used purely because of its known effects on the body's normal coordinate frame of reference according to which sensory inputs and motor outputs are integrated. In neglect, not only is this egocentric reference frame biased to the right, but also the neck vibration can temporarily correct this imbalance. What we see in the Schindler *et al.* (2002) paper is that, when combined with systematic visual search training, and when systematically applied for 15 treatment sessions over 3 weeks, temporary effects become long lasting and hence therapeutically important.

An important difference between CIT and neck vibration treatment for neglect is that the latter has not been subject to the same number of replications, and does not, to our knowledge, have brain-imaging data to indicate at least partial mechanisms for recovery. Are there ways in which

standardization and dissemination of candidate protocols could be fostered? We believe that CIT provides an excellent model for other types of cognitive neurorehabilitation: if standardized protocols based on good theoretical models are developed, then opportunities for replication and multicenter trials will multiply, along with the funding and credibility for the field that will inevitably follow. As mentioned above, a major challenge for the field is how to facilitate the development of such protocols and to channel resources in such a way that critical mass of basic and evaluative research is attained.

One possibility is that the institutionalization of an accreditation or regulatory system such as exists for medical devices and pharmaceuticals be devised for cognitive neurorehabilitation methods. Given how small the field of cognitive neurorehabilitation is, and the adaptability of most interventions to a variety of care-delivery systems, an international effort may be the best approach. Even the most cursory glance at the reviews of evidence for the effectiveness of cognitive neurorehabilitation presented in Part V will reveal that there are very few candidate neurorehabilitation methods that would meet most likely sets of criteria. What might some of the elements of a list of such criteria look like? Let us return to the definition of cognitive neurorehabilitation given at the beginning of the chapter: *Structured, planned experience derived from an understanding of brain function which ameliorates dysfunctional cognitive and brain processes caused by disease or injury and improves everyday life function.*

A possible set of criteria for an acceptable science of cognitive neurorehabilitation might be captured in this definition, as follows:

(a) *Structured, planned experience.* Implicit in this element of the definition is that cognitive neurorehabilitation methods should be instantiated in detailed protocols with or without assistive technologies, that allow for replication of evaluation studies;

(b) *. . . derived from an understanding of brain function.* This element implies that there should be at least some theoretically articulated and empirically supported model underlying the intervention;

(c) *. . . which ameliorates dysfunctional cognitive and brain processes.* Implicit in this part of the definition is that effective cognitive neurorehabilitation should be able to demonstrate changes both in cognitive function and in brain function as measured by one or more imaging or associated methods (MRI, fMRI, PET, ERP, MEG, EEG, TMS);

(d) *and improves everyday life function.* Cognitive neurorehabilitation should be able to demonstrate effects in the everyday life of the individual.

A further criterion may be added to this definition, namely that methods should be *tested in large multicentered phase III clinical trials* (without the array of participant exclusion and selection criteria often seen in small trials). Finally, treatment delivery and outcome assessment must be independent of one another.

As can be seen from the chapters in this book, there are very few studies of cognitive neurorehabilitation that meet all of these criteria, though progress has been made over the last few decades. One study of cognitive training with normal elderly serves as an example of a theoretically motivated approach, strongly based on cognitive and neuroscience research (Stuss *et al.*, 2007). Healthy subjects experiencing age-related cognitive declines showed meaningful changes in everyday performance as rated both by the participating subject and by caregivers. Future studies with this protocol should identify possible mechanisms of improvement through imaging measures and they must also determine whether the findings are robust enough to hold up in the clinical trials arena with individuals experiencing cognitive decline as a result of injury or disease. If the next phase of preclinical research is promising the protocol needs to be shaped for a multicenter, double-blinded, randomised, controlled clinical trial. Ultimately, of course, the real goal is to have a finding robust enough to be useful in everyday clinical practice.

These are the examples of the sorts of challenges facing all cognitive neurorehabilitation protocols if research is truly going to be translated into widespread clinical practice.

If, as we believe, anatomical and functional brain imaging is to be important to the future evaluation of cognitive neurorehabilitation, then there are a number of important factors that may bear on the future of cognitive neurorehabilitation, in particular raised in Chapter 10 by Corbetta.

Among other things, Corbetta reviews evidence that better language production recovery in aphasic disorders is associated with an apparent reactivation of left hemisphere language systems, while less optimal recovery is associated with right hemisphere activations. Furthermore, it appears that in some cases, inhibitory rTMS applied at the chronic stage to right hemisphere frontal regions produces some limited but persistent gains of naming in patients with severe aphasia. In contrast, however, with respect to speech comprehension, Corbetta shows that right hemisphere activity alone may also lead to good outcome, possibly due to a more bilateral representation of comprehension mechanisms.

This implies that our indices of brain imaging will have to become more sophisticated and theoretically informed. More is not necessarily better, and successful neurorehabilitation may be indexed as much by certain decreases in brain activation as by increases. This is particularly true when the extent of diaschisis in certain types of lesion is observed – for instance in the case of unilateral neglect following right hemisphere stroke – where widespread suppression of blood flow is observed even in certain distant regions of the brain. Corbetta raises the intriguing possibility that activity spreads in sensory and motor systems differently, with a lesion to the former blocking a "spreading" activation to widely distributed networks of areas. In contrast, lesions to motor areas may operate quite differently because – he speculates – motor signals may require greater focusing onto the appropriate response mechanism, which may involve the inhibition of other response areas. Lesions to motor areas may therefore lead to a decrement of inhibition and a consequent over-activation of motor areas. Corbetta argues that the principal mechanism for recovery is reorganization of widely distributed neural networks, and cognitive neurorehabilitation has yet to take on board this complexity in its models of treatment.

Cognitive neurorehabilitation has yet to be considered in the light of new technologies for altering brain function such as deep brain stimulation, repetitive transcranial magnetic stimulation, or neural transplantation and related procedures. There can be no doubt that the precision and neuroanatomical specificity of these methods will present bracing challenges to the science underpinning cognitive neurorehabilitation. An important area of research will be how useful they are in restoring meaningful function useful to patients in their everyday lives. But it is early days, and it is most likely that technological approaches and behavioral approaches will continue to be tested, refined and evaluated. There equally can be no doubt that if cognitive neurorehabilitation rises to these challenges, then its potential – both alone and in combination with these emerging therapies – for improving the lot of the tens of millions of people worldwide suffering from impaired brain function will be very high indeed.

Practical recommendations for the future of cognitive neurorehabilitation

(1) Establish an international clinical trials network so that promising neurorehabilitation interventions tested in research laboratories and on small groups of patients can quickly be scaled up for trials on large numbers of patients in diverse environments.

(2) Develop a mechanism whereby clinical outcome information is made readily available to researchers so that a continuous improvement communication loop is created.

(3) Create convenient and readily accessible training and professional development tools for clinicians.

(4) Establish a shared repository of validated outcome measurements that can be easily applied in the clinical setting but are ecologically valid and reflective of real world improvements.

(5) Develop diagnostic tests guiding the selection of potential therapies.

Summary: some questions for the future science of cognitive neurorehabilitation

The authors of this chapter are optimistic that the vision for the future of the science of cognitive neurorehabilitation can be realized. We acknowledge that there are elements missing, and even that there may be visions departing significantly from the one suggested here. We find it unlikely, however, that a scientific approach to cognitive neurorehabilitation grounded in an understanding of brain function, cognitive science and behavior challenged by a serious commitment to improving everyday performance will not succeed. In summary, we leave you with some questions we believe the science of cognitive neurorehabilitation can answer in the near term and when it does, the impact on patient care will be measurable.

(1) What are the neural, cognitive, behavioral and environmental factors that contribute to the observed disconnect between an individuals' cognitive function as measured with neuropsychological tools and their observed performance in everyday life? (See Chapter 14 by Dawson and Winocur.) Understanding this disconnect will reveal important interactions among these different levels and the ways by which each contributes to everyday performance.

(2) In what ways do alterations in cognitive function impact behavioral performance in the short and near term? What is the impact of altered behaviors on the functioning of cognitive systems? In other words, what are the feedforward and feedback links between cognition and behavior? It might be worth knowing if the inability of an individual to engage in certain behaviors could further "decondition" cognitive

functions. For example, how might the effects of early brain injury manifest throughout an individual's lifespan? Similarly, how might brain injuries acquired in mid-life interact with natural aging processes?

(3) Could understanding the dynamic interplay whereby neural and cognitive dysfunction reduce an individual's capacity for altering/reacting to/modifying his or her environment hold promise for the treatment and cognitive neurorehabilitation of certain neuropsychiatric diseases?

(4) How can we successfully exploit combinations of pharmacologic, technical and behavioral interventions? The appeal of engineered smart prosthetics and cellular replacement therapies will be difficult to fulfill unless we know much more about how computations are performed and actions represented by neural circuits. Pursuing the development of highly technical or cell-replacement treatments will command

significant financial investments. In the absence of a science of cognitive neurorehabilitation as envisioned in this chapter, such enterprises may become little more than intellectual exercises.

REFERENCES

Schindler, I., Kerkhoff, G., Karnath, H. O., Keller, I., & Goldenberg, G. (2002). Neck muscle vibration induces lasting recovery in spatial neglect. *Journal of Neurology, Neurosurgery and Psychiatry*, **73**, 412–419.

Staines, W. R., McIlroy, W. E., Graham, S. J., & Black, S. E. (2000). Bilateral movement enhances cortical activity associated with the paretic hand in acute stroke: A functional magnetic resonance imaging (fMRI) study. *Stroke*, **31**, 16.

Stuss, D. T., Robertson, I. H., Craik, F. I. M. *et al.* (2007). Cognitive rehabilitation in the elderly: a randomized trial to evaluate a new protocol. *Journal of the International Neuropsychological Society*, **13**, 120–131.

Index